For three decades *Pears Medical Encyclopaedia* has been a popular guide to health and medicine, its clear language,  approach making it an all-round family adviser.

The original work was written by the late James Alexander Campbell Brown, MB, B.Chir. (1911–1964) who, after studying medicine at Edinburgh and in several European countries, became a specialist in social psychiatry and psychology and was the author of several books, including *The Distressed Mind* (1946), *The Evolution of Society* (1947), *The Social Psychology of Industry* (1954), *Freud and the Post-Freudians* (1961) and *Techniques of Persuasion* (1963). Since it was first published in 1962 by Pelham Books, *Pears Medical Encyclopaedia* has been revised and updated several times to take account of new methods and techniques. The present edition has been rewritten by Dr Michael Hastin Bennett MA, MB, B.Chir., FRCS, who has had wide experience as a surgeon and family practitioner in this country, West Africa and the Oman.

Pears Medical Encyclopaedia is truly international, covering many tropical diseases and conditions, and providing advice for the world traveller.

The aim of *Pears Medical Encyclopaedia* is to encourage co-operation between doctor and patient, to present sensible articles about many controversial topics and to provide laymen with up-to-date information on many common conditions that may affect their health.

PEARS
Pocket
MEDICAL
ENCYCLOPAEDIA

J.A.C. BROWN, MB, BChir

**Revised by
A.M. HASTIN BENNETT,
MA, FRCS**

LITTLE, BROWN AND COMPANY

A LITTLE, BROWN BOOK
First published in Great Britain by Pelham Books Ltd
in association with Rainbird Reference Books 1962
Published by Sphere Books Ltd 1977
Reprinted 1977, 1979, 1981, 1983, 1986, 1988
Completely revised and updated edition published 1991
Published by Warner Books in 1992
Reprinted 1993, 1994, 1996, 1997

This edition published by Little, Brown and Company (UK) 2000
Reprinted 2001 (twice)
Copyright © J.A.C. Brown 1962, 1963, 1965
Copyright © Pelham Books Ltd and Rainbird Reference Books Ltd 1971
Copyright © A.M. Hastin Bennett 1991
The moral right of the author has been asserted.

Printed and bound in Finland

ISBN 1-85605-546-9

Companies, institutions and other organizations wishing
to make bulk purchases of this or any other books
published by Little, Brown, should contact their local
bookshop or the special sales department at the address below.
Tel 0207 911 8000. Fax 0207 911 8100.

Little, Brown and Company (UK)
Brettenham House
Lancaster Place
London WC2E 7EN

Weights and Measures: in 1960 units of scientific measurement were agreed as the *Système International d'Unités*, the International System of Units, abbreviated to SI units. They are now used in medicine. The basic units are: second (s) for time, metre (m) for length, kilogram (kg) for mass, Kelvin (K) for absolute temperature, ampere (A) for electric current, candela (cd) for luminosity, mole (mol) for amount, radian (rad) for plane angles and steradian (st) for solid angles. Defined in terms of these basic units are derived units, of which the most frequently used in medicine are: for force newton (N), for pressure pascal (Pa), for energy joule (J), for power watt (W), for temperature Celsius ($^{\circ}C$), for radioactivity becquerel (Bq), for absorbed dose of radioactivity gray (Gy), for magnetic flux density tesla (T) and for frequency hertz (Hz). Some equivalents are: 1 kg force = 10 N, 1 mm mercury = 133 Pa, 1 calorie (energy) = 4.2 J, and 1 kilocalorie (rate of work) = 70 W. In order to avoid a number of figures before or after decimal points, metric prefixes are used, if possible representing 10 raised to a power that is a multiple of three. Examples are: tera (T) 10^{12}, giga (G) 10^{9}, mega (M) 10^{6}, kilo (k) 10^{3}, hecto (h) 10^{2}, deca (da) 10, deci (d) 10^{-1}, centi (c) 10^{-2}, milli (m) 10^{-3}, micro (μ) 10^{-6}, nano (n) 10^{-9}, and pico (p) 10^{-12}. The term mole is applied to ions, molecules and atoms; it is abbreviated mol, and the definition is the amount of a substance which has a mass in grams equal to its relative molecular weight. In medicine the unit of volume is the litre although it is not part of the SI system. It is used for the sake of convenience, and the abbreviation is l.

Decimal multiples of the kilogram are written by using the SI prefix with g, for gram, and not kg. e.g. milligram (mg) although the gram is not a basic SI unit. A concentration may therefore be expressed in grams per litre, g/l, milligrams per decilitre, mg/dl, or moles per litre, mol/l.

Blood pressures are still given in mm mercury.

Temperature: °C signifies degrees Celsius or centigrade, a scale in which 0° is the temperature at which water freezes and 100° the temperature at which it boils. Anders Celsius was a Swedish mathematician (1701–44). °F signifies degrees Fahrenheit, in which the melting point of ice is 32°F and the boiling point of water 212°F. Gabriel Fahrenheit was a German physicist (1686–1736). To convert °F to °C subtract 32 and multiply by 5/9. Normal body temperature is taken to be about 37°C or 98.6°F.

Introduction

This book is designed for laymen, assuming no medical knowledge on their part, but since its aim is to be scientific, and within the limits imposed by space to be reasonably detailed, it may also prove useful to nurses and others who wish to refresh their memories or refer to something outside their own immediate field. It has been written in the belief that so far as possible all knowledge should be available to anyone who seeks it, and that in the particular case of medical information those who feel it can be harmful are wrong because the choice is no longer between some knowledge or none at all but between correct and incorrect information.

The *Encyclopaedia* cannot take the place of a doctor's opinion and care. The experienced physician never seeks to heal himself. How much less should laymen, relying not on a lifetime's skill and knowledge but on the pages of a small book, try to diagnose and treat their own illnesses. No book can be a substitute for a doctor, for diagnosis and treatment are not mechanical matters but depend in great part upon the doctor's estimate of the patient's total condition, including the character, personality and circumstances.

It follows that the patient must always be frank with the doctor, answering all questions carefully although they may not at first seem relevant. There must be no false modesty about any sort of examination that may be required.

Conversely, the doctor must be worthy of the patient's trust, and answer all questions truthfully. If the patient wants a second opinion the doctor should arrrange for one; if the patient does not trust the family doctor, the time has come for a change.

Laymen should never believe what they hear from non-medical sources, and never give medical advice to others. Nevertheless, there is every reason why we should all try to understand something of what goes on inside our bodies and, if there is something wrong, have a good idea of the nature of the malady and what treatment to expect. It is the aim of the *Encyclopaedia* to help laymen to co-operate with the family doctor in dealing with the everyday problems of health and disease by providing an accurate source of general medical information.

Where drugs have been mentioned in the *Encylopaedia*, generic or approved names have been used rather than proprietary names which may be more familiar.

A

Abdomen: that part of the trunk between the thorax (chest) and the pelvis. It is separated from the thorax by a muscular partition called the diaphragm, but is continuous below with the cavity of the pelvis. It is well protected behind by the bone of the vertebral column and the lower ribs, but is vulnerable in front and at the sides where the abdominal contents are covered only by muscular layers – the transverse, internal and external oblique muscles at the sides, and the vertical rectus abdominis muscle in the midline. The structures which make up the abdominal wall are skin, fat of varying thickness, muscle, another layer of fat, and the thin, slippery membrane called the peritoneum which lines the abdominal cavity. The peritoneum, which is rather like wet cellophane, covers all the internal organs in the abdominal cavity. The principal contents of the abdominal cavity are the organs of the digestive system: the stomach, small and large intestine with the appendix and caecum, and the liver and pancreas. The end of the intestine, the rectum, lies in the pelvis. The kidneys lie at the back of the abdomen, up under the lower ribs at each side of the spinal column. Tubes called ureters run down the back wall of the abdomen from the kidneys to the bladder, which is in the pelvis. On the left side, up under the diaphragm, lies the spleen, corresponding roughly in position to the liver on the right. The liver is much larger than the spleen, which is pushed back and up by the stomach. At the back, running down in front of the spinal column, are the biggest artery and vein in the body – the abdominal aorta and the vena cava; and on each side of the spinal vertebrae runs the abdominal autonomic nervous system with its chain of ganglia. The prostate gland in the male and the uterus, ovaries and Fallopian tubes in the female are in the pelvis below the abdominal cavity. Diseases of the abdomen and pelvis are dealt with under the various systems affected or under their commonly known names.

Abdominal Injuries: although the front of the abdomen is relatively unprotected (*see above*) serious abdominal injuries affecting the internal organs are relatively rare in civilian life. They occur most often in car accidents, crushing accidents and falls from a height, when the liver or spleen may be ruptured. If a large blood vessel is torn the bleeding may be so severe that the patient dies before operation is possible. Penetrating wounds of the abdomen, however slight they may appear, must always be taken seriously, for the external appearance of the wound may bear little relation to the extent of internal damage. The kidneys are sometimes damaged by a blow in the flank, and in such a case the urine may be blood-stained. If the condition is very severe, or does not improve, operation may be needed. In the interval between the occurrence of the injury and the arrival of skilled help the victim should be kept warm and still, and moved as little as possible. Nothing should be given by mouth.

Abortion: the death and expulsion of the foetus before it is viable. It may be accidental or procured. Accidental abortion, or miscarriage, is dealt with under that heading. Procured abortion may be lawful or criminal. The Abortion Act of 1967 has been amended by the Human Fertilisation and Embryology Act 1990, and now states: Medical termination of pregnancy.

1 (1) Subject to the provisions of this section, a person shall not be guilty of an offence under the law relating to abortion when a pregnancy is terminated by a registered medical practitioner if two registered medical practitioners are of the opinion, formed in good faith –

(a) that the pregnancy has not exceeded its twenty-fourth week and that the continuation of the pregnancy would involve risk, greater than if the pregnancy were terminated, of injury to the physical or mental health of the pregnant woman or any existing children of her family; or

(b) that the termination is necessary to prevent grave permanent injury to the physical or mental health of the pregnant woman; or

   (c) that the continuance of the pregnancy would involve risk to the life of the pregnant woman, greater than if the pregnancy were terminated; or

   (d) that there is a substantial risk that if the child were born it would suffer from such physical or mental abnormalities as to be seriously handicapped.

(2) In determining whether the continuance of a pregnancy would involve such risk of injury to health as is mentioned in paragraph (a) or (b) of subsection (1) of this section, account may be taken of the woman's actual or reasonably foreseeable environment.

(3) Except as provided by subsection (4) of this section, any treatment for the termination of pregnancy must be carried out in a hospital vested in the Minister of Health or the Secretary of State under the National Health Service Acts, or in a place for the time being approved for the purposes of this section by the said Minister or the Secretary of State.

(3a) The power under subsection (3) of this section to approve a place includes power, in relation to treatment consisting primarily in the use of such medicines as may be specified in the approval and carried out in such manner as may be so specified, to approve a class of places.

(4) Subsection (3) of this section, and so much of subsection (1) as relates to the opinion of two registered medical practitioners, shall not apply to the termination of a pregnancy by a registered medical practitioner in a case where he is of the opinion, formed in good faith, that the termination is immediately necessary to save the life or to prevent grave permanent injury to the physical or mental health of the pregnant woman.

The Act does not extend to Northern Ireland.

In other countries the law is different, and in the USA the laws differ from State to State.

Abrasion: an abrasion is the area from which the surface layer of the skin has been rubbed, for example by contact with a rough surface, as when a boy falls off his bicycle and his knee hits the road. When a very large area is affected it is obviously best to consult a doctor, but a minor graze may be dealt with by careful washing with soap and water to clear away any foreign matter. The abrasion will heal most quickly if it is left open to the air without any dressing, but it may have to be covered to keep it from contact with clothes. A piece of antiseptic gauze kept in place by porous adhesive tape is convenient; if it becomes dirty it should be changed, but the less interference the better. If the abrasion is contaminated with soil it is wise to go to the doctor at once for an injection against tetanus.

Abreaction: a technique in psychiatry. The doctor brings to the patient's conscious attention details of an incident partially or completely suppressed in the memory. The process can often be made easier by the use of a very light anaesthetic; just enough is used to produce drowsiness. During abreaction the patient may become very excited, feeling again the strong emotion that caused the memory to be suppressed in the first place.

Abscess: an abscess forms in the tissues as the result of irritation, usually because of bacterial infection. Increased blood flow leads to effusion of fluid into the tissue spaces and the collection of a great number of white blood cells. The area of infection becomes cut off from the healthy tissue and in time the dead white blood cells, bacteria and exuded fluid form pus. The earliest outward sign of abscess formation on the surface of the body is a painful and tender area of redness. As the abscess becomes localised and pus forms, so the area of redness becomes more sharply defined, and its centre begins to soften. Usually the pus tracks to the area of least resistance, which in the case of a surface abscess or boil is the surface of the body, and points. If left, the abscess will eventually burst and discharge, but often much pain and illness can be avoided if it is lanced or incised as soon as it has localised and pus has formed. It is worse than useless to incise an abscess, or stick a needle into a pimple, before the inflammation has become localised and pus has formed because this will only spread the infection. In the early stages, it may be possible to abort the formation of an abscess by using antibiotics, but once it has localised and pus has formed antibiotics are liable to interfere with the natural course of events and prolong resolution and healing. It is sensible to ask for skilled advice on the treatment of all but the smallest abscesses. When it has started to discharge the abscess will heal quickly, provided that drainage is free and the affected part is kept at rest. Use plain dry dressings to cover the discharging abscess, and change the dressings frequently. While abscesses on the surface of the body are caused by infection entering through a small cut or abrasion, through the tiny lubricating glands of the skin or hair follicles, internal abscesses can be caused by the entry of a foreign body as in the case of knife or bullet wounds, or, in the lungs, by the accidental inhalation of food or a tooth. Other internal abscesses are caused by the spread of local infections, as in a burst appendix which causes a pelvic abscess, or the spread of infection from the middle ear to the brain. *See* Inflammation.

Acarus: a genus of very small creatures called mites which often live as parasites on the external surface of larger animals. They cause various skin diseases such as itch and mange. *See* Mites.

Accidents: figures given by the Medical Commission on Accident Prevention show that there are 40 deaths attributed to accidents every day in the United Kingdom. Of these, one-third are caused by road traffic accidents and one third by accidents in the home. Traffic accidents cause 1% of deaths at all ages, but of all *male* deaths between the ages of 15 and 24 no less than 38% are attributable to road traffic accidents. Most fatal accidents in the home occur among children and the elderly. The average number of beds in NHS hospitals occupied every day by patients following injury is 13,500. While advances in treatment over the last 20 years have resulted in the overall death rate from accidents falling from 400 to 300 per million of the population, and deaths from road traffic accidents falling from 155 to 102 per million, it is obvious that much more action must be undertaken in the prevention of accidents generally. The Royal Society for the Prevention of Accidents lists these causes of road accidents as most common:
1. Speed too fast for the conditions.
2. Overtaking improperly.

3. Turning without due care.
4. Misjudging speed, distance or intended direction of movement.
5. Loss of control (e.g. skidding).
6. Vehicle defects such as faulty tyres or brakes.
7. Vehicles crossing carelessly at junctions.
8. Alcohol or drugs.
9. Lack of experience.
10. Jay-walking by pedestrians or thoughtless misuse of the roads.

In 1983 the Road Traffic Act made it compulsory for front-seat occupants of most motor vehicles to wear seat belts. The use of seat belts increased from under 40% to over 90%, and in the first year the number of deaths of those involved in accidents while sitting in the front seats of cars fell by 21% and the number of serious injuries by 24%. A great deal of thought is going into the design of motor cars to try to lessen the injurious effects of accidents, but it is obvious that once a person ventures outside the 'natural envelope of performance' or the natural environment there must be a risk. If you hit something at a speed greater than you can run, if you fall from a height greater than you can jump, if you venture into reduced or increased atmospheric pressure, indeed if you stay under water longer than you can hold your breath, sooner or later you are going to have an accident.

Accommodation: the lens of the eye is made of elastic tissue so that its shape can be altered by contraction of the ciliary muscle which surrounds it. When the muscle contracts the lens becomes more convex, and as it relaxes the lens becomes less convex. The result is that images can be brought to a sharp focus on the retina at the back of the eye at varying distances. The process is called accommodation. As we get older the lens loses its elasticity so that the power of accommodation is diminished.

Acetone: a substance found in the urine, primarily in severe cases of diabetes, sometimes in chronic wasting diseases such as cancer, and after prolonged vomiting. It has a characteristic smell which can often be detected in the breath of patients in diabetic coma.

Acetylcholine: a substance normally found in many parts of the body. It is used in the transmission of nervous impulses between nerve endings and the muscles and in the workings of the parasympathetic nervous system (see Nervous System). Normally it is broken down in the body by the substance cholinesterase. If the amount of cholinesterase is lowered, for example by poisoning by phosphorus insecticides, the effect is to increase the amount of circulating acetylcholine and therefore to produce too much stimulation of the parasympathetic nervous system. The action of the heart is slowed down, the muscles become weak, and the patient suffers from nausea, giddiness, headache and disturbance of vision (the pupils of the eyes contract). If the condition is not relieved by the injection of atropine, which counteracts the excess of acetylcholine, the patient develops colic and more severe symptoms which eventually end in convulsions and coma. Drugs which compete with acetylcholine at the neuro-muscular junction are used in anaesthetics to produce controlled relaxation of the muscles, thus easing the task of the surgeon. They also relax the vocal cords and allow the passage of an endotracheal tube. There are several of these drugs, which are based on the action of curare.

Acetylsalicylic Acid: *see* Aspirin.

Achalasia: the term means 'no relaxation' and is applied to a condition of the oesophagus in which the mechanism of swallowing is disturbed. Food normally stimulates the muscle of the wall of the gullet to begin a series of contractions which pass the food towards the stomach in waves. Where achalasia is present this does not happen, nor does the muscle surrounding the junction of the oesophagus with the stomach relax to allow food to pass. The muscle only opens when the column of food which builds up in the oesophagus is heavy enough to force its way through, which occurs when the column is about 20 cm high. The patient is troubled by discomfort rather than pain, and complains of food sticking in the throat. Young people of both sexes are affected; the treatment may have to be surgical.

Achilles Tendon: according to Greek myth, Achilles' mother dipped him in the river Styx to make him invulnerable. She held him by the back of the ankle, and the heel was the only part of the hero which remained dry. Not until he was struck in the heel could he be wounded: it was his only weak point. The tendon, which runs from the great muscles of the calf to the calcaneum, the bone which forms the heel, draws the foot downwards about the hinge of the ankle. It is the tendon we use to stand on tiptoe. It is liable to become inflamed and very painful, sometimes without obvious cause, but often because it has been irritated by the heel of an ill-fitting shoe or boot. It is difficult to rest it, because it is used in walking, but normally if the shoe is changed and undue exercise is avoided the condition resolves in a few days. The Achilles tendon becomes the weak point of some athletes as they get older, and if it is suddenly put under strain it may rupture partly or completely. It is repaired by surgical operation.

Achlorhydria: the absence of normally occurring hydrochloric acid in the stomach. It is found in 4–5% of normal people in whom it produces no ill effects, but it is the rule in cancer of the stomach and pernicious anaemia.

Achondroplasia: a form of dwarfism which is inherited, of unknown cause, and unalterable. The trunk is of normal size while the arms and legs are abnormally short and the head relatively large. Most of the dwarfs seen in circuses are of this type; the less frequently seen dwarf of the 'Tom Thumb' type who has perfectly proportioned limbs and body is suffering from a defect of the pituitary gland (q.v.) resulting in a deficiency of the growth hormone. Treatment is, in these cases, possible if undertaken early enough.

Acidity: a term sometimes used to signify excess of acid in the stomach, thought to be the cause of gastric pain. As a diagnosis it leaves a lot to be desired, and commonly occurs in advertisements for mildly alkaline medicines.

Acne Rosacea: more often known as rosacea, and formerly described as 'grog-blossom', this condition of the skin of the face is primarily dependent upon changes in the small blood vessels of the skin. They become enlarged, and the result is a red, greasy and coarsened area shaped like a butterfly spreading across the nose and extending out over both cheeks. Associated with this may be chronic dyspepsia or gastritis, and in some cases a meal, hot drink or alcohol will make the butterfly area flush. The name 'grog-blossom' arose from the belief that rosacea was invariably associated with chronic indulgence in alcohol; but this is less than kind to the commonest type of sufferer who is a middle-aged lady of blameless habits except, perhaps, for addiction to numerous cups of strong tea. It is true that in former times such people as coachmen who were exposed both to the elements and to the temptation of frequent noggins of hot grog tended to develop red noses and cheeks, but the alcoholic of today is no more likely to bear such stigmata than the teetotaller, for rosacea is associated with anything that leads to frequent flushing of the face – prolonged exposure to harsh weather, the change of life in women, hot foods such as curries, and hot and irritant drinks which produce gastritis when consumed in excess, such as strong and stewed tea. Treatment includes the cure of gastritis, and possibly the correction of any hormonal imbalance in women; as in the case of acne vulgaris (*see below*), the use of tetracycline is often very helpful.

Acne Vulgaris: a chronic skin disease affecting the sebaceous (grease) glands of the face, shoulders, back or chest. It occurs most often in people between the ages of 14 and 20, and the typical 'blackheads' and pimples may cause a great deal of embarrassment at an age when people tend to be particularly sensitive about their personal appearance. A plug forms in the canal through which the sebaceous gland normally discharges its secretion to the surface of the skin, and the top of the plug becomes hard and black. Sometimes the gland goes on secreting although the canal is blocked, and a cyst forms containing glandular secretion. The sebaceous plug contains vast numbers of the acne bacillus, but it may become infected by other bacilli whereupon pus is formed and the area becomes inflamed. The medical name for a blackhead is comedo;

comedones are found not only in the acne of puberty but also as a result of exposure of the skin to oil and grease. They may also form when susceptible people are given bromides or iodides by mouth, and when workers in industry are exposed to some compounds containing chlorine. Treatment in the first place must be aimed at keeping the skin and hair thoroughly clean; the hair shampooed twice a week with a simple shampoo and the face washed frequently with soap and water. Blackheads may be expressed with a special comedo expressor from the pharmacist, but must not be touched if they are inflamed, very large or have no 'head': they are then best left alone, since squeezing them often leads to infection. Locally applied lotions usually produce some irritation when they are first used. Older remedies include sulphur, which may cause the skin to peel. It may be combined with salicylic acid or benzoyl peroxide in a number of proprietary preparations, or benzoyl peroxide may be used by itself to clean and sterilise the skin. Hydrocortisone cream or ointment should not be used. The best treatment for severe cases is tetracycline by mouth, used in small doses e.g. 250 mg twice a day taken on an empty stomach. It will be necessary to get a doctor's prescription for this antibiotic, and it must be taken regularly over some months. Resistant cases may have to be referred to a dermatologist. Studies have shown that diet has little effect on the condition, although it is commonly thought that chocolate makes it worse.

Acoustic Nerve Tumour: the acoustic nerve is one of the cranial nerves (q.v.); it connects the brain with the ear. Upon it there may rarely form a fibrous tissue tumour which, as it grows, presses upon the brain stem and on the other cranial nerves which originate there, for on one side of the tumour is the hard temporal bone which contains the inner ear and on the other side the soft brain tissue. Giddiness, double vision, deafness, weakness of one side of the face, and various other signs point to the presence of an acoustic nerve tumour. The only treatment is removal; recent advances in early diagnosis and neurosurgical technique have greatly improved the outcome.

Acrocyanosis: a condition found especially in younger women in which there is coldness and blue discoloration of the skin of the hands and feet, spreading sometimes to the nose and ears. The underlying cause is undue tendency to spasm of the arterioles and arteries; it may occur in warm as well as cold weather. It is not amenable to treatment, but is not in any way dangerous. *See* Raynaud's disease.

Acromegaly: a state produced by over-secretion of the pituitary growth hormone, commonly as the result of a tumour of the gland. When this occurs in early life, before the bones have stopped growing, the result is increased height or gigantism: after the bones have ceased to grow the patient develops a prominent forehead and cheekbones, a large lower jaw, hands and feet, a bent back and general coarsening of the features with a hollow deep voice. Other symptoms such as disorders of vision or impotence may be present. Although the appearance of an acromegalic patient may suggest great strength the opposite may be true. Treatment is directed towards restoring the level of growth hormone to normal and preventing further growth of the pituitary tumour, and may be by radiotherapy, surgery or the use of the drug bromocriptine.

Acromion: the point of the shoulder, formed by the outermost part of the spine of the scapula or shoulder-blade.

ACTH: abbreviation for adrenocorticotrophic hormone, or corticotrophin, a secretion of the pituitary gland which has the function of stimulating the adrenal gland cortex, increasing among other things the secretion of cortisone. ACTH was first isolated in 1933, but was not used in medicine to any extent until 1949, when it appeared to be useful in the treatment of rheumatoid arthritis. It is now rarely used, being superseded by corticosteroids (q.v.).

Actinomycosis: a chronic disease caused by the 'ray fungus', *Actinomyces israelii* in man and *Actinomyces bovis* in cattle. Infection commonly takes place through the mouth, and there is usually a history of injury or removal of a tooth. The infection attacks the face and neck giving rise to a painful swelling with pus formation which discharges both into the mouth and outwardly. The infection may spread to the lungs, intestine or liver. Diagnosis depends on bacteriological investigation; the outlook for treatment has been revolutionised by penicillin, which has to be taken in large doses for some weeks. Resistant cases usually respond to other antibiotics, notably tetracycline. The organism *Actinomyces bovis*, which produces 'lumpy jaw' or 'wooden tongue' in cattle, is not dangerous to human beings.

Acupuncture: a method of treatment used in Chinese medicine for the treatment of pain, to produce anaesthesia, or to treat various general illnesses. It consists of puncturing the surface of the body with needles at traditionally established sites. The needles may be rotated, vibrated or electrically stimulated. The reported success of the method has produced increasing interest in the West, but it is not possible to reconcile the Chinese system of medicine with that followed by Western doctors. Consequently in the West acupuncture is not used as a complete system, but is tested by the effect of needling at certain points. Nevertheless, there is evidence to suggest that pain can be relieved by acupuncture, and an explanation sought in Western terms is that needling has been shown to increase blood levels of naturally occurring substances called endorphins, which are known to be concerned in the relief of pain. Some workers have shown that pressure over the acupuncture point P6 has relieved morning sickness in pregnancy. This point is about an inch above the skin crease at the wrist, between the first two tendons that can be felt on the thumb side, and in the reported cases pressure was applied for five minutes on four successive mornings and repeated at four-hourly intervals. Others have found that wearing wrist bands with a button exerting pressure at this point on both wrists ameliorated postoperative nausea. Whatever the explanation of the successes of acupuncture may be, it remains a harmless method of treatment which merits careful consideration.

Acute: in medicine, any process which has a sudden onset and runs a relatively severe short course is called acute.

An example is the acute pain one suffers on being struck on the shin. The opposite is 'chronic', a term applied to a permanent or long-lasting illness or pain.

Acute Abdomen: the patient who is suffering from acute pain in the abdomen (or pelvis) – a pain of sudden onset and considerable severity – is said to have 'an acute abdomen'. Such cases include appendicitis, perforated ulcers, and acute inflammation of the gall-bladder. There is an old surgical rule which states that an acute abdomen which does not get better within six hours is a surgical case; and it is a good rule to call the doctor about any abdominal pain which does not improve in a few hours. In the more severe cases it quickly becomes obvious that professional help is needed. Until medical help arrives, the patient should be kept as still as possible, and given only enough water to keep the mouth moist. Laxatives should not be given in cases of abdominal pain except on medical advice.

Acyclovir: a drug active against certain virus infections through its action as an inhibitor of DNA synthesis. It is active against the virus of herpes simplex, HSV, but less so against the virus of herpes zoster, V-Z (*see* Herpes).

Adaptation: the process by which the eye is able to adjust to varying intensities of light. If we come into a shady room from the bright sunlight at first everything seems dark, but after a little while the light is perfectly adequate. Any photographer will have found that the human eye has far greater powers of adaptation than film: a good exposure requires the use of a light meter, for the eye is so flexible that it is a bad judge of the level of light. Even those infallible men, first class cricket umpires, have had to resort to light meters to back up their judgement of light.

Addiction: the word implies that those who indulge in the over-use of alcohol or take drugs, notably opium derivatives, have become slaves to the substance. During the nineteenth century, at a time when medicine was becoming based on science, and disease entities were increasingly differentiated by the growing knowledge of pathology and physiology, the concept was advanced that addiction was a physical disease beyond the control of the will. The effects of withdrawal of opium derivatives were thought to be so severe in their physical manifestations that the addict was forced to continue taking the drug; but in fact the physical effects of withdrawal even when undertaken without help are unpleasant but no worse than a severe attack of flu, providing that the patient is in a reasonable state of general health. The psychological effects of withdrawal are however a different matter, for in a chronic case taking the drug has become the whole object of life. This can be true of many substances – hallucinogens, cocaine, solvents involved in glue sniffing – indeed, an Expert Committee of the World Health Organization (WHO) said 'there is scarcely any agent which can be taken into the body to which some individuals will not get a reaction satisfactory or pleasurable to them, persuading them to continue its use even to the point of abuse.' The conception of addiction as a disease overpowering the will is being modified, and treatment of addiction recognises this. Instead of there being one definite method of treatment, as there is in the case of an established disease, many methods of treatment are in use, but all pay the greatest attention to the addict's mental state. The habits of drug takers may be such as to lead to grave deterioration in their general as well as mental health, which may make treatment doubly difficult.

Addison's Disease: first described by Dr Thomas Addison (1793–1860), the disease is due to insufficiency of the secretion of the adrenal glands. Addison's own account cannot be bettered: 'Anaemia, general langour or debility, remarkable feebleness of the heart's action, irritability of the stomach, and a peculiar change of colour in the skin.' The discolouration begins first on exposed areas – the face and hands – and ranges from yellow to dark brown or even black as it spreads over the rest of the body. Extreme weakness on slight exertion, fainting attacks or giddiness and noises in the ears due to low blood pressure, palpitations, nausea with or without actual vomiting, and sometimes diarrhoea complete the picture. The cause is destruction of the suprarenal glands due to auto-immune disease (q.v.), tuberculosis or tumours leading to loss of the hormones which are essential to life. The disease is rare in childhood or old age. Treatment was formerly not possible, but the necessary hormones are now known and can be manufactured. Hydrocortisone and fludrocortisone are given by mouth; as this is a form of substitution therapy, like the use of insulin in diabetes, it must be continued permanently.

Adenitis: inflammation of a gland. Usually applied to inflammation of the lymphatic glands (q.v.).

Adenofibroma: a tumour composed of connective tissue with glandular elements. *See* Breast Disease (benign tumours).

Adenoids: lymphatic glandular tissue present at the back of the nose in children, which may become enlarged as the result of chronic infection and obstruct the free passage of air. This leads to mouth breathing and snoring. In severe cases the obstruction may cause infection of the middle ear or sinusitis; the child may be hard of hearing. Infection and enlargement of the adenoids is associated with chronic tonsillitis and recurrent colds. Treatment may have to be surgical, but removal of the tonsils and adenoids is not now advised as often as formerly.

Adenoma: a tumour, usually benign, composed of glandular tissue.

Adenovirus: a virus first isolated from human adenoid tissue, responsible for many upper respiratory and conjunctival infections.

Adhesions: many structures in the body are normally separated by tissues which are free to move over each other. The lung is separated from the chest wall by the pleural membrane; the inside of the joints is covered by slippery synovial membrane; and the abdominal organs move over each other easily because they are covered by the peritoneal membrane. Sometimes these membranes become inflamed, often because of disease in the organs they cover, and in the course of inflammation and recovery fibrous tissue may form and stick the normally slippery membranes together so that adhesions are formed. Adhesions in the joints may make the joint stiff and require physiotherapy, but adhesions in the abdomen can lead to obstruction of the gut or twisting of the bowel. If the condition is severe, surgical operation may be unavoidable, but this in its turn may lead to further adhesions.

Adipometer: an instrument for measuring the thickness of a fold of skin, so that some indication can be gained of the efficacy of a reducing or, on occasion, a fattening diet.

Adiposis: an abnormal accumulation of fatty tissue in the body.

Adolescence: the period between puberty and the end of bodily growth. It is the time during which a child matures into an adult. Rapid physiological changes may produce difficulties in psychological development, leading to turbulent behaviour. It is often a time of particular difficulty for parents, who may have to call on all their reserves of tolerance and understanding.

Adrenal Glands: over the upper part of each kidney lies an adrenal gland, weighing about 5 g, shaped like a cocked hat and coloured yellow. Each gland has two parts separate in function and development. The outer part, the cortex, is derived during development from mesoderm, like the gonads, while the inner part, the medulla, arises from nervous tissue. The gland has a capsule separate from that of the kidney and takes its blood supply from the aorta, renal artery and the arteries running to the diaphragm. The medulla secretes the hormones adrenaline and noradrenaline (*see below*) which are together referred to as the catecholamines; their action was in 1916 described by Walter Cannon (1871–1945) as preparation for 'fright, flight or fight'. The modern physiologist might be more likely to say that the hormones are released in situations of stress. The cortex of the gland, which is under the control of the pituitary gland, secretes the corticosteroid hormones (q.v.).

Adrenaline: one of the hormones secreted by the adrenal medulla, the other being noradrenaline. These hormones are also released at the endings of the nerves of the sympathetic nervous system, which is therefore described as adrenergic. The function of the hormones is to prepare the body for action: the pulse is speeded up, the blood pressure raised, the flow of blood diverted from the guts and skin to the muscles, and glycogen in the liver is transformed to glucose, an immediate source of energy. The pupils of the eyes and the air passages in the lungs dilate. Adrenaline was first prepared by Takamine in 1901 from the adrenal glands of animals, but is now produced synthetically. It is used in medicine for relieving severe attacks of asthma, in cardiac arrest, and in severe allergic reactions. It is combined with local anaesthetics, particularly in dentistry to control local bleeding. Adrenaline cream is sometimes rubbed into the skin over painful muscles or joints, but whether the relief obtained is due to the cream or the rubbing is a matter of opinion.

Adverse Drug Reactions: the large number and great potency of the drugs available in modern medicine mean that from time to time, quite unexpectedly, patients may suffer unwanted, unpleasant and even dangerous reactions. Although every effort is made to ensure that drugs are tested thoroughly before they are released for general use, people differ considerably in their reactions to the same drug, and it is not possible for the doctor to know precisely what will happen in every case when he issues his prescription. In many cases when a drug is chosen for its main effect on an organ or system, the doctor knows that it is likely to have some unwanted or side effects, and can warn the patient about them – although it is possible that the warning itself can produce the side-effect; but in rare cases there will be unexplained effects. If this should happen the doctor will want to know at once, and will report the happening, in the UK to the Committee on Safety of Medicines. If by any chance you are prescribed a medicine that has in the past produced an adverse reaction do not hesitate to let the doctor know.

Aerophagy: the neurotic habit of swallowing air, usually unconsciously, which is the cause of much gastric flatulence and 'wind'. It may be cured by carrying a cork between the teeth.

Aerosol: a suspension of very finely divided liquid or solid particles in a gas. In medicine aerosols may be used for destroying insects such as fleas, flies or mosquitoes which carry disease, for attempting to combat disease caused by droplet infection in public places, and for the administration by inhalation of drugs in cases of disease of the lungs. The method of administration may be by a hand-operated spray or nebuliser, a specially designed inhaler, or the common pressurised container. Aerosols are very effective against insects provided they are used in a confined space. Antiseptics delivered into the air by a spray will certainly kill infective organisms in a bottle, but whether they remain in the air in sufficient concentration to be effective against droplet infection spread by people coughing is another matter. Aerosols are extremely useful in cases of asthma and other conditions in which the airways are obstructed, carrying drugs directly to the place where they are needed. The technique of using pressurised aerosols is usually easily acquired, but some, particularly older people with arthritis and small children, may find it difficult. Inhalers using powder, which depend on the patient's breathing, may be easier, but may cause coughing. Nebulisers usually overcome such difficulties. The introduction of aerosols has transformed the lives of many sufferers from asthma, but it is important for patients to follow instructions with care; the drugs used are powerful, and it is easy to take an overdose.

Affective Disorders: in psychiatry, changes from the normal in emotion, mood or feeling. Examples are mania and depression.

Afterbirth: placenta and membranes expelled in the third stage of labour. *See* Placenta, Labour.

Agar: a vegetable jelly made from seaweed. It resists the digestive action of bacteria, and is therefore used by bacteriologists to make a medium on which cultures can be grown. It is commonly combined with broth or blood for this purpose. It can be used to make soups or jellies, particularly in the East; it has also been found effective as a laxative.

Ageing: *see* Geriatrics.

Agglutination: the coming-together of small particles in a solution to form clumps. It is brought about by the action of antibodies on antigens carried, for example, by red blood cells or bacteria, and is therefore used in identifying blood groups and bacteria. Blood of incompatible groups when mixed will produce clumping of the red blood cells; the serum of a patient containing antibodies to typhoid will produce clumping in a solution containing typhoid bacilli, a phenomenon first described by the French bacteriologist Georges Widal (1862–1929).

Agoraphobia: an uncontrollable sensation of anxiety at the thought of leaving home and being out in crowded places. Patients suffering from agoraphobia often feel that they will faint or have a heart attack if they go out. They may panic at the thought of crossing the road, and in the end become unable to leave the house. Treatment by a psychiatrist is usually successful.

Agranulocytosis: a serious but not common condition in which there is a diminution in the number of granulocytes (one type of white blood cell) in the circulation. It may be accompanied by mouth ulcers and a sore throat, and a much reduced resistance to infection. It has been found associated with many drugs, but the commonest are those used in the chemotherapeutic treatment of cancer. Other drugs are those used in the treatment of rheumatism, for example gold and penicillamine; phenylbutazone (Butazolidine) was an offender, but is no longer in general use, being best reserved for horses. The list is long, but a doctor prescribing a drug that is known to produce the condition will carry out regular blood counts on his patient. If the offending drug is withdrawn immediately there is any suspicion that the white cell count has dropped, recovery should only take a couple of weeks. Overexposure to radiation causes the white cell count to drop, as may the excessive consumption of alcohol, and several diseases have the same effect, such as glandular fever and malaria.

Agromania: the opposite condition to agoraphobia – an abnormal desire to be alone, to wander in open fields.

Ague: a vague and outdated term for a fever with shivering, which came to be applied in the main to malaria.

AIDS: Acquired Immune Deficiency Syndrome. A disease caused by a retrovirus, Human Immunodeficiency Virus, referred to as HIV. Unrecognised before 1981, its precise origin is unknown, but the most severely affected part of the world is Africa. It is transmitted sexually; originally identified in the USA among homosexuals, it is now clear that it can be transmitted from man to man, man to woman, woman to man and by an infected mother to her unborn child. It can be transmitted by the transfusion of infected blood or blood products or by the use of dirty needles, as when needles are shared between intravenous drug abusers. It has a long incubation period: it is not yet clear how many showing a positive blood test will eventually develop the disease, but it is thought that between 10% and 30% of those infected will do so within three to five years. Infectiousness is high during a short period early after infection, before and during the time when antibodies are developed in the blood, and again much later when the disease begins to affect the immune system. But those who have a positive blood test seem to remain infectious to some degree indefinitely. The worst feature of the disease is that there is as yet no cure, and it is almost invariably fatal because of its destructive action on the cellular immune system (q.v.), which leaves the victim open to any sort of infection, common among them being *Pneumocystis carinae* pneumonia and Kaposi's sarcoma, which is due to a virus. The only drug so far found to influence the disease is zidovudine.

It cannot be stated too strongly that there is no risk of infection through normal social contact. The means of transmission are strictly limited. People will remain free from infection if they remain constant to one sexual partner. If this is not possible, a condom should be used. Users of intravenous drugs must not share syringes or needles. Blood transfusions and blood products are not now infectious. The World Health Organization (WHO) estimates that the number of people in the world carrying the AIDS virus is between eight million and ten million, and that the disease will kill three million women and children during the 1990s and leave ten million children orphans. Worst affected is sub-Saharan Africa, with about five million people infected, one adult in every 40. In Asia at least half a million people are infected. The WHO estimate for the year 2000 is between 15 million and 20 million infected people, but this could increase.

Ainhum: a condition found mainly among Negroes in Africa. A constriction appears in the skin covering a toe, commonly the fifth, which runs round the affected part so that as it gets worse the blood supply is progressively diminished. The toe eventually falls off.

Airsickness: *see* Motion Sickness.

Air Travel: in general, those who are fit to walk to the aircraft are fit to travel in it. If there is any doubt about fitness to travel by air the doctor will advise. Those disabled who find it difficult to get about should let the airline know in good time and they will help. The number of people who should not travel as ordinary airline passengers is small: active tuberculosis is a bar to flying, and so is a recent heart attack or severe anaemia. A moderate degree of anaemia with a haemoglobin of over 8g/dl is no bar to flying, but in sickle-cell anaemia the fall in partial pressure of oxygen can bring on a crisis. Patients should not travel after a recent abdominal operation nor after a recent operation on the eyeball nor, obviously, if they are suffering from an infective disease. Epileptics and diabetics will take care that their condition is well controlled. The cabin of a passenger-carrying aircraft is pressurised to 8000 feet, which represents a considerable fall from the atmospheric pressure at ground level, so that any gas trapped in the body will expand. Those with a pneumothorax should not fly, nor those with any considerable cyst in a lung. Very severe asthma may cause trouble, but most people with obstructive respiratory disease are able to cope with the changes in pressure for the climb to altitude and the descent normally takes place over about thirty minutes. Colostomy patients are advised to take an extra supply of bags to cope with an increased flow due to the possible expansion of gas in the intestine. Those with severe colds or hay fever should take some decongestive preparation with them for the variation of air pressure inseparable from flying may cause pain in the sinuses or the middle ear. One unexpected place where air may be trapped is under the filling in a tooth; the resulting pain has a name, aerodontalgia. Most airlines decline to take expectant mothers after the eighth month. Healthy infants can travel by air after they are seven days old. Be sure that they do not get dry by slightly increasing their intake of fluid, and wake them up for the descent as the pressure changes.

Airway: in medical use airway means the path by which air enters and leaves the lungs – the mouth, throat, trachea or windpipe, and the air passages in the lungs themselves. In anaesthetics the term is transferred to mean a device for ensuring the free and unobstructed passage of air in and out of the lungs. It is as important in an accident case to make sure that the airway is clear, and is kept clear, as it is to stop bleeding. The easiest way of doing this is to turn the patient over onto his side, or onto his face with his head to one side; secretions or vomit will run out of his mouth and not into his lungs. Pressure forwards on the angles of the jaw will stop the tongue from obstructing the airway. Be very careful how you move a patient if there is any possibility that there is a broken bone; support the injured limb. Do not move a patient if there is a possibility of neck or back injury; if necessary keep the mouth open and the jaw forward by pressure behind the angles of the jaw.

Albumin: a protein which enters into the composition of all living organisms, and is the commonest protein found in the blood serum. It is mainly responsible for keeping the osmotic pressure constant in the circulation, and facilitates the transport of fats, hormones, haptens and drugs. Albumins vary in their composition, but all contain carbon, hydrogen, nitrogen, oxygen and sulphur. The main ones found in food are egg albumin (sometimes spelt albumen) in the white of egg, fibrinogen and haemoglobin in the blood, myosin in meat, caseinogen in milk, casein in cheese, and gluten in flour. Albumins show the following characteristics: they are colloidal and do not pass, as salts do, through parchment membranes or the membranes of normal living cells; they are coagulated by heat, following which they become insoluble in water until treated with caustic alkalis or mineral acids; they are precipitated by various chemicals such as alcohol, tannin, nitric acid and mercury perchloride.

Albuminuria: albumin is not normally found in the urine, for it does not pass through the kidney cells unless they are damaged by, for example, nephritis or inflammation of the kidneys. However, its presence in the urine does not necessarily mean that the kidneys themselves are damaged, for albumin can be found in any inflammation of the lower part of the urinary tract where pus or blood is produced, for example pyelitis, cystitis and urethritis (q.v.). Heart disease, many fevers, severe anaemia and the administration of drugs or poisons may be accompanied by albuminuria, the significance of which is as serious as the disease causing it. Despite what has been said above, albumin is sometimes found in the urine of a small proportion of perfectly normal people, usually in youth. This condition is described as cyclic, postural or orthostatic albuminuria, as it disappears when the individual lies down, only to reappear on standing upright. It has no pathological significance. During pregnancy the urine must be tested regularly, for albuminuria may indicate the presence of complications which can be dealt with if they are discovered in time.

Alcohol: the name given to a large class of organic chemical compounds, the only ones relevant to medicine being methyl or wood alcohol, and ethyl alcohol which is the compound found in alcoholic drinks. Methyl alcohol is poisonous and when drunk leads to blindness, neuritis and death. Methylated spirits contains ethyl alcohol, 10% methyl alcohol, a little paraffin oil, and an aniline dye, the idea being to make it undrinkable; similarly denatured alcohol, or surgical spirit, contains acetone or methanol.

Being theoretically undrinkable and intended for industrial or household use, these alcohols carry no excise duty and are therefore very cheap, an unfortunate fact which attracts people who are impervious to the disagreeable taste and drink them neat or mixed with cheap wine, a potentially lethal habit. Ethyl alcohol when free of water and other impurities is called absolute alcohol. Its chemical formula is C_2H_5OH, and it is used in medicine as a solvent, in the preparation of tinctures, essences and some elixirs, to remove grease from the skin or to clean it before making an injection, and to harden the skin in those confined to bed for long periods where its use lessens the risk of bedsores. Internally there are no conditions for which alcohol need be prescribed, but for those accustomed to its use a drink before a meal, wine during a meal or a nightcap of whisky no doubt play their part in aiding digestion by quelling nervous tension or inducing sleep. So-called tonic wines are useless. Spirits should never be given to those who are in a fainting or collapsed state; they are more likely to choke than revive.

Alcoholism: addiction to alcohol. A condition in which there is chronic or periodic drinking of a compulsive nature. It is often both a cause and a reflection of emotional and social difficulties. Abuse of alcohol leads to a great deal of misery, marital unhappiness and broken homes, a certain amount of crime, and produces physical and mental disease, both directly and indirectly: directly, by the physical effect of alcohol on the body, and indirectly by the fact that those in a drunken state are more likely to contract venereal disease, succumb to ordinary illnesses such as pneumonia if they are chronic addicts and, of course, to endanger the lives of themselves and others by causing motor and other accidents. On the other hand there can be no doubt that some people can drink very considerable quantities of alcohol throughout a long life without showing any apparent ill effects whatever, and that in most cases alcoholism is a symptom rather than a disease. Thus although alcohol may be the immediate cause of a broken home, it is extremely likely that adjustment problems of long standing have antedated the obvious problem of alcoholism and perhaps contributed to it. Similarly it could well be argued that if the evil effects of alcohol are constantly discussed, its good effects in oiling the wheels of social intercourse and reducing tension have usually been ignored, and it might be said with more than a grain of truth that moderate amounts of alcohol have kept some people going who would otherwise have found it difficult to carry on reasonably good relations with their families or friends. Painstaking statistical study carried out in the USA has demonstrated that, if heavy drinking considerably lowers the average expectation of life, the moderate drinker has a higher than average expectation.

The general (although by no means universally accepted) belief today among those who have studied the subject scientifically is that both the alcohol itself and the malnutrition to which it leads produce the physical effects seen in alcoholism. The repeated consumption of strong spirits especially on an empty stomach leads to a chronic gastritis and probably inflammation of the intestines which interfere both with the appetite and the absorption of food substances, notably vitamins of the B group; this in turn damages the nervous system, causing alcoholic neuritis and injury to the brain cells, thus leading to certain forms of insanity. The liver may be severely affected: fatty change, hepatitis or cirrhosis may ensue.

The alcoholic is not necessarily the sort of person who becomes obviously drunk on frequent occasions; he or she may be the man or woman who drinks steadily throughout the day, often without any effect being apparent to others. Later, however, symptoms which are partly due to the physical changes, partly to the underlying neurosis which is at the root of the trouble in most cases, and partly social, begin to show themselves. The person eats less and drinks more, often begins the day with nausea or vomiting which necessitates taking the first drink before he can appear in public, his work suffers, he forgets to keep appointments and becomes indifferent to social responsibilities, his craving for drink becomes worse, and when he is unable to get it he becomes shaky, irritable and tense. As he is ashamed of his condition he tries to hide it and often, instead of drinking openly, hides bottles throughout the house. The emotions are poorly controlled and he gets angry or tearful readily, tells facile lies, and a minor illness or cessation of drinking may even lead to an attack of delirium tremens. In another type, there may be no craving for alcohol for quite long periods, until a sudden impulse makes it seem absolutely necessary to have a drink; in a few hours the sufferer becomes dead drunk and uncontrollable. This form of alcoholism is less frequent than the other and is known as dipsomania. In very severe cases the alcoholic may die from liver damage – although this is not as common a result of drinking as it used to be – or an attack of pneumonia, or some other infection not ordinarily fatal to healthy people may be so to him; in other cases there may be gradual mental deterioration with loss of memory (Korsakoff's psychosis).

Nearly all cases of chronic alcoholism need specialist treatment, and may need admission to an institution or nursing home accustomed to such cases. The principles of treatment are: complete abstention, psychotherapy to treat the psychological causes of the condition, and attention to general health. Concentrated injections of vitamins may be given, and in some cases drug treatment designed to create revulsion from alcohol may be used. The drug disulfiram (Antabuse) if taken regularly causes the patient to feel so ill after taking even the smallest amount of alcohol that it may turn him against the habit permanently. Unfortunately, when left to themselves, some patients are more likely to give up Antabuse than alcohol.

Aldomet: proprietary name for methyldopa, a drug used in the treatment of high blood pressure.

Aldosterone: one of the two hormones secreted by the adrenal cortex; the other is hydrocortisone. Its function is to control the salt balance of the body, promoting by its action on the kidney the retention of sodium and water and the excretion of potassium.

Alkalis: substances, usually oxides, hydroxides, or carbonates and bicarbonates of metals which neutralise acids to produce salts. Weak solutions of household alkalis – ammonia or washing soda – are useful to alleviate the discomfort of insect bites or stings, but strong ammonia, caustic soda or potash and washing soda are caustic poisons. The main use of alkalis in medicine is to neutralise acid in the stomach. The chief agents used are: sodium bicarbonate, calcium carbonate (chalk), magnesium carbonate, magnesium trisilicate and aluminium hydroxide. They may be used alone or in mixtures. Although there is no harm in using sodium bicarbonate (baking soda) from time to time when nothing else is available, its regular use is unwise because it tends to produce gas in the stomach, and it is so strongly alkaline that it may upset the acid–alkali balance in the body. Magnesium trisilicate and aluminium hydroxide are the safest in this respect, but it is important to emphasise that prolonged dyspepsia should be medically investigated and not self-treated.

Alkaloids: a large group of alkaline substances found in plants. They are extremely potent and widely used in medicine. Insoluble to a greater or lesser degree in water, but soluble in alcohol, those given by mouth are usually made up in tablets or tinctures, i.e. alcoholic solution. They are frequently given by injection. Most of them have a bitter taste and are poisonous if taken in excess of the correct dosage. Common alkaloids are atropine from the belladonna plant, cocaine from coca leaves, caffeine from tea and coffee, morphine, codeine and other drugs from the opium in poppy juice, nicotine from tobacco, quinine and quinidine from Peruvian bark, strychnine from nux vomica seeds. It will be noticed that alkaloids have names ending in -ine; certain drugs with similar properties but no alkaline reaction have names ending in -in, for example ouabain.

Allantotoxicon: a poison formerly supposed to be found in sausages. Fortunately there is no evidence that it exists.

Allergy: all mammals possess an immune system, which is a means of defence against potentially harmful micro-organisms such as bacteria, viruses, parasites and fungi which might invade the body and lead to disease. The system brings into action a process designed to neutralise, kill and get rid of the invader. The body recognises as foreign any substance which differs from that occurring naturally in the organism, even if the difference is minute. The foreign matter carries an antigen, which is a small

35

chemical group included in a larger molecule forming part of the structure of the foreign body. The antigen stimulates the formation of an antibody, an immunoglobulin, IgE, in the blood of the invaded organism which is specific to the antigen. The tissues of the body contain cells called mast cells, mostly below the skin and mucous membranes which line interior structures within the body. The mast cell has an affinity for IgE which has been formed elsewhere and collects antibodies upon its surface, which becomes sensitised to substances which have previously given rise to the formation of antibodies. When the antigen comes into contact with the mast cell, a series of reactions follows. Histamine (q.v.) is released, with a range of other substances which set up an inflammatory reaction, cause spasm or relaxation in smooth muscle, and change the permeability of small blood vessels so that fluid leaks into the tissues.

All this is very well if the foreign invader is a pathogen, that is, an organism which can set up a disease; but in some people there is an inherited tendency to produce antibodies to protein substances which are not liable to cause disease. The term allergy was coined in 1906 by von Pirquet (1874–1929) to describe the altered reactions which ensue when such a person is exposed more than once to a specific foreign substance: allergic conditions include asthma, hay fever, skin reactions such as urticaria or swelling and eczema. In recent years there has been a tendency to attribute a great number of conditions to 'allergies', and sometimes the condition is difficult to diagnose with certainty. In a true case the condition is based on the reaction described above; particularly in so-called food allergies this cannot often be demonstrated, and other explanations must be sought, such as a deficiency in enzymes, the effect of toxic ingredients or even an unrecognised disease.

Treatment includes the use of drugs and sometimes the use of vaccines derived from the precipitating agent, such as pollen in hay fever, bee sting venom in cases of severe allergic reaction to the insect stings, and house dust mites in certain cases where they are found to be the allergen. The vaccine is given in graded doses, starting with a low concentration; but the injections can be unpleasant and the procedure can itself give rise to severe reactions, to such an extent that a course of desensitising vaccine should only be undertaken in a hospital. The most useful drug in the case of a severe reaction is adrenaline given by injection, repeated if necessary. There are a number of antihistamine drugs which can be used in cases of hay fever, insect stings and skin reactions; but they have a slight drawback in that they may produce drowsiness.

In recent years increasing understanding of the immune system has made possible the formulation of new drugs which act on the allergic response, such as sodium cromoglycate, which stabilises the mast cell membrane and so prevents the release of the substances which produce the allergic symptoms. Sodium cromoglycate must be taken regularly, and in the case of allergic asthma is delivered directly to the lungs by an inhaler. In hay fever it can be used in eye drops or in a nasal spray. Corticosteroids reduce the action of antibodies, and are therefore useful in the treatment of allergies. They may be used as an aerosol for inhalation, in a nasal spray or drops, or in the case of eczema in an ointment or cream. In severe cases of asthma they are given by mouth or by injection.

Allopathy: a term used to describe treatment by drugs opposed to manifestations of the disease concerned. Originally used to signify treatment used by orthodox medical practitioners as opposed to the methods of homeopathy, it has come to mean the methods of conventional doctors as opposed to any 'alternative' form of treatment.

Allopurinol: a drug used to reduce the formation of uric acid in the treatment of gout (q.v.).

Alopecia Areata: a form of baldness brought about by factors which are not understood. As the hair grows back again in time, letters written to makers of 'hair restorers' by grateful customers are usually written by those suffering from this condition.

Alphafetoprotein: protein made by the foetus as it develops. If an excess is found in the amniotic fluid there is a defect in the developing nervous system of the growing foetus such as spina bifida or anencephaly (q.v.). Samples of the amniotic fluid can be taken by the process of amniocentesis (q.v.) early in the second three months of pregnancy in cases where it is thought to be advisable, and analysis carried out. Alphafetoprotein is also found in increased quantities in the blood of adult patients suffering from certain malignant tumours.

Alternative Medicine: the term applied to systems of treatment which cannot be accepted by orthodox medical practitioners because they cannot be ratified by accepted scientific methods. Many doctors would like to see studies that compare alternative, or complimentary, systems with conventional medical practice in order to be able to compare the effectiveness of treatment, but those using such methods of therapy find this a difficult and inappropriate approach. *See* Acupuncture, Homeopathy, etc.

Aluminium: compounds of this element are used in medicine as antacids and astringents. Aluminium hydroxide is widely used to relieve the symptoms of dyspepsia, and aluminium acetate can be used in ear-drops to clear up a weeping inflammation of the outer ear or in a lotion to help an infected area of eczema or a wound. Poisoning by aluminium has been found to produce encephalopathy, disorder of the brain, and researchers have found a difference in blood concentrations of aluminium between sufferers from Alzheimer's disease and Down's syndrome and those with dementia following a stroke. The significance of this is not yet clear.

Alzheimer's Disease: pre-senile dementia. A common and most distressing condition, at the outset characterised by failing memory and increasing difficulty in concentration. It occurs in people in their fifties and beyond, and is progressive, affecting the speech and the ability to read; later patients lose the ability to look after themselves. They become confused, especially at night, and tend to wander about. The disease runs its course in about six years. It is not distinguishable from the dementia of old age, both showing atrophy of the brain and characteristic changes in the brain tissues. It has been suspected that the accumulation of aluminium in the brain might be a cause, but this seems uncertain. It has however been demonstrated that some cases are hereditary. No treatment has yet been found. The condition was first described by the German physician Alois Alzheimer (1864–1915).

Amaurosis: blindness, in particular the type of blindness that is caused by disease of the optic nerve, the brain or the retina, so that the blind eye looks outwardly normal.

Amblyopia: dimness of vision without apparent abnormality in the eye.

Amenorrhoea: absence or stoppage of the menstrual flow. The commonest cause of amenorrhoea is pregnancy. *See* Menstruation.

Aminophylline: drug used to dilate the air passages in cases of reversible obstruction such as asthma. Used as a sustained-release preparation, it can be given by mouth every 12 hours. It is particularly useful used as an intravenous injection in the relief of acute severe attacks of asthma.

Ammonia: a gas with the chemical formula NH_3. It is soluble in water, and is used in solution for domestic purposes. It is very irritating to the lungs, and if inhaled can cause distressing symptoms. Inhalation of the vapour arising from a solution of ammonia, while uncomfortable, is not dangerous, but inhalation of the gas can cause oedema of the lungs and bronchitis; this is rarely serious. Ammonia can also cause burns.

Amnesia: loss of memory, a symptom occurring in a number of brain disorders such as early Alzheimer's disease or increased pressure from a tumour. Korsakoff's syndrome (q.v.) resulting from alcoholism has this effect. Some strokes will damage the memory, as will a prolonged period of oxygen deprivation or severe convulsions. It is common for a severe blow on the head, severe enough to cause unconsciousness, to result in a loss of memory for events both before and after the period of unconsciousness. The loss of memory of events leading up to the injury is called retrograde amnesia, and in time the memory returns, often completely. The loss of memory after the injury, which includes the period of unconsciousness, is called post-traumatic amnesia. There is a form of amnesia which lasts only for a matter of hours during which the subject is quite conscious and seems normal except for mild confusion. There is a loss of memory for past events, perhaps for years; but the person can carry out quite complicated tasks, such as driving or mowing the lawn. On recovery the memory is regained except for the period of the attack. The condition is called transient global amnesia; the cause is not understood, but there is usually no underlying illness and the attack does not recur. There remain cases of poor memory or loss of memory which are of psychological origin, being found in anxiety states and hysteria.

Amniocentesis: the withdrawal of amniotic fluid from a pregnant uterus *via* a needle introduced through the skin of the abdominal wall. The technique is used in the antenatal detection of Down's syndrome and other abnormalities in the foetus early after the third month of pregnancy. It carries a slight risk of miscarriage, between 0.5 and 1%. *See* also Chorionic Villus Sampling.

Amoeba: a single-celled microscopic organism belonging to the group of protozoa. The common amoeba is found in pond water and is just visible to the naked eye; it is harmless. Other harmless amoebae are found in the human intestinal tract; there is however an amoeba, *Entamoeba histolytica*, which infects about one-tenth of the world's population, mainly in tropical countries, and can produce severe dysentery with dangerous complications. Amoebic dysentery is treated with the drug metronidazole or, in severe cases, emetine hydrochloride or dehydroemetine. Travellers to tropical countries should be careful to observe simple hygienic measures, for the disease is spread by contamination of food by flies or the handling of food by those infected by the amoeba.

Amoxil: a derivative of ampicillin better absorbed by mouth.

Amphetamine (Benzedrine, Dexedrine, Methedrine): this drug acts as a stimulant to the central nervous system. It produces feelings of excitement, elation and alertness. High doses make the subject anxious, restless, tremulous, clumsy and talkative. The temperature may rise, and there may even be a collapse. Because of their stimulating action amphetamines have in the past been used to treat depression, to combat fatigue and to depress the appetite in the obese, but unfortunately they have proved to be drugs of addiction upon which the susceptible can easily become dependent, and it is known that brain damage can result from continued high doses. The use of amphetamines in medicine has therefore been given up, and they now have no place in treatment except in the rare case of narcolepsy.

Ampicillin: a penicillin with a wide range of action.

Amputation: the removal of part of the body, usually a limb.

Amylase: an enzyme concerned with the breakdown of starch. It is found in the salivary glands and the pancreas.

Amyl Nitrite: a clear yellow fluid which evaporates easily. Its action is to relieve spasm of smooth muscle and dilate the arteries. Dispensed in a glass capsule, it has been used to relieve the pain of angina pectoris (q.v.); the capsule is crushed and the vapour inhaled.

Amylobarbitone: proprietary name Amytal. A drug formerly used as a sedative and an aid to sleep. *See* Barbiturates.

Amyloid: in some patients with chronic diseases such as tuberculosis, rheumatoid arthritis, leprosy, ulcerative colitis and others, a peculiar substance is deposited in the walls of blood vessels, in connective tissue and in the organs themselves, called amyloid from a fancied resemblance to starch. According to the organ affected, illness is produced, for which the only cure is successful treatment of the causal disease. There is a rare hereditary form of amyloidosis.

Anabolic Drugs: one of the effects of the male hormone testosterone is to increase the weight and strength. It has been argued therefore that patients who need building up should be given male hormone, but a drawback is that whereas it is all very well for debilitated men to grow hair on their chests it is not so good for women. Various steroids similar to testosterone but without its virilising effects have been synthesised and are offered for use in convalescence from severe illness to increase growth and appetite, but there is considerable difference of opinion as to their value. They are called anabolic steroids because of their tissue-building properties. They have been abused by some athletes, although their value as body-builders is in doubt; in any case it is now illegal for athletes – or racehorse trainers – to use them.

Anaemia: a reduction of the concentration of haemoglobin and the number of red cells in the circulation. The WHO recommends that men with a haemoglobin level below 13 g/dl and women with a level below 12 g/dl should be considered anaemic. There are very many causes of anaemia, but roughly two main types: that in which the circulating red blood cells are smaller than usual, called microcytic anaemia, and that in which they are larger, called macrocytic anaemia. The diagnosis is made by means of a blood count. The mere fact that somebody looks pale is no proof that anaemia exists; although it is often used as an explanation when an individual feels generally run-down, is nervous, has a poor appetite and so on, it leads to these symptoms much less frequently than is generally believed. There is no point in self-medication with 'iron tonics' or pills. It is true that many cases of anaemia are treated with iron, but only after the doctor has established the presence and the cause of the condition can he say that iron should be used. In general the causes of microcytic anaemia are iron deficiency in the diet, chronic disorders including those causing continuous blood loss, such as peptic ulcers or menorrhagia, inadequate absorption of iron from the digestive tract, kidney disease or malignant disease. Drugs, chemicals or parasitic infestation can also be to blame. Iron therapy is often needed during pregnancy. The commonest cause of macrocytic anaemia is deficiency of vitamin B_{12} and folic acid. *See* Pernicious Anaemia, Sickle-cell Disease and Thalassaemia.

Anaesthesia: the primary meaning is a loss of feeling (particularly of the senses of pain and touch) found in organic diseases where damage to the sensory nerves, the spinal cord or the brain has occurred, or in certain psychological states. More generally it is applied to the deliberate induction of partial or total insensibility for the purpose of performing surgical operations.

In ancient times opium, hemp and alcohol were variously used to produce partial anaesthesia for such surgical operations as could be carried out, but none of these drugs could do more than reduce the pain. Surgery was a bloody and brutal business up to the introduction of modern anaesthetics in early Victorian times, and the rapid advances in surgery of the last hundred years are due as much to the discovery and refinement of anaesthesia as to increased knowledge of physiology and pathology. In 1785 Dr Pearson, an English physician, suggested the inhalation of ether for asthmatic attacks, and in 1800 Sir Humphrey Davy observed the anaesthetic effects of nitrous oxide (laughing gas). He proposed the use of nitrous oxide in surgical operations, and in 1818 Faraday and several American physicians noted the anaesthetic effects of ether, but it was left to the American dentist Horace Wells of Hartford, Connecticut, to use nitrous oxide as an anaesthetic in 1844, and to another American dentist, Dr Morton of Boston, to use ether in 1846. In the same year Liston carried out the first operation in Britain under ether anaesthesia, and during 1847 J.Y. Simpson of Edinburgh used ether in childbirth for the first time. Simpson discovered the use of chloroform as an anaesthetic a few months later. Until quite recent times the main general anaesthetic drugs such as ether or chloroform were given by inhalation through a mask, which made them moderately unpleasant for the patient; but the introduction of intravenous anaesthetics has made induction of a general anaesthetic no more distressing than a pinprick.

The modern anaesthetist has a number of drugs at hand, and will administer several drugs with different actions.

After the use of an intravenous agent to render the patient unconscious, anaesthesia is maintained by another drug given by inhalation, and a tube is passed into the trachea to ensure that the airway is clear. Further drugs may be given by injection to relax the muscles or drop the blood pressure as required. In cases where it is necessary to relax the muscles of respiration, the breathing will be assisted by hand or by a breathing machine. Before an operation the anaesthetist will make sure that the patient is as fit as possible and take note of probable difficulties, such as a history of previous sensitivity to an anaesthetic drug. Premedication, that is drugs to be given before the operation, will be prescribed to lessen the salivary and bronchial secretions, to sedate the patient, and to help the action of subsequent anaesthetic agents.

After the operation the anaesthetist will be responsible for the patient's condition until the return of consciousness, when it may be necessary to prescribe postoperative drugs for the relief of pain or anxiety. This responsibility continues if the patient is postoperatively in intensive care.

Local anaesthetics act by blocking nerve impulses in the nerve supply of the part of the body to be anaesthetised, and are applied to the surface of the body, or by injection either at the site of operation or into the sensory nerves supplying the part. There are a number of drugs used for local anaesthesia which vary in their action, enabling the operator to choose the most suitable for each operation. Cocaine was at one time used on the mucous membranes of the nose, throat and larynx, and on the eye, but its use has now almost ceased in favour of lignocaine or, in the case of the eye, amethocaine or oxybuprocaine. Infiltration of the skin to anaesthetise the nerve endings at the site of operation is called field block, and injection of the sensory nerves that supply a particular area, for example the brachial plexus for the arm, is called regional nerve-block. Local anaesthetics can sometimes be usefully combined with a light general anaesthetic.

Anaesthesia of the lower part of the body can be produced by injection of a local anaesthetic into the fluid in the space round the spinal cord and the nerves which issue from it, a technique called spinal anaesthesia, or into the space just outside the dura mater which envelops the spinal cord (epidural anaesthesia). The latter technique is useful in childbirth. Finally, it may be comforting to know that nobody ever gives away any secrets when anaesthetised.

Analgesia: the relief of pain in the conscious patient. Many drugs can be described as analgesics, from aspirin to morphine, and it often needs considerable skill to prescribe suitable drugs; people vary in their appreciation of pain and in their reaction to analgesics.

Anaphylaxis: a most severe and possibly fatal sudden reaction to the injection or the ingestion of a substance to which the victim has become abnormally sensitive. The precipitating factor can be the venom of a bee or wasp, a food or a drug, or the injection of a vaccine. Reactions to insect stings are thought to account for four deaths each year in the United Kingdom. The mechanism is the same as that involved in allergic reactions (*see* Allergy) but there is a virtual explosion of the reacting cells and consequent collapse, with failure of the circulation and swelling of the air passages. The only treatment likely to help is the immediate injection of adrenaline. People who are known to be sensitive to bee and wasp stings should carry adrenaline either as an inhaler or in an emergency kit with an ampoule of 1:1000 adrenaline for injection with a syringe and needle.

Anastomosis: communication between two hollow organs, blood vessels or spaces in the body. Communication between blood vessels – veins or arteries – is a feature of normal anatomy; anastomotic communication between two hollow organs, for example the cut ends of the bowel after the removal of a diseased segment, may be made by the surgeon in the course of an operation; rarely an anastomosis may be the result of disease or injury.

Anatomy: the study of the structure of the body and its parts. In ancient times physicians and surgeons could only make a superficial study of human anatomy (possibly on the battlefield) because of religious and other restraints and based many of their ideas on the examination of animals. It was, for example, believed that the uterus was double, as in the sow. Not until the Renaissance did scholars begin to study human anatomy in detail, but even then, for many years, their difficulties were made greater by the attitude of the Church. Few bodies were available; dissection had to be carried out quickly because means of preserving bodies were lacking. Students of anatomy attended demonstrations held in anatomy theatres, but had no chance of dissecting bodies for themselves. In recent times things have improved so that students have the chance of dissecting the body in detail. The provision of bodies has always been difficult, and even today the supply is often unequal to the demand. It is therefore sensible to consider leaving one's body for anatomical study, and those who wish to do so are advised to consult the professor of anatomy in the nearest university or medical school.

Androgen: a substance which causes masculinisation. The testes secrete the hormone testosterone which is partially responsible for male sexual development, and is the chief androgen. Used in the treatment of male castration and in retarded development of male characteristics due to pituitary or testicular malfunction, it is useless in the treatment of impotence unless there is accompanying deficiency of hormonal secretion. It is both useless and dangerous as an aphrodisiac. Androgens have the effect of increasing the use of protein in the body, and have therefore been used when this effect is wanted, for example in convalescence after a severe illness; but this use is limited because of the virilising action in women. See Anabolic Drugs.

Anencephaly: congenital abnormality where the upper part of the skull is missing, and the brain beneath defective or absent. It is not compatible with life.

Aneurysm: abnormal swelling of the wall of an artery, sometimes forming a sac, sometimes elongated or fusiform. It may be congenital, the result of injury, or formed by disease of the vessel wall, such as atherosclerosis or syphilis.

A false aneurysm is formed when blood has escaped from a damaged vessel and is outside it but contained in fibrous tissue. Disease of the vessel wall may result in a dissecting aneurysm, where the blood tracks between the layers of the wall of the artery, eventually bursting out. This occurs in people with a high blood pressure.

The commonest site for an aneurysm is in the abdominal aorta. If it leaks or bursts the patient develops acute pain in the upper abdomen or the back, and shock. It may give rise to symptoms without bursting, when the enlarged aorta can often be felt on examination of the abdomen. Occasionally an aneurysm is found in the abdominal aorta which has given rise to no symptoms at all. Aneurysms also occur in the thoracic aorta where they are usually found on a chest X-ray taken for some other condition, but they may give rise to chest pain or produce symptoms by obstructing the trachea, oesophagus or superior vena cava. Often the first sign of their presence is sudden death caused by rupture, for the thoracic aorta is the most common site of dissecting aneurysm. An aneurysm can occur in the popliteal artery, which is behind the knee. Here it can be felt as a pulsating swelling. Other sites of aneurysm formation are in the femoral artery in the thigh, and the arteries to the kidney and spleen. Aneurysms are also found in the brain, where they can press on the nerves to the eye and cause blindness or on the brain and cause paralyses; a burst aneurysm here causes sudden blinding headache, unconsciousness and possibly death. A slow leak causes headache and signs of irritation of the meninges, the membranes covering the brain (*see* Subarachnoid Haemorrhage).

Treatment is surgical, but difficult and in the case of abdominal and thoracic aortic aneurysms dangerous, especially if the aneurysm has burst. The intention is to introduce a graft, usually of knitted or woven dacron. In the case of aneurysms within the skull, many cases are successfully treated, the intention here being to obliterate the aneurysmal sac.

Angina: originally meaning choking or suffocating pain, the word is now applied to the disease causing the pain, for example Vincent's angina, an infection of the mouth and throat which may make breathing difficult, and angina pectoris, dealt with below.

Angina Pectoris: patients with disease of the coronary arteries of the heart may suffer from characteristic pain which is brought on by effort, particularly at the beginning of the day, after large meals and in cold weather. The pain is suffocating, and is often described as gripping or pressing. It is felt behind the breastbone and it spreads into the neck, into both sides of the chest, into the left arm and down over the upper abdomen. It may be very severe, but it is not usually sharp – sharp pains in the chest are more often due to indigestion than to heart disease. Anginal pain is caused by reduced blood supply to the heart muscle, which sends out distress signals when the circulation is too poor to cope with the work the heart is required to do. The pain produced stops the patient in his tracks; a particularly effective alarm system, for when the patient rests the load is taken off the heart, the circulation becomes just adequate, and the pain goes. Anginal pain that persists when the patient is at rest is a sign of serious disease. The diagnosis is made on the basis of the characteristic nature of the pain and confirmed by an electrocardiogram (q.v.).

Treatment calls for rest and relief of anxiety and fear, and the patient must learn to live inside the 'envelope of performance' defined by the pain. Smoking must be stopped, but there is no objection to alcohol in moderation. Those who are found to have a high blood cholesterol (above 6.5 mmol.) should alter their diet (*see* Cholesterol). Raised blood pressure needs treatment, and any tendency to excess weight should be controlled. The most effective drug for swift relief of anginal pain is glyceryl trinitrate taken in tablets dissolved beneath the tongue or in an aerosol spray; the effect lasts for about half an hour. The drug may be taken to relieve an attack or before exertion likely to provoke an attack. The tablets only last for eight weeks, then need renewing. Adhesive plasters containing glyceryl trinitrate can be used on the skin of the chest; the effect lasts for 24 hours, and a different site should be used each time the plaster is renewed. Ointment to be applied to the skin is also available. Longer-acting drugs are isosorbide dinitrate and isosorbide mononitrate which can be taken two or three times a day. Other drugs used in the treatment of angina are a group called calcium-channel blockers; they reduce the force of the heartbeat, slow down the conduction of electrical impulses in the heart, and dilate the blood vessels. They may be used in conjunction with another group of drugs called beta-blockers (q.v.).

Angiography: radio-opaque substances injected into the blood vessels render them visible on X-ray examination. The resulting angiograms demonstrate the outline and course of the vessels so that abnormalities and displacements can be seen.

Angioma: a tumour or swelling made up of a cluster of abnormal blood vessels. Angiomas may occur in the internal organs, especially in the brain where they may bleed dangerously or give rise to epileptic attacks, or on the surface of the skin in the form of naevi or birthmarks. Treatment is indicated when they are inconvenient or ugly; small angiomas can be cauterised with the electric needle, larger ones are removed under local or general anaesthetic. Angiomas are not malignant or cancerous. *See* Birthmark.

Angioneurotic Oedema: also called giant urticaria, this produces large swellings of the subcutaneous tissues particularly of the face and hands. Occasionally the swelling involves the air passages of the nose and throat so that there is obstruction to the breathing. The condition is an immunological reaction (*see* Allergy); some families are particularly prone to it. Young people are particularly affected, often those of a sensitive and nervous disposition (the condition sometimes appears after emotional stress). Treatment is by antihistamine drugs; obstruction to breathing requires immediate injection of adrenaline.

Aniline Poisoning: aniline is amino-benzene, and the term aniline poisoning is taken to include poisoning with nitro- as well as amino- compounds of benzene and chlorbenzene, for example nitro-benzene and tri-nitro-toluene (TNT). The substances are absorbed through the skin or mouth, and produce dizziness, headache, nausea and difficulty in breathing. The patient may go blue. Jaundice may follow because of liver damage, especially with TNT. In acute cases the diagnosis may be easy because the patient is known to have been in contact with the poison, but in chronic cases where the poison has been slowly absorbed over a period of time it is more difficult to recognise what is wrong. The patient feels weak and tired, gets out of breath easily and may complain of indigestion; he may become jaundiced In an acute case the whole body must be washed clean, and if there is difficulty in breathing the patient may need oxygen. He must be put to bed; alcohol is dangerous and must not be given. During convalescence anaemia may develop and need treatment with iron. There is no specific antidote to aniline poisoning.

Animals Causing Disease: *see* Zoonoses.

Ankylosing Spondylitis. inflammation of the joints of the spine eventually leading to rigidity of the spine. Occurring mostly in young males, the disease is familial, and is associated with the tissue type antigen HLA B27. The exact mechanism producing the disease is unknown; it starts in the sacro-iliac joints, where it may give rise to low back pain, worse after rest and improved by exercise. In time the spine becomes stiff; the normal curve in the lower back becomes straight, and the thoracic curve more pronounced. The process can stop at any time. X-ray examination of advanced disease shows characteristic changes described as 'bamboo spine'. Treatment is aimed at reducing pain by the use of NSAI drugs (q.v.) and physiotherapy to keep the posture as normal as possible. Expectation of life is not lessened.

Ankylosis: fixation or near-fixation of a joint normally freely movable, brought about by disease, injury or surgical operation. Common causes of ankylosis are tuberculosis, rheumatoid arthritis or septic arthritis, in which conditions the bones become bound together by scar tissue. Joint deformities caused by fractures can result in ankylosis, and fixation of a joint may follow if it is kept immobilised for a long time. Ankylosis of a joint can be achieved by gross hysterics who maintain that it is paralysed, or by mystics who hold a limb in the same position for years as part of their religious devotions. Sometimes the surgeon deliberately causes ankylosis of a painful joint with restricted movement in order to relieve chronic pain.

Ankylostoma: the hookworm, a parasite found in the tropics, parts of Western Europe, and the southern States of the USA. In temperate lands it is usually found in damp and insanitary places like tunnels and sewers. *See* Hookworm.

Anopheles: a genus of mosquito, some species of which can carry from man to man the parasite of malaria (q.v.). The female anopheline mosquito bites an infected person and takes up in the blood the sexually differentiated forms of the parasite, which couple in the mosquito and produce many hundred asexual parasites. These the mosquito passes on to the next person it bites. The female anopheles is identified by its posture at rest; the body makes an angle with the surface on which it alights, while the culicine mosquito, which does not transmit malaria, rests with its body parallel to the surface.

Anorexia Nervosa: first described in 1868, the 'slimmer's disease' is a complex condition made up of psychological disturbance, nutritional deficiency and hormonal upset. Occurring mainly in girls between the ages of 14 and 17, the patient takes to a slimming diet under the impression that she is too fat, although her development is in fact quite normal. The avulsion to food is taken to extremes; she becomes progressively thinner, irritable and restless, and her periods cease. She will deny that there is anything wrong, and persist in the belief that if she eats a reasonable diet she will become too fat; she is not able to see that she has become too thin. Treatment is dependent upon the doctor and attendants gaining the confidence of the patient, and sympathetically persuading her to eat normally. Often she will need to be admitted to hospital, and the attendance of a psychiatrist may be essential, although many patients will not admit to any psychological disturbance. The introduction of a normal diet must proceed slowly, and the patient's progress followed by regular weighing. Successful treatment results in a return to normal weight in a month or two, but there is a tendency to relapse; the disease may last for up to three years or longer and requires continuing sympathetic support from family and friends. Unfortunately about a quarter of the patients tend to relapse into a chronic state with continuing psychological disturbance and increasing malnutrition, and in some cases the outcome is fatal. The disease is uncommon in young males.

Anosmia: absence of the sense of smell.

Anoxia: lack of oxygen, which may be relative or absolute.

Antabuse: proprietary name of disulfiram. *See* Alcoholism.

Antacids: medicines for counteracting gastric acidity. *See* Alkalis.

Antenatal Diagnosis: *see* Amniocentesis, Chorionic Villus Sampling.

Anterior Tibial Syndrome: unaccustomed exercise may produce severe pain and swelling in the shins on one or both sides, due to swelling of the anterior tibial muscles. The pain may become chronic, coming on after the slightest exercise, and in such a case the fibrous membrane (fascia) which encloses the muscle may have to be opened surgically.

Anthelmintics: drugs used to kill or drive out parasitic worms from the body. They include mebendazole, active against threadworms (pinworms), roundworms, hookworms and whipworms, piperazine for threadworms and roundworms, niclosamide for tapeworms, and bephenium for hookworms. *See* Worms.

Anthracosis: deposition of carbon or coal dust found in the lungs of miners. It may be present in city-dwellers from the inhalation of soot; there is no evidence that it does any harm.

Anthrax: an infectious disease caught from herbivorous animals, usually from carcases or hides. Farmers, veterinary surgeons and butchers are liable to contract anthrax, which is also known as woolsorter's disease, rag-picker's disease, and malignant pustule. Workers in industries dealing with bones, hides, hair and bristles are at risk. The disease is caused by a bacillus, *Bacillus anthracis*, and is most common in Australia, Russia and South America. It is not common in the United Kingdom. There are two types of anthrax, external and internal. The external type can occur by infection through cracks and cuts in the skin, even from hides long removed from the animal; a 'boil' appears in the area, often on the face, neck or arm, and the inflamed area spreads and the centre ulcerates to produce a black scab. Internally, breathing in the spores of the bacillus perhaps from wool or eating infected flesh gives rise to acute pneumonia or gastro-enteritis. Examination of scrapings from the external ulcer will disclose the presence of the anthrax bacillus, but diagnosis of the internal disease is difficult and may be impossible. Fortunately the anthrax bacillus is sensitive to antibiotics, and benzyl penicillin is the drug of choice; but because of the difficulty in recognising the internal form of the disease, treatment may be too late or not possible at all, and the condition then proves fatal. Prevention includes destruction by burning of all hides and bodies thought to be infected, disinfection of premises, and prevention of grazing in the infected area. Free ventilation of factories will stop the spread of respiratory or gastro-intestinal anthrax, and preventive clothes may be worn by workers. It is possible to immunise both animals and human beings against anthrax.

Antibiotics: collective name for a class of substances produced by living organisms which are capable of destroying or stopping the growth of pathogenic organisms, i.e. organisms causing disease. It is also used to cover similar synthetic compounds which have the same function. The best-known is penicillin, found by Fleming in 1928 and introduced into clinical use by Florey and Chain in 1941. Research has since produced a large number of antibiotics, but as each comes into general use it stimulates the growth of resistant organisms. The problem of resistance has been made more difficult by the indiscriminate use of antibiotics. Ideally, they should never be used in trivial illnesses: their use should be confined to infections in which the causative organism has been identified and shown to be sensitive, but this is a counsel of perfection and in practice they tend to be prescribed for almost any condition in which there is a remote possibility that they might help. They are unfortunately useless against viruses.

Antibody: *see* Allergy.

Anticoagulants: drugs which reduce the formation of clot in the blood. They are used to prevent the formation of clots in the veins after operation and, in cases where it is known that clotting has occurred, to prevent further extension of the clot. They are used in vascular surgery and in renal dialysis. There are two types of anticoagulants: those that can be given by mouth, and those given by direct infusion into the blood vessels. Heparin is given by intravenous infusion; its action is quick and its effect short-lived and therefore controllable. Warfarin is the drug most commonly used by mouth. Its action is slow, and it takes 36 or 48 hours to reach its full effect. The dosage is regulated by laboratory tests on the blood, undertaken at regular intervals. Patients who are taking anticoagulants should carry a card with them giving the name of the drug and the dose, and show it to any doctor who is unfamiliar with their case, for there are a number of drugs such as aspirin which alter the action of anticoagulants. Warfarin – the name is taken from the Wisconsin Alumni Research Foundation – has been used widely as a rat poison.

Antidepressants: drugs used to control the psychiatric illness of depression. *See* Mental Illness.

Antidote: substance given to counteract the effect of a poison. *See* Poisons.

Antihistamines: histamine is one of the substances liberated by the cells of the body in cases of allergy (q.v.); it produces the symptoms of various allergic diseases. Antihistamines are drugs which counteract the effects of histamine; they are used in the treatment of hay fever, urticaria, allergic and itching rashes, insect bites and stings and drug allergies. They are not useful in asthma. There are a number of antihistamines, and it can be sensible to try to establish which one suits a particular person best. With most of them there is the drawback that they make people drowsy, and this may interfere with the ability to drive or operate machinery. The effect of alcohol is intensified. These adverse actions are not as likely to occur with newer compounds such as astemizole or terfenadine. It must be pointed out that it is not a good idea to use antihistamine creams locally on insect bites and stings, for not only are they likely to have little effect but they may themselves set up a hypersensitivity. Antihistamines can be useful in the treatment of nausea and vomiting, and may be used in the care of children for their sedative action (promethazine, trimeprazine).

Antimony: a metal similar in its effects to arsenic. Formerly used in the treatment of fever and bronchitis, and in the form of tartar emetic as an emetic (for which it is not to be recommended). It is very poisonous to protozoa and is therefore used in the treatment of some tropical diseases such as sleeping sickness, bilharzia and leishmaniasis (q.v.).

Antiphlogistics: substances used to treat inflammation, usually used to mean poultices applied to the surface of the body, the most familiar being the kaolin poultice.

Antipyretic: a substance or method of treatment to reduce fever, e.g. aspirin in adults or paracetamol in children.

Antiseptics: strictly speaking, substances that destroy or arrest the development of the bacteria which cause putrefaction. A disinfectant destroys the organisms causing disease; but the two terms have been so often confused that they are now virtually synonymous. Although Louis Pasteur (1822–95) first discovered the fact that bacteria could cause disease, the Hungarian obstetrician Ignaz Semmelweis (1818–65), while working in Vienna in 1846, had demonstrated that contamination of the hands of attendants could spread childbed fever. He tried to make his colleagues understand that this was so, but the profession would believe neither him nor Oliver Wendell Holmes of Boston (1809–94) who had maintained that puerperal fever was contagious in 1843. It was left to Lord Lister (1827–1912) to realise that Pasteur's work accounted for the fact that infection was so common in surgical wounds, and in London in 1865 he introduced carbolic acid as an antiseptic in his operating theatre. Gradually the use of antiseptics in surgery was supplanted by aseptic techniques (*see* Asepsis) in which everything used in an operation is sterile so that infecting bacteria are kept away rather than killed on arrival. Nowadays antiseptics are used to clean the skin or to clean dirty wounds. They have to be used carefully because they can delay healing; many surgeons believe that the best and mildest antiseptic is soap and water, and this is true of the cuts and abrasions of everyday life.

Antiserum: serum from an animal that has been infected with a disease naturally or artificially and has formed antibodies which are contained in the serum. Unfortunately the use of animal serum to combat diseases such as tetanus in man has in the past given rise to severe, sometimes fatal, reactions (*see* Allergy, Anaphylaxis, Serum Sickness) and the use of such preparations has been given up in favour of human immunoglobulins prepared from the blood of people with an immunity to the disease in question. It is best, however, to be immunised actively against such diseases as tetanus and diphtheria, for the use of immunoglobulins which give immediate protection confers only a passive immunity which does not last.

Antispasmodics: drugs to counteract the spasm which may occur in hollow organs such as the gastro-intestinal tract or the ureter. Ureteric pain, which can be caused by the passage or the arrest of a stone, can be very severe and requires the injection of atropine or hyoscine. Spasms of the smooth muscle of the stomach or intestine can be helped by dicyclomine and other preparations, while spasm of the lower bowel is often relieved by mebeverine.

Antitoxin: antibody formed in the blood in response to the presence of a toxin, which may be from an animal, e.g. bee or wasp, a bacterium or a plant.

Antrum: used in anatomy to mean a cavity, especially in a bone. The maxillary antrum lies in the upper jawbone between the palate and the eye-socket, and the mastoid antrum lies behind the ear.

Anuria: condition in which no urine is produced by the body. It can be caused by failure of the kidneys, low pressure in the renal arteries, or blockage of the ureters.

Anus: end of the alimentary canal, where the rectum opens to the exterior. It is controlled by two sphincters or rings of muscle.

Anxiety: *see* Neurosis.

Aorta: main artery of the body. Beginning in the chest at the left ventricle of the heart, it curves up, over and down to pass through the diaphragm into the abdominal cavity, where it ends opposite the fourth lumbar vertebra, dividing into the left and right common iliac arteries. During its course it gives off many branches through which the body is supplied with oxygenated, or arterial, blood.

Aperients: *see* Constipation.

Apgar Score: in 1952 Dr Virginia Apgar (1909–74) introduced in the USA a method of assessing the condition of a newborn infant by observing a number of physiological factors such as heart rate and denoting their functional state by reference to an agreed scale, from which could be derived an inclusive judgement expressed as a number.

Aphakia: condition in which the lens is missing from the eye.

Aphasia: loss of the power of speech or the understanding of speech, reading and writing, caused by damage to the parts of the brain concerned with these functions. Dysphasia is a lesser degree of the same defect. Aphasia can be sensory or motor, for the main parts of the brain concerned with language are divided into the afferent or sensory side and the efferent or motor side. The sensory side is in the upper part of the temporal lobe, and is responsible for the understanding of words both written and spoken. The motor area is in the lower rear part of the frontal lobe of the brain above the sensory area, and in front of it. The 'speech centre' is in the dominant side of the brain – in right-handed people on the left side, in those left-handed the right. Damage to the sensory area produces word deafness, where the words cannot be understood although the power of hearing is intact, and word blindness where the patient is not blind but cannot read written words. If the motor area is disturbed, the patient suffers from motor aphasia, when the attempt to speak produces only unintelligible noises, and agraphia where the function of the hand is apparently normal but writing impossible. In practice, word deafness affects the power of speech, for if the patients cannot hear themselves speak, understandably speech relapses into nonsense. Moreover, injuries and diseases of the brain nearly always affect a mixed area and produce a mixture of symptoms. Because we think largely in words, serious aphasia may lead to a degree of confusion.

Aphrodisiac: substance which gives rise to sexual desire or increases the potency. Unhappily genuine aphrodisiacs have so far defied detection; but much practical research has been pursued into the matter. *See* Cantharides, Impotence.

Apical Abscess: a abscess forming at the tip of the root of a tooth as a result of disease of the tooth. The abscess may extend and cause the face to swell. It may present itself as a localised swelling in the mouth – a gum boil. Treatment involves a course of antibiotics and a visit to the dentist.

Apnoea: cessation of breathing.

Apollonia, St: patron saint of dentists. She was burned at the stake after her teeth had been struck out.

Apomorphine: an alkaloid drug derived from opium, used as an emetic when given by mouth. It has a violent and unpleasant action on the vomiting centre.

Apoplexy: a stroke. The condition is caused by a sudden accident (haemorrhage, thrombosis or embolism) occurring in a diseased blood vessel responsible for part of the blood supply to the brain, resulting in loss of consciousness, paralysis or death. Strokes are not uncommon in the later part of life. If a patient suddenly becomes unconscious and lapses into coma the chances are that it is a stroke; the smell of alcohol on the breath can be confusing, but must not be misleading. While strokes usually occur in the middle-aged or elderly, if the apoplexy is caused by a burst cerebral aneurysm (q.v.) it can happen to younger people. Sometimes warning signs precede a stroke, especially when clotting begins in a smaller branch and spreads back into the main artery; tingling or clumsiness of a limb can be followed by paralysis and loss of consciousness. If the stroke is due to clotting in the internal carotid artery (the main artery supplying the brain) there may have been previous attacks of weakness, difficulty in speech or confusion. Sometimes a severe headache gives warning of an impending stroke, but those due to an embolism (blocking of an artery by a clot formed elsewhere) are quite sudden.

Immediate treatment must ensure that the patient can breathe freely and easily and is kept warm. Do not try to give alcohol or indeed anything to drink or eat. Patients who are going to recover begin to regain consciousness within a day or two, being at first confused and restless. As they become more aware of their surroundings it becomes possible to tell how much paralysis the stroke has caused. The convalescence may be complicated by pneumonia or the development of bedsores, and the nursing is hard work. Over the weeks recovery begins to take place, but unless the paralysed limbs are moved through their full range at least four times a day they will stiffen irrevocably and become painful. The limb muscles must not be allowed to contract; it may be necessary to use splints to prevent the limbs flexing at the joints. Convalescence can be long and hard, especially if the patient is left with difficulty of speech and comprehension, and demands courage from the patient and determination and patience from the attendants. The only sort of apoplexy that is likely to respond to active treatment at the outset is that due to bleeding from an aneurysm, but occasionally it is possible to evacuate a large clot from the brain. Both these conditions are revealed by angiography.

Apothecary: the old term for one who prepared and sold medicines, the activity now carried on by pharmacists. Eighteenth-century apothecaries were also medical practitioners, and the Apothecaries Act of 1815 requiring apothecaries to have been licensed by the Apothecaries Society after five years' training was the first attempt to lay down a standard for medical practice in England and Wales.

Apothecaries' weights were once used in compounding medicines. They are now obsolete; they were:

20 grains or minims	= 1 scruple
3 scruples	= 1 drachm
8 drachms	= 1 ounce
12 ounces	= 1 pound

Liquid measure:

60 minims	= 1 fluid drachm
8 fluid drachms	= 1 fluid ounce
20 fluid ounces	= 1 pint

Appendicitis: inflammation of the vermiform appendix, a vestigial structure attached to the caecum at the point where the small intestine joins the large intestine. A bacterial infection, appendicitis is not caused by swallowing fruit stones, an idea produced by the concretions (faecoliths) looking like fruit stones found in a diseased appendix. Although appendicitis accounts for about half the acute abdominal emergencies occurring between the ages of 10 and 30, it was not recognised until the last quarter of the nineteenth century. Inflammation of this part of the gut was called perityphlitis, which means inflammation around the caecum. One of the first operations for appendicitis was carried out on King Edward VII in 1902, and after this it became fashionable.

The pain of appendicitis is often first felt about the navel; it later moves down to the right lower part of the abdomen. The pain may be preceded by general discomfort in the abdomen, indigestion, diarrhoea or constipation; nausea is common, and the patient may vomit once or twice. The appetite is lost. The tongue and the mouth are dry and there is often foetid breath. Diagnosis is sometimes difficult, especially in the elderly patient, but in a straightforward case the abdomen is tender, especially in the right lower quadrant, where a resistance is felt because the muscles over an inflamed appendix become tense as the overlying peritoneum becomes involved. This is known as guarding or rigidity. Internal examination discloses tenderness in the pelvis, and is very important in diagnosis. If the appendix perforates, peritonitis, at first local, is set up and the signs are intensified; the tenderness is greater, the muscles rigid, the temperature rises and the patient becomes shocked, pale and clammy as the peritonitis spreads. If the infection arising from the ruptured appendix is successfully localised by natural processes, an appendix abscess may be formed.

The best treatment of appendicitis is removal of the appendix at the earliest possible stage. If an abscess has formed it is drained, and the appendix may be removed later. Peritonitis is treated by antibiotics, as are cases where operation is not possible. The diagnosis of 'grumbling' appendix is not made now as often as it once was, for it is recognised that recurrent pain in the right lower abdomen with irregular bowel action, loss of appetite and mild nausea is more likely to be due to other conditions such as the irritable bowel syndrome (q.v.). While it is possible that a patient may suffer from recurrent attacks of mild inflammation of the appendix short of the acute state, only to be terminated by removal of the organ, many surgeons doubt the existence of 'chronic' appendicitis. In any case a diagnosis of grumbling or chronic appendicitis is only to be made when a diligent search has failed to demonstrate any other cause for pain in the right lower abdomen.

Approved Names: non-proprietary names for drugs, otherwise known as generic names. These names are those used in the British National Formulary in the United Kingdom, and are agreed by the British Pharmacopoea Commission. In general the use of generic names in prescribing rather than brand names is more economical.

Arachnoid: one of the membranes covering the brain, named for its resemblance to a spider's web.

Arbovirus: a virus transmitted by insects and spiders. Examples are the viruses of dengue fever, sandfly fever and yellow fever.

Areola: round coloured area surrounding a raised centre, e.g. the red area around a pustule. The areola of the breast is the pink area surrounding the nipple which becomes brown in women who have borne children.

Argyll Robertson Pupil: named after Douglas Argyll Robertson (1837–1909), the Scottish ophthalmologist who first described it, this is a condition in which the pupil of the eye does not contract when a light is shone into it, but does contract on accommodation; that is, when a patient looks at something far away and then something very near. The affected pupil is small and irregular, and characteristically is found in syphilitic infection of the central nervous system.

Arm: designed to put the hand where it is needed, the arm is capable of remarkable flexibility of movement. The bone of the upper arm is the humerus, which at its upper end makes a ball-and-socket joint with the shoulder-blade, the scapula, and at its lower end a hinge joint with the bones of the forearm, the radius and ulna. The scapula is able to move in relation to the thorax and swivel so that the arm can be moved above the head (*see* Shoulder), the shoulder girdle being supported by strong muscles running from the chest wall. The ball-and-socket joint between the humerus and the scapula has a free range of movement forwards, backwards and sideways. The movements at the elbow (q.v.) are flexion and extension. The bones of the forearm can twist round each other; the ulna is fixed at the elbow, the radius at the wrist, and they move so that the palm of the hand can face up or down with the elbow bent and forwards or backwards with the arm at the side. Rotation of the whole arm takes place at the shoulder joint.

The artery of the arm is the brachial artery, a branch

of the subclavian artery; it branches at the elbow into the radial and ulnar arteries. The deep veins run with the arteries, but superficial veins show on the back of the hand and up the forearm, and are accessible at the elbow. The vein running up the outside of the arm is the cephalic vein, and that on the inner side the basilic vein. They communicate through the median cubital vein at the front of the elbow. The lymphatic vessels of the arm run into nodes at the elbow and in the armpits. The return of fluid from the arm depends on the pumping action of the muscles, and if the hand, elbow or shoulder are immobilised and the limb allowed to hang down it becomes swollen unless the muscles are exercised.

The nerves supplying the arm come from the cervical nerve roots 5, 6, 7, 8, and the first thoracic root, which form a plexus, the brachial plexus, from which the separate nerves take origin. The principal nerves are the median, which supplies muscles of the forearm and some in the hand, the ulnar, which supplies most of the small muscles of the hand and two of the forearm, and the radial, which supplies many muscles of the arm and forearm.

Arrythmia: term describing any irregularity in the rhythm of the heartbeat.

Arsenic: metallic element which, when given in big enough doses, irritates the stomach and intestines and blocks the action of enzymes. It is not used in modern medicine, although small doses are said to revive the appetite and make the hair shine. Before penicillin it was used in the treatment of syphilis in the form of Salvarsan. It is a traditional poison, and used as such causes nausea and faintness, followed by violent vomiting and diarrhoea, cramps, convulsions and coma. Although it may be available, it is not recommended to the murderer, for it is readily identified. The antidote is dimercaprol, given by injection. It is possible to build up an immunity to the effects of arsenic; the arsenic eaters of Styria took amounts that would kill several normal men, but prolonged exposure to arsenic is said to predispose to cancer of the skin or other organs.

Arsine: arseniuretted hydrogen, a chemical formed by the interaction of compounds containing arsenic and hydrochloric acid. It has a smell rather like garlic, and has been implicated as a cause of industrial poisoning. Victims suffer faintness, weakness and nausea and a severe headache followed by abdominal pain, pain in the muscles and loins and shivering. These symptoms may develop some hours after exposure to arsine, and they are succeeded by jaundice, passage of blood pigment in the urine, anaemia and anuria. Although arsine is essential in some industrial processes, its dangers are well known and adequate precautions are taken.

Arterial Disease: because the arteries are solely responsible for bringing to the vital organs and other parts of the body oxygen and nourishment without which they die, death and disease are often determined by the state of the arteries. The commonest cause of death in the over-forties is insufficient circulation to the brain or heart caused by arterial atherosclerosis. This begins as a fatty streak on the inner lining of the artery, which proceeds to the formation of a fibrous patch or plaque. As the plaque grows it begins to obstruct the artery, and clots may form on it. Eventually the artery may become blocked. Factors encouraging the development of atherosclerosis are smoking cigarettes, obesity, high blood pressure, diabetes and excess of cholesterol (q.v.) in the blood. There may be a family history of arterial disease. Treatment of the condition has recently become much improved through advances in vascular surgery, for treatment with drugs has never been very satisfactory. The best way to discourage the onset of arterial disease is to eschew smoking, take exercise, and keep an eye on the weight.

Arteries: the blood vessels that carry oxygenated blood round the body. The exceptions are the pulmonary arteries which carry deoxygenated blood from the right side of the heart to the lungs. The aorta carries blood pumped from the left side of the heart and gives off the main arteries, which divide into ever smaller branches ending in tiny arteries called arterioles, taking blood to the capillary vessels of the tissues. Blood is pumped from the heart at a considerable pressure – the blood pressure – and the walls of the arteries are pulsatile and relatively thick, containing elastic tissue and smooth muscle. The arterial system has many connections between its branches, so that interruption of one artery does not mean that all the blood supply to a part is cut off: the circulation can be carried on through various anastomoses (q.v.).

Arthritis: inflammation of joints or a joint. In general applied to osteoarthritis, a degenerative condition usually seen after the age of 50. *See* Gout, Osteoarthritis, Rheumatic Fever, Rheumatoid Arthritis.

Arthrodesis: surgical abolition of movement in a joint in order to stop pain or to make the joint stable.

Arthroplasty: the opposite of arthrodesis: the surgical formation of a moving joint, possibly by the construction of an artificial one.

Arthroscopy: examination of the interior of a joint through an endoscope (*see* Endoscopy). It is now possible to carry out certain operations on the knee through an endoscope.

Artificial Insemination: introduction of semen into the vagina by artificial means. This procedure has been used for years in the breeding of animals (except racehorses) and is available for families in which the husband is unable to impregnate his wife in the ordinary way because there is some impediment to intercourse. His semen, obtained by masturbation, is injected by a syringe high into the vagina in the middle of the menstrual cycle, which is about the time of ovulation. This is known as AIH (Artificial Insemination by Husband). If the husband is sterile it is possible to obtain semen, possibly frozen, from an anonymous donor (AID). This is regarded as morally wrong by most religious bodies, and is specifically forbidden by the Roman Catholic Church. *See* Assisted Conception.

Artificial Kidney: the function of the kidney is to filter the waste products of metabolism from the blood and to keep the chemical balance of the body within normal limits. In severe kidney disease the kidney fails to do this, and the patient becomes very ill; death may ensue from the accumulation of waste products and disturbance of the blood chemistry. It is possible to withdraw blood from the circulation, remove the waste products from it and return it to the body again by using an artificial kidney. In principle the blood is passed over a membrane on the other side of which is a specially formulated solution. Waste products pass across the membrane, so that the composition of the blood is gradually rectified. The process has to be carried out regularly and by its use patients otherwise doomed can be kept alive indefinitely or until it is possible to carry out a kidney replacement operation. The technique is called renal dialysis (q.v.).

Artificial Respiration: mouth-to-mouth artificial respiration is the method of choice. First the airway must be clear, and the first step in reviving those who have ceased to breathe naturally is to remove all obstructions, such as dentures or dental plates, from the mouth. The tongue must be well forward and the head back. Pinch the patient's nose with the left hand, keep the jaw well forward with the right, and blow into the mouth until the chest wall rises. Let the air come out of the lungs by itself before blowing again. The first 10 breaths should be as rapid as possible, and after that the rate of artificial respiration should be between 12 and 20 times a minute; it should be continued until the patient starts breathing or is obviously dead. In cases of electrocution artificial respiration should go on for two hours before hope is abandoned. Some people may find the idea of mouth-to-mouth artificial respiration aesthetically unattractive, but it is possible to carry it out successfully through a handkerchief placed over the patient's mouth and nose.

Other more modern – see 2 Kings 4:34 – techniques of artificial respiration are the Holger–Nielsen method and Eve's rocking method. In the Holger–Nielsen technique the patient is laid flat on the ground face downwards with false teeth and any other obstruction from the mouth or throat removed. The arms are placed forwards on each side of the head and the elbows bent outwards so that the hands lying palm downwards, one on top of the other, are beneath the forehead. The back is then smacked hard to bring the tongue forward. The operator kneels on his right knee in line with the patient's head and facing his back, the left leg being placed with the heel near the patient's right elbow. The hands are placed on the patient's shoulder-blades and the operator leans forward until the arms are vertical, forcing the air out of the patient's chest. This should take $2\frac{1}{2}$ seconds; the hands are then moved along the patient's arms as far as the elbows, and the arms and shoulders lifted up until the weight of the chest is felt. The chest or head should not be moved. This should cause inspiration for $2\frac{1}{2}$ seconds. The elbows are then lowered and the operator's hands move back to the shoulder-blades to repeat the cycle.

In Eve's rocking method the patient is rocked up and down while lying secured to a stretcher on a pivot, the tilt up and down being 45 degrees from the horizontal. This rocking is carried out 10 times a minute, and has the advantage of stimulating the circulation as well as the breathing. Nevertheless, the best method of artificial respiration is the mouth-to-mouth.

In some cases the heart has stopped beating or is beating so feebly that there is no pulse. If this is so, carry out cardiac massage (q.v.) giving about eight impulses to the heart to every respiration. The most important thing in starting artificial respiration is speed. Don't wait – get on with it.

Asbestosis: the lungs of workers who inhale asbestos fibres are liable to react to the inhaled dust by becoming fibrous. The symptoms are breathlessness, cough, loss of appetite and weight. Pneumonia may develop; worse, asbestosis is associated with the development of malignant growths of the lung and pleura. Protection against inhaling dust containing asbestos fibres is therefore of great importance to all who may come into contact with the substance. *See* Pneumoconiosis.

Ascaris Lumbricoides: roundworm, looking rather like an earthworm, which may infest human beings, usually children. Drugs used in treatment include mebendazole and piperazine. *See* Worms.

Ascites: an accumulation of fluid within the peritoneal cavity of the abdomen. It makes the abdomen swell in such conditions as heart, kidney or liver disease which bring about exudation of fluid from the blood vessels. If the accumulation of fluid becomes large it can be drawn off by a needle passed under local anaesthetic through the abdominal wall, an operation called paracentesis abdominis.

Ascorbic Acid: vitamin C. Deficiency causes scurvy, lowered resistance to infection and slow wound healing. There is no evidence to support the belief that large doses are useful in treating the common cold.

Asepsis: in modern surgery infection is prevented by excluding bacteria from the operating area rather than by destroying them after they have gained entry (*see* Antiseptic). In theory the operating theatre is sterile, but everybody who goes in there is of course covered with germs. All staff working in operating theatres should change their clothes before they go in; spectators or visitors must cover their clothes with a gown and discard their outdoor shoes. Masks must cover the mouth to catch infected droplets from the nose and throat, and caps cover the hair completely. The surgeon and assistants wash their hands thoroughly and wear sterile gloves and gowns; they touch nothing that is not sterile, and even then touch sterile instruments as little as possible. Everyone who enters an operating theatre must submit to the discipline of asepsis: there can be no room for sloppiness or carelessness.

Asphyxia: suffocation. It can be brought about by obstruction to the air passages, by lack of oxygen in the air, or by gases which interfere with the use of oxygen by the body, such as carbon monoxide (q.v.). Those asphyxiated by obstruction to the airway or lack of oxygen go blue, but victims of carbon monoxide poisoning retain the pink colour of the lips and mouth. Sometimes the difficulties of rescuing those overcome by fumes is very great, and it must be remembered that two casualties are worse than one. If breathing apparatus is not to hand, then at least the rescuer should have a rope tied round him in case he too is overcome.

Aspiration: withdrawal of fluid, etc., from the body, for example from the joint in the case of effusion into the knee, or the sucking out of mucus from the trachea.

Aspirin: proprietary name invented by the Bayer Drug Company for acetylsalicylic acid, first discovered in Germany in 1899. The name has since passed into general use. It is a mild analgesic, lowers the body temperature when raised by a fever, and has an important effect in reducing the swelling which accompanies inflammation. It is extremely useful in the treatment of rheumatic fever and arthritis; it also has an action in preventing the clotting of blood, and in small daily doses has been used after cerebral or cardiac thromboses to prevent further attacks. Unfortunately it has a tendency to cause bleeding in the stomach, and has been implicated as a factor in the causation of Reye's disease (q.v.); its use in children under the age of twelve is not now recommended. It may produce urticaria in sensitive people and in asthmatics may precipitate an attack.

Assisted Conception: assisted conception is conception occurring in those who have not been able to conceive without medical treatment. Methods used include artificial insemination, where sperm from the husband (AIH) or from a donor (AID) is placed in the vagina or in the cervix of the uterus by a syringe; sperm may be washed and introduced directly into the body of the uterus, a procedure called intrauterine insemination (IUI), or it may be injected through the top of the vagina to lie near the opening of the Fallopian tubes (direct intraperitoneal sperm insemination, DIPI). In-vitro fertilisation and embryo transfer (IVF/ET) involves collecting eggs, oocytes, recovered from the ovary, fertilising them in a culture medium at 37°C with spermatozoa, and transferring the embryos into the uterus one or two days later. They may be transferred into the Fallopian tube (zygote intra-fallopian transfer, ZIFT). In gamete intrafallopian transfer (GIFT), oocytes and sperm are placed together in one or both Fallopian tubes so that fertilisation occurs *in vivo*, or they may be placed in the peritoneal cavity near the opening of the Fallopian tubes (POST). The production of oocytes may be assisted by the administration of human chorionic gonadotrophin or the use of clomiphene, a drug which stimulates the secretion of gonadotrophic hormone. The surgical manoeuvres necessary in these procedures are carried out through the laparoscope or with the aid of ultrasound. Assisted conception may be of great help in preventing the birth of abnormal babies; if parents are known to carry a disease such as cystic fibrosis, and wish to have a child, it may be possible to test the fertilised eggs produced by in-vitro fertilisation and only to replace in the mother those that are found to be healthy. The Human Fertilisation and Embryology Act of 1990 now exists to control and supervise all research into human embryos, and those types of assisted conception which involve the creation of a human embryo outside the body or partly inside and partly outside, or the use of donated embryos or gametes (egg and sperm). *See* Ovary, Menstruation.

Asthenia: debility, loss of strength.

Asthma: disease of the respiratory system producing attacks of difficulty in breathing. The difficulty is caused by narrowing of the airways in the lungs in response to a precipitating agent, or spontaneously, being more common in children, often males. The malady may last into adult life or it may disappear after puberty; it may be seen for the first time in middle age. Children with the usually inherited condition known as atopy are prone to develop hay fever, asthma and eczema. It is thought that a severe virus infection at an early age predisposes to asthma, and it is sometimes observed that asthmatic attacks follow a respiratory virus infection in adults. Agents precipitating an attack may include a large number of substances breathed in, such as house mite dust, pollen, dust coming from feathers or animals, and the sulphur dioxide present in polluted air. Exercise may induce an attack, or eating shellfish, nuts or fruit; alcohol, aspirin and beta-blockers (q.v.) are all known to bring on an attack, as can emotional stress. Workers in some industries may develop asthma, including woodworkers, those working with plastics or paints containing isocyanates, and millers and bakers.

In an attack the patient coughs and wheezes and complains that it is difficult to breathe. The severity ranges from mild to dangerous, when the pulse races and the patient becomes exhausted, possibly even blue. Such a state demands the administration of a large dose of corticosteroids, the use of a nebuliser to give salbutamol or terbutaline and possibly the intravenous injection of aminophylline and the use of oxygen. Urgent admission to hospital is imperative. Less severe attacks may be controlled by the inhalation of salbutamol or terbutaline, with corticosteroids by mouth at first in large doses, gradually reducing over subsequent days. Mild attacks can usually be controlled by salbutamol or terbutaline, perhaps with corticosteriods by inhalation. It is often the case that the patient becomes very anxious, and sympathetic reassurance goes a long way towards helping the breathing. There is no doubt that the best way to treat asthma is to prevent the attacks. The regular inhalation of sodium cromoglycate may be valuable; the drug has no action in dilating the air passages, and is therefore no use during an attack, but can be used regularly for prophylaxis. Regular inhalations of salbutamol or terbutaline may be needed, with the addition in some cases of inhaled corticosteroids. The use at night of long-acting preparations of theophylline often controls nocturnal asthma and wheezing.

Astigmatism: if the refracting surfaces of the cornea and lens are not truly spherical, objects seen will be distorted in one axis (a circle, for example, will look oval). Correction is by glasses with a cylindrical lens.

Astragalus (or talus): the bone of the ankle that forms the link between the bones of the foot and those of the leg, the tibia and fibula.

Astringents: substances that cause contraction of mucous membranes and broken areas of skin, and so stop bleeding or discharge of a minor degree. Examples are aluminium acetate lotion and potassium permanganate solution.

Astrocytoma: brain tumour of varying malignancy.

Asystole: absence of heartbeat.

Ataxia: inability to co-ordinate movements of the muscles, either motor, due to disturbance of the cerebellum or inner ear, or sensory, when there is a defect in the part of the sensory system normally concerned with detecting and signalling the position of the muscles and joints. It results in unsteadiness of gait, speech, posture and movements.

Atelectasis: failure of the lungs to expand at birth. Sometimes used to mean collapse of part of the lung in adults.

Atenolol: beta-adrenoceptor blocking drug. *See* Beta-blockers.

Atheroma: disease of the arterial wall in which there is thickening of the wall with deposition of fatty matter in the thickened part. The fatty patches are yellow.

Atherosclerosis: disease of the walls of arteries in which they become thick, stiff and swollen following the deposition of atheromatous material. *See* Arterial Disease, Cholesterol

Athlete's Foot: fungus infection of the feet. The infecting fungus, *Tinea pedis*, lives in the horny, or keratinous, layer of the skin, and is usually found in the clefts between the toes, particularly between the third, fourth and fifth toes. The skin becomes white and sodden, and itches. The infection may spread and give rise to eczema. Acute attacks may be painful. If there is added infection this is treated first, and the fungus infection controlled by the use of topical application of an imidazole or triazole preparation. The infection is often chronic and very difficult to eradicate, but can be controlled by keeping the feet dry, clean and cool, and using imidazole or triazole cream as necessary. Cotton socks are best, changed twice a day. Severe chronic infections may be treated with griseofulvin by mouth, but the course of treatment may be long.

Atopy: hereditary hypersensitivity state which may cause hay fever, asthma and eczema.

Atresia: incomplete development resulting in the obliteration of a passage such as the anus or oesophagus.

Atria: the two smaller chambers of the heart which receive blood from the veins and pump it into the ventricles. Often called the auricle, but this is, properly speaking, only an appendage of the atrium, not the whole structure. Atrial flutter is a condition in which the contractions of the atrium, while regular, are at the abnormal pace of about 300 a minute, which is far too fast for the conduction of impulses normally controlling the beating of the ventricles, which react to only the second, third or fourth impulse, and take up a rhythm accordingly. In atrial fibrillation the contractions of the atrium are rapid and irregular, and in consequence the ventricular rhythm is also rapid and irregular. *See* Heart.

Atrophy: wasting away or shrivelling up of a part of the body as the result of lack of nutrition or use.

Atropine: an alkaloid found in the plant deadly nightshade. It opposes the action of the parasympathetic nervous system, and therefore dilates and paralyses the pupil of the eye, dries up the secretions of the mouth and the air passages of the lungs, relaxes the smooth muscle of the gut and ureters, and increases the heart rate. It is used as a premedication and in the treatment of renal colic, and is the antidote to poisoning by organophosphorous insecticides. It is also the antidote to nerve gases.

Audiometry: measurement of the power of hearing. Each ear is tested in turn through earphones. The subject is asked to listen to pure tones of different frequencies, and the intensity is altered to find the quietest sound that can be heard. The frequencies are altered to cover the range normally heard by the human ear, and the results plotted as an audiogram. They can be compared with the results found when the sounds are transmitted by bone conduction, and the result shows whether a deafness is due to disturbance of the conduction of sound in the middle ear or abnormal function of the auditory nerve, i.e. conductive or perceptive deafness.

Aura: a sensation felt when the subject is about to have an epileptic fit.

Auricle: the external ear; also used to denote the lesser chambers of the heart, properly called the atria.

Auscultation: a method of examining the body by listening. Mostly used in the chest, where the doctor can listen to the sounds made by the heart and by the air passing through the passages of the lungs. In ancient times the ear was applied directly to the chest wall, but at the beginning of the nineteenth century the French physician Théophile Laennec (1781–1826) invented the stethoscope, at first a rolled-up piece of paper, then a wooden cylinder; gradually the modern instrument was evolved with two ear-pieces and a separate chest-piece connected by rubber tubing. Beside sounds in the chest, sounds can also be picked up from the arteries, intestines, the developing foetus, and elsewhere.

Autism: a disorder of behaviour in children, who look quite normal but are entirely self-centred. Usually the disturbance is present at birth, but it can become apparent in the second year after an apparently normal initial development. The child is backward in speech and understanding; some begin to speak at about five, but always they keep to themselves and are solitary, showing apparently purposeless actions of a repetitive pattern. The cause of the condition is not known.

Autoclave: in the autoclave, steam under pressure sterilises instruments, dressings, etc., to be used in surgery. A valve regulates the steam pressure and therefore the temperature just as it does in a domestic pressure cooker.

Autogenous: self-generated: term applied usually to vaccines prepared from organisms found in the patient's own body, for example in recurrent boils or bronchitis, and used in treating the disease.

Auto-immune Disease: individuals normally react to the introduction of foreign tissues or proteins into the body (*see* Allergy). In some cases it seems probable that people produce an immune reaction to one of their own tissues in consequence of changes that are not understood, and the autoantibodies set up inflammation which damages the organ or tissues involved. A growing number of diseases are thought to be produced by this mechanism, among them blood disorders such as pernicious anaemia and some kinds of haemolytic anaemia, myasthenia gravis, nephritis, ulcerative colitis, and rheumatoid arthritis. Some diseases of the thyroid gland appear to be produced this way.

Autologous Blood Transfusion: the transfusion of a patient's own blood. Most patients who are to have an elective operation can safely deposit an amount of their blood in the blood bank less than four weeks before the operation, to be used if necessary, thus avoiding any risks associated with homologous transfusion, the use of other people's blood. In major vascular surgery, or other operations in which there is no risk of infection, the blood shed during the operation can be collected by a special device, an anticoagulant added, and two or three litres re-infused during the operation.

Autonomic Nervous System: that part of the nervous system that regulates those aspects of body function that are not under conscious control, for example the heartbeat, movements of the intestines, the size of the pupil of the eye, and to some extent the activity of the glands. It has two divisions, the sympathetic and the parasympathetic, whose actions are opposed to each other; roughly speaking, the sympathetic system prepares the body for action, the parasympathetic for rest. *See* Nervous System.

Autopsy: the examination of a body after death, made so that physicians can see for themselves the effects of injury or disease, arrive at a true diagnosis of the cause of death, and gather observations for use in the future.

Avascular Necrosis: a fracture or other injury to a bone may disrupt an artery so that the blood supply to a part of the bone is cut off and the cells die. One of the bones most liable to this process is the femur, and fracture of the neck of this bone, a common accident in the elderly, may lead to avascular necrosis of the head of the bone.

Avomine: the proprietary name for promethazine theoclate, which is effective in the prevention of travel sickness. It causes sleepiness and increases susceptibility to alcohol.

Axon: the long extension from a nerve cell along which nerve impulses run. A nerve is made up of a bundle of axons.

Azathioprine: an immunosuppressant drug used in transplant surgery to prevent rejection of the transplant, and in a variety of auto-immune diseases.

Azotaemia: excess of nitrogenous compounds in the blood, such as urea. It may occur in kidney failure. *See* Uraemia.

B

Babinski Reflex: if the outer part of the sole of the foot is firmly stroked, the toes will clench – the great toe goes down and the other toes curl. Before the infant starts to walk, and if the nerve tracts that connect the brain with the motor nerves (the corticospinal tracts) are damaged, the response is altered and the great toe goes up while the other toes fan out. This reflex, the extensor plantar reflex, was described by Joseph Babinski (1857–1932) in 1896.

Bacillus: the name originally used in bacteriology to mean a rod-shaped as opposed to a round micro-organism. It is now properly used to denote only one genus of which the bacillus of anthrax is the sole organism harmful to man, but old usage dies hard.

Back Pain: although four out of five people experience pain in the back at one time or another, it remains one of the most difficult complaints to deal with. Disregarding those cases in which a definite cause can be found, there are a large number left for which only vague diagnoses can be made, ranging from undefined structural defects to psychogenic disorder. The commonly invoked 'slipped disc' is comparatively rare: disc protrusion can only be definitely diagnosed if there are signs in the nervous system such as sciatica to go with the back pain. A number of cases have a definite history of accidental damage, but it is still difficult to be sure of the precise nature of the condition. The complicated structure of the backbone and the muscles acting on it, allied to the strain that it has to bear in a creature walking upright, leaves room for any number of explanations. A full examination will exclude any serious underlying condition, and if the severity of the case warrants it an X-ray will show such causes as arthritis of the spine, congenital abnormalities, ankylosing spondylitis or other bone disease.

It is generally believed that rest on a hard bed – if necessary, with boards underneath the mattress – until the pain has gone, followed often by a course of physiotherapy, is the best treatment, but even that is open to argument, some believing that physiotherapy or manipulation is indicated in acute cases. Posture is responsible for much of the trouble. The back should be as far as possible extended; straight or hollow rather than bent forwards. Bending forwards to pick up anything weighty is a recipe for back pain; squat and let the legs do the work. Sit upright in a straight-backed chair, and when driving slip a cushion behind the small of the back. Many kinds of work tend to lead to bending forwards, but the seat and the height of the work should be adjusted to avoid this as far as possible.

Many sufferers consult practitioners of complementary medicine such as chiropractors and osteopaths, who have a great deal to offer in the way of manipulative treatment; cases suited for such treatment are those in which there is no suspicion that the back pain is part of a general illness, in which there are no signs that the nervous system is involved, and in which X-rays have been used if necessary to exclude serious bone disease. Part of the success of treatment depends on the personal involvement of the practitioner and the patient, and in some cases this is more evident with a complementary medical practitioner than in a hospital department, although the hospital may have more physical resources than a practitioner. Complementary medical practitioners should be members of a recognised professional association. In qualified hands, acupuncture may have a distinct role in the management of back pain.

Bacteraemia: the condition of having bacteria in the bloodstream.

Bacteria: single-celled microscopic organisms usually classified with plants rather than animals, but distinct from plants. Smaller than yeasts but larger than viruses, they were discovered by the Dutch microscopist Anthony van Leeuwenhoek (1632–1723), but it was left to Pasteur and Koch in the last century to elucidate the part bacteria play in the production of disease. By no means all bacteria are harmful: many are actively useful, for example the nitrogenous bacteria of the soil. They can be classified by their shape: cocci are round, bacilli like rods, vibrios are curved like a comma, and the spirillum is wavy. Staphylococci are cocci arranged in bunches, streptococci are arranged in chains, diplococci in pairs. Further classifications of bacteria are based on their reaction to the staining method invented by the Danish physician Gram (see Gram's Stain) or whether they produce disease (pathogenic) or not (non-pathogenic).

BAL: British Anti-Lewisite, a substance otherwise called dimercaprol, discovered during the Second World War as an antidote to the war gas Lewisite which contains arsenic. Dimercaprol is used by injection as an antidote to poisoning by heavy metals – lead, arsenic, antimony, gold, mercury and bismuth.

Balanitis: inflammation of the parts beneath the foreskin.

Baldness: hair normally grows at the rate of of about 1 cm a month, and lasts for two or three years before it is shed. It grows from a little pit in the skin called a hair follicle, which has associated with it a sebaceous gland. In very many men and some women it ceases to grow on the head as the years pass, thinning first at the temples and forehead and then at the top of the head. The amount lost seems to run in families, and is dependent on the male hormone, for eunuchs do not go bald. Baldness in men is accompanied by increased growth of hair on the chest: it is a matter of argument whether it is also accompanied by potency. The rate of loss varies considerably, but both men and women in their eighties lack a full head of hair. Various diseases lead to hair loss, as does the use of cytotoxic drugs in the treatment of malignant disease, when fortunately it grows back again. Alopecia areata is a condition of unknown cause in which the hair falls out in patches, but again the tendency is for it to grow again after a few months. Treatment for baldness is not encouraging. Hair transplants may be taken in punch grafts from the occipital region at the back of the head and inserted into the area to be covered, but are liable to be disappointing. Minoxidil, a drug used in the treatment of high blood pressure, has been found to produce hairiness, and it is offered as a lotion for the scalp, but it is expensive and neither its safety nor its effectiveness have yet been established.

Ballismus: violent involuntary movement of the limbs. It usually affects only one half of the body, when it is called hemiballismus. The cause is damage to a nucleus in the brain, the corpus Luysi, which lies below the thalamus in the midbrain.

Balsam: vegetable resin combined with oil, for example Canada balsam, used in preparing slides for microscopy, which comes from the balsam fir of North America; or balsam of Gilead, made from a tree which grows by the Red Sea. Friar's balsam is benzoin, from the *Styrax benzoin*

Bandage: piece of material used for binding up wounds or keeping dressings and splints in place. Roller bandages are made of long strips of loosely woven fabric wound into a firm roll, but are now only used in special cases, e.g. where the patient is sensitive to adhesives or, as in the case of the lower jaw, an adhesive bandage is not practical. Otherwise they have been supplanted to a great extent by adhesive tape or by seamless tubular gauze made in various sizes, which can incorporate elasticated threads. Crêpe bandages are still useful for support and pressure over injured joints, particularly the knee or ankle.

Barber's Itch: *see* Sycosis Barbae.

Barbiturates: derivatives of malonyl urea or barbituric acid. Once used widely for their depressant effect on the central nervous system, they were found to have addictive properties which are particularly dangerous because tolerance to the drugs is easily acquired, and while the effects of sedation and intoxication become less marked, the effects on the vital centres remain unaltered. It therefore becomes easy to take an overdose. Barbiturates are now controlled drugs under the Misuse of Drugs Regulations and should be prescribed only for epilepsy and use as anaesthetic agents. Severe addiction to barbiturates should be treated in hospital, for the withdrawal syndrome resembles that of alcohol, involving a state which can resemble delirium tremens.

Barium: barium sulphate is insoluble in water and radio-opaque – that is, it shows up on X-ray examination because radiations do not pass through barium. It is therefore made up into fluid mixtures which are taken by mouth to outline the stomach and upper intestine, or given as an enema to outline the lower intestine.

Barotrauma: an injury caused by pressure. In aviation, the pressure of the atmosphere falls as the aeroplane ascends. Although the cabin of a civil airliner is pressurised, usually to 565 mm Hg (8000 feet), the pressure differential between the middle ear and atmospheric is sufficient to cause trouble if the Eustachian tube between the back of the nose and the middle ear is inflamed, as it may be in the common cold. The tube, although allowing the pressures to equalise during the climb, acts as a non-return valve during the descent, causing a painful deformation of the ear-drum inwards as the atmospheric pressure rises and the pressure in the middle ear stays low. In the same way if the communications between the sinuses and antra and the nose are blocked a pressure differential arises with painful consequences. It is therefore inadvisable to fly with a bad cold or sinus trouble; if you must, take a decongestant. In the same way, a diver may run into trouble with the middle ear or sinuses as he descends and the ambient pressure rises.

Barrier Nursing: when a patient is suffering from a serious infective disease, it is necessary to adopt a technique of nursing which prevents the harmful bacteria from being carried out of the patient's room into the general wards. In cases where the patient's normal immune defences are compromised, the reverse is necessary, and nursing technique is aimed at preventing any bacteria from outside reaching the patient.

Bartholin's Glands: named after the Danish anatomist, Caspar Bartholin (1655–1738), who first described them, they are a pair of glands lying on each side of the opening of the vagina. They sometimes become infected and cause a painful abscess.

BCG (Bacillus Calmette-Guérin): used in the preparation of a vaccine against tuberculosis invented in 1908 by the French bacteriologists Leon Calmette (1863–1933) and Camille Guérin (1872–1961) and consisting of an attenuated strain of the bacillus of bovine tuberculosis. It may be given to infants who are especially exposed to the risk of tuberculous infection and to young people who have been shown by the tuberculin skin test to have no natural immunity to the disease, and to hospital workers. In the United Kingdom mass inoculation of susceptible children between 11 and 13 is undertaken. The vaccine is given by injection into the skin, and in a few cases an ulcer develops at the site; but this is of little consequence and heals naturally.

Beat Elbow, or Knee: the term applied by miners to swelling and inflammation of the joints arising from constant pressure and ingrained particles of dirt.

Bed Bug: *Cimex lectularius*, a wingless blood-sucking insect which hides by day in cracks in walls or floors, or in the bedclothes, emerging at night to feed on human beings and leave irritating bites.

Bedsores: may form in those confined to bed who cannot change their position often and regularly. They are most common over the heels and sacrum, for here unrelieved pressure on the skin quickly interferes with the blood supply and causes necrosis or death of the tissues. Bedsores can also form on the shoulders, elbows and ankles. The affected part first goes blue and then ulcerates to form a black slough which comes off leaving an open sore likely to become bigger. The most important measure in treatment is prevention. Two-hourly changes of position and a dry skin are essential and should be ensured in all bedridden people. The skin must be washed at least once a day, dried carefully, rubbed with spirit and dusted with powder. An air bed in which alternate portions are slowly inflated can be used, and the patient can lie on a fleece. Treatment of established bedsores is a matter for the surgeon.

Bed-wetting: children normally learn to control the passage of urine by day during the second year and by night during the third year. Bed-wetting may go on until the fourth or even fifth year without the child being abnormal. About one in ten children over five years old who wet the bed are found to have some disease to account for the trouble; deep sleep and failure to be aroused can cause a wet bed, but in some cases the trouble is psychological. The less fuss that is made about it the better. It is possible to use electrical devices to sound an alarm if the bed is wet, or the child may be woken up regularly to pass urine. If the trouble persists after seven, drug treatment may be tried, the most commonly used drug being amitryptilene, but this should not go on for more than three months without a full investigation being carried out which may include an electro-encephalogram (q.v.). A change of circumstances, particularly one likely to give rise to feelings of insecurity, may precipitate a later recurrence of the trouble.

Belladonna: a preparation of *Atropa belladonna*, or deadly nightshade, which contains atropine and therefore relieves spasm of involuntary muscle. One of the actions of atropine eye-drops is to dilate the pupil of the eye, and a widely dilated pupil is, or was, thought by some to be an attractive attribute of a beautiful lady. Belladonna can therefore produce beauty not only in the eye of the beholder; but unfortunately it produces blurred vision as well as that far-away look.

Bell's Palsy: first described by the Scottish surgeon Charles Bell (1774–1842), it is the commonest cause of paralysis of one side of the face. The facial nerve enters the face just below the ear, having passed through a canal in the petrous temporal bone on its passage from the brain stem. In Bell's palsy the nerve becomes swollen inside its canal and is unable to transmit impulses. The cause of the swelling is obscure: it may be a virus infection, but the onset of the paralysis is sudden. The condition is benign and as a rule recovery is complete. Treatment recommended by some is the administration of corticosteroids at the onset of the attack; as the eye is commonly affected and unable to blink it may be sensible to cover it against dust. A wire splint can be arranged to hold up the corner of the mouth. Operations have been carried out to relieve the pressure on the nerve in its bony canal when recovery is delayed, but the necessity for this is by no means universally accepted. In the rare case where recovery is not complete, plastic operation can improve the appearance of the paralysed side of the face.

Bends *see* Caisson Disease.

Benzene: not to be confused with benzine, benzene is used in various industries. Acute benzene poisoning, possibly by inhalation of the vapour, causes headache, giddiness and restlessness, sometimes confusion, muscular twitching and even convulsions. Chronic benzene poisoning resulting from exposure over a number of years causes aplastic anaemia and agranulocytosis (q.v.) by interfering with the formation of blood cells in the bone marrow.

Benzodiazepines: a group of drugs that have superseded barbiturates as the most commonly used to combat anxiety and sleeplessness. Known generally as tranquillisers, they are safer because they have fewer toxic effects, being less likely to give rise to dependence and less dangerous in overdose. They do however sometimes give rise to symptoms on withdrawal, which include anxiety and loss of sleep – symptoms similar to those for which they were originally given – which may lead to them being prescribed again. Withdrawal therefore has to be gradual and may take a long time. It is recommended that courses of benzodiazepines should for the most part be short, whether given for anxiety or sleeplessness. Those commonly used for sleeplessness include nitrazepam, flurazepam and temazepam, and those given for the relief of anxiety diazepam, chlordiazepoxide, lorazepam and oxazepam. The last two have a shorter-lasting action.

Berger Rhythm: in 1924 Hans Berger (1873–1941), a neurologist in Jena, described electrical activity in the brain showing itself as a wave rhythm between 8 and 13 times a second. The source of these waves is obscure, but it is a matter of observation that the rhythm only occurs in normal subjects when they close their eyes. *See* Electro-encephalography.

Beriberi: a vitamin deficiency disease due to lack of vitamin B_1, or thiamine. At one time prevalent among those rice-eaters in the East who used polished rice, the husk with the vitamin-containing embryo being removed in the milling process, it was common in the Japanese prison camps of the Second World War. It may be found in chronic alcoholics who develop gastritis that not only interferes with the absorption of vitamins but also takes the appetite away. There are two main types of beriberi, the 'wet' and the 'dry'. In the wet type, the heart muscle becomes flabby and the patient weak and oedematous (i.e. with swelling of the legs and abdomen due to excess fluid leakage into the tissues), and in the dry the main damage is to the nerves supplying the limbs so that the patient is unable to walk properly and suffers from numbness. The treatment is to give thiamine, which is found in all living cells and therefore in most natural foods.

Beryllium Poisoning: workers with beryllium, especially beryllium oxide, may find their eyes irritated and weeping, and develop a severe cough and sore throat. If they are removed from the metal the lung reaction will improve, but corticosteroids may be advised when recovery is delayed. Another reaction to beryllium produces dermatitis and ulcers in the skin, but this is probably due to sensitivity rather than poisoning.

Beta-blockers: adrenaline, the substance by which the sympathetic nervous system transmits impulses and so stimulates the tissues over which it has control, has two types of receptors at the nerve endings, called alpha and beta. Beta-blocking drugs interfere, in a manner which is not precisely understood, with the transmission of impulses at the beta-type sympathetic nerve terminals.

These impulses normally excite the heart, increasing the rate and force of the beat, dilate blood vessels in the muscles and constrict those in the skin and intestines, dilate the air passages in the lungs and aid the breakdown of glycogen in the liver to glucose. Beta-blockers are therefore used in the treatment of high blood pressure, angina, some abnormalities of heart rhythm such as tachycardia where the pulse rate is too high, and can be used to diminish some types of anxiety. The group of drugs includes propranolol, atenolol, oxprenolol and others, but all have the unfortunate effect of precipitating attacks of asthma in susceptible subjects.

Biceps: a muscle with two heads arising at the shoulder and running down the front of the upper arm to be fixed to the radius, one of the two bones in the forearm. It flexes the elbow, and also supinates the forearm – that is, it helps turn the screwdriver. The tendon below the shoulder is sometimes subject to a painful inflammation, and occasionally the tendon ruptures so that the muscle forms a lump in the upper arm. This, however, has surprisingly little effect on the use of the arm.

Bile: a greenish-brown fluid secreted by the liver. It is partly a secretion which helps in the digestion of fats (the bile salts), partly an excretion of substances resulting from the destruction of old red blood cells (the bile pigments), and it also contains cholesterol and various electrolytes. The bile duct runs from the liver to the duodenum, and the bile can run directly into the small intestine, but between meals it is diverted through the cystic duct into the gall-bladder where it is concentrated and stored. Bile in the gall-bladder has more mucus in it than when it comes from the liver, and contains a greater concentration of cholesterol, bile pigments, salts and calcium. This may result in the formation of gallstones, especially if there is any infection of the gall-bladder. Many substances excreted in the bile are reabsorbed in the gut, circulating from the liver to the intestine and back again. 'Biliousness' is an imaginary disease; the symptoms are usually caused by eating and drinking too much. The vomiting of bile is popularly considered to have a sinister significance, but any attack of repeated vomiting may result in the vomit being discoloured by bile whether the cause is trivial or serious. *See* Gall-bladder.

Bilharzia: infestation by flukes of the genus *Schistosoma*, one of which, *Schistosoma haematobium*, was first found by the German anatomist Theodor Bilharz (1825–62). It is a disease found widely in the world, principally in Africa, South America and the Caribbean, and Asia. It can affect the liver, spleen, lungs, intestines and the urinary system. The fluke is picked up from infected water by bathing or wading in it, or by drinking it. The parasites make their way through the skin, sometimes causing a rash called swimmer's itch. They then migrate to the portal vein through the bloodstream and the lungs, and in the ramifications of the portal vein in the liver they become mature adults and copulate. They then move off to various destinations, and the female lays her eggs, many in the bladder or intestines whence they pass out of the body. If an egg reaches water it turns into a miracidium, in which form it can swim; it searches for a water snail, for it is only in a water snail that the fluke can develop into the next stage, the cercaria. The cercariae live in the water until the next unwary person comes along, and the cycle starts again.

Symptoms of the disease begin to show some weeks after the original invasion, which may have been accompanied by the rash mentioned above, and include fever, headache, cough and diarrhoea. Later the liver and spleen become enlarged, and in time, as the eggs pass out, blood is seen in the urine. Eggs that remain in the tissues give rise to swellings called granulomas which may damage the liver, spleen and urinary tract. *S. haematobium* is more likely to affect the urinary system, *S. mansoni* the colon, and *S. japonicum* the portal and alimentary systems. All are treated by the drug praziquantel. Without water snails the flukes cannot survive, so that prevention requires the eradication of the snails, provision of a clean water supply and adequate sanitation. None of these measures is easy to ensure or, in many places, practical. Boots for use when wading in water and the boiling of water will prevent a certain amount of infection; it has been suggested that mass chemotherapy of children is the most likely way to control the disease.

Binet–Simon Test: the earliest form of intelligence test, devised in 1905 by the French psychologist Alfred Binet (1857–1911) and his collaborator Théodore Simon (1873–1961). Questions for children of various age groups were standardised according to the average performance of the age group in the population as a whole. According to the questions a child could answer compared with the average ability of the age group his mental age was estimated, and this gave his Intelligence Quotient (IQ) which was calculated by dividing the mental age by the chronological age and multiplying by 100. The test has since undergone several revisions.

Bioassay: the biological effect of an unknown drug, or a known drug in an unknown concentration, when compared with the effect of a standard preparation, enables the pharmacologist to identify the drug and measure the strength of the solution.

Biochemistry: the chemistry of living things.

Biofeedback: a technique in which a subject is given information about his current heart rate or blood pressure and asked to try to alter the pressure or the pulse. The results have been equivocal. The technique has also been used with the electro-encephalogram in epileptic patients to endeavour to control abnormal electrical activity accompanying fits.

Biopsy: examination of fragments of tissue taken from a living creature. Usually applied to the microscopical examination of fragments of tissue taken from a patient in order to make a diagnosis, for example in the case of a tumour.

Biotin: a member of the vitamin B group, required for many functions in metabolism. Also known as vitamin H.

Bird Breeder's Lung: an allergic reaction taking place in the lung after inhalation of the dried droppings of birds. *See* Farmer's Lung.

Birth: the average baby weighs 7 lb (3.2 kg) at birth. A stillborn child is 'any child which has issued from its mother after the 28th week of pregnancy and which did not at any time after being completely expelled from the mother breathe or show any other signs of life'. Premature birth is one which takes place before the natural time but in which the child is capable of surviving. A birth which takes place so prematurely that the child must necessarily die is known as an abortion or miscarriage. *See* Labour.

Birth Control: *see* Contraception.

Birthmark: the commonest is the strawberry naevus, which is a collection of dilated and overgrown blood vessels. Developing shortly after birth, it normally needs no treatment; growth slows after the first year, and then over the course of a few years the blemish gradually disappears. Port wine naevi are present from birth, and persist for life. They are harmless. They may be treated by the dermatologist.

Bismuth: a metal used as bismuth subgallate in the treatment of haemorroids. It has a mild astringent action. It is also used as a chelate in the treatment of peptic ulcers, where it promotes healing. During treatment milk should not be taken by itself.

Bistoury: a type of knife once used in surgery. It was long and narrow and could have a straight or curved blade.

Bites and Stings: simple dog bites are only serious if the dog has rabies. If the dog is healthy, the bite is treated like any other wound: it is cleaned and dressed, and precautions are taken against tetanus if the patient is not already covered by vaccination within the last five years. If the dog is likely to have rabies an immunoglobulin is available, and active immunisation by vaccine should be started at once. Bites from rhesus monkeys may be dangerous, for they may carry a herpes virus; they need urgent medical attention.

In Europe, only the adder or viper is poisonous, and although about a hundred people are bitten a year in Great Britain there have been only 14 deaths reported in the last 100 years. In North America the most deaths, between 9 and 14 a year, are caused by the diamond-back rattlesnake. There are about 200 species of deadly venomous snakes in the world, in all countries except Antarctica, and islands such as Ireland, Iceland, New Zealand, the Caribbean, and others in the Atlantic and Pacific Oceans. Treatment of a snakebite should be in hospital. It is important to realise that most people who think they have been been bitten are very frightened and need a great deal of calm reassurance. They should be kept still, and a bitten limb splinted or otherwise immobilised. The use of a tourniquet is only necessary with very venomous snakebites, and any interference with the wound is not likely to help. If possible the snake should be killed and taken with the patient so that it can be identified, for anti-snakebite serum is available for use in severe cases. The most important thing to remember if bitten by a snake is: keep still.

Weever fish stings are very painful but not dangerous, and the best treatment is to put the painful leg in hot water at about 50°C. If a sting is present it should be removed. Stings from the Portuguese man-of-war are best treated with baking soda and water.

Bee and wasp stings are only dangerous if they produce severe allergic reactions, and if they do the patient needs an immediate injection of adrenaline; people who know that they are unduly sensitive to stings should carry with them a loaded syringe of adrenaline during the summer. When it stings, the bee leaves the sting in the wound, and this should be removed by scraping rather than squeezing for it has a venom sac still attached to it. Ice-packs will help the pain, and antihistamines by mouth will help excessive swelling. Do not use antihistamine creams, for they are disappointing in their results and can lead to sensitisation. Calamine is better.

In the USA the Black Widow spider is responsible for a number of fatal bites; it has a habit of spinning its web and laying its eggs in outdoor latrines, with obvious results.

The only dangerous spider seen in the British Isles is the banana spider, which is known to have been imported in bunches of bananas from South America.

Blackheads: *see* Acne Vulgaris.

Black Motions: known medically as melaena, black motions are caused by altered blood from bleeding peptic ulcers or disease of the intestine. They can also be caused by iron taken for anaemia or by drinking heavy red wine.

Blackwater Fever: the passage of haemoglobin in the urine in severe cases of malignant tertian (falciparum) malaria, with low blood pressure and ensuing coma.

Bladder, Urinary: the bladder lies in the pelvis, guarded in front by bone – the symphysis pubis. In the male, the rectum lies behind the bladder, and the prostate gland below it; in the female the vagina and the neck of the uterus lie behind it. The uterus in its normal position is separated from the upper surface of the bladder by a pouch of peritoneum in which may lie intestine. The bladder normally holds upwards of 300 ml of urine, which enters the bladder near its base through two tubes called ureters running down from the kidneys. Near them in the midline another tube called the urethra takes the urine to the exterior. The wall of the bladder is muscular to enable it to expel its contents, and the muscle when relaxed expands more if the bladder is filled slowly than if it is filled quickly. Sudden distension of the bladder leads to an urge to urinate. A nervous reflex controls the mechanism of passing urine, which can normally be over-ridden by the conscious mind; the reflex is set in motion by distension of the bladder or by irritation of its most sensitive part, the triangle at the base where the two ureters enter and the urethra leaves. The nerves concerned in the reflex are part of the autonomic nervous system which reach the bladder from the pelvic plexus and the pelvic splanchnic nerves; the pudendal nerves supply the muscles which close the urethra or relax it to let the urine pass. The centre for the reflex is in the sacral segments of the spinal cord, and conscious impulses to control the reflex travel through the spinal cord from the brain. All these structures have to be intact for the act of passing water to be carried out normally.

Bladder Disease: congenital deformities of the bladder occur, such as ectopia vesicae in which the anterior wall of the bladder and the abdominal wall fail to close; hypospadias, where the urethra fails to run the length of the penis, opening short to the exterior; and failure of the urachus, the duct which runs from the bladder to the umbilical cord in the embryo, to close. These conditions all fall into the province of the urological surgeon. Inflammation of the bladder is very common, and is considered under the heading of cystitis (q.v.). Tumours occur, the first symptom of which is painless passage of blood in the urine. Ultrasound, contrast radiography where a radio-opaque substance is introduced into the urinary system, and direct examination through a cystoscope may be used in making the diagnosis. Again the treatment is surgical, and ranges according to the severity of the case from coagulation of the tumour through the cystoscope to removal of part or the whole of the bladder, with the ureters being implanted into an artificial bladder made from a portion of the intestine. Radiotherapy is used before or after surgery; in some cases it is the only practical treatment. Injury to the bladder is uncommon, but may occur in cases where the pelvis is fractured or where a penetrating knife wound in the lower abdomen has been sustained. Stones may form in the bladder, and cutting for the stone is an operation of very considerable antiquity, going back at least to the time of Hippocrates, who disapproved of the operation. The surgeon no longer has to cut to remove stones in the bladder, as they can be broken up through the cystoscope and the fragments washed out. Foreign bodies have been found in the female bladder ranging from hairpins to pencils, having been introduced through the urethra. Damage to the nervous system from injury or disease can interfere with the proper working of the bladder, and produce dysfunction ranging from incomplete control to automatic emptying or complete paralysis.

Blastomycosis: infection with the yeast *Blastomyces dermatitidis* found in North America. It affects the lungs, where it gives rise to many small abscesses, and the skin where it causes pustules and ulcers. The treatment is the drug amphotericin B.

Bleeding Time: the time needed for a small wound (pinprick) to stop bleeding. The normal time is between four and five minutes; anything over seven minutes indicates an abnormality of the blood-coagulating mechanism.

Blepharitis: an inflammation of the eyelids usually from a staphylococcal infection in which small abscesses develop in the hair follicles of the eyelashes, especially in children. The common name for a localised abscess is stye. There is pain and swelling of the eyelid until the stye discharges. Chloramphenicol eye ointment is commonly used for such infections.

Blepharospasm: a distressing recurrent involuntary closure of the eyelids, which may occur only on one side. No efficacious treatment has been found.

Blindness: may be congenital or acquired, the result of congenital abnormality, disease or injury affecting any of the structures in the visual pathway – the eye, the optic nerves, their connections with the brain, or the visual cortex. In the United Kingdom a blind person was defined in the National Assistance Act of 1948 as one 'so blind as to be unable to perform any work for which eyesight is essential'. In the case of children the term includes not only those totally blind but also those who cannot be taught by visual methods, even by the use of large print, blackboard writing, or lenses for magnifying print. Particulars of welfare services for the blind can be obtained from the Royal National Institute for the Blind.

Blistering and Counter-irritants: formerly blistering was carried out by the application of small hot irons or cauterising substances to provide counter-irritation intended both to relieve existing pain by producing irritation in the skin of the area and to increase the flow of blood to the part. Counter-irritants, now often called rubefacients, are still used in cases of pain in the examples being oil of wintergreen, turpentine and white liniments. Many proprietary preparations are available.

Blood: fluid composed of plasma, a pale slightly yellow liquid, containing red and white blood cells which separate from the plasma on standing. The cells are present in the blood in fairly constant numbers: variations from the normal are a sign of disease. In males the red cell count is normally between 4.4 and 6.5 million per cu mm and in females between 3.9 and 5.6 per cu mm. There are between 150,000 and 400,000 platelets (q.v.) per cu mm, and between 4000 and 11,000 white cells per cu mm. They may be divided according to appearance and staining characteristics, and a differential count shows neutrophil polymorphs 40–75%, basophil 0–1%, eosinophil 1–6%, monocytes 2–10% and lymphocytes 20–40%. (*See* Leucocytes.) Many chemical determinations and analyses can be carried out on the blood to give an accurate picture of the state of the individual in health and disease. The blood circulates throughout the body in the arteries, veins and capillaries. Its functions are:

1. Transport of oxygen, which is carried in combination with the haemoglobin in the red cells.
2. Removal of carbon dioxide from the cells of the body, formed as the tissues use oxygen, and carried by haemoglobin.
3. Transport of food substances to the cells and the removal of waste products.
4. Heat exchange: the blood removes excess heat from deep structures and carries it to the surface where it can be dissipated.
5. Control of many vital processes by the transport of hormones and other substances.
6. Defence of the body against infection by the transport of antitoxins, antibodies and white cells to the infected part.

The normal volume of blood in an adult is between four and five litres.

Blood Diseases: *see* Agranulocytosis, Anaemia, Christmas Disease, Haemolytic Disease of the Newborn, Haemophilia, Hodgkin's Disease, Polycythaemia, Purpura, Sickle-cell Disease, Thalassaemia.

Blood Groups: early attempts to transfuse blood from one man to another were sometimes successful, but often ended in death. The reason was not understood until 1900, when the Austrian pathologist Landsteiner (1868-1943) discovered the blood groups. All human beings of whatever race belong, in respect of their blood, to one of several groups classified according to the power of the serum of one person's blood to cause the red cells of another to agglutinate, or clump together. The reaction depends on the presence of antibodies called agglutinins in the serum, and antigens called agglutinogens on the surface of the red blood cells. The make-up of the blood is inherited, and there are many antigens carried by the red blood corpuscles, but those of the greatest importance to medicine are two that Landsteiner called A and B. It is possible for one or the other to be present, both together, or neither. The groups are therefore called A, B, AB and O. The antibodies in the serum are in group A, anti-B, in group B, anti-A, in group AB, none, and in group O, anti-A+B. If therefore blood of the wrong group is transfused the red cells of the donor will react with the serum of the recipient. The exception is group O, for the red cells will not react with the other groups' serum, having no antigen. Nevertheless group O blood can contain enough antibodies to react with the recipient's red cells. Except in the case of dire emergency, when group O blood may be transfused to patients of other groups, cross-matching is carried out between the recipient's serum and the red cells of the donor before all transfusions.

A further very important group was discovered in 1940 by Landsteiner and Wiener. They found that they could prepare an antibody by using the red cells of a rhesus monkey as the antigen. Those whose red blood cells were agglutinated by this antibody they called Rh-positive, and those whose cells did not were called Rh-negative. If an Rh-negative woman had a transfusion with Rh-positive blood she would produce antibodies, and if she had a child these could cross the placenta and cause severe anaemia, called haemolytic disease of the newborn. The same thing could happen if the father was Rh-positive and the mother Rh-negative, for the child may be Rh-positive. The mother will produce antibodies and in a subsequent pregnancy the child will be affected. It is however possible for the mother to be given by injection an anti-Rh immunoglobulin to prevent her becoming sensitised.

Blood Poisoning: a term used to signify the presence in the blood of bacteria, their toxins, or infected matter. Bacteraemia is the result of an infection with organisms virulent enough to invade the bloodstream and multiply there, septicaemia the presence of their toxins, and pyaemia the release of fragments of an infected clot or pus into the blood. The treatment is antibiotics according to the infection, and the condition is no longer as dangerous as once it was.

Blood Pressure: blood is driven through the arteries at a considerable pressure; if there were no pressure there would be no circulation. It is highest when the heart contracts (systole) and lowest when it relaxes (diastole). In a healthy young male adult the normal pressure at systole is 120 mm of mercury, and the pressure at diastole 80 mm. It is often a little lower in the female. The pressure is expressed as 120/80; the difference is the pulse pressure. The blood pressure tends to rise with age. *See* Hypertension.

Blood Spitting: *see* Haemoptysis.

Blue Baby: some congenital abnormalities of the heart or the great vessels associated with it allow venous blood, which is dark, to bypass the lungs and mix with the oxygenated red arterial blood from the left side of the heart to join the general circulation. The parts of the skin and mucous membranes which are normally pink then show a blue tinge. *See* Fallot's Tetralogy.

Boils: staphylococcal infections of the hair follicles of the skin. A painful red nodule appears, often where the clothes rub, for example on the back of the neck, which grows bigger and then breaks down in the middle for pus to appear. In a few days it discharges and heals. It must not be squeezed in order to express the pus, for this only spreads the infection. A simple dressing is all that is needed. The use of antibiotics is limited, for they interfere with the normal process of inflammation and often delay healing. An interconnecting collection of boils is called a carbuncle. Recurrent boils may require the use of skin disinfectants such as chlorhexidine; they may be associated with diabetes mellitus.

Bone Disease: *see* Cystic Fibrosis, Osteitis, Osteomalacia, Osteoporosis, Osteosarcoma, Paget's Disease, Periostitis, Rickets, Tuberculosis.

Bones: bones support and protect soft tissues, and by acting as hinged rods and levers make it possible to use the arms and legs. They are made of varying amounts of fibrous tissue and a hard crystalline mineral called calcium hydroxyapatite. A child's bones are nearly two-thirds fibrous tissue, while an old man's are two-thirds mineral; the child's bones bend while the old man's break. The bones are covered by a membrane called the periosteum, and can be classified according to their shape as long, flat, irregular and short. Long bones have a tubular shaft and the ends are covered with cartilage to form the joints. The interior consists of spongy, or cancellous, bone, made of plates which develop according to the mechanical strain which will be put upon them. They are covered by an outer layer of compact hard bone. The limb bones are long bones. Flat bones, for example the bones of the vault of the skull, are made of inner and outer plates, or tables, of compact hard bone with a layer of spongy bone between them. Irregular bones, for example the vertebrae or the bones of the base of the skull, also contain spongy bone and are covered by compact hard bone. The short bones, for example of the fingers, have the same structure as the long bones. The periosteum which covers the bones is pierced by small holes through which blood vessels reach the interior. After growth has stopped, a further supply of blood is derived from the periosteum itself.

At birth the marrow of all the bones is red, because it is a factory for the production of blood cells, but gradually the active marrow recedes until in the adult it is fatty and yellow, and red active marrow is confined to the vertebrae, the skull, the pelvis, the ribs and the breast bone, although the marrow of the long bones remains capable of making blood cells in a crisis – for example after a serious loss of blood.

Bones develop from membranes in the case of certain flat bones or from cartilage in the case of most bones. The cartilage persists at the ends of the bones as they grow and is called the epiphyseal plate, which goes on producing bone and thus lengthening the bones until growth is complete. Bones are formed during growth by two special sorts of cell – the osteoblasts, which lay down bone, and the osteoclasts which remove and so shape it. In childhood and adolescence more bone is laid down than is absorbed; in mature adults the amount of bone is kept constant, although there is continual absorption and deposition of bone so that there is a complete change in 20 years; and in old age there is more absorption than deposition, which leads to rarefaction. *See* Fractures.

Borborygmi: gurgling and rumbling sounds arising from the passage of liquid and gas in the intestines.

Bornholm Disease: first described as occurring on the Danish island Bornholm, it is also called devil's grip, because there is severe pain round the lower chest and sometimes round the abdomen. It is caused by infection by the Coxsakie virus B, and usually lasts about a week; there may be fever with a headache and sometimes a sore throat. It is not dangerous, and no treatment is needed beyond analgesics. It may occur in epidemic form.

Botulism: a very rare but often fatal form of food poisoning, caused by the toxin of *Clostridium botulinum*, which may grow in tinned, fermented or smoked food. It is found in the soil, and its spores are resistant to heat, surviving for short periods at up to 100°C; they are also resistant to very low temperatures. Nearly all the cases are traced to domestic canning or bottling, for commercial interests are continually on their guard against the possibility of any contamination of their products. The toxin is the most powerful known, and is absorbed in the gut and taken up by the nervous system where it eventually produces paralysis of the muscles of respiration. It is destroyed by heating for 10 minutes at 90°C.

Bougie: an instrument used for dilating strictures in natural passages, for example the urethra.

Bowels: the intestines.

Bow-Legs (genu varum): the legs are bowed outwards, the opposite of knock-knee. Formerly found as the consequence of rickets, it is now more commonly found in children without obvious cause, and tends in such cases to be self-correcting. Bow-legs can be acquired by people who spend a lot of time on horseback.

Brachial: pertaining to the arm.

Brachycephalic: short-headed. A term applied by anthropologists to those races with skulls the breadth of which is at least four-fifths of the length. (Cf. Dolichocephalic, where the breadth of the skull is less than four-fifths of the length.)

Brachydactyly: a condition in which the fingers and toes are abnormally short.

Bradycardia: slow pulse, i.e. below 60 a minute.

Brain: *see* Nervous System.

Branchial Arches: at an early stage in the development of the human embryo six 'visceral arches' form just below the head. The first arch corresponds to the lower jaw of a fish, the second to the gill cover, and the last four, which are called the branchial arches, to the arches of the gills. Between the arches are clefts, and from the arches and the clefts develop the structures of the neck and the lower jaw as well as part of the ear. All vertebrate embryos go through the stage of development where they have 'gills', but only in the fish do these structures go on to form part of the breathing apparatus. Sometimes in human beings the final development of the branchial arches is abnormal, and cysts or slits, like rudimentary gills, persist in the neck.

Breast: mammary glands are typical of a group of highly developed animals which suckle their young and are known as mammals. In the adult human female there are normally two breasts, the tissues of which are divided into 12–20 compartments containing systems of branching tubes which secrete milk. The tubes in each compartment, or lobe, join to form one duct which opens to the surface at the nipple, which lies in the lower outer quadrant of the breast near the centre surrounded by an area of pink skin called the areola. During the first pregnancy the colour of the areola darkens to become brown. In pregnancy the breasts enlarge under the influence of a number of hormones, among them prolactin, oestrogens, and progesterone. After birth the oestrogen level falls and the breast secretes milk about the third day, under the influence of the pituitary hormone prolactin. The milk is preceded by the secretion of a yellowish fluid called colostrum, which contains much protein and many antibodies. Suckling is itself a powerful stimulus to milk production, and by reflex action stimulates the secretion of prolactin; this hormone also inhibits ovulation, so that further conception is unlikely in a nursing mother. The average yield of human milk is about a litre a day. Accessory breasts may develop anywhere along a diagonal line running from the armpit to the lower abdomen (the milk line), but if they are unsightly or embarrassing they can easily be removed. At puberty boys sometimes suffer slight enlargement of the breasts or one breast which normally settles down, and at a more advanced age men being treated with oestrogens for carcinoma of the prostate undergo enlargement of the breasts. Only very rarely is enlargement of the breast in men associated with testicular deficiency.

Breast Disease: the breast may be the site of cancer, benign tumours, cysts and inflammation. Cancer of the breast is the commonest cause of deaths from cancer in women, accounting for some 20% of cancer fatalities. The cause is unknown, but there is evidence to suggest a hormonal basis, for the likelihood of developing it is less in those who have their first baby as young women, although the number of children is not important. This may mean that the age at which the first lactation is stimulated is the important factor, although again the length of time the baby is breast-fed is not significant. It is not certain that the contraceptive pill has any effect on the development of cancer, but present evidence suggests that it does not. Early detection is very important, for the earlier the treatment the more likely it is to be effective. Monthly examination of the breasts, together with regular mammography (X-ray examination of the breast) should be the aim; mammography at three-year intervals for those aged 50 to 65 is at present recommended. The detection of a lump will require examination by a surgeon, who may undertake a biopsy often by the use of a needle. If the lump is found to be malignant there are a number of possibilities in treatment, which are varied according to the needs of each case; removal of the lump or the breast – the operation of radical removal of the breast and surrounding tissues once widely used is now much less often thought necessary – combined with radiotherapy and possibly chemotherapy is the usual course of action. The prolonged use of tamoxifen, which is an antagonist to oestrogen, is commonly advised after initial treatment. In advanced cases secondary deposits of malignant cells may affect the bones, particularly those of the vertebral column or pelvis. It is possible, but much less common, for cancer to develop in the male breast, and treatment will be as outlined above.

Benign lumps are common in the breast, and are usually composed of fibrous tissue with a variable amount of gland tissue. They are known as fibro-adenomas, and are treated by simple surgical removal. Cysts also occur and may be aspirated or removed. They are often found in association with a condition called chronic mastitis which is not in fact due to inflammation, as the name suggests, but is probably dependent on hormonal factors, for it occurs during the child-bearing period of life and produces discomfort which varies with the menstrual cycle. Breasts which are affected by chronic mastitis may be firm and nodular, often with discrete nodules: the breast is sometimes described as 'lumpy'. The condition does not appear to have any relation to malignant disease. Acute inflammation of the breast is not uncommon in those who are breast-feeding infants; there is pain and redness of the breast with fever. If left untreated, an abscess forms, but the use of penicillin is possible for it does not harm the infant. The affected breast should have the milk expressed by hand, but there is no need to abandon breast-feeding entirely.

Breathalyser: an instrument for determining the amount of alcohol excreted in the breath. It is illegal in the UK to drive a car with a blood alcohol concentration of more than 80 mg/100 ml, or with a greater amount of alcohol in the breath than 35 mg/100 ml.

Breathlessness: may occur in any condition in which there is a deficiency of oxygen in the blood. It may therefore result from a deficiency of oxygen in the inspired air, obstruction to the air passages, diminution of the area of lung tissue able to carry out exchange of carbon dioxide for oxygen between the blood and the air, diseases of the heart which prevent adequate circulation of the blood, or diseases of the blood in which its capacity to carry oxygen is reduced.

Breech Delivery: normally a child being born lies upside down with its head being presented first for delivery, but it can happen that the position is reversed and the buttocks are presented first. *See* Labour.

Bright's Disease: acute nephritis (q.v.).

Bromides: salts of bromine were formerly used as sedatives, but they unfortunately have objectionable features: rashes develop in those who are sensitive, and the consumption of bromides over a long period results in mental dullness and sometimes even confusion. There is, however, no foundation in the belief once prevalent in the British Army that bromides were put in the soldiers' tea.

Bromidrosis: the secretion of offensive sweat. *See* Perspiration.

Bromocriptine: a drug which acts on the pituitary gland to inhibit the secretion of prolactin and the growth hormone. It is therefore used to stop the secretion of milk and to treat acromegaly. It may also be used in the treatment of Parkinson's disease (q.v.), for it has a stimulating action on dopamine receptors in the brain.

Bronchiectasis: permanent abnormal dilation of the bronchi, the air passages in the lung. It arises from chronic inflammation after pneumonia, particularly that caused by measles and whooping cough in childhood, from obstruction of the airways by an inhaled foreign body, and in association with tuberculosis and cystic fibrosis as well as other less common conditions. The advent of mass immunisation against measles and whooping cough has greatly diminished the occurrence of the disease, as has the use of antibiotics. The condition is characterised by coughing, the spitting of blood, and the production of a quantity of sputum which may smell foul. Diagnosis is aided by X-ray appearances, which may if necessary be made more accurate by the introduction of radio-opaque substances into the air passages to make a bronchogram. Treatment is by the use of antibiotics. Excessive sputum may be removed from the lungs by postural drainage, where the patient is positioned with the affected part of the lung uppermost and natural drainage is assisted by gravity. Judicious percussion of the chest will aid the effectiveness of the process, which may be carried out in the morning and at night. In cases troubled by difficult breathing the inhalation of salbutamol or similar bronchodilators may help. In a few cases, where the disease is localised, it is possible that surgery might be advised.

Bronchitis: inflammation of the bronchi, the air passages in the lungs. It can be acute or chronic. In acute cases, the infection may be caused by bacteria or a virus; in a considerable number of cases virus infection is followed by bacterial invasion. It is not uncommon for this to be followed by asthma, which may last for some weeks or even longer. While the bacteria are susceptible to treatment with antibiotics, viruses are not, but they will disappear in time. Commonly, acute attacks of bronchitis are exacerbations of a pre-existing state of chronic bronchitis, a state in which there is excessive secretion of mucus in the bronchi. It is not necessarily associated with bacterial infection but can be caused by smoking or air pollution. There is no doubt that smoking is the cause of most cases of chronic bronchitis, and the chronic productive cough, often worse in the morning, is accepted as 'smokers' cough' and regarded as the natural consequence of smoking. It may be accompanied by shortness of breath, due to the partial obstruction of the airways by excessive mucus. Smokers are liable, particularly in the winter, to chest infection which shows itself by increased coughing; the colour of the sputum changes from grey to yellow-green, and the patient feels ill. These attacks of acute-on-chronic bronchitis can be treated with antibiotics as they are usually due to bacterial infection. The only treatment likely to improve chronic bronchitis is avoidance of the irritating factor. In the case of smoking it is obvious; with the control of industrial smoke in recent years air pollution has markedly decreased, but there are still places where it is prevalent and if possible they should be avoided. In patients who suffer from bronchitis, any change in 'the usual cough' should be investigated, for there may be an underlying cause.

Bronchogram: an X-ray examination of the bronchial tree or a portion of it after the introduction of a radio-opaque substance.

Bronchopneumonia: the extension of infection from the bronchi to the lung tissue resulting in a combined inflammation of the air passages and the lung itself. It often occurs during the course of another illness, particularly when the condition is severe and the patient bedridden. It has been called 'the old man's friend', for it can be the terminating factor in a distressing long-drawn-out illness.

Bronchoscope: an instrument for examining the air passages of the lungs. With the development of fibre-optics the bronchoscope has become flexible, and the examination can be more extensive than once it was.

The instrument is passed between the vocal cords into the bronchi and an inspection of the interior of the air passages is carried out, and if necessary a biopsy taken.

Bronchus: the trachea (windpipe), after its passage through the neck, divides in the chest into two main bronchi – the air passages to the right and left lungs, which in turn divide into smaller branches. These smaller bronchi again branch to form the bronchial tree; when the branches are less than about 0.2 mm in diameter they are called bronchioles. The bronchioles divide still further until they end in minute air sacs called alveolar sacs, which are lined by the alveoli, small pockets in which the exchange of gases takes place between the blood and the air. *See* Lungs.

Brucellosis (Malta fever, undulant fever): a disease caused by the micro-organisms of the genus *Brucella*, identified by the Scottish bacteriologist David Bruce (1855–1931) in 1886. The species of *Brucella* that produce disease in humans are usually *Brucella abortus*, *Brucella melitensis* and *Brucella suis*. All are parasites of mammals. The natural hosts of *B. abortus* are cows, of *B. melitensis* goats and sheep, and of *B. suis* pigs, caribou and reindeer. In some parts of the world *B. canis*, found in dogs, can produce human brucellosis. The disease can be acute or chronic, and has an incubation period of between two weeks and some months. In the acute form, there is a high fever, with headache, muscular pains, and generalised weakness. There may be pain in the chest accompanied by an irregular pulse, and confusion; occasionally there is pain in the abdomen. Convalescence is slow, and patients complain of a general lack of strength and energy for months. In the chronic form of the disease, recurring fever with headaches and sweating, accompanied by tiredness and lack of energy, leads to depression; often there is low back pain, which makes work even more difficult. This may be due to involvement of the bones of the spine in the disease process, which can produce inflammation of the vertebrae and the intervertebral discs. Infection can involve the lining of the heart and the aorta, and give rise to meningitis, inflammation of the testicle and gall-bladder disease. Brucellosis is a disease of farmers and of associated occupations such as slaughtermen and butchers. It can be spread by raw infected milk and milk products, but in Britain in 1971 it became compulsory for infected animals to be slaughtered, and in 1981 all dairy herds were declared to be free of brucellosis. Eradication has been achieved in many countries. The treatment of the disease is with tetracyclines and rifampicin or streptomycin. Co-trimoxazole has also been used in treatment.

Bruise: an escape of blood from damaged vessels into the surrounding tissues causes discoloration of the skin, which at first goes red, then black and blue, then as the blood pigments break down turns yellow until in time the colour disappears. Usually bruises show in the area where the injury has been sustained, so that a blow in the eye leads to a black eye; but there are times when blood from a deeper injury tracks along muscles and the planes of connective tissue to show under the skin in a different place, so that black eyes can result from a fracture of the base of the skull, and a fracture of the upper arm produces bruising at the elbow.

Bubo: the swelling of a lymphatic gland or group of glands, particularly in the groin or the armpit. *See* Plague.

Bulbar Palsy: the medulla oblongata, which is part of the brain stem, is sometimes called the spinal bulb, and paralysis of the motor cranial nerves which take their origin from nuclei in this area is called bulbar palsy or paralysis. It causes difficulty in speaking, coughing and swallowing, as it affects the muscles of the mouth, lips, tongue, larynx and pharynx.

Bulimia: a depressive illness linked to anorexia nervosa (q.v.), characterised by bouts of over-eating and a craving for food. It is associated with a fear of becoming fat, which leads to self-induced vomiting and excessive purging, with intervals of starvation between the bouts of over-eating. The cause of the illness is imperfectly understood, the treatment difficult.

Bunions: a common deformity of the foot is deviation of the great toe towards the outer side of the foot. This is called hallux valgus, and in this condition the joint between the great toe and the first metatarsal bone of the foot becomes prominent. Pressure of the shoe on the joint sets up chronic irritation and inflammation of the tissues with the formation of an adventitious bursa (q.v.) which in this situation is called a bunion. Treatment is to wear wide shoes which do not press on the prominent joint; if the bunion becomes very painful it can be removed surgically, and the deformity of the joint can be set right.

Burns and Scalds: scalds are caused by boiling water or steam, and burns by dry heat, flames, electricity or chemicals. Both damage the skin, and are divided into groups according to the damage suffered, which may be simple reddening of the skin with blistering, partial thickness destruction of the skin, or destruction of the whole thickness of the skin with damage to underlying tissues. Burns of the first group are painful but not dangerous, but extensive burns of the second and third groups are dangerous and require skilled treatment; much tissue fluid leaks from the burned surfaces and salts and water are lost. In addition there is shock and the risk of infection. First aid treatment is to cover the burns with a sterile or clean cloth, keep the patient warm and give hot drinks. If immediate aid is not forthcoming the cloths may be soaked in weak salt water and bound in place, or the patient put into a warm bath with a teaspoonful of salt to each pint of water. It is not sensible to try to put any kind of antiseptic on the burns. Minor burns are best treated by covering them with gauze; do not interfere with blisters if they form. In dealing with burns careful cleanliness is essential, for infection complicates healing even in the simplest burn.

Bursa: a closed sac lined with synovial membrane containing fluid placed where there may be friction between structures such as tendons and bones so that they can move easily over each other. Sometimes they become inflamed, as the result of either injury or infection, a condition called bursitis. An example of this is housemaid's knee, where as the result of incessant kneeling the bursa overlying the kneecap becomes inflamed and swollen.

Byssinosis: a lung disease found in workers in the cotton and jute industries who are exposed to fine dust containing vegetable matter, moulds and cotton fibres. They develop a cough with wheezing and breathlessness, which is worse going into work on Mondays after the weekend rest (Monday fever), deteriorating over a period of years. If exposure to dust continues, the condition progresses to chronic bronchitis and emphysema (q.v.).

C

Cachexia: extreme debility produced by serious chronic illness.

Cadmium Poisoning: exposure to the fumes from this metal, which is used in several industries, produces acute and severe irritation of the lungs, developing sometimes over several hours and requiring hospital treatment. Chronic poisoning, resulting from exposure to cadmium fumes or dust over years, produces damage to the lungs, the nose and the kidneys.

Caduceus: the wand of Hermes or Mercury, messenger of the gods, consisting of a winged staff with two serpents entwined round it. The staff of Aesculapius, the legendary Greek physician, has one serpent, and is used, surrounded by a laurel wreath, as the badge of the Royal Army Medical Corps. The serpent is widely associated with regeneration and healing, for it grows a new skin and sloughs off the old.

Caecum: the blind sac at the beginning of the large intestine where it joins the small intestine. It lies in the lower right-hand side of the abdominal cavity, and may be the seat of inflammation, ulceration or cancer. *See* Appendicitis.

Caesarean Section: the delivery of a child by an incision through the abdominal wall and womb, named after an ancient Roman law which laid down that if the mother died the child was to be removed from the womb and buried separately. Once a serious operation only performed when natural childbirth had proved impossible or the mother was dead, it is now done for a number of reasons, for example disproportion, when the pelvis is too small to accommodate the baby's head; cases where the placenta is placed right over the internal opening of the uterus (placenta praevia); some cases of breech presentation in older women; distress of the foetus or mother during delivery, and other emergencies. Up to 10% of babies are born this way, for the operation has become well understood and in the average case is not particularly difficult or dangerous.

Caffeine: an alkaloid found in tea and coffee; cocoa contains the related alkaloid theobromine. It is a weak stimulant to the central nervous system, counteracting tiredness. The dose is about 100 mg or two cups of freshly ground coffee. About twice this amount is needed to get the same effect from instant coffee. Caffeine acts on the kidneys, increasing the flow of urine, and on the heart, which it stimulates to the extent of producing palpitations after over-indulgence. It also increases gastric secretions, and can lead to gastritis. Caffeine was once popular with students who used it before examinations, although it was more likely to produce an uncomfortable bladder than counteract the serious effects of not knowing enough. It has no place in modern medicine; from time to time it is suspected of being responsible for undue anxiety in those who take too much coffee, and even of being addictive, but the only withdrawal symptom noted is the development of headaches.

Caisson Disease: decompression sickness, found in those working in compressed air in a chamber under water (a caisson) during the construction of a bridge in the last century. The same condition is now found in divers, following too rapid ascents from a depth. The length of time a diver can spend under pressure varies with the depth to which he descends; pressure exerted by the water is about 1 atmosphere for each 10 metres depth of sea water, and commercial diving takes place at pressures up to 35 atmospheres. The symptoms are pain in the joints and chest, with breathlessness and in very severe cases paralysis. The reason is that under increased pressure, gases, mainly nitrogen, go into solution in the blood, and when the pressure falls come out of solution as bubbles in the circulation. In the joints they produce pain, the 'bends', in the lungs pain and breathlessness, the 'chokes', and in the brain bubbles in the small blood vessels may produce the 'staggers' – giddiness, double vision, dimness of vision and even convulsions. In the spinal cord the bubbles may bring on paralyses. There may also be pain in the abdomen, nausea and vomiting, deafness and the 'itch', irritating red patches in the skin. The only cure is to recompress the diver in a compression chamber to the pressure to which he was originally subjected and to decompress slowly over a period of hours according to the treatment tables. The rate of ascent must be strictly controlled to allow the dissolved gases to disperse slowly without forming bubbles.

Calamine: zinc oxide with 0.5% ferric oxide, made up into a lotion or ointment to relieve itching conditions of the skin.

Calcaneum: the heel-bone or os calcis.

Calciferol: vitamin D_2, made by irradiating ergosterol, which is found in yeast and fungi. Vitamin D occurs naturally in milk, butter, cheese, eggs and liver, particularly fish liver. Lack of the vitamin in children produces rickets, a disease of poverty and sunless cities, for vitamin D can be produced by the irradiating action of sunlight on sterols in the skin. Overdose of vitamin D is dangerous for it can lead to high levels of calcium in the blood and abnormal formation of bone.

Calcification: the abnormal deposition of calcium in the tissues, for example in the scars left by tuberculosis in the lungs.

Calcium: a metallic element of great importance in the body. Not only are the bones made of calcium, but it is essential for proper blood clotting, for the functioning of muscles and nerves, and for the efficient action of the heart. The balance of calcium in the body is regulated by several hormones, the chief among them being the parathyroid hormone and the thyroid hormone calcitonin. Vitamin D is essential for the absorption of calcium and also for its normal availability in the body. The amount of calcium needed daily is about 1 g, present in a normal diet. Lack of calcium, the consequence of vitamin D deficiency, leads to malformation of the bones (*see* Osteomalacia); low levels in the blood produce tetany, which is involuntary contraction of muscles caused by high irritability of muscular tissue – not to be confused with tetanus. Chronically low levels may lead to brittle ridged nails, dry hair, eczema of the skin, mental disturbances and even fits. Symptoms produced by excess of calcium in the blood include pain in the bones, loss of appetite, nausea and vomiting, fatigue and thirst, and mental changes. Stones are commonly formed in the kidneys.

Calcium Antagonists: or calcium channel-blockers, a group of drugs recently developed that interfere with the action of calcium on heart muscle, the impulse-conducting cells in the heart and on the smooth muscle in blood vessel walls. Some reduce the tone in the arteries and therefore dilate the coronary system which supplies the heart, some slow the heartbeat and reduce its output. They are used in the treatment of angina and high blood pressure and some disorders of heart rhythm.

Calculus: a hard stony concretion formed by precipitation from natural secretions and fluids in the kidneys, gall-bladder, urinary bladder, or salivary glands. Calculi are usually referred to as stones.

Caldwell–Luc: an operation designed to drain a chronically infected maxillary antrum permanently by making an artificial opening through the upper jaw opposite the second molar tooth. (George W. Caldwell, 1834–1918 and Henry Luc, 1855–1925)

Calipers: external metal splints designed to take the weight of the body off a diseased or fractured leg bone when the patient stands or walks. The word also means an instrument resembling a large pair of compasses with curved legs for measuring distances and thickness, used for example by an obstetrician to measure the size of the pelvis.

Callosity: an area of thickening of the horny layer of the skin caused by chronic pressure or friction.

Callus: when a bone is broken blood collects between the broken ends, and in it cells called osteoblasts multiply and lay down a mass of irregular bone which knits the two ends together. This is the callus; it takes about four weeks to calcify, after which it becomes tougher and bone is absorbed as well as laid down until the original structure of the bone is largely replaced and its strength restored.

Calomel: mercurous chloride. Formerly used as a purgative and in the treatment of syphilis, it is, like most mercury compounds, poisonous and its use has been abandoned. One of its uses was in teething powder given to infants, where it gave rise to pink disease in which the hands and feet became pink and painful; the disease remained a mystery until it was realised that calomel was at fault and cases are now very rarely seen.

Calorie: the small, gram or standard calorie is the amount of heat required to raise 1 g of water 1°C in temperature. The large or kilogram calorie used in dietetics is the amount of heat needed to raise 1 kg of water 1°C. Although these measurements are still largely used in medicine, they have been replaced as units of energy under the SI system of 1960 by joules and megajoules. The joule is defined as the work done when a force of 1 newton acts over a distance of 1 metre; 1 calorie is the equivalent of 4.1868 joules, and 1 megajoule the equivalent of 239 kilocalories. *See* Weights and Measures.

Campylobacter: *Campylobacter jejuni* and *Campylobacter coli* are micro-organisms which cause watery diarrhoea in human beings; they are found in birds, including chickens, and other animals such as domestic cats and dogs. Unlike salmonella, they do not multiply in infected food. The organisms are spread in contaminated food, milk or water, and the incubation period is three or four days; there is fever and general malaise, and the diarrhoea is accompanied by colicky abdominal pain. Severe diarrhoea lasts only a few days, but malaise and milder diarrhoea may last for a week or so. Treatment when needed is with erythromycin; the organisms are resistant to ampicillin.

Cancer: a malignant tumour, that is one made of cells which multiply in a disorderly and uncontrolled way, invade surrounding tissues, and can give rise to secondary growths in parts of the body remote from the original tumour. Cancer has been recognised since antiquity, but it was not until the early nineteenth century, when the microscope revolutionised the study of human tissues, that cellular pathology laid the foundations of our knowledge of abnormal growth of cells. By the end of the century classification of cancers based on the type of cell involved, its site of origin, its appearance and the likely progression of the disease had been achieved, and at the turn of the century cancer research units began to function. Since then an enormous amount of knowledge has accumulated, but the precise nature of the change that cells undergo when they become cancerous still eludes understanding. Nevertheless, the treatment of cancer and measures for its prevention have advanced remarkably. At first advances in surgery made it possible to undertake ever wider removal of the growth and surrounding tissue; then the use of X-rays for limiting cell growth increased and became better understood between the two World Wars, and advances in nuclear physics during the Second World War led to the use of cobalt-60 and the linear accelerator; and now rapid advances are being made in the understanding and use of chemotherapy, the aim of which is to use drugs to affect the growth of cells. Modern treatment of cancer may employ a combination of all three approaches designed to meet the individual needs of each patient. A further line of treatment relies on the fact that tumours of the breast and the prostate gland are to some extent dependent on hormones, so that the use of stilboestrol affords a period of relapse for prostatic cancer, and the drug tamoxifen, with an anti-oestrogen effect, aids in keeping cancer of the breast quiescent. Many substances are known to bring about cancerous changes in the tissues, ranging from soot, observed by Percivall Pott (1714–88) in 1775 to be responsible for cancer of the scrotum in sweeps, to tobacco smoke, responsible for cancer of the lung today. The most easily avoided cause of cancer is smoking tobacco. Otherwise avoid obesity, be moderate in the use of alcohol, increase dietary fibre and eat more vegetables and fruit. For women it is important to examine the breasts for lumps once a month, to have a cervical smear every three or four years up to the age of 65, and over the age of 50 to seek regular mammography, at present recommended at three-yearly intervals. Substances used in industry which are known to produce cancer are carefully controlled, and new substances are examined as they are introduced.

Candidiasis: *Candida albicans* is a fungus commonly present in the mouth and on the skin in health which may produce an infection of the mouth in infants or those treated for a long time with antibiotics, or of the vagina in women, again especially after a course of antibiotics. The infection produces white patches in the mouth, and irritation and a white discharge from the vagina. Nystatin is effective, used as a suspension or pastilles in the mouth or as a cream or pessaries in the vagina. The imidazole drugs are also effective: fluconazole or itraconazole are given by mouth except in the case of children and pregnant women. It is sensible for treatment to be offered to the marital partner, for the infection can be transferred to affect the penis in men.

Cannabis Indica: Indian hemp, hashish, bhang or gan-ja, marihuana or pot, is derived from the leaves and flowers of the plants *Cannabis indica* or *Cannabis sativa* which flourish in Asia and America. Together with opium, hashish is one of the earliest known drugs and was used in early medicine to produce drowsiness and relative insensitivity in the treatment of pain and the performance of surgical operations. It has no medical use today, but is illegally taken in the form of cigarettes, when it leads to a cheerful mood with a sense of exhilaration without delirium or excessive excitement. Visual hallucinations may occur, but the most typical results of hashish are prolongation of the senses of space and time; because of the latter effect it is used by players of popular music, for it appears to improve the control of rhythm. The limbs may feel heavy and the eyes look bright; there is no hangover effect although a feeling of unreality may persist for some hours. Like any form of narcotic, hashish is best avoided, although it rarely leads to addiction or any ill effects in normal people. Possibly its worst effect is the sort of company into which its use may lead.

Cantharides: a powder made from the dried bodies of the beetle Spanish fly, *Lytta vesicatoria*. It contains an active principle, cantharidin, which has a powerful blistering action on the skin, and was used at one time as a counter-irritant. Together with bay rum, cantharides is still used as a hair tonic. It has since ancient times had a reputation as an aphrodisiac, founded on the fact that if it is taken internally and excreted in the urine it irritates the urethra so badly that it produces priapism (q.v.). As the kidneys may be permanently damaged, and the irritation of the urethra greatly exceeds any advantage gained in the sexual field, it is perhaps safer for the impotent to see a psychiatrist.

Capillary: the smallest blood vessels in the circulation are called capillaries, although their size is considerably less than a hair. They join the arterioles and venules, and have about the same diameter as a red blood cell. It is in the capillaries that the blood and the tissue fluids exchange gases, food and waste products. The blood cells normally remain inside the capillaries, as do the larger molecules, e.g. proteins

Carbohydrate: a substance with a formula which includes only carbon, oxygen and hydrogen, the oxygen and hydrogen being in the proportions two of hydrogen to one of oxygen, the proportion which forms water. There are many carbohydrates, and they form the sugar and starchy components of food; they are the principal substances broken down to furnish energy, being metabolised to water and carbon dioxide.

Carbolic Acid: phenol, one of the first antiseptics introduced by Lord Lister in 1867 (*see* Antiseptics). It is still used as a standard by which to test other germicides, but has little application in modern medicine beyond its use, well diluted, as a mouthwash and as an oily injection in the treatment of haemorrhoids. It is a corrosive poison.

Carbon Dioxide: when oxygen is burned in the body, carbon dioxide is formed in the tissues. It is removed in the blood and excreted through the lungs in the air breathed out. In anaesthetics carbon dioxide may be used in combination with oxygen to stimulate respiration, for the body detects the excess of carbon dioxide and speeds up the breathing in an effort to get rid of it and maintain the essential balance between oxygen and carbon dioxide in the blood – the acid–base balance. Carbon dioxide is also used in medicine in its frozen form as carbon dioxide snow, which forms when the gas under pressure is allowed to expand quickly; it is used to burn off warts.

Carbon Monoxide: a deadly gas, without odour or colour, formed by the incomplete burning of fuels containing carbon, and present in car exhaust gas, smoke and coal gas, but not natural gas. Its deadliness arises from the fact that it combines with the haemoglobin of the blood 200 times more readily than oxygen; moreover the combination is irreversible, so that any appreciable amount of carbon monoxide in the air leads to a concentration in the body and chemical asphyxia, for no longer can the tissues be supplied with haemoglobin carrying oxygen. A concentration of 0.2% in the air is dangerous, 0.4% fatal in under an hour. Poisoning is insidious, and may not be detected if it comes from, for example, a faulty heating stove with insufficient ventilation. A brazier of coke has on occasion proved fatal to a watchman on a cold night, and motorists have been overcome by fumes from a faulty exhaust system. First aid obviously depends on removal to fresh air, but do not go without help into a confined unventilated space where a person has already collapsed. Artificial respiration may be needed until the arrival of the ambulance with oxygen. Carbon monoxide must not be confused with carbon dioxide (q.v.).

Carbon Tetrachloride: a volatile solvent used in industry, and formerly for dry cleaning and in fire extinguishers. Its use has been restricted, for its vapour is readily given off and is poisonous, affecting the liver, the kidneys and the central nervous system.

Carbuncle: an interconnected mass of boils, commonly occurring on the back of the neck. It is usually caused by infection with *Staphylococcus aureus*, and is particularly prone to arise in diabetics.

Carcinoma: a malignant tumour arising from the epithelial cells. *See* Epithelium.

Cardiac: pertaining to the heart or the upper part of the stomach. A 'cardiac heart', like a 'gastric stomach', is a tautology but not a cause of ill health.

Cardiac Asthma: shortness of breath owing to failure of the left side of the heart and therefore of the circulation of blood through the lungs. Occurring in intermittent attacks, it often appears at night, and may be relieved by sitting up.

Cardiac Catheterisation: the passage of a catheter under radiographic control through an artery or vein until it reaches the heart. The technique is used in the diagnosis and study of heart disease.

Cardiac Massage: external cardiac compression. If the heart stops suddenly, as it may after a heart attack, it may be possible to start it beating again. The interval between the cessation of circulation and its restoration should not exceed three minutes, so that swift action is necessary. Lay the patient flat, face upwards, note the time, and kneel beside the subject. Put the heel of one hand on the lower part of the breastbone, the other hand on top of it, and press straight down using all your weight so that the breastbone gives. Release the pressure and let the breastbone come up. Do this 60 times a minute. If possible get an assistant to give mouth-to-mouth artificial respiration, one breath for every five to eight pressures over the heart, but if you are alone start the pressure on the chest and stop it every eight to ten pressures to blow up the lungs. Keep up the resuscitation as long as you can – recovery has been achieved after as long as an hour.

Cardiogram: a tracing made by a cardiograph, an instrument for recording the action of the heart. Usually used to signify an electrocardiogram (q.v.).

Caries: decay and death of a bone, usually applied to the teeth.

Carminatives: substances which allegedly aid digestion, relieve spasm or colic, and expel flatulence. Among these are: cloves, nutmeg, cinnamon, lemon, pepper, ginger, cardamoms, oil of lavender, peppermint, aniseed, coriander, dill and gentian. There is no evidence that anything aids digestion unless there is something lacking in the stomach, such as the necessary enzymes, no evidence that these substances relieve colic or spasm, and since flatulence is usually the result of swallowing air, no evidence that they will help here. It is, however, likely that such spices may aid the appetite and set the salivary secretions flowing.

Carotid Artery: the great artery of the neck which supplies the head and brain with blood. Arising in the chest as the common carotid artery, it divides in the neck into the internal branch, which supplies the brain, and the external branch which goes to the outside of the skull. Disease of the carotid may make it increasingly narrow (carotid stenosis) and so decrease the flow of blood to the brain that the cerebral circulation is impaired and the function of the brain disturbed. The narrowing of the artery may be associated with a clot which may throw off small emboli and cause a stroke. It is possible in some cases to improve circulation in the carotid by surgical operation.

Carotid Sinus and Carotid Body: just above the division of the common carotid artery into internal and external branches there is a slight swelling of the internal branch called the carotid sinus, and between the two branches of the artery lies a small structure called the carotid body. The carotid body is concerned with the chemical balance of the blood, and so with respiration, and the carotid sinus with the maintenance of the blood pressure. Both derive their nerve supply from the glossopharyngeal and vagus nerves. Pressure on the sinus may slow the heart rate, and even produce fainting.

Carpal Tunnel Syndrome: as the median nerve runs down from the forearm to the hand, it passes over the wrist (the carpus) between the bones and the transverse ligament which overlies the nerve and the tendons passing into the palm. At this point it may become irritated and swollen, with consequent tingling of the index and middle fingers and discomfort in the wrist and forearm, followed by weakness of the thumb and in advanced cases flattening of small muscles of the thumb. Examination of the electrical reactions of the muscles is used to make the diagnosis, and the condition is treated by surgical division of the transverse ligament.

Carpus: the wrist.

Carrier: a person who unknowingly carries the organisms of a disease without suffering from its symptoms, although capable of passing the disease to others.

Cartilage: a special type of supporting tissue which with bone makes up the skeleton. Most of the bones are originally formed from cartilage, and as the foetus develops and the child grows the process of ossification takes place until the only cartilage left is at the ends of the bones where it forms the articular surfaces of the joints, more slippery than ice. The only other parts of the adult skeleton made of cartilage are at the ends of the ribs, where they join the breastbone, the framework of the ear, part of the nose, and the rings of the trachea or windpipe.

Cascara: *Cascara sagrada*, or 'sacred bark', is the bark of the Californian buckthorn. An extract is used in liquid or solid form as a purgative; it acts in 6–8 hours.

Caseation: a process found principally in tuberculosis in which the dead central part of a chronically infected area, instead of turning into pus to form an abscess, changes into a cheesy mass which may later be replaced by fibrous tissue or undergo calcification and turn into chalk.

Castor Oil: oil squeezed from the seeds of the Indian castor oil plant, *Ricinus communis*. The seeds themselves are poisonous, but castor oil is soothing when applied to the skin, as in zinc and castor oil ointment. When it is taken by mouth it is changed by digestion into ricinoleic acid, which is a violently irritating purgative and acts with fairly explosive effect in three or four hours.

Castration: the removal of the testicles; sometimes applied also to the removal of the ovaries in women. This is generally done for disease of the organs, but in cases of carcinoma of the prostate gland the growth progresses more slowly in the absence of the hormone testosterone which is secreted by the testis. Consequently castration has been used as a treatment in this condition, but more generally stilboestrol, the female sex hormone, is given by mouth with the same effect. The results of castration vary with the age at which it is carried out; before puberty the operation prevents the development of the male sexual characteristics. The voice remains high-pitched, the figure takes on female outline, the beard fails to grow, and the subject does not grow bald with age. After puberty there are only very gradual changes; the subject is completely sterile, but not necessarily impotent.

CAT (computerised axial tomography): X-rays are held up by different tissues to a different extent, but ordinary radiography is only able to show these differences when they are very great. The introduction of this technique by the English physicist Sir Godfrey Hounsfield in 1973 means that small differences can be picked up, fed to the computer, and presented as a reconstructed image. Originally used to examine the brain, the method has since been extended to the whole body and, in conjunction with the use of special substances developed to throw target structures into greater contrast, has proved of inestimable value.

Catalepsy: an old-fashioned word used to describe a form of suspended animation characterised by immobility and lack of movement. The limbs remain in whatever position they are placed. It is a symptom of gross hysteria, and rare since hysteria became unfashionable. It may also be found in advanced schizophrenia.

Cataplasm: a poultice.

Cataplexy: sudden attacks of muscular weakness which may cause the patient to fall to the ground. The attacks are brought on by emotional stimuli such as anger or laughter, fear or surprise. The condition is associated with narcolepsy (q.v.).

Cataract: an opacity in the lens of the eye which obscures vision. Children may be born with cataracts, some of which may be inherited, others due to a virus infection during early pregnancy, most commonly rubella or German measles; but the most common cataract is that which forms in later life. This is caused by the gradual deterioration of the blood supply in the eye; the lens becomes hard and shrinks, and opacities develop. Cataracts can also develop in association with diabetes, after injury, after long exposure to heat as with glass workers, and after exposure to ionising radiation. The opacities increasingly interfere with vision. Spots may be seen before the eyes which, unlike those seen by perfectly normal people when they pay attention to them, do not move; bright lights may be seen double, and later on vision in twilight may be better than in full daylight since more light is admitted to the eye through a dilated pupil. An obvious greyish-white discoloration is eventually seen in the lens behind the pupil. The treatment is surgical. The surgeon removes the opaque lens from its capsule; a recent advance in technique may enable him to replace it with a plastic lens, otherwise spectacles can compensate for absence of the lens.

Catarrh: Hippocratic word meaning discharge from an inflamed mucous membrane, particularly from the mucous membranes lining the nose and the air sinuses and antra. As a diagnosis 'catarrh' is entirely unspecific and unsatisfactory, but it tends to linger.

Catatonia: in some types of schizophrenia the patient may show a disturbance of movement; there may be complete immobility, and the patient stays exactly in the same position without reacting to any stimuli. The limbs may be held in any position to which they are moved (*flexibilitas cerea*).

Catgut: catgut is not made from the guts of a cat, but from the intestines of sheep. The fibrous tissue is sterilised and split into threads which are woven to give various thicknesses and strengths; it can be treated with chromic acid to make chromic catgut, which stays intact in the tissues for up to three weeks instead of being absorbed like plain catgut in a week. It is the fact that it is absorbed which makes it so useful, for it can be used for ligatures or stitches in places where persisting material might carry the risk of infection or chronic irritation. It is not normally used to stitch skin for such stitches can easily be removed and catgut causes a reaction.

Cathartics: purgatives.

Catheter: a tube made for introduction into a body cavity, usually the bladder. Originally made of metal, the introduction of rubber and later plastics made them flexible and revolutionised their use. They are now made in all kinds of sizes and shapes, from cardiac catheters which are long and of small bore to those designed to be self-retaining in the bladder. It was once the urogenital surgeon's habit to carry a catheter rolled up in his top hat; with modern disposable ready-sterilised instruments it is once again possible.

Cat-scratch Fever: a disease in which there is fever and swelling of the local lymph glands after superficial damage to the skin, often but not necessarily from a cat-scratch. The organism responsible is not known, but the disease is mild, runs its course in a week or two, and no treatment is required.

Cauda Equina: the spinal cord is one-third shorter than the spinal column in which it lies, but the nerves issuing from the cord run out one by one between the vertebrae. The consequence is that the nerves in the neck run out almost straight from the cord to the spaces between the vertebrae, but as the discrepancy in length becomes greater the nerves take on a more slanting course, until the cord ends opposite the second lumbar vertebra. By then it has given off the nerves that are going to run through the spaces between the lower lumbar and sacral vertebrae, and they continue downwards as a leash of nerves that is called the cauda equina, the horse's tail.

Cauliflower Ear: a blow on the ear may cause bleeding between the cartilage of the ear and the membrane which covers it, the perichondrium. If the blood is left it may not be absorbed, as there is no pressure on the ear and no movement to break up the clot. In consequence it may become fibrous so that the ear is distorted as scar tissue forms and contracts.

The result is a cauliflower ear. It may be prevented if the blood is let out while it is still liquid and a pressure bandage used to prevent it collecting again.

Causalgia: a very severe burning pain which may develop after injury to one of the major nerves supplying the arm or the leg. Incomplete division of the nerve is most likely to lead to this distressing complication, but the precise cause is not known. The nerves most likely to be affected are the median nerve or other branches of the brachial plexus in the arm, and the sciatic nerve in the leg. A few weeks after the injury the patient notices that the hand, the foot or the leg is beginning to tingle, and then the sensation turns into a burning pain which may be set off by the slightest touch. The affected area turns red and sometimes moist. Treatment is difficult, but the condition may respond to removal of the sympathetic nervous plexus supplying the affected limb.

Cautery: an instrument by which heat is applied in the process of cauterisation, the burning of tissue to destroy it or stop bleeding. Once a heated metal instrument, it is now the electric cautery which is widely used in surgery. The term is also used to describe the burning of tissue by the application of caustic chemicals.

Cell, the unit of which the body is made. Some primitive organisms are made up of one cell, but the most complicated animals, the mammals, are made of many million cells of different types. Study of the cell is basic to an understanding of the function and chemistry of living creatures, and it has been carried on ever since optical microscopes were invented; the electron microscope has given an enormous impetus to the work, as has the technique of tissue culture. The cells found in man are of all sizes and shapes, from the cells of the nervous system, which may give off processes which extend for two or three feet, to the smallest cell of all, the blood platelets or thrombocytes, which have a diameter of 2–4 mm. A cell usually contains the following structures: outer lining membrane, cytoplasm and nucleus. The nucleus consists of the envelope, nucleoplasm, and the nucleolus; it is concerned with cell division and inheritance. It contains deoxyribonucleic acid (DNA) which is responsible for the synthesis of protein and carries the genes which are the basic units of heredity. The nucleolus is concerned in the synthesis of ribonucleic acid (RNA). The cytoplasm of the cell consists of a matrix, endoplasmic reticulum, the mitochondria, lysosomes, Golgi apparatus, peroxysomes, ribosomes and centrioles. The cell membrane is made of protein, carbohydrate and fatty molecules, and in life is in incessant motion. It regulates the passage into and out of the cell of chemical substances, and carries on its outer surface antigens which identify it (*see* Allergy). Cytoplasm is the name given to all the material inside the cell except the nucleus; it is seen by the electron microscope to be organised into many definite tubes, circles and other structures, called the endoplasmic reticulum. Parts of the endoplasmic reticulum have been named – the Golgi apparatus, concerned in the formation of glycoproteins, peroxysomes which are concerned with oxidation processes, ribosomes concerned in the synthesis of proteins from amino-acids, lysosomes which contain enzymes, mitochondria which are concerned with the metabolism of the cell and the synthesis of adenosine triphosphate (ATP), and the centrioles, which are concerned with cell division. Each type of cell is different, and each has special features which vary according to its function.

Cellulitis: inflammation which is not localised by the reaction of the infected tissues may spread into the surrounding connective tissues. The overlying skin becomes red, painful and swollen. The infecting organism is usually a streptococcus, and treatment of this serious condition is by antibiotics.

Cellulose: carbohydrate which forms the skeleton of most plants and some fungi. It is not digestible by man, although it is by herbivorous animals, and it therefore provides the bulky part of the intestinal contents and plays a part in the treatment of cases of constipation where it is thought that an increase in the volume of the contents of the large bowel might help evacuation. As methyl cellulose it has been used in the treatment of obesity, for taken with water it swells up in the stomach and so quells the pangs of hunger.

Its advantage is that it has no action whatever either as drug or nourishment; its disadvantage that people often imagine that they have to take it in addition to their normal diet.

Celsius: the Swedish astronomer (1701–44) who devised a scale of temperature based on the melting point of ice, which was 0°, and the boiling point of water, taken to be 100°. The scale, now in universal use, is called the Celsius or Centigrade scale.

Central Nervous System: the brain and spinal cord. *See* Nervous System.

Cephalosporins: a group of broad-spectrum antibiotics with an action against Gram negative and positive bacteria, useful in treating infections resistant to other antibiotics, especially urinary tract infections.

Cerebellum: that part of the brain which occupies the posterior fossa of the skull, behind the brain stem. It is concerned with balance, muscle tone and co-ordination of movement.

Cerebral Abscess: an abscess occurring in the brain, arising from middle ear disease, frontal sinus infection, local injury, or infection carried in the blood from the lungs in chronic disease such as bronchiectasis. The treatment is surgical.

Cerebral Cortex: the grey matter which forms the outer layer of the cerebral hemispheres, the biggest part of the brain; the two cerebral hemispheres lie in the vault of the skull. *See* Nervous System.

Cerebral Haemorrhage and Thrombosis: *See* Apoplexy.

Cerebral Tumour: a tumour arising within the skull. Such tumours may arise in the brain matter itself, in the covering membranes of the brain, in the structures associated with the brain, or may be metastatic, that is, spread by the bloodstream from malignant tumours elsewhere in the body, commonly the breast, lung or kidney. They produce their symptoms by interfering with neighbouring structures and by raising the pressure within the skull.

Cerebrospinal Fever: *see* Meningitis.

Cerebrospinal Fluid: the fluid in which the central nervous system lies, contained by the meninges, the covering membranes. Abbreviation CSF. *See* Nervous System.

Cerebrovascular Accident: a stroke; commonly abbreviated to CVA. *See* Apoplexy.

Cerebrum: properly the largest part of the brain, the two linked cerebral hemispheres, but sometimes used for the brain as a whole.

Cerumen: waxy secretion normally found in the outer passage of the ear, which if present in excess may block the passage and cause deafness. It is easily removed by syringing, but it is dangerous for uninformed people to try to get it out, for there is a risk of damage to the ear-drum.

Cervical: pertaining to the neck, as in cervical vertebrae or cervical nerves. Also concerned with the cervix uteri, the neck of the womb.

Cervical Disc Disease: the cervical nerves and spinal cord may be damaged by protrusion of the intervertebral discs. Protrusion of a cervical intervertebral disc is usually found at the levels C5–6 or C6–7. It may be sudden, and may follow an injury. When the protrusion is on one side, the disc presses on the nerve as it emerges between the vertebrae, producing pain in the neck with limitation of movement. The pain spreads down the arm and there may be changes of sensation in the skin supplied by the affected nerve, but only in severe cases is there any interference with function. The condition improves with rest and is helped by wearing a cervical collar. Only where the protrusion is central is the spinal cord itself compressed, and then paralysis may follow, which must be relieved by operation.

Cervical Smear: the cells lying on the surface of the cervix uteri are removed by gently scraping it with a special spatula through a vaginal speculum, stained, and examined under the microscope. In this way it is possible to detect any change from normal which might indicate pre-malignant or malignant disease before the development of symptoms, and institute appropriate early treatment. It is used as a routine examination on women before the age of 65, and should be carried out every three or four years.

Cervical Spondylosis: a degenerative disease of the cervical spine, with bulging of the intervertebral discs and osteophyte formation, that is the development of spurs of bone characteristic of arthritis at the edges of the vertebrae. It may be the result of an old injury. The symptoms are much the same as in cervical disc disease (q.v.), and may be helped by wearing a supporting collar.

Cetrimide: used for cleaning and disinfecting the skin, this preparation has useful detergent properties.

Chalazion: a small round swelling of the eyelid, caused by blockage of the duct of one of the sebaceous glands with consequent formation of a retention cyst. It may easily be removed surgically.

Chancre: the primary ulcer of syphilis, usually occurring on the genitals, starting a week or more after exposure to infection as a painless small lump which ulcerates, the ulcer having a hard raised edge. It takes some weeks to heal if left untreated and leaves a scar.

Chancroid: an ulcer on the genitals caused by infection with Ducrey's bacillus, transmitted by sexual contact. It is found mainly but not exclusively in tropical countries, and is known as soft sore in contrast to the hard chancre of syphilis. It responds to tetracycline and sulphonamides.

Change of Life: *see* Menopause.

Cheiropomphylix: a condition of the skin in which tiny blisters appear on the palms of the hands or soles of the feet. There may be intense itching. The rash may be a reaction to irritants, it may develop in association with eczema, or it may be a sensitivity reaction to fungus infection in another part of the body. Attacks of athlete's foot (q.v.) are often the exciting cause. Corticosteroid ointment is used in the treatment.

Cheloid: *see* Keloid.

Chemotherapy: the treatment of infections or other conditions by chemical agents specifically designed to act on organisms or abnormal cells. In 1910 Paul Ehrlich (1854–1915) introduced arsphenamine (Salvarsan) which killed the organisms of syphilis, but this has now been abandoned for penicillin. In 1935 sulphonamides were introduced, followed by penicillin and an avalanche of synthetic and semi-synthetic antibiotics. But the term is now used mainly to mean treatment with cytotoxic drugs used in the treatment of cancer, of which there are upwards of 20. Ideally, these drugs would only interfere with the growth of malignant cells, but this ideal is not yet attainable, and the drugs interfere with normal as well as malignant cells. Nevertheless, while the drugs interfere with the process of cell division in all cells, some normal cells are more resistant to the drugs than others, and some malignant cells are more susceptible than others. In some instances the difference between the normal and malignant cells is just enough to make treatment worthwhile; moreover, after cells have been damaged by cytotoxic drugs, normal cells recover more quickly than malignant cells. In practice the use of the drugs has to be finely balanced so that the greatest possible number of malignant cells are killed without destroying so many normal cells that life is endangered. It is inevitable that severe general disturbance will occur to normal cells, and this must result in considerable disturbance to the well-being of those being treated with cytotoxic drugs. But the combination of surgery, radiotherapy, chemotherapy and in suitable cases hormone therapy offers continually improving hope in the treatment of cancer, and as our understanding of the cell advances so will widely effective and relatively harmless chemotherapy become possible.

Cheyne–Stokes Breathing: a type of breathing found in those in deep coma and the dying. The breathing rhythm is in cycles, starting with shallow breaths, which gradually increase in depth until having reached a peak they die away again. The breathing may stop altogether between cycles. (John Cheyne, 1777–1836, and William Stokes, 1804–78)

Chicken-pox (varicella): a common infective disease usually in children. It is caused by the varicella-zoster (V–Z) virus, and has an incubation period of two or three weeks. A rash appears as tiny red spots on the trunk and face, which become blisters and eventually scab over. The child has a headache, is irritable and has a slight temperature. If the rash is scratched it may become infected, but calamine lotion is usually sufficient to take care of the irritation, and in children there are few complications. In adults, however, the symptoms are more severe, and the patient can feel very ill. A second attack of chicken-pox is very rare. The infective period extends from five days before the rash to one week after it appears.

Chilblains: cold injury of the hands and feet, and sometimes of the thighs. The skin becomes red and swollen, and begins to burn and itch. The condition is most often seen in young people, and is caused by poor circulation and exposure to cold; curiously it is not found in really cold climates because protection from the cold has to be taken seriously, but in the United Kingdom it is common during the winter.

Chill: a meaningless term better avoided.

Childbirth: *see* Labour.

Chimney Sweep's Cancer: cancer of the scrotum, caused by irritation of the skin by soot.

Chiropody: profession concerned with the care of the feet.

Chiropractic: an independent branch of complementary

medicine which specialises in the diagnosis and treatment of mechanical disorders of the joints, particularly those of the spine and their effects on the nervous system. X-rays are often used in diagnosis, and a chiropractor carries out treatment by specific manipulation. Drugs and surgery are not used.

Chlamydia: a genus of micro-organisms classified as bacteria, but behaving like viruses because they cannot multiply except within cells. They are responsible for a number of diseases, principally trachoma (q.v.), urethritis in men, cervicitis and salpingitis in women, lymphogranuloma venereum, and psittacosis (*see* Ornithosis). The organism is sensitive to tetracyclines and erythromycin.

Chloral Hydrate: an old-fashioned but still useful hypnotic for children and the elderly.

Chloramphenicol: a powerful broad-spectrum antibiotic which has, unfortunately, toxic properties, for it interferes with the action of the bone marrow in making blood cells. Its systemic use is therefore limited to certain dangerous conditions, e.g. typhoid and *Haemophilus* meningitis; but it can be used on the surface of the body without danger in eye and ear drops for local infections such as conjunctivitis and otitis externa.

Chlorhexidine: a disinfectant used for cleaning the skin. It may also be used in a mouthwash.

Chlorine: a yellow poisonous gas, an element widely distributed in natural compounds. Chlorinated solutions are used to disinfect the skin, wounds and ulcers, for chlorine kills bacteria, fungi and viruses. Such solutions are chlorinated lime and boric acid solution (Eusol) and sodium hypochlorite solution. Chlorine is widely used to disinfect water for drinking, and used in swimming pools. It is also used for bleaching, and some household bleaches may contain hypochlorites. The action of the gas, which was first used in war in 1915, is to irritate the eyes, nose and throat, and to irritate the lungs, causing difficulty in breathing and pain in the chest. Severe poisoning may cause waterlogging of the lungs and need hospital treatment. If breathing apparatus is not available, a passable gas mask is a cloth soaked in water. Chlorine gas is heavier than air and it remains at ground level.

Chloroform: introduced as an anaesthetic agent in 1847, and used for many years by inhalation as a general anaesthetic, it has now been superseded by safer means, for it could damage the liver and upset the action of the heart.

Chlorophyll: the green pigment of plants, similar in structure to haemoglobin except that it has magnesium in place of iron. It enables plants to form carbohydrates from carbon dioxide and water under the influence of light (photosynthesis). It has been thought to sweeten the breath and when taken internally to prevent what is known in the advertising trade as body odour, but there is no evidence to support this hope.

Chloroquine: an antimalarial drug of considerable potency, used both for cure and prophylaxis. While it is still used in the treatment of benign malaria (infections with *P. vivax, ovale* and *malariae*), strains of the organism *P. falciparum* which causes malignant malaria are becoming increasingly resistant to the drug, particularly in Central and South America, South-East Asia including India, and East, Central and West Africa. Other antimalarials have therefore to be used. Chloroquine is used prophylactically in a dose of 300 mg once a week, and should be taken a week before travelling and for four weeks after returning. When travelling to areas where resistant *P. falciparum* is prevalent, proguanil 200 mg daily should be added, except for South-East Asia, Western Pacific and Oceania where one tablet of Maloprim weekly with 300 mg chloroquine is advised. Mefloquine has recently been introduced for the treatment and prophylaxis of resistant strains of the malarial parasite; up-to-date information may be obtained from the doctor or the travel agent. Chloroquine is also used in certain cases of rheumatoid arthritis and lupus erythematosus, but only under medical supervision, for in long-term use it may have unwanted effects, particularly on the retina of the eye.

Chlorpromazine: chemically related to the antihistamine drug promethazine, its use in mental disorders as a 'tranquilliser' is said to have resulted from the observation that the use of allergy-suppressing drugs in the mentally ill was often accompanied by a sedative effect and an improvement in mental symptoms. It is now used with great effect in the treatment of schizophrenia, the emergency control of severe behavioural disorders, and in severe anxiety states.

Choanae: the posterior nasal apertures, by which the nasal cavity communicates with the upper part of the pharynx. They are divided by the bony part of the nasal septum.

Choking: the gullet and windpipe divide in the upper part of the throat behind the tongue, and there is a mechanism to shut off the windpipe when food is being swallowed. If this mechanism fails, rarely because of nervous disease (*see* Bulbar Palsy), more often because the individual is laughing or talking or taking a breath at the same time as trying to swallow, food or drink or other things such as chewing-gum can 'go down the wrong way'. An involuntary gasp can have the same effect. As soon as anything reaches the sensitive lining of the windpipe the muscles go into spasm and it becomes difficult to take a breath. The victim tries to cough but cannot. It may be possible to dislodge the offending matter by a smart blow on the back, or in the case of children to turn them upside down and smack the back, but if choking continues stand behind the sufferer, embrace the lower chest with the hands locked together in front, and squeeze sharply. The outward rush of air should dislodge the obstruction.

Cholangiogram: X-ray examination of the biliary apparatus after the introduction of a radio-opaque compound. The contrast medium can be given by mouth, to be excreted and concentrated in the bile ducts and gall-bladder, or introduced through a needle passed into a bile duct in the liver, or introduced into the bile duct by using a fibre-optic endoscope passed through the stomach into the duodenum.

Cholangitis: inflammation of the bile ducts, usually associated with gallstones, giving rise to upper abdominal
pain, vomiting, fever (usually intermittent), and later
jaundice, itching, dark urine and pale motions. The
infection is brought under control with antibiotics, and
later investigation of the biliary tract may well lead to
surgical treatment.

Cholecystitis: inflammation of the gall-bladder, which
may be acute or chronic. In an acute attack there is upper
abdominal pain, which can radiate through to the back and
be felt in the right shoulder-blade and at the tip of the right
shoulder, nausea and vomiting. In the majority of cases
the cause is a gallstone lodged in the cystic duct, by which
the gall-bladder normally empties into the duodenum.
Once the diagnosis is established (*see* Cholangiogram) the
treatment is conservative, unless signs of complications
develop, in which case urgent operation may be needed.
In the majority of cases, surgery is postponed until the
acute inflammation has resolved. Chronic cholecystitis is
more common, and again results from the presence of
gallstones. It may follow an acute attack. Usually the
symptoms are somewhat vague, with discomfort rather
than acute pain in the abdomen, flatulence, 'indigestion',
worse after eating fatty food, and a feeling of distension of
the abdomen. Plain X-rays may show the stones, as may
ultrasound. Treatment is usually surgical.

Cholelithiasis: the presence of stones in the biliary tract.
Stones in the gall-bladder are common and are of three
types: cholesterol stones, bile pigment stones, and mixed
stones, containing cholesterol, bile pigments and calcium.
Stones composed of bile pigments may be hard or, more
rarely in Europe, soft. The reasons for the formation of
stones are not entirely understood, but include infection,
the influence of age and sex – stones are more common
in women – and obesity. They may be silent and give
rise to no symptoms, or they may lodge in the bile
ducts and produce colic, cholangitis, or acute or chronic
cholecystitis (*see above*). They may be seen on plain X-ray
plates if they contain calcium, shown up by ultrasound, or

by computerised tomography. More precise information may be gained by a cholecystogram (q.v.). Treatment in the majority of cases causing symptoms is surgical removal of the gall-bladder (cholecystectomy) and stones, but cholesterol stones can sometimes be dissolved by giving chenodeoxycholic acid or ursodeoxycholic acid by mouth, or by lithotripsy (q.v.).

Cholera: an acute disease caused by infection by the *Vibrio cholerae*. Originating in Bengal, it spread from India during the nineteenth century along the trade routes. In 1817, it reached Japan and Astrakhan in Russia; in 1826 it was in Moscow, in 1831 Berlin, and by 1832 it had been taken to Paris and London. There have been seven pandemics of cholera in the world, the last extending from Indonesia in 1961 through Asia and Africa to the Mediterranean in Europe and the Gulf Coast of the USA. The disease spreads by contamination of water supplies, and contamination of food. The infecting organism multiplies in the small intestine, producing a toxin which damages the wall of the gut so that it pours out fluid containing electrolytes essential for life: sodium, chloride, bicarbonate and potassium. There is painless fluid diarrhoea, vomiting, and in severe cases muscle cramp and prostration. The condition worsens in proportion to the amount of fluid lost. To be successful, treatment must replace the fluid and electrolytes; the World Health Organization recommends for intravenous use a solution of 4 g sodium chloride, 6.5 g sodium acetate, and 1 g potassium chloride in 1 litre of sterile distilled water. If the thirst which accompanies the loss of fluids is slaked by plain water, the body salts are only diluted further, but the WHO recommends a solution of 3.5 g sodium chloride, 1.5 g potassium chloride, 2.9 g sodium citrate, and 20 g glucose in 1 litre of water to be taken by mouth. This solution may be used to treat patients whose condition is not bad enough to demand intravenous fluid, but 1.5 volumes of the solution is needed to replace every volume of fluid lost. Although patients will recover if fluid and electrolyte losses are made up, tetracycline may be used as well to eradicate the infecting organisms. Prevention of cholera rests on adequate sanitation and clean water supplies, and where this is not possible scrupulous personal hygiene and careful preparation of food are essential. Immunisation with standard vaccines provides some protection for a few months, but it cannot be entirely relied upon.

Cholesterol: a steroid alcohol found in animal tissues, essential for life. It is a constituent of cell membranes, and is used in the synthesis of steroid hormones – the sex hormones and cortisone – bile salts and vitamin D. It is supplied in the diet, principally in dairy products such as butter and cheese, and is also synthesised in the cells, principally of the liver. It forms some gallstones and is found in the atheromatous patches of arterial disease, and a relationship has been found between high levels of cholesterol in the blood and heart disease, although the precise mechanism remains unclear. It is at present generally agreed that the level of cholesterol in the blood should be below 6.5 mmol/l. High levels of cholesterol are in many instances an inherited characteristic, or they may be associated with thyroid deficiency disease, diabetes or excess intake of alcohol. Reduction of high blood cholesterol involves in the first instance attention to any predisposing condition, and then a diet; those overweight should take a reducing diet and exercise, which in itself will help; otherwise a reduction in the amount of animal fat and dairy products is advisable. Oily fish such as mackerel are particularly useful; more poultry can be eaten, and more bread, cereal, rice, potatoes and pasta to make up for the reduced fat intake. Cooking oil should be vegetable (corn, sunflower or olive). In most cases simple attention to the diet will reduce the blood cholesterol to a reasonable level; in cases which prove refractory there are a number of drugs which can be used.

Choline: a substance found in egg yolk and fat. It plays an important part in the metabolism of fats in the body, and also in the working of the nervous system in the form of acetylcholine. It is sometimes included in the vitamin B complex.

Chondroma: a benign and harmless tumour of cartilage.

Chorea: a condition in which there is incessant involuntary jerky movement involving the whole body, including the limbs, face and tongue. It occurs in a number of diseases of the central nervous system, but when the term is unqualified it refers to one of two conditions: Sydenham's chorea or Huntington's chorea. Thomas Sydenham (1624–89) was an English physician who described chorea associated with rheumatic fever, which affects children suffering from a throat infection with a group A haemolytic streptococcus. It has become relatively rare during the last 50 years. The child becomes restless, irritable and tired; the involuntary movements are first taken for clumsiness, and then recognised for what they are. The face may be affected, so that the child grimaces and sticks its tongue out; the movements of the limbs may be confined to one half of the body. In about one-third of cases the heart is also affected, and this is of great importance, for while the chorea will in a few months recover, the heart may not.

The American physician George Huntington (1850–1916) described in the last century an inherited disease which develops characteristically in middle age, although it may affect children and the aged. The disease shows itself by a progressive dementia, allied to increasing chorea, and deteriorates to its end over about 14 years. Children of a parent with Huntington's chorea have a one in two chance of developing the disease, and their children carry a one in four risk.

Chorion: the outer of the two membranes enclosing the embryo. From it develops the foetal side of the placenta. Occasionally it is the site of abnormal change, which develops at the expense of the foetus into a hydatidiform mole (q.v.). Very rarely there may be a malignant change in the chorion following a hydatidiform mole or even more rarely following a normal pregnancy. The malignant tumour that results is called a chorio-epithelioma or trophoblastoma.

Chorionic Villus Sampling: a small portion of the placenta including the foetal chorion is removed by aspiration through the cervix of the uterus or, increasingly, through the abdominal wall under ultrasonic guidance. The maternal tissue is removed, and the foetal tissue subjected to DNA and chromosome analysis. It can also be cultured for biochemical investigation. The sampling is carried out between the eighth and the tenth week of pregnancy; it carries a very small risk of miscarriage, slightly higher than that of amniocentesis, and is used in prenatal diagnosis of genetic diseases or malformations.

Choroid: *(1)* The middle pigmented and vascular coat of the eye (q.v.). *(2)* Choroid plexus of blood vessels, three of which lie in the brain, one in each lateral ventricle and one in the third ventricle. They secrete the cerebrospinal fluid.

Christmas Disease: a blood disease similar to haemophilia in which the power of coagulation is impaired and bleeding readily occurs. Like haemophilia, it is inherited. Named after the surname of the first case investigated in England, it can only be distinguished from classical haemophilia in the laboratory, and is sometimes called haemophilia B. The missing factor in the blood of classical haemophilia is factor VIII; in Christmas disease factor IX is absent.

Chromium: used widely in industry, chromium and its salts can produce dermatitis. Long-term exposure can result in the formation of indolent ulcers which may penetrate deeply into the skin and underlying tissues. Calcium edetate ointment 10% is used in treatment. In the chromate-producing industry there is an increased incidence of carcinoma of the lung.

Chromosomes: threadlike structures made of protein and deoxyribonucleic acid which are found in pairs in the cell nucleus. Each species has a characteristic number of chromosomes; man has 46, or 23 pairs. The spermatozoa and the ova have half that number, one member of each pair. Chromosomes carry segments of DNA called genes, which control the inherited characteristics of the organism. *See* Cell, Heredity.

Chrysotherapy: treatment with gold, used in rheumatic disease in the form of sodium aurothiomalate for injection or auranofin by mouth.

Chyle: the contents of the chief lymph vessel, the thoracic duct, which carries an emulsion of fat absorbed from the intestines by the lymph vessels of the intestinal wall, the lacteals, to the jugular vein in the neck.

Chyme: the contents of the stomach – partly digested food.

Cicatrix: a scar.

Cilia: the hairs growing on the eyelid: the eyelashes. Also the small processes like eyelashes which are present on the outer surface of certain cells, which by an undulating action sweep matter along passages in the body, for example the air passages in the lungs.

Cimetidine: the effects of histamine in the body are mediated by two sorts of receptors, H_1 and H_2. Histamine receptors in the gut, lungs and blood vessels which are blocked by antihistamine drugs (q.v.) are of the H_1 type; those in the stomach, which are responsible for the secretion of acid and pepsin, are H_2, and are unaffected by antihistamines. They are however blocked by cimetidine and the similar drug ranitidine, which, by decreasing the secretion of acid, heal peptic ulcers (q.v.).

Cinchona: a genus of trees growing in South America, in the bark of which is present the quinoline alkaloids; quinine is still used in the treatment of malaria, and quinidine has an action on abnormal rhythms of the heart. Cinchona bark was known as Jesuit's bark, for it was the Spanish priests who observed its use against malaria by the native people during the Spanish invasion of Central and South America. It is said to have been brought to Europe from the New World in 1640 by the wife of the Viceroy of Peru, the Countess of Cinchon, from whom it derives its name.

Circulation of the Blood: the fact that the blood circulates through the body was demonstrated by the English physician William Harvey (1578–1657). He did not, however, understand how the blood flows from the arteries into the veins, and assumed that it must percolate through 'pores' in the flesh. This gap in knowledge was filled 30 years later by Marcello Malpighi (1628–94) of Italy who, with the new microscope, was able to find the minute capillary vessels which join the arterial and venous systems.

The course of the blood through the body is as follows: arterial blood comes from the lungs into the left side of the heart, enters the left atrium, and is pumped by the contraction of the atrium through the mitral valve into the left ventricle. The left ventricle contracts, the mitral valve closes, and the blood, which cannot run back into the atrium, is pumped through the aortic valve into the aorta, the great artery of the body. The arterial system branches into many separate arteries, and the blood is carried to all parts of the body. The arteries branch into smaller arterioles, which in turn branch into many capillaries. These are very small indeed – much smaller than the hairs after which they are named – and in them the bright arterial blood gives up its oxygen to the tissues, receiving in return waste products and carbon dioxide and becoming dark venous blood. This is carried back to the heart through the venous system, which includes a special arrangement (the portal system) by which blood from the intestines, carrying the products of digestion, goes to the liver through which it passes before joining the venous blood from the rest of the body. The dark venous blood, exhausted of oxygen, passes through the superior and inferior venae cavae to reach the right side of the heart. Entering the right atrium, the blood is pumped through the tricuspid valve into the right ventricle; from the right ventricle it is pumped through the pulmonary valve into the pulmonary artery, and so into the lungs. Here the vessels branch again into many progressively smaller channels until in the capillaries the venous blood is only separated from the air in the alveoli – the air sacs – by an extremely thin membrane. The blood exchanges gases with the air, and leaves the lungs full of oxygen, to flow into the left side of the heart and to begin circulating through the arterial system again.

Circumcision: the removal of the foreskin of the penis, possibly the oldest surgical operation. There are few medical indications for such an operation, but it is a religious rite of great antiquity. It is found in many parts of the world, and was practised among others by the ancient Egyptians, the Coptic branch of the Christian religion which copied it from the Egyptians, the primitive Arabs and the Aztecs of South America; it is obligatory among Moslems, Jews and the aborigines of Australia. Its religious significance is not clear, but presumably it was both a form of sacrifice and a distinctive tribal mark. Female circumcision, involving the removal of the larger part of the external genitals, is still practised by a few primitive peoples; unlike male circumcision, which is a trivial procedure medically, this is a cruel, barbaric and dangerous rite.

Cirrhosis: the development of fibrous tissue in an organ with consequent scarring, hardening and loss of function. The term is commonly used to mean cirrhosis of the liver, otherwise called 'hobnail liver'. There are a number of causes for this condition, but pre-eminent is chronic alcoholism. Chronic hepatitis B, or non-A, non-B hepatitis, account for a number of cases, as do gallstones and cholangitis, certain metabolic diseases, and chronic right heart failure. The condition develops over a long time, and the causative factor must act continuously or intermittently for cirrhosis to ensue. The patient feels ill, becomes easily tired, is nauseated, loses appetite and weight, the abdomen feels bloated and there may be pain. Jaundice is common. The skin shows changes; there may be spider naevi (small collections of dilated blood vessels) over the upper part of the chest, and redness of the hands except in the palms. There may be swelling of the ankles. The outlook is grave, but much improved in alcoholics if they stop drinking. Treatment of the causal disease in other cases may be possible.

Claudication: limping, from a Latin word – the Emperor

Claudius was a cripple. Intermittent claudication is a condition in which poor circulation of blood in the legs leads to the development of a cramping pain when the patient walks a certain distance; the pain wears off at rest, but recurs when the patient has walked the same distance again.

Claustrophobia: an irrational fear of enclosed spaces. It may be a symptom of neurosis, but many otherwise normal people have this feeling from time to time.

Clavicle: the collar-bone, so called from its fancied resemblance to an ancient key. *See* Collar-bone.

Claw Hand: a condition of the hand following paralysis of the ulnar nerve; the wrist is flexed, the knuckles extended and the fingers flexed. Also called 'main en griffe'.

Cleft Palate: the nose, upper lip and palate are formed in the embryo by three separate blocks of tissue. Growing downwards from the region of the forehead is the fronto-nasal process, and growing forwards towards the midline from each side are the right and left maxillary processes. The fronto-nasal process forms the middle of the upper lip, the nose and forehead, and the very front part of the hard palate. The two maxillary processes form the cheeks, the two sides of the upper lip, and the rest of the hard and soft palate. If development is abnormal the following deformities may ensue:

1. Cleft face, where the maxillary process fails to unite with the fronto-nasal process. There is a cleft in the face running from the inner angle of the eye to the side of the mouth.
2. Bilateral or unilateral cleft lip, or hare lip; here one or both maxillary processes have failed to fuse with the fronto-nasal process below the nose, so that the outer part of the lip is separated from the middle part.
3. If the two parts of the maxillary processes that grow in towards each other to form the roof of the mouth fail to meet and join, a cleft palate is the result; the defect may be in the hard or soft palate. If the failure extends to include failure of fusion with the fronto-nasal process, there is a complete cleft palate and a hare lip on one

or both sides. The treatment is by plastic surgery.

Climacteric: *see* Menopause.

Clostridium: a genus of bacilli found in the soil; they live without oxygen, and form spores – inactive forms which lie dormant and can survive conditions which would kill the active organisms. Under the right circumstances they can be very dangerous, for the genus includes the organisms of tetanus, botulism and gas gangrene.

Clotting: *see* Coagulation of the Blood.

Cloxacillin: an antibiotic effective against penicillin-resistant staphylococci. Neither cloxacillin nor flucloxacillin are affected by the enzyme penicillinase, produced by penicillin-resistant organisms to destroy penicillin. These antibiotics are therefore reserved for use against such organisms; but strains of *Staphylococcus aureus* have started to appear that are resistant to cloxacillin.

Clubbing: in certain conditions which interfere with respiration, notably chronic diseases of the lungs and heart disease, the soft tissues over the ends of the fingers are the site of tissue overgrowth, so that the ends of the fingers become club-shaped, with the root of the nail lifted in a characteristic way.

Club-foot (talipes): a deformity of the ankle and foot which renders the patient unable to stand with the sole of the foot flat on the ground. It is congenital, rarely being acquired through nervous or muscular disease such as poliomyelitis or scarring after severe injury. It is classified by description of the deformity. In talipes equinus, the heel is pulled up so that the patient walks on the toes like a horse; in talipes calcaneus, the toes are pulled up so that the heel is on the ground; in talipes varus, the sole of the foot is turned inwards, and in talipes valgus the sole of the foot is pulled outwards. Combinations of these basic varieties are usually present, and the commonest are talipes equino-varus in which the toes are on the ground and the foot is twisted inwards, and talipes calcaneo-valgus where the heel is on the ground and the foot is twisted outwards. Treatment is a matter for the orthopaedic surgeon and the physiotherapist.

Clyster: an archaic name for enema. The phrase was to 'throw up a clyster'.

Coagulation of the Blood: a very complicated process. Essentially, a substance circulating in the blood called fibrinogen is converted into an insoluble substance, fibrin, which forms the framework of the clot. So far 13 factors necessary for the production of a clot have been identified, and if all of them function properly a circulating substance, prothrombin, is changed by tissue juice liberated by injury, or by platelets adhering to an injured surface, into thrombin, which acts on fibrinogen to produce fibrin. Calcium is necessary for the process to be successful. Platelets play a large part in the formation of a clot, for they collect at the site of an injury to a blood vessel wall and form a plug to stop minor leaks, as well as liberating substances necessary for the formation of the clot. It is clear that once a clot begins to form something must keep it within bounds, or else it might spread to fill the whole of the vascular system; and in fact there is a substance in the blood called antithrombin, which binds to thrombin and neutralises it. There is also a substance called plasminogen, which in the presence of damage to blood vessels is changed to plasmin, an enzyme that breaks up fibrin. As soon as a clot begins to form because of damage to a blood vessel it is attacked by plasmin produced by the same injury and kept under control; during the course of a day many small reactions of this sort must occur in the body. In such a complicated mechanism there is room for many accidents and deficiencies, and there are a number of conditions in which the abnormalities produce symptoms. The best known disease affecting the coagulation of the blood is haemophilia (q.v.).

Coarctation: abnormal narrowing forming a constriction. Coarctation of the aorta is a congenital abnormality of the aorta cutting down the blood supply to the lower part of the body, and increasing the blood pressure in the head, neck and arms. The treatment is surgical refashioning of the aorta.

Cobalt 60: radioactive isotope used in the treatment of malignant tumours by radiotherapy, following a technique developed in Canada in 1951.

Cocaine: an alkaloid derived from the leaves of the South American shrub *Erythroxelon coca*. It stimulates the central nervous system and induces feelings of alertness, euphoria and lack of fatigue. An overdose produces symptoms of poisoning – confusion, excitement, headache, fever, rapid pulse, irregular respiration, sweating, collapse and sometimes convulsions. Cocaine is a local anaesthetic; applied to mucous membranes it causes constriction of the blood vessels. It has virtually no use in medicine now, but has become notorious as a drug of addiction, together with its derivative 'crack' (q.v.). It is used by sniffing up the nose, or injecting a solution into the veins. Smoking cocaine powder is relatively ineffective. It may be taken in combination with other drugs such as heroin.

The cocaine addict is anxious, thin, depressed and irritable, and often impotent; the pupils of the eyes may be dilated. There is narrowing of the coronary arteries, leading to acute or chronic damage to the heart muscle, narrowing of the arteries of the brain, and loss of reasonable behaviour. Sometimes there are hallucinations, visual and auditory, and a feeling of insects crawling beneath the skin (the 'cocaine bug'). Following a dose of cocaine the addict appears to become cheerful, witty and inexhaustible, but the exhilaration is soon followed by depression. Dementia may follow the chronic use of cocaine, which is the most self-reinforcing drug known. Because cocaine constricts blood vessels, the blood supply to the placenta is reduced in regular users of the drug who are pregnant; this leads to abortion, stillbirth, prematurity and a stunted baby. Effects of cocaine on the heart and brain may last for 10 days after withdrawal of the drug, which may be very difficult to achieve even after a limited exposure. Antidepressive drugs such as imipramine and desipramine have been found useful, and research is continuing into the use of bromocriptine, which, it is hoped, may reduce the addict's craving for cocaine.

Coccus: bacterium shaped like a sphere, arranged in various groups, the staphylococcus in bunches like grapes, the streptoccus in chains, the diplococcus in pairs. Many varieties are the source of disease.

Coccydynia: severe pain in the region of the coccyx, the small bone at the lower end of the spinal column. It follows injury to the coccyx by a kick, a fall on the bottom, or sometimes in childbirth, and the discomfort is very hard to treat successfully, sometimes lasting for months.

Cochlea: part of the inner ear, and shaped like a snail shell, the cochlea contains the organ of Corti, the essential organ of hearing, in which the sound waves transmitted through the ear-drum and the small bones of the middle ear are transformed into impulses in the auditory nerve. The cochlea has $2\frac{3}{4}$ turns and lies in the petrous temporal bone.

Codeine: or methyl morphine, has the same formula as morphine with the addition of a methyl group; it is one of the opium alkaloids, but from its action one would not recognise it as so nearly related to morphine. It has an action in relieving pain, but it is not very powerful and certainly not suitable for serious pain. It has in addition a useful constipating action, and an action on the coughing centre, and is consequently used in cases of diarrhoea and in cough mixtures. It is not suitable for continuous use, as both tolerance and a measure of dependence may develop.

Cod Liver Oil: a rich if nauseating source of vitamins A and D which can be given to infants to ward off the possibility of rickets. The smaller the children the less they appear to dislike the taste. It is possible to give too much vitamin D, and the dose of cod liver oil emulsion should not exceed 5 ml a day (about 2.5 ml cod liver oil).

Coeliac Disease: a condition found in childhood in which the small intestine is unable to absorb food properly. It is due to sensitivity to gluten, a protein found in wheat and other grain. After the addition of cereals to the diet of an infant between six and nine months old, the child, previously healthy, begins to lose weight, becomes irritable and passes large pale offensive motions. After a time the abdomen begins to protrude, the limbs waste and the child may even develop the deficiency diseases anaemia and rickets. If, however, all food containing gluten is avoided the child will quickly recover. Special flour without gluten is on the market, and gluten-free bread can be bought already baked. Our understanding of this condition is a case of good coming out of evil, for during the Second World War the Dutch physicians H.A. Weijers (1914–72) and J.H. van der Kamer noticed that children suffering from coeliac disease improved when bread became unobtainable, and from this observation the truth about the malady emerged.

Coil: a type of intrauterine contraceptive device.

Colchicine: *Colchicum autumnale*, the meadow saffron or autumn crocus, yields from its bulb the alkaloid colchicine, which is an ancient remedy against gout. The drawback is that in effective doses it may well produce nausea, vomiting and diarrhoea, with abdominal pain.

Cold: the common cold, otherwise called acute rhinitis or acute coryza, is a virus infection of the upper respiratory tract. Any one of about 10 or 11 viruses can be involved, each of which have numerous strains which are pathogenic; the commonest are the rhinoviruses, the second most common the cornaviruses. The infection usually occurs in winter or autumn, more often in children than adults. It begins with an irritation in the nose, with sneezing; the nose begins to run, the patient may feel ill and shiver, and there is an unproductive cough. The throat feels sore, and the eyes may be red. Cold sores may break out on the lips. If the swelling in the nose is bad enough it may block drainage from the sinuses and produce pain in the face, or may block the Eustachian tube and lead to discomfort in the ear and mild deafness. In an uncomplicated case recovery takes the inside of a week, but it may leave sinusitis or ear infection. No treatment is possible beyond aspirin or paracetamol; a solution of soluble aspirin in water may be used as a gargle to ease a sore throat, and the inhalation of steam with or without menthol may help. Antibiotics are of no value except where there is secondary infection. A cold is infectious for about 24 hours before the symptoms appear, and for 4 or 5 days afterwards. The incubation period is between 1 and 4 days, and the infection is spread by droplets of infected material in the air. Immunisation is not possible because of the number of different strains of the viruses involved; the rhinovirus has more than 90 different strains, any of which can produce a cold.

Cold Abscess: one which develops slowly, with little reaction of inflammation and hardly any redness or heat in the surrounding tissues. Usually due to tuberculosis.

Colectomy: the removal of part of the colon or large intestine (partial colectomy), half of the colon (hemicolectomy) or the whole of the colon (total colectomy). The operations may be performed for the removal of tumours or the radical cure of ulcerative colitis (q.v.).

Colic: characteristic pain felt in the abdomen as the result of spasm of the smooth muscle surrounding one of the hollow tubular structures – intestines, ureters and bile ducts. This may be produced by a blockage such as a stone, when the muscle contracts to expel it but cannot, or when the lining of the gut is irritated by infection or toxic food. The pain of colic is intermittent, coming on suddenly and rising to a peak and then dying away to leave an ache. The spasms may come at irregular intervals and be of great intensity The pain is reduced by atropine and hyoscine, which relax smooth muscle

Colitis: *see* Ulcerative Colitis.

Collagen Diseases: a group of diseases affecting the collagen fibres which help to make up the fibrous supporting tissues of the body. These diseases may affect the heart, joints and subcutaneous connective tissue and are: polyarteritis nodosa, rheumatic fever, rheumatoid arthritis, lupus erythematosus, scleroderma, dermatomyositis and others. The cause of this group of diseases is poorly understood.

Collapse Therapy: at one time tuberculosis of the lungs

was treated by collapsing the lung so that the diseased area was at rest. The introduction of drugs effective against tuberculosis has entirely changed the pattern of treatment so that collapse therapy has fallen into disuse, and artificial pneumothorax, the most common method of collapsing the lung, is hardly ever performed.

Collar-bone: the clavicle, which keeps the shoulder propped out away from the rib cage, runs from the upper part of the breastbone, the sternum, to the outer part of the shoulder-blade, the scapula. It is often fractured, usually by a fall onto the shoulder or the outstretched hand, and usually at the junction of the middle and outer thirds. Immediate treatment is to tie a bandage round the wrist and then round the neck so that the wrist is kept as near to the neck as possible. A figure of eight bandage, passing round each shoulder and crossing over the back, may be used to keep the shoulders braced back and the bone ends in good position, or the arm may be carried in a sling. The fracture heals well in about three weeks in the majority of cases.

Colles' Fracture: a common type of fracture of the wrist often caused by falling on the outstretched hand. The radius, the outer bone of the forearm, is broken about 2 cm above the wrist joint, and the fragment is pushed backwards. The fracture is recognised by its appearance which is described as a 'dinner fork' deformity. When the fracture has been reduced, the forearm and wrist are enclosed in a light plaster cast with the fingers free to move. It is important to be on guard against the shoulder becoming stiff while the forearm is out of action, for once a shoulder becomes stiff it is very difficult to get it moving properly again. (Abraham Colles, Irish surgeon 1773–1843)

Collodion: a clear solution of pyroxylin in ether and alcohol (pyroxylin is the product of the action of sulphuric and nitric acids on cotton). The addition of castor oil makes flexible collodion, which can be used as a covering for minor cuts and wounds.

Colloids: literally, substances like glue. A colloid system

149

consists of a dispersion medium in which matter larger than an atom or molecule, called the disperse phase, is distributed. In suspension colloids, the disperse phase is composed of insoluble matter, for example metal, and the dispersion medium is gas, liquid or solid; in emulsion colloids the dispersion medium is liquid, usually water, and the disperse phase complicated organic matter such as starch or albumin.

Colon: the main part of the large intestine. Starting in the right iliac fossa, the right lower part of the abdominal cavity, where the small intestine joins the caecum at the ileo-caecal junction, the ascending colon passes upwards to turn and travel to the left across the upper part of the abdominal cavity as the transverse colon. It bends downwards on the left of the abdomen in front of the spleen to become the descending colon, and after forming a loop in the pelvis called the sigmoid colon it joins the rectum.

Colostomy: a loop of colon is brought up to the abdominal wall, to which it is secured, and an opening made to the surface. The intestinal contents are collected in a special receptacle. A colostomy is used when there is an obstruction to the large intestine, or when a portion of it is removed. It may be temporary or permanent, but if it has to be permanent there is no reason why it should be more than a minor nuisance. The practical difficulty is in regulating the bowel movements, for the patient has no control over them; but methods have been worked out to overcome this handicap, for the number and timing of the motions is fundamentally controlled by the food the patient eats, and can be regulated by a suitable diet. A colostomy does not prevent a patient from leading a substantially normal life.

Colostrum: a clear yellow fluid produced by the breast in the first two or three days after childbirth. It is rich in proteins and contains many antibodies.

Colour Blindness: the theory of colour vision depends on the fact that any colour in the spectrum can be matched by a mixture of three pure spectral colours of variable intensity but fixed wavelength. If this is so, then the presence of three pigments in the eye will enable it to carry out the matching of any colour in the spectrum. The visual pigment rhodopsin, visual purple, has been identified in the rods of the retina, and its function is to do with the recognition of light, which bleaches it. It plays no part in colour vision; research has therefore been concentrated on finding three further pigments in the cones of the retina (*see* Eye). There are indications that such pigments are there, but the mechanism of colour vision is still far from clear. However, theory based on the hypothetical normal presence of three pigments accounts for the types of colour blindness found in the general population. Colour blindness is quite common, commoner in men than in women. It is found in about 8% of all men and 0.4% of women, and is inherited. Complete absence of colour vision resulting from absence of cones in the retina is very rare, but has been reported. Colour blindness that would result from the absence of two pigments and the presence of one is extremely rare. Absence of one pigment leading to dichromatic vision – perception only of green and red, or more commonly blue and yellow – exists, but most common is the condition of anomalous trichromatopsia, where all three pigments are present but of an intensity different from normal. Anomalous trichromats see all the colours but have difficulty in distinguishing between red, green and yellow, or blue, green and yellow. The first is the red–green type of colour blindness, the second the blue–yellow type. Most colour-blind people are ignorant of their abnormality until it is demonstrated by special tests (Ishihara test), but there are some situations in which it may be important to be able to distinguish special colours quickly so that for some jobs perfect colour vision is essential.

Colporrhaphy: a surgical operation to repair prolapse of the vaginal wall.

Coma: a state of deep unconsciousness in which even the reflexes are lost, for example the eyeball can be touched without making the patient blink. There is no response to the most painful stimuli; the patient cannot be roused.

Community Medicine: the responsibilities of the Community Health Physician include 'medical administration, environmental health, preventive medicine in the Community and epidemiology. . . .the Community Physician has a unique role in the planning of comprehensive health care for the community as a whole' (Merrison Report, 1979). A new specialty, with wider scope than the old Local Health Authority Medical Officer of Health, it came into being with the reorganisation of the NHS in 1974.

Comminuted: broken into pieces; used to describe fractures where the bone is in fragments.

Compensation Syndrome: some patients injured in accidents for which financial compensation may be received may make a recovery which is slower than usual, or even produce symptoms which are not strictly referable to their injury. It is often found after head injuries, when the patient for example may develop a headache which will not respond to treatment, or after injuries to the back which lead to continuing discomfort. The syndrome is very difficult to deal with; it will not improve until litigation is complete, and unfortunately it is not uncommon for it to persist after compensation has been settled.

Compositor's Disease: lead-poisoning found in those who handle lead type.

Computerised Axial Tomography: usually abbreviated to CT, or CAT (q.v.).

Conchae: the bony plates covered with mucous membrane which project from the lateral walls of the nasal cavity. There are three conchae on each side, superior, medial and inferior, and they are called conchae from their resemblance to shells. They are also known as the turbinate bones.

Concussion: a violent shock, produced for example by an explosion or a heavy blow, and by extension the state produced by such a blow especially on the head. In this sense, concussion means a loss of consciousness, partial or complete, which recovers after a limited period, usually within 24 hours. Any severe blow on the head accelerates the brain in relation to the skull, for the brain floats in the cerebrospinal fluid within the skull; the brain undergoes shear, or twisting, forces and also comes into contact with the skull, especially with the floor of the skull in the frontal and temporal regions where the bone is irregular. The shear forces cause damage to a greater or lesser degree to the substance of the brain, and contact with the skull bruises the the surface of the brain, the cortex. The result, if the force applied is great enough, is a loss of consciousness; the higher centres become inactive, although the lower brain centres essential to life continue to function. It is probable that the injuries to the brain in concussion differ in degree rather than kind from the more severe injuries that lead to coma, a more profound and longer-lasting loss of consciousness. Patients suffering from concussion need attention first to the maintenance of an adequate airway; when that is established it is important to make sure that there are no signs of other injuries, and until that has been done they should not be moved. If possible they should not be moved without skilled help. It is important that patients who have lost consciousness should be admitted to hospital for observation, for although an uncomplicated case of concussion will regain consciousness within 24 hours, and be none the worse for it, in some cases there are dangerous sequels which develop in the hours following the injury (*see* Head Injury). After recovery from concussion there is usually a period of retrograde amnesia (*see* Amnesia).

Condyloma: a large warty accumulation of tissue near the anus or vulva, found in secondary syphilis (*condyloma latum*) or in infection by a sexually transmitted virus (*condyloma acuminatum*).

Congenital: a word meaning 'present at birth', which has become erroneously almost synonymous with 'hereditary', which means a condition handed on from parents to offspring in the germ cells. Hereditary diseases are congenital; congenital diseases are not necessarily hereditary.

Congenital Dislocation of the Hip: a deformity resulting from developmental abnormality, which if untreated prevents the child from walking properly. It is recognised by routine examination of infants, and treated by special splints.

Conjunctiva: the thin translucent membrane covering the exposed portion of the eyeball.

Conjunctivitis: inflammation of the conjunctiva, which becomes red and sometimes so swollen that it protrudes over the eyelids. The eyes itch and become painful; rubbing them makes the condition worse. It can be caused by a variety of agents, from infective organisms to irritation from chemicals or ultraviolet light (arc eye). Allergic conjunctivitis is common in hay fever. Infection may be caused by bacteria or viruses; treatment for bacterial infection is by eye-drops or ointment, usually containing chloramphenicol or gentamicin. The use of eye ointment, especially at night, prevents the eyelids sticking together. Infection by the herpes virus is treated with acyclovir or idoxuridine drops; allergic conjunctivitis by sodium cromoglycate eye-drops. For the conjunctivitis of trachoma the treatment is tetracycline eye ointment together with sulphonamides or erythromycin by mouth. Chemicals splashed into the eye must be washed out with sodium chloride eye lotion or, in an emergency, tap water from the mains. Arc eye is usually caused by welders omitting to use their goggles and looking directly at the welding arc; it is painful, and may need the use of dark glasses and chloramphenicol or similar eye-drops to prevent secondary infection. Infective conjunctivitis is spread by touching infected objects and touching the eyes, so that an infected child can spread the infection on towels, face-flannels, or by bodily contact, and the spread of an infection is often fast. The sticky eyes of infants may be due to chlamydial infection from the mother, in which case tetracycline drops or ointment should be used, or occasionally may be due to staphylococcal or even gonococcal infections which respond to antibiotics.

Constipation: infrequent or absent movement of the bowels. This may be due to disease, causing complete or partial blockage of the intestine, or to a variety of other causes. In the case of obstructive disease the diagnosis becomes clear, and treatment is surgical. Constipation in infants is often due to lack of sufficient fluid, allowing the motions to become hard and difficult to pass, especially in hot weather; milk-fed infants need water as well as milk, perhaps four or five times during the day. It may be due to pain arising from a fissure-in-ano, but this can be detected by a gentle examination of the anus and treated. The addition of a little sugar to milk feeds will often ease constipation, or after weaning the amount of vegetable and fruit in the diet can be increased. In older children the habit of voiding the bowels at a set time after a meal, usually breakfast, must be encouraged; for it is the neglect of this habit which leads to the majority of cases of constipation in later life. Although it is not necessary to have a bowel movement every day, the impression fostered by the makers of laxatives that it is so has led to widespread unnecessary use of such medicines. It is far more important that a regular habit should be formed at whatever intervals suit each individual. Diet obviously plays a part in the regulation of the bowels, but not a very great part. Nevertheless if a regular bowel habit is lost, it is often possible to restore it by taking a 'bulking' agent such as unprocessed bran or methyl cellulose granules; stimulant laxatives, for example senna, may be used, but only to try to restore a regular habit. Osmotic laxatives, which act by keeping fluid within the bowel by osmotic action, should be reserved for occasional use; they include magnesium sulphate and lactulose, and require a good fluid intake while they are being used. Not a few cases will improve considerably by taking more water daily without the salts. In old age decreased muscle tone and inactivity may result in constipation with, in some cases, diarrhoea set up by a hard impacted mass of faeces. Here treatment is, if possible, prevention by the use of bulking agents, an adequate intake of fluids, osmotic or mild stimulant laxatives, or even regular enemas. If the condition has gone too far, manual removal of the faeces may be necessary. It must not be forgotten that the use of analgesics containing codeine (methyl morphine) has a constipating action, as does morphine itself and other related drugs.

Contact Lens: lenses can be worn on the eyeball to cover the cornea, with various advantages; they are nearly invisible, so that people who do not like to be seen wearing glasses can use them; they do not steam up; they can be worn to play quite violent games; and in certain disturbances of vision they give better results than ordinary lenses. On the other hand, some people cannot tolerate them as they prove too irritating and uncomfortable, and they find the process of inserting and removing them unpleasant. They are not suitable for all visual defects. The choice of contact lenses must be made with the help of an expert. Contact lenses may be used under specialist supervision for the treatment of disease of the cornea; visual improvement is then a secondary consideration.

Contraception: artificial prevention of pregnancy following copulation. There are six main methods: the use of spermicidal chemicals in the form of creams, pessaries, jellies or foam; the use of mechanical occlusive devices such as a rubber sheath for the man or a rubber diaphragm for the woman; the use of permanent intrauterine devices; the use of sex hormones taken by mouth to suppress ovulation; the use of 'natural' methods such as coitus interruptus and the 'safe period'; and sterilisation of the man or woman. The first of these methods should be combined with the second to give maximum protection. The diaphragm should be fitted at a birth control clinic. The third, an intrauterine device (IUCD), takes various forms, and can be fitted at the birth control clinic or by a doctor skilled in such matters. Although the precise action is obscure, it is a very effective method and the only common reason for its failure is that the device has been expelled without its absence being noticed. The doctor who fits the device will explain how to check that it is in place. The disadvantage of the IUCD is that it may produce increased menstrual bleeding, and it is less suitable for women who have not borne children because there is a risk of pelvic infection and consequent infertility.

The most popular and the easiest method is that of taking synthetic hormones to prevent ovulation, and it is very effective. The most widely prescribed is the combined pill containing an oestrogen and progestogen, which is taken for three weeks out of every four. The amounts of the hormones needed are the least that will control the cycle best and produce the least unwanted effects, such as headache, nausea and tenderness of the breasts, and vary from patient to patient, so that prescriptions must be written on an individual basis. There are a large number of preparations available. The beneficial effects of the combined hormone pill are that it is very efficient if taken regularly, it improves such menstrual disorders as dysmenorrhoea and menorrhagia, it suppresses the formation of ovarian cysts and benign cysts in the breast, and it appears to reduce the likelihood of cancer of the ovary or the body of the uterus. Against that must be set the increased risk of thrombosis of the veins, and possibly strokes and heart attacks. There have been reports in the past suggesting that there is an increased risk of cancer of the breast, but this is far from certain; however, research continues in the matter. Taking the contraceptive pill does not produce subsequent infertility, although pregnancy may not follow at once after stopping the pill. It is often advised that women over 35, especially those who smoke, should not continue to take the contraceptive pill, but should adopt an alternative method of birth control.

It is possible to use the combined hormonal pill for contraception after unprotected intercourse; in such a case two pills containing 250 µg levonorgestrel and 50 µg ethinyloestradiol should be taken within 72 hours, followed by another two after 12 hours; this may give rise to nausea and vomiting. Medical follow-up is necessary. It should be noted that some drugs interfere with the efficiency of the contraceptive pill: the most commonly encountered are the antibiotics ampicillin and tetracycline and the anti-fungal drug griseofulvin but there are others.

Methods of contraception being developed include combined depot injections, hormone-releasing intrauterine devices, the use of immunisation, and drugs to prevent spermatogenesis in the male. The 'natural' methods of coitus interruptus and the so-called safe period are mentioned only to be condemned.

Convulsions: spasmodic involuntary muscular contractions, such as occur in epilepsy (q.v.). They may occur in young children as the result of a high temperature; if this does happen while waiting for the doctor, parents should make sure that the child's airway is clear, and take measures to reduce the temperature such as opening the window, taking the bedclothes off, and sponging the child with tepid water. The occurrence of such convulsions does not mean that the child is epileptic.

Corn: a small localised thickening of the skin of the foot which is painful. Larger areas of thickening are called callosities, and are usually protective; but the corn, commonly produced by friction from badly fitting shoes, is most uncomfortable and is best treated by the chiropodist. Verrucas, small painful warts on the sole of the foot, may be mistaken for corns.

Cornea: the transparent part of the eyeball which lies over the pupil and iris, through which we see. If it becomes scarred by injury or disease, vision is disturbed or lost, although the eye may be otherwise intact. It is possible to graft part of another individual's cornea into the defect left after cutting out the scar, for the cornea has very little blood supply and therefore immunological reactions leading to rejection of the graft are weak or absent. The graft can be taken from an eye removed at operation for another reason or from a dead body within six hours of death. As long as the eye is taken with full aseptic precautions, the cornea can be stored in a 'bank' until it is needed. It is possible to leave one's eyes for use in this way, but strictly speaking this is no more than a wish and if a surviving relative or the person who is legally in charge of the body objects the eyes will not be used. Age is no bar: the eyes of an old person are entirely suitable for corneal grafting. With modern tissue-typing techniques a satisfactory result is achieved in some 75% of cases.

The cornea is concerned in the refraction and focusing of light in the eye, and alteration of its curvature alters the depth of focus in short and long sight. It has been found possible to correct these abnormalities of vision by using laser light to modify the shape of the cornea, but the technique is not yet in general use, and the risks of the operation have to be put against the simplicity of correcting the vision by glasses.

Coronary Arteries: arteries supplying the heart muscle. There are two main arteries, right and left, which take origin from the aorta as it leaves the heart. The left divides into an anterior interventricular branch which, as its name suggests, passes downwards between the ventricles to the apex of the heart, and a left circumflex branch which runs round between the left atrium and ventricle and then descends on the rearward surface of the heart. The right coronary artery runs round between the right atrium and ventricle and supplies the right ventricle and the sinu-atrial node, the pacemaker of the heart. The branches of the coronary arteries form limited anastomoses, which are of practical importance in that the freer the anastomotic flow the less likely it is for a blockage in a branch to produce symptoms by starving a portion of the heart muscle of blood.

Coronary Artery Disease: the coronary arteries of the heart may be affected by arteriosclerosis (*see* Arterial Disease) which narrows the interior of the arteries and so decreases the flow of blood. The commonest site is the first part of the descending branch of the left coronary artery, the next most common the first part of the right coronary artery, and in about a quarter of the cases the first part of the left circumflex branch is affected. A block sufficient to cause the supply of oxygen to the heart muscle to fall short of the demand will provoke pain, as will spasm of the diseased artery. This pain is brought on by exercise, and is felt in the chest, the throat, the left arm, and even the back, and is called angina (q.v.). The state of the coronary arteries is investigated by electrocardiography, the record of the electrical changes set up by the contractions of the heart muscle, by echocardiography using ultrasound, and by angiography, X-ray examination after the introduction of a radio-opaque substance through a catheter introduced through the femoral artery up to the root of the aorta and so to the origins of the coronary arteries. Treatment of coronary insufficiency ranges from the drug treatment of angina to bypass surgery, where a graft of a blood vessel is used to bypass the narrowed part of the coronary artery. The graft is commonly taken from the long saphenous vein of the leg; it is also possible to use an internal mammary artery from the chest wall. The results of bypass surgery are good. It has lately become possible to use a technique called transluminal angioplasty, in which a balloon is fastened to the tip of a catheter which is passed along a fine guide wire introduced as in coronary angiography into the narrowed coronary artery. When the balloon is in position it is inflated and the artery is opened up. *See also* Myocardial Infarct.

Coronary Thrombosis: *see* Myocardial Infarct.

Coroner (in Scotland, Procurator Fiscal): Coroners are appointed by the County Council to enquire into certain deaths occurring in the area. A coroner must be legally or medically qualified, and deaths falling into the following categories must be reported by the Registrar of Births and Deaths:

1. Where the dead person has not been seen by the doctor within 14 days of the death, or after death.
2. Where the cause of death is uncertain or unknown.
3. Where the death is thought to be unnatural, or caused by accident, violence, neglect, poisoning, or abortion, or there are suspicious circumstances.
4. Where death occurred under a general anaesthetic or in the course of an operation.
5. Where the death is thought to have occurred as the result of an industrial disease or poisoning.
6. If the Registrar cannot obtain a medical certificate of death.
7. If, in the case of a reported stillbirth, the Registrar has reason to think that the child was born alive.

The majority of cases are reported to the coroner by the registrar, but some are reported by the doctor, some by the police, and some by the officials of certain places such as prisons who must report deaths in their institutions. A member of the public who thinks that there has been an unnatural or unexplained death should report it to the coroner or the coroner's officer, who is a police officer. The coroner can only take action when he has a report of a death. He may or may not decide to hold an inquest, except in certain cases such as deaths by violence or unnatural causes, or deaths in prison, where it is required by law. It is not necessary for him to summon a jury. In many cases he will order an autopsy to determine the cause of death, and issue a death or cremation certificate without an inquest.

In Scotland, the Procurator Fiscal is a lawyer appointed by the Lord Advocate whose duty it is to prosecute criminal offences. His enquiries are carried out in private, but if he finds that it is necessary he reports to the Crown Office, and the Lord Advocate may order a public enquiry with a jury; this is however not often done, except where there has been a fatal accident in industry. The fiscal does not have to find a medical cause for death, but must satisfy himself with expert medical aid that there has been no negligence or criminal activity involved. In the USA arrangements vary from State to State, but most rely on a Medical Examiner who is a pathologist appointed to enquire into sudden or unexplained deaths, or those which are suspicious or the result of crime.

Corpuscle: a small body or cell, generally used to describe the red blood cells.

Corpus Luteum: the yellow mass of cells that fills the ovarian follicle after the ovum has been shed (*see* Ovary). It produces the hormone progesterone, which prepares the lining of the uterus for the implantation of a fertilised ovum. If implantation does not occur, it degenerates and the prepared lining of the uterus is lost at menstruation; if pregnancy develops, it persists and becomes larger, continuing to secrete hormones.

Cortex: the outer layer of an organ or other structure such as bone, brain, suprarenal body or kidney.

Corticosteroids: aldosterone and cortisol (hydrocortisone), steroid substances of physiological importance formed from cholesterol by the cortex of the adrenal glands. Since their discovery, similarly acting synthetic compounds have been made which are also called corticosteroids. Aldosterone is known as a mineralocorticoid and cortisol as a glucocorticoid from their actions; the first is concerned with the balance of sodium, potassium and fluid in the body, the second with the metabolism of carbohydrates, fat and protein, as well as the maintenance of the blood pressure, the formation of red blood cells, and the strength of muscles. Cortisol has some mineralocorticoid action, but most importantly it reduces the reaction of inflammation and reduces antibody formation. It or its synthetic analogues are therefore used widely in medicine in the treatment of allergic conditions such as asthma, skin reactions, and in immunosuppression for transplant surgery. The action in suppressing the inflammatory reaction is used in the treatment of rheumatoid arthritis, rheumatic fever, ulcerative colitis, sarcoidosis and other diseases.

Possibly the widest use of the corticosteroids is in ointments or creams for the skin, where they relieve non-infective eczematous disorders; they are divided into groups ranging from mild to very potent. While the mild preparations such as hydrocortisone 1% ointment rarely produce unwanted effects, the very potent group has to be used carefully, for not only can they be absorbed into the body but can also lead to changes in the skin itself. A further trouble is that they do not cure the condition, but only suppress the symptoms, so that when they are discontinued the condition may well recur.

As with any powerful drug, corticosteroids taken by mouth can be dangerous, and where possible they are used locally, for example as injections into joints, inhalations into the lungs, and enemas. If it is necessary to give them by mouth the smallest effective dose is used, and as the course is finished it is tapered off slowly. In cases where they have to be given for any length of time, the unwanted effects may include a rise in blood pressure, weakness of the muscles, loss of potassium and retention of sodium with consequent water retention and oedema; in children growth may be retarded, and in older people the bones may become soft (osteoporosis) which may result in collapse of a vertebra. Diabetes is a danger, the face becomes round and swollen, and there are mental changes ranging from over-cheerfulness to paranoia, depression and suicidal tendencies. The body's reactions to infection are altered so that severe disease may escape detection. Prolonged treatment with corticosteroids diminishes the secretion of corticotrophin, the hormone by which the pituitary gland stimulates the secretory activity of the suprarenal glands, so that the natural supply of the essential steroids may be lost, an effect which may last for years. All patients on steroids should carry a card with them to warn doctors of the fact, for in the case of illness or accident the dose may have to be increased, and even when the course has been finished they should be careful to tell doctors they have not seen before that they have been on steroids, particularly if they have to have an operation.

Corticotrophin: the activity of the suprarenal glands depends on a hormone secreted by the pituitary gland at the base of the brain, called ACTH, or adrenocorticotrophic hormone, otherwise known as corticotrophin. Without this the suprarenal glands cannot secrete corticosteroids (*see* above).

Coryza: inflammation of the nasal mucous membrane producing a running nose. *See* Cold.

Cosmetic Surgery: also called aesthetic surgery, is that branch of plastic surgery concerned with restoring to normal an abnormal appearance, and by doing so to treat the psychological distress caused by self-consciousness, which may be considerable and unrelated to the degree of disfigurement.

Cot Death: a tragic occurrence; a baby previously in good health is found suddenly dead for no apparent reason. In some cases a cause can be found, but in others the breathing seems to have stopped for no reason at all. The babies are often between three and four months old, but can be up to a year old. There is an association to help parents who have suffered this terrible loss, and research into the matter continues; it has recently been suggested that one factor is excessive heat, and another sleeping face downwards.

Cough: the air passages are lined with cells which secrete mucus; when they are infected or irritated the secretion of mucus increases and there is an urge to cough. This is a complicated action which may be voluntary or involuntary; the breath is drawn in, the glottis closed, the muscles contract to build up pressure in the chest, and then the glottis is suddenly opened so that there is an explosive discharge of air which sweeps through the air passages carrying with it the excess secretions. The treatment of a cough first depends on the underlying cause which may range from severe respiratory disease to cigarette smoking, but is often part of a minor illness. Cough mixtures abound, but the effects are disappointing. One of the best remedies is the inhalation of steam, with or without a flavouring such as benzoin tincture. A soothing linctus can be made out of honey with lemon juice in water.

Counter-irritants: *see* Blistering.

Cowpox: pox of cows' udders caused by a modified form of the virus responsible for smallpox. *See* Vaccination.

Coxalgia: pain in the hip joint.

Coxa Vara: a deformity of the femur or thigh-bone in which the angle between the neck of the bone and the shaft is decreased. In coxa valga the angle is increased.

Coxsackie Virus: an enterovirus originally isolated from patients in a town in New York State. There are two types, A and B; they can produce upper respiratory infections, muscular pains, Bornholm disease (q.v.), meningitis and encephalitis, and in children skin rashes and hand, foot, and mouth disease, a mild condition in which small ulcers develop in the mouth, with a red, blistering rash on the palms of the hands and the soles of the feet.

'Crack': the popular name for a derivative of cocaine made by dissolving cocaine hydrochloride, the form in which it is exported, in water and heating it with baking soda. The resulting crystals can be smoked; cocaine hydrochloride is ineffective when smoked. The effects of smoking 'crack' are felt very quickly, last for about ten minutes or slightly longer, and are at their height in one to five minutes. There is an intense feeling of well-being, strength and increased mental powers, with resistance to pain and fatigue. As the effects wear off they are succeeded by anxiety and depression.

Frequent use brings hallucinations with after-feelings of persecution and even suicidal inclinations. There may be fits. Although the habit is said to be dangerously addictive, only less than half of those who try the drug are inclined to continue with it, but those who do may take to crime to obtain money to pay for the drug. *See* Cocaine, Addiction.

Cramp: the painful involuntary contraction of a muscle; when it occurs in the smooth muscle of the internal organs it is described as colic (q.v.). It can be caused by exercise when the blood supply to a muscle is insufficient because of disease, as in intermittent claudication (q.v.); or in swimmers when the body is cold and exhausted, a state which may be compounded by a minor injury to a muscle such as torn fibres which cause the muscle to contract uncontrollably. Similar trouble can overtake athletes, particularly when training has not been sufficient. Loss of salt from the body in excessive sweating because of hot surroundings may lead to cramps, as may diseases such as cholera in which there is a loss of salt and in such cases replacement of the lost salt is necessary. Cramps sometimes attack the elderly in the night, and may be relieved by taking quinine before sleep. An attack of cramp can usually be stopped by stretching the muscle for a few seconds; for example, if it is in the calf, by standing up. The muscle should not be contracted again for as long as possible. Pains described as cramp sometimes affect people who have to carry out repetitive and delicate movements of the hands and fingers, such as writers, violinists, tailors, typists and others; but it is thought that there is a psychological factor here, for while the discomfort prevents the sufferer from carrying out the job, it is not associated with any bodily disease that can be demonstrated, and it does not prevent other activities such as using a knife and fork.

Cranial Nerves: twelve nerves which arise from the brain and brain stem within the skull. They are usually denoted by Roman numerals: I *Olfactory nerve*, the nerve of smell running from the nose to the brain. II *Optic nerve*, which conducts impulses from the eye to the brain. III *Oculomotor nerve*, which supplies muscles which move the eyeball, control the size of the pupil, alter the shape of the lens, and lift the upper eyelid. IV *Trochlear nerve*: this leaves the back of the brain stem and runs round it to pass forward and supply the muscle which moves the eyeball downwards and outwards (the superior oblique muscle). V *Trigeminal nerve*, which is mostly sensory but has a small motor part. The sensory root has three branches: first, which supplies the upper front part of the head – eye, nose, forehead and scalp up to a line joining the ears; second, which supplies the upper lip, the cheek, the upper teeth and the roof of the mouth; third, which supplies the lower lip, the chin, the temple, the lower teeth and the floor of the mouth. The motor part supplies the muscles used in chewing. VI *Abducent nerve*, which supplies the muscle that turns the eyeball outwards (external rectus muscle). VII *Facial nerve*, which supplies the muscles of the face. VIII *Auditory nerve*, which carries to the brain impulses from the ear. It has two parts: one carries signals from the organ of hearing, the other signals from the organ of balance. IX *Glossopharyngeal nerve*, which carries impulses to the brain from the middle ear, the Eustachian tube, the back of the tongue, the tonsil and side of the throat and the soft palate. It also supplies branches to the parotid gland and the small mucus-secreting glands of the tongue and part of the throat. X *Vagus nerve*, called 'the wanderer' because it travels so far. It sends branches to the pharynx, the larynx, and to the muscles moving the vocal cords, and brings parasympathetic fibres (*see* Nervous System) to the heart, the stomach and the lower part of the oesophagus, the whole of the small intestine and half the large intestine. XI *Accessory nerve*: this gives a branch to the vagus nerve, and then leaves the skull to supply two muscles in the neck, the sternomastoid and the trapezius. XII *Hypoglossal nerve*, which supplies the muscles of the tongue and the muscles which act on the tongue although they are separate from it.

Craniotomy: the operation of opening the skull.

Cranium: the skull.

Cremation: the disposal of a dead body by burning. In the United Kingdom, cremation requires a special certificate signed by two doctors, one of whom has signed the death certificate. This doctor must have been seen and questioned by the other who must have been qualified for at least five years. The doctors must not be partners. Both doctors must have seen and examined the body. The certificate is then seen by another doctor, the Referee, who must be satisfied that all is in order before the cremation can take place.

Crepitus: the noise or sensation of grating. Felt when the ends of a broken bone are moved against each other, it is a sign of fracture.

Cretinism: deficiency in secretion of the thyroid gland in the newborn results, if left untreated, in cretinism – stunted growth and mental deficiency. The infant does not feed properly and tends to be constipated, but at first looks normal. If the condition is allowed to progress the appearance gradually becomes characteristic: a cretin looks thickset and stunted, with dry skin, coarse features and a disproportionately large tongue with deep fissures which protrudes from the mouth. The mental age of a cretin is that of an infant. If however the condition is recognised early and treated with thyroid hormone, development is normal; the later treatment is started, the worse the result. Babies can be screened for thyroid deficiency in the week after birth. Thyroid deficiency in later life results in myxoedema. *See* Goitre, Thyroid Gland.

Creutzfeldt–Jacob Disease: a rare degenerative disease of the brain which can be transmitted to susceptible animals. The disease is fatal, and is characterised by a spongiform degeneration of the grey matter of the brain; material from such a brain has proved to transmit the disease when injected into the brain of a chimpanzee, and rodents have been found to be susceptible in the laboratory. It has also been transmitted in corneal transplantation in human beings, and in injections of growth hormone. The infective agent is not visible under the electron microscope, nor can it be cultured; it is thought to be similar to the agent of scrapie, a disease of sheep and goats, and of kuru. *See* Kuru, Scrapie.

Crisis: apart from its use implying a state of emergency, in medicine the word may be used to mean a sudden intensification of symptoms in the course of a disease, or a sudden turn for the worse or the better.

Crohn's Disease: *see* Ileitis.

Cross-infection: the infection of patients in hospital by organisms derived from other patients. Unfortunately this can be a problem, despite strict adherence to the principles of asepsis, and control requires constant vigilance from the medical and nursing staff.

Cross-matching: the process of ensuring before transfusion that the blood of the donor and of the recipient are compatible. *See* Blood Groups

Croup: occurring mostly in children, croup is caused by an obstruction in the larynx which produces a brassy cough and a high-pitched noise, or stridor, as the child tries to draw breath. It is usually the result of a virus infection which makes the vocal cords swollen, and in the majority of cases responds to steam inhalation from a kettle kept on the boil in the room. Only in a very few cases is it necessary to take further measures such as the use of oxygen. It is distinguished from whooping cough by the absence of the whooping noise and coughing attack; diphtheria, which used to affect the larynx, is now rare because of mass immunisation. It must not be forgotten that the inhalation of a foreign body can obstruct the larynx.

Cryosurgery: the production of surgical lesions by the application of cold; growths can be removed from the skin by using liquid nitrogen, and it is possible to produce localised areas of destruction in tissues such as the brain by using special instruments that freeze the desired area.

Cryotherapy: treatment by the use of cold.

Cryptorchidism: imperfect descent of the testicle, so that it remains in the abdominal cavity. The normal male child should have both testicles descended by the age of five, and if no testicle can be identified in the scrotum or the inguinal canal hormonal treatment may be tried. If this is not successful, surgical exploration may be carried out, for there is known to be an increased risk of malignant change in testicles left in the abdomen. Incomplete descent of the testicle when it can be identified in the inguinal canal is a different matter, and the testicle can be brought down if necessary by operation.

Culicine Mosquitoes: important carriers of disease. They do not transmit malaria, but are responsible for the spread of yellow fever, filariasis, dengue fever and various types of encephalitis. Culicine mosquitoes at rest hold their bodies parallel to the surface on which they are resting, unlike anophiline mosquitoes, responsible for the spread of malaria, which incline their bodies to the surface with the head down. The most important culicine mosquito is *Aedes aegypti* which spreads yellow fever and dengue fever. It is a black mosquito with silver markings, living near houses.

Culture: the process of growing micro-organisms or other living cells in artificial circumstances on suitable material such as agar mixed with blood or broth. 'Culture' is also used to mean the growing colony of micro-organisms or cells.

Cupping: a technique once but no longer popular, in which diseases thought to be caused by the congestion of underlying tissues were treated by measures designed to draw blood to the surface. A cupping glass was applied to the skin, and suction induced whereby the blood was drawn up. In wet cupping the skin was first scarified to increase the flow of blood and lymph.

Curare: an extract made from various plants by South American Indians, with which they tipped their arrows to paralyse their prey. It contains tubocurarine, which when injected paralyses the muscles by acting on the junction between motor nerves and muscle fibres, where it interferes with the function of acetylcholine (q.v.). It has therefore been widely used in anaesthesia as a muscle relaxant, but recently has been overtaken by newer muscle-relaxing drugs. These drugs may also be used in the treatment of tetanus.

Curette: an instrument used for scraping the walls of a body cavity in order to remove unwanted material, growths or specimens for microscopical examination. Also used to refer to the act of using such an instrument. The most common operation carried out with the curette is performed on the interior of the uterus; it is usually combined with dilatation of the neck of the uterus and is called dilatation and curettage – D & C.

Cyanides: hydrogen cyanide is extremely poisonous, and with its derivatives is widely used in industry for many purposes, among them being the production of synthetic rubber, insecticides, fertilisers, electroplating solutions and rat poisons. Cyanides are liberated by burning polyurethane foam, a substance used in upholstering a great deal of furniture. Inhalation of cyanide fumes or the consumption of cyanide may prove quickly fatal; it can be absorbed by splashes on the skin. The symptoms of poisoning are sore throat and running nose, breathlessness, headache, sickness, giddiness and weakness of the arms and legs, which may progress to unconsciousness, cessation of breathing and collapse of the circulation. Chronic poisoning leads to unsteadiness, loss of vision and deafness. Treatment is removal from the poisoned atmosphere, administration of oxygen, and intravenous injection of dicobalt edetate, followed if this is not successful by intravenous injection of solutions of sodium nitrite and sodium thiosulphate. These antidotes are normally kept in hospitals and in places where there is a known risk of cyanide poisoning.

Cyanosis: a blue tinge of the skin and mucous membranes. It is the blood that gives pink skin its colour, and normally the circulating blood is red. If however it is carrying less oxygen than it should it becomes blue, the colour of venous blood, and pink skin is darkened. Cyanosis is found in respiratory diseases in which the function of the lungs is depressed so that the blood cannot take up the normal amount of oxygen, and in heart disease when the circulation is impaired and the amount of blood passing through the lungs is less than it should be. If the circulation to a particular part of the body such as a limb is cut off or impeded the part will become blue as the blood gives up its oxygen to the tissues; it may happen in the skin when the circulation stagnates because intense cold makes the arterioles contract.

Cyclopropane: an anaesthetic gas, which has no colour but a sweet smell; it is explosive when mixed with air or oxygen, and must therefore be used in a closed rebreathing circuit. Its value lies in the fact that it acts quickly and is quickly excreted, and it can be mixed with large quantities of oxygen without losing its anaesthetic properties; but the risk of explosion has greatly curtailed its use.

Cyst: a hollow swelling, especially one containing fluid.

Cysticercosis: the tapeworm *Taenia solium* has a life-cycle involving the pig, and if infected pork is not sufficiently cooked in countries where the tapeworm is found (which include Europe, South Africa, Latin America, parts of India and South-East Asia), man can become infected by the worm. Larval cysts are present in the muscles of the pig, and when they are eaten they develop into the adult form of the worm in the intestines. It can sometimes happen that a person harbouring a worm can infect themselves or others by transferring the worm's eggs to food, perhaps by the hands, and then the cystic larval form of the worm develops in the muscles and also in the brain, where the cysts can give rise to epilepsy and other symptoms. The treatment if possible is surgical removal of the cysts and the use of the drug praziquantel.

Cystic Fibrosis: a hereditary disease in which there is abnormally thick secretion of mucus in the body, affecting the lungs, intestines and pancreas in particular. It is found mainly among Europeans and those of European descent, and is of autosomal recessive inheritance; both parents carry the gene but do not show the disease, although their children have a one in four chance of being affected. The disease makes the sweat glands secrete more sodium and chloride than is normal, a fact that is used as a diagnostic test in infants. A sign of the disease is repeated infection of the lungs, for the bronchioles become blocked with the thick secretions and full expansion of the alveoli, the air sacs, is not possible. In such circumstances bacteria thrive, and treatment with antibiotics must be energetic. The pancreas is affected, and children have fatty diarrhoea and fail to thrive; pancreatic enzymes must be given by mouth. Changes may also develop in the liver and intestine, but the most dangerous feature of the disease is the involvement of the lungs. With skilled treatment four-fifths of the children found to have the disease survive to become adults. Occasionally the disease is not recognised until patients are adolescent, or even later. It has recently become possible to diagnose the presence of the disease before birth by the examination of foetal cells obtained by chorionic villus sampling (q.v.).

Cystitis: inflammation of the bladder, usually due to bacterial infection by *Escherichia coli*, but other organisms may be involved. Women are particularly prone to the infection, for it is thought to occur because the organisms ascend the urethra which in women is short. Rarely, tuberculous infection occurs, and in countries where bilharzia (q.v.) exists *Schistosoma haematobium* may cause chronic cystitis. The symptoms are frequency of passing water, pain on doing so, pain in the lower part of the abdomen, and a constant desire to pass water. The urine may be offensive and blood-stained. Infection may be accompanied by fever and malaise. The presence of infection is confirmed by microscopy and culture of a specimen of urine, by which the organism and its sensitivity to antibiotics can be identified; but this takes time, and the symptoms are usually too urgent to postpone treatment; it is therefore sensible to use the antibiotics to which the infection is usually sensitive, namely amoxycillin or co-trimoxazole, straight away and not to wait for the results of the culture. If treatment is not successful, it can be modified in accordance with the laboratory report. In children investigation of the urinary tract must be carried out after the first episode of infection, for it is often associated with abnormalities; in men, it may be associated with enlargement of the prostate gland, tumours of the bladder or stones; but in women it is uncommon to find any abnormality of the urinary tract, although recurrent infections must be investigated.

Cystoscope: an endoscope for examining the interior of the urinary bladder. It is passed into the bladder through the urethra, and through it the surgeon can not only examine the interior of the bladder but can carry out various operations, and can pass thin catheters up the ureters into the pelvis of the kidney.

Cystotomy: the surgical operation of opening the bladder.

Cytology: the study of the function and structure of cells.

Cytotoxic Agents: agents which damage or kill cells, used in the treatment of cancer. *See* Chemotherapy.

D

Dacryocystitis: inflammation of the tear sac at the inner angle of the eye. *See* Eyelids.

Dandruff: scales formed by dead cells of the skin of the scalp, which collect in the hair.

D & C: *see* Curette.

Dangerous Drugs and Poisons: the Poisons Act of 1972 regulates the supply and sales of toxic substances, and the Misuse of Drugs Regulations of 1985 lay down the conditions under which drugs likely to cause dependence may be prescribed and supplied. The Food and Drugs Act of 1972 enables the Minister to regulate substances that may be used as food additives, and the Health and Safety at Work Act of 1974 enables the government to make sure that poisonous substances used in industry, including pesticides used in agriculture, are properly controlled. Drugs on the market for supply on prescription or for sale without are controlled by the Medicines Committee, who advise the Minister of Health, and there are two further committees, one on the Safety of Medicines and the other on the Review of Medicines. Any unexpected or adverse reactions to drugs are reported to the Committee on Safety of Medicines by the doctor observing them. In the USA the supply of drugs is controlled by a Federal Agency called the Food and Drug Administration.

DDT: dichlorodiphenyltrichlorethane. First synthesised in 1874, its insecticidal properties were not recognised until 1940. It owes its undoubted efficiency to its chemical stability and the fact that it is physically inert, so that it has considerable staying power. Although this has made it a great blessing to people who live in countries infested by mosquitoes, lice, fleas, flies, bed bugs and all the host of insects that carry crippling if not fatal diseases such as plague, malaria, typhus, cholera and enteric fevers, the fact that DDT persists unchanged has meant that in the end it has figured involuntarily in the diet of man. If taken in large doses it affects the nervous system, producing tremor, convulsions and even paralysis, and it may interfere with the formation of blood corpuscles. However, there are now other efficient insecticides, notably the organophosphorus compounds, and DDT is slowly being phased out.

Deafness: inability to hear has several causes. The ear has three parts: the outer ear, the pinna, is the visible ear and its canal, the external auditory meatus, leads to the eardrum and the middle ear; the middle ear contains a chain of three small bones which transfer vibrations of the drum to the inner ear, where lies the organ which transforms the vibrations into nerve impulses (*see* Ear). Deafness may occur when the outer canal is blocked, as can happen if sufficient wax accumulates; this can be seen through a simple instrument, the otoscope, and washed out with a syringe after it has been softened by appropriate ear-drops. It is not sensible to try to clear the wax out yourself by using anything poked down into the ear, as this can be dangerous to the drum, as well as packing the wax in more densely. Infection of the middle ear, especially in children, can interfere with the movement of the drum and the small bones it contains; treatment with antibiotics is in most cases successful, but some children are found to have a persistent sticky effusion into the middle ear, known as glue ear, and in such cases the eardrum is opened and a grommet inserted to ventilate the ear, allow the secretion to disperse, and the pressure on each side of the drum to equalise. In time the grommet is usually discharged, the drum heals and the child can hear normally.

Perforation of the eardrum can occur in the course of an infection, or through injury; it usually heals, but if it persists the drum can often be repaired. Free movement of the eardrum relies on the air pressure being equal in the outside atmosphere and the middle ear, and this is normally ensured by the Eustachian tube, which runs from the cavity of the middle ear to the upper throat. It may become blocked, often by a cold, and the hearing is affected; it may take some time before it clears.

Movement of the small bones, the ossicles, in the middle ear is impaired by the disease otosclerosis, which may run in families. The stapes becomes bound to the surrounding bone and cannot transmit the vibrations of the drum. Surgical operation can be very successful.

However, cases of deafness due to malfunction of the organ of Corti (Alfonso Corti, 1822–76) in the inner ear, by which vibrations are turned into nerve impulses -- perceptive rather than conductive deafness - are not amenable to surgery but may be helped by hearing aids. Such a deafness may be induced by continual exposure to loud noise, which can lead to inability to perceive certain tones. The type and extent of a loss of hearing is defined by an audiometer, which can produce tones of varying pitch and amplitude. According to what is found, a hearing aid which matches as far as possible the lost frequencies can be prescribed, but as it can only amplify sound it sometimes cannot help those who have a perceptive deafness. It has, however, recently become possible to convert sound into electrical impulses that can be used by the cochlea, the sound being picked up and converted outside the body; the lead carrying the electrical impulses is implanted into the cochlea. It is always worth seeking an expert opinion in cases of deafness.

Death: it was always accepted that a person is dead when the breathing stops and the heart is still. Now that it is possible for machines to take over the function of the lungs and keep the blood full of oxygen in the absence of natural breathing, while the heart continues to beat strongly, keeping the body alive although the brain may have ceased to function except at its lowest levels, the determination of death is not so easy. But if there are signs that the higher functions of the brain are irretrievably lost: if, for example, there is no detectable electrical activity in the electro-encephalogram and angiography shows no circulation in the brain, then the patient may be said to be brain dead, and when the breathing machine is turned off the body will cease to function. In such a case death may be equated with irreversible damage to the brain resulting in permanent deep coma, paralysis of the muscles of respiration, and cessation of cerebral circulation and electrical activity; although the breathing machine may be oxygenating the blood and the heart is still beating, the patient is dead. This is a matter of great importance in transplant surgery, when the organ to be transplanted has only a relatively short time of survival outside the body. Opinions must differ, but modern reason argues that it is proper to keep the body 'alive' after brain death if there is a chance that organs might be successfully transplanted by doing so.

Decompression: a surgical operation designed to release or relieve pressure on an organ or structure, for example removal of part of the skull to relieve the pressure inside the head of a tumour which cannot be removed, removal of bone pressing on the spinal cord in the case of a fracture, or division of the transverse ligament at the wrist to relieve pressure on the median nerve in the carpal tunnel syndrome. The word is also used to mean the decrease in atmospheric pressure on divers as they ascend from the deep, or on aviators as they ascend into the sky. *See* Caisson Disease.

Defibrillation or Cardioversion: after a sudden disaster overtaking the respiration or the heart, as for example a myocardial infarction, or electrocution, the heart may cease to beat effectively. This may be due to an abnormality of rhythm, either a very rapid beat, tachycardia, or fibrillation, where the muscle fibres instead of contracting together contract in an uncoordinated way which prevents the heart beating. This is detected by electrocardiography, a recording of the electrical activity of the heart, and may be treated by the application of an electric shock to the heart. This stops the abnormal rhythm and allows the heartbeat to start again at its natural pace and strength. The electric shock is delivered by a defibrillator: two electrodes are placed on the chest wall, one over the base of the heart, the other over the apex, and a shock of short duration but high energy applied. In a case of ventricular fibrillation the first charge is 200 joules; if this is not successful, the energy may be increased to 300 or 400 joules. The technique may also be used where drug treatment has failed to control fibrillation or flutter of the atrial muscle (*see* Heart). Where a defibrillator is not immediately available, it is necessary to start cardiac massage and artificial respiration if the heart stops beating for this can keep the patient alive for upwards of 20 minutes after a heart attack.

Deformity: the distortion of the normal shape and size of the body or its parts, occurring congenitally or acquired by accident or disease.

Degrees and Diplomas: in the United Kingdom medical degrees are conferred by universities, and diplomas are granted by the Royal Colleges of Physicians and Surgeons of England, Scotland and Ireland, and the Society of Apothecaries in London, which can be legally registered by the General Medical Council, the statutory body responsible for keeping the Medical Register. On first passing the final examinations, registration is provisional; full registration is granted after a further period of a year's work in a recognised hospital. This enables the holder to sign prescriptions for dangerous drugs and poisons and to sign death certificates and statutory certificates and to hold a public office. In the United States medical degrees are given by universities and diplomas, or board certificates by specialty boards. A medical degree entitles the physician to apply for a licence to practise medicine in the State chosen, and he or she may have to pass examinations designed to ensure competence before being given a licence to write prescriptions for dangerous drugs, to treat individuals seeking the services of a physician and to sign death certificates. As in the United Kingdom, further degrees and diplomas are earned by postgraduate training and examination in the particular branch of medicine wherein the doctor wishes to specialise.

Dehydration: lack of water in the body. This can be caused by insufficient water to drink, by excessive loss of water as in severe vomiting and diarrhoea, or by excessive sweating. In infants the consequences of dehydration are rapid and dangerous and cases of diarrhoea and vomiting are to be taken seriously. Salts as well as water are lost, and the infant should be given a solution of oral rehydration salts which consists of sodium chloride 3.5 g/l, potassium chloride 1.5 g/l, sodium citrate 2.9 g/l and anhydrous glucose 20 g/l (WHO formulation) in appropriate quantities. If vomiting is too severe for this to be retained it will be necessary to provide the water and salts by intravenous infusion. The same solution is used in the treatment of gastro-intestinal infections such as cholera (q.v.). Excessive sweating may be unnoticed in very hot conditions, and can lead to heat exhaustion, from which the patient will recover once he or she has drunk enough water (*see* Heat Stroke). In conditions where the supply of water is short, a person can live on 500 m/l of water a day taken in three portions; if conditions are desperate, there is a good chance of survival on half that amount. Despite some opinions to the contrary, it is dangerous to drink sea water even in the most severe conditions because it contains a higher concentration of salts than the kidney can excrete.

Delhi Boil: cutaneous Leishmaniasis; Oriental sore, Baghdad sore, Aleppo sore, etc. An infection of the skin with *Leishmania* (q.v.). It is found in tropical and subtropical countries in the Old World and the New. Starting as a small itching papule, it is usually scratched until it ulcerates. Left alone, healing in the Old World infections takes months and leaves a scar, but some New World infections need surgical treatment. *Leishmania* are sensitive to a pentavalent compound of antimony, sodium stibogluconate.

Delirium: a Latin word meaning 'off the track'. It signifies confusion and excitement combined with hallucinations, illusions, and delusions. There are many causes including intoxication with various drugs, severe diseases, heat exhaustion and high fever. Examples of diseases are meningitis, heart failure, alcoholism and typhoid fever. The patient is restless, suspicious, anxious and may have feelings of persecution; consciousness may be impaired, and the condition may be worse at night. While the underlying cause is being treated the patient may have to be sedated by a suitable drug such as chlorpromazine, and kept in quiet surroundings. The delirium of alcoholism is self-limiting and lasts for three or four days; other types of delirium usually respond to treatment of the underlying disorder.

Delirium Tremens: delirium produced by excessive consumption of alcohol over a period of years. It may follow the sudden withdrawal of alcohol. *See above.*

Delta Waves: abnormally slow waves seen in the electroencephalogram (q.v.) in certain diseases of the brain, for example, some sorts of epilepsy and deep brain tumours.

Delusions: false beliefs or judgements usually taken to be a sign of severe mental illness. However, one must be cautious; a person, for example, may exaggerate the significance of a true belief (such as the fact that there is a mole on the face) by supposing that everybody notices it as an ugly blemish (which may not be true at all) without being insane. Similarly a delusion must be taken in its social and cultural context: an East African who thinks that he is ill because he has been cursed by a witch-doctor may have a belief which, although untrue, is quite usual in the circumstances, whereas an educated European who thought the same would probably be deluded in the sense that he was mentally ill.

Dementia: loss of intellectual functions, resulting in deficient memory, concentration and thought; the condition is progressive and may lead to self-neglect, irrational behaviour, rambling talk, and incontinence. There are a number of causes, ranging from thyroid deficiency to chronic infections in the elderly, where there is a hope of successful treatment; but many cases are due to degenerative processes which cannot be set right. Sometimes no cause can be found, but in all cases investigations should be undertaken if only to exclude the possibility of treatment.

Dengue Fever: an acute fever found in tropical and subtropical countries, caused by a virus transmitted by the bite of a mosquito, commonly *Aedes aegypti*, the yellow fever mosquito. The incubation period is about a week, and the symptoms are reddening of the skin and eyes, headache, sore throat and severe pain in the joints and bones which gives it the popular name 'breakbone' fever. About the fourth day a rash may appear. The condition is self-limiting and usually takes a week or so to recover. There is no specific treatment. There is a much more dangerous form of the disease called dengue haemorrhagic fever, in which after an acute onset and the development of what looks like dengue fever, in a few days or a week there is a drop in temperature and the patient becomes shocked; there is a drop in blood pressure, there may be spontaneous bleeding and loss of plasma into the pleural cavity or the abdomen, and immediate intravenous saline or plasma is required. It may be necessary to give blood. After about 48 hours recovery begins. Most of the cases have been in children. Like other virus diseases, dengue fever may be followed by a period of depression.

Depression: *see* Mental Illness.

De Quervain's Disease: Fritz de Quervain (1868–1940), a Swiss surgeon, described a painful tenosynovitis (q.v.) affecting the thumb.

Dermatitis: inflammation of the skin. The dividing line between dermatitis and eczema is not clearly drawn, but dermatitis can be used when the skin is injured by an external agent, and eczema when the cause is within the body. In general terms dermatitis and eczema appear to be roughly synonymous. There are about as many possible external causes of dermatitis as there are substances which can touch the skin, and it is not sensible to try to set them all down here. There are over 50 items in a standard battery of patch tests used to identify substances to which patients may be sensitive. The skin may be damaged by irritants such as acids or alkalis, by oil, antiseptics, cleaning agents and so on, or by simple wear and tear. It can become sensitive to substances after exposure to them over a period of time, or be sensitive at the first touch. A very common cause of sensitivity reaction is nickel, which is found in many applications from metal buttons to costume jewellery; cosmetics can set up sensitivity reactions, as can plastics, cement, plants, and detergents.

However the reaction is set up, the first part of treatment is the identification of the substance causing it, but unfortunately this is often easier said than done. If it is identified then it must be avoided but if this is impossible, as it may be in industry, cleanliness, ventilation and care, and the use of appropriate skin creams such as aqueous cream or a barrier cream will help. In many instances topical steroids are useful, but the lowest possible strength must be used such as hydrocortisone 1% ointment for the shortest possible time.

Some types of dermatitis can be misleading, for dermatitis affecting the hands or feet can set up reactions in other places, the common affliction of athlete's foot can produce eczema of the hands. To make the difficulty greater, the ointment or cream used to soothe the dermatitis can itself set up reactions if it contains substances such as wool fat or fragrances. It may be best to try simple remedies, such as emulsifying ointment, cetomacrogol cream or aqueous cream, which will often prove successful. *See* Eczema.

Dermoid Cyst: resulting from the inclusion of ectoderm (q.v.) in the wrong place during development, may be found in a number of sites, but most commonly in the ovary where the cyst may contain hair and even teeth. The tumour is not in most cases malignant, but in the ovary may be associated with haemolytic anaemia. Ectoderm may also be driven deep to the skin by an injury and form a small cyst, an inclusion dermoid. Both types of cyst are removed surgically.

Desensitisation: the attempt to prevent allergic responses by injecting small but increasing doses of the antigen to which the patient is sensitive. Up to recently it was commonly used in cases of hay fever, but the injections may provoke anaphylactic reactions, and the method is now used only in places where there is a full range of equipment ready to deal with such an emergency. The results are not uniformly successful. *See* Allergy.

Dexamphetamine: *see* Amphetamine.

Dextran: a complex carbohydrate of large molecular size. Solutions of dextran can be used for intravenous infusion when plasma or blood is not available to maintain or increase the blood volume in cases of shock or burns. It may interfere with subsequent blood typing, and if it is to be used a specimen of blood should be taken first.

Dextrocardia: a congenital abnormality where the heart is on the wrong side of the chest. It may be associated with a similar abnormal position of the abdominal organs, when the condition is called *situs inversus*.

Dextrose: also known as glucose (q.v.).

DFP (Dyflos): a poisonous organophosphorus compound which interferes with the action of acetylcholinesterase in breaking down acetylcholine, as do all such compounds. It has been used in solution in arachis oil as eye-drops in the treatment of glaucoma (q.v.) because it has a powerful miotic action, that is, it causes the pupil to contract and so decreases the pressure inside the eyeball. It has a prolonged action, which may last for a week. Unfortunately its use may lead to the development of cataracts, and the vapour of dyflos is very toxic although solutions in vegetable oil are stable. *See* Organophosphorus Compounds.

Diabetes Insipidus: a condition in which the patient passes a large quantity of dilute urine, owing to deficiency of the hormone vasopressin, also known as ADH, the antidiuretic hormone, secreted by the posterior part of the pituitary gland. The condition is treated by use of the ADH analogue desmopressin, which is given in nasal drops or spray.

Diabetes Mellitus: 'sugar' diabetes. There is a loss of the ability to oxidise carbohydrates which may be due to deficiency in the secretion of insulin in the pancreas or a decreased ability to use insulin in the body. There is an excess of sugar in the blood and urine, passage of increased amounts of urine, and symptoms of hunger, thirst, loss of weight and weakness. There is impaired metabolism of fats and protein which may interfere with the body chemistry. There may be itching, particularly of the vulva in women, and in men inflammation of the foreskin. There may also be an increased liability to infection, often causing recurrent boils. A severe untreated case may lose consciousness and fall into a diabetic coma. There are two main types of diabetes mellitus: in the first, the main deficiency is in the secretion of insulin, and the disease is found mostly in young people. In the second, there is some insulin present, but a resistance to its use in the body. This type is found in older people, and may be linked to obesity. There are other types of diabetes but they are not common.

The long-term effects of diabetes include an increased tendency to atherosclerosis and heart disease, changes in the retina of the eye and cataract which interfere with vision, changes in the kidneys which lead to the passage of protein in the urine and, if untreated, may end in kidney failure, and damage to the nervous system, particularly of the legs, which produces sensations of tingling and numbness.

Diabetes mellitus is diagnosed by the presence of sugar in the urine and high glucose levels in the blood, and treatment varies according to the type of diabetes. In the first group the diet is regulated with the help of the dietician, and it aims for a high carbohydrate content, high fibre content, low fat with increased polyunsaturated fat, and no quickly absorbed carbohydrate. The food should be spaced well out during the day in three larger meals and three snacks. In addition insulin is used by injection in the form and quantity needed by each individual. There are a large number of preparations of insulin available which vary in their length of action, and each individual will vary in requirements.

In the second group the obese individual will be advised to lose weight, and in some cases this will be sufficient. Initially in all cases efforts will be made to control the disease by an appropriate diet, but if this fails sulphony-lureas are given by mouth; if these fail it is possible to use metformin hydrochloride. In rare cases it may be necessary to use insulin by injection.

In all cases it is important for the patient to understand the disease as far as possible, for the treatment must be controlled by its effects. Methods of monitoring the effects include the simple testing of urine to assess the sugar content by means of a test strip, and the estimation of blood glucose, which can be carried out in the laboratory or at home by a test strip used on the blood drawn from a pinprick. It may happen that a patient who is taking insulin fails to cover the dose with food, or the balance is affected by exercise, and the blood sugar then falls to a level low enough to cause unconsciousness. The warning signs are restlessness, faintness, palpitation, cold sweats and hunger. Usually the symptoms are recognised and can be cut short by taking sugar, but patients should carry a card on them stating that they are diabetic in case they should collapse. The treatment is the administration of glucose.

The long-term consequences of diabetes are less likely to occur if control of the disease has been good, but vigilant continuing follow-up is necessary, for the earlier any changes in the retina or kidney are detected the more likely it is that they can be treated. The feet in older diabetics can be a source of serious trouble, for the combination of deteriorating circulation and damage to the nervous system can cause even a trivial injury to result in gangrene; regular attention from a chiropodist is very important. *See* Insulin.

Diagnosis: the determination of the nature of a disease in a given case.

Dialysis: the process of separating colloids from crystalloids in a solution by their different rates of diffusion through a semipermeable membrane. The process is used in renal dialysis (q.v.).

Diaphoretics: it used to be thought that in certain cases of fever it was advisable to promote a flow of perspiration, and substances used for the purpose were called diaphoretics.

Diaphragm: the muscular and tendinous partition between the thoracic and abdominal cavities. The fleshy outer part of the diaphragm takes origin from the lower six ribs and their cartilages, the lowest part of the breastbone in front and the upper lumbar vertebrae behind. The general shape of the diaphragm is like a dome, convex upwards, and when the outer muscle contracts it pulls the tendinous central part of the diaphragm down and flattens the dome, so that the volume of the thoracic cavity is increased at the expense of the abdominal cavity and the lungs expand. The diaphragm is supplied by the phrenic nerve which itself originates in the cervical part of the spinal cord (the reason is developmental) so that damage to the cervical cord in the neck caused by disease or accident can paralyse the diaphragm and interfere with breathing. There are large openings in the diaphragm through which pass the oesophagus, the aorta and the vena cava, and the thoracic duct. The superior epigastric arteries pass through it in front. It is possible for the upper part of the stomach to protrude upwards through the diaphragmatic opening, a condition known as diaphragmatic hernia or hiatus hernia (q.v.).

Diarrhoea: frequent passage of loose motions. Acute diarrhoea in infants is common, and is usually due to virus infection. Since 1970 electron microscopy has shown a number of viruses to be involved; as the condition is usually self-limiting, and electron microscopy the only way of detecting a virus in the motions, the virus is not routinely identified in many cases. No specific treatment is available, but attention must be paid to the possibility of dehydration and loss of essential salts, for these are the only dangerous features of the condition especially if it is accompanied by vomiting. Replacement of water and salts is accomplished by giving oral rehydration salts; there are a number of proprietary preparations available, and for the WHO formula *see* Cholera.

The disease is spread by contamination of food with infected material or by contaminated hands; viruses can be spread by coughing or sneezing. Acute diarrhoea in adults is usually due to infection from contaminated food; the type quickest in onset is that due to the toxin made by colonies of staphylococci growing on food infected by contamination during preparation. The attack comes on suddenly in a matter of a few hours, and may be accompanied by vomiting and abdominal pain; it is while it lasts very unpleasant, but usually passes off in a day or two. No treatment is possible beyond rehydration, for the trouble is due not to the organism itself but to the toxin present in the food.

A common type of food poisoning is due to the organism *Clostridium perfringens*, which is liable to contaminate meat or poultry. A dish is prepared and then allowed to stand at room temperature for some hours, perhaps a day, and then served cold or poorly heated. The infection is common in places where catering has to take care of a number of people, such as schools or institutions. Diarrhoea starts after 12 hours or so, and lasts for a day; the disease is self-limiting.

Other infecting organisms are *Salmonella typhimurium* and *Salmonella enteritidis*, which are present in a large number of animals. The organisms are only likely to cause diarrhoea if they are present in large numbers, and correct preparation and handling of food prevents them multiplying; but if they are allowed to do so by less than scrupulous attention to hygiene, infection shows itself in a day or two by the onset of headache, abdominal pain, nausea and diarrhoea, which may last for two or three days or longer and be accompanied by a fever and shivering. Unless the condition is severe, and this is unusual except at the extremes of age, specific treatment is not needed, but as in all cases of diarrhoea the danger is loss of water and salts. In mild cases of diarrhoea kaolin mixtures can be useful for their action in encouraging more formed motions, but they do not restrict water and salt loss. Loperamide is useful for reducing the intestinal secretions and so reducing the diarrhoea, but it should not be used for children under four.

Cases of diarrhoea that are due to food poisoning should be reported to the Community Physician, for control of hygiene in restaurants and other catering establishments is a responsibility of that post. Normally the doctor will do this, but in mild cases of food poisoning it may not be felt necessary to get medical advice. It is best, however, to ask for medical advice in cases of diarrhoea that last more than a week, for it may be a sign of a number of diseases.

Traveller's diarrhoea is common, and apart from the

causes mentioned above, can be due to strains of *Escherichia coli*. Most cases improve in a few days, and the only treatment needed is attention to making up the loss of water and salts. In severe cases tetracycline, trimethoprim or co-trimoxazole can be used, but their action may be disappointing because of the presence of organisms that are not sensitive to these antibiotics. In such cases ciprofloxacin may be useful, but it should be reserved for treating infection resistant to other drugs. It is not recommended for children.

Diastole: that part of the heart's cycle when the chambers dilate and fill with blood. The mitral and tricuspid valves relax to allow this to happen; when the heart contracts, the atria contract just before the ventricles; the left atrium delivers about 60–100 ml of blood into the ventricle, and at the end of contraction there is about 20–50 ml remaining in the ventricle.

Diathermy: if a rapidly oscillating current is passed through the tissues they heat up because of the resistance they offer to its passage. This effect can be used in surgery, where a large indifferent electrode is fastened to the leg and the other electrode is a needle or the point of a pair of fine forceps. The tissue in contact with the point of the needle or forceps will heat sufficiently to make the needle cut or an artery caught by the forceps coagulate. A dampened oscillating current is used for coagulating, and undampened current for cutting soft tissues. In physiotherapy diathermy is used to engender heat in deep tissues, but insufficient energy is used to heat to the point of harm. Short-wave diathermy is the application of high frequency electromagnetic radiation.

Diazepam: one of the benzodiazepine group of drugs used for the relief of anxiety, perhaps better known by its trade name Valium. It has a sustained action, and may produce drowsiness; the effect of alcohol is increased. Taken in the lowest effective dose for the shortest possible time the drug can be very useful, but it is possible to become dependent upon it.

Dieldrin: a chlorinated hydrocarbon used as a rapidly acting insecticide with a wider range than DDT. It is poisonous to man and animals and its use is restricted.

Digestive System: the digestive system is responsible for breaking down food into compounds which can be absorbed into the body. It begins in the mouth, where saliva secreted by the salivary glands – the parotid in front of the ear, the submandibular under the jaw, and the sublingual under the tongue – mixes with the food and acts by its enzyme ptyalin to break down starch into maltose and dextrose. When the food reaches the stomach, secretion of acid has started in response to the beginning of a meal, and this acid is accompanied by the secretion of intrinsic factor which makes the absorption of vitamin B_{12} possible and by the gastric enzyme pepsin which breaks down protein into polypeptides. Distension of the stomach by the meal increases the flow of secretions, and the mass becomes liquid. The main function of the stomach is to store the food which it receives at irregular intervals, liquefy it and pass it on at regular intervals in suitable amounts to the small intestine in which the main processes of digestion and absorption take place. Over the next two hours or so the digesting meal, called chyme, reaches the duodenum, the first part of the small intestine, and turns alkaline in the intestinal secretions. In the duodenum bile and pancreatic enzymes are added through the bile duct and pancreatic duct which discharge through the duodenal papilla. Bile, secreted in the liver and concentrated in the gall-bladder, is concerned with the emulsification of fats and makes fatty acids more soluble in water. The secretion of the pancreas is alkaline and helps to neutralise the acid chyme, and it contains the enzymes trypsin, chymotrypsin, amylase and lipase. Trypsin breaks down proteins into polypeptides and amino-acids; chymotrypsin curdles milk; amylase converts polysaccharides into disaccharides; and lipase breaks fats into free fatty acids. Leaving the duodenum, the food, now breaking down into its absorbable constituents, enters the jejunum and ileum, the second and third parts of the small intestine, where the breakdown is completed and carbohydrates, fats, amino-acids and peptides are absorbed. Water and salts are also absorbed

DIGITALIS

in the small intestine, with water and fat-soluble vitamins and minerals. Waste material passes from the small into the large intestine, the colon, where further absorption of water takes place, and so through the rectum to the exterior.

Food and chyme are passed through the gut by a combination of movements: segmentation, which is alternate contraction and relaxation of the muscle of the intestinal wall; peristalsis, which is a slow wave of contraction passing along the intestines at about 2 cm/second; and pendular movement which is a wave of contraction passing backwards and forwards along the intestine. In the colon, waste is passed along by alternate contraction and relaxation of the muscular walls. Food normally passes through the small intestine in about four hours, and waste products are excreted in a day or two. The absorbed constituents are passed through the walls of the intestines and carried away by the blood through the portal system, and by the lymph which passes through lymph vessels to the cisterna chyli and so through the thoracic duct into the left subclavian vein in the neck.

Digitalis: prepared from the dried leaves of plants of the species *Digitalis*, such as the purple foxglove, this substance has been used for many years in the treatment of heart disease. It contains a number of active principles, named cardiac glycosides, and because preparations of digitalis vary in strength these have been isolated and are now used instead of the crude drug. The most commonly used are digoxin and digitonin, and their actions are to increase the strength of the heartbeat and to decrease the conductivity of its tissues. They are therefore useful in cases where the cardiac rhythm is abnormal, especially in atrial fibrillation, and in some cases of heart failure.

Dimercaprol: BAL, British Anti-Lewisite (q.v.).

Dinitro Compounds: used less now as pesticides, they are sometimes used as washes on fruit trees and in warm weather as defoliants. They stain the skin yellow, and can be absorbed through the skin or by mouth. They interfere with metabolism and speed it up, and toxic symptoms are tiredness with an inability to sleep, yellow discoloration of the whites of the eyes, excessive sweating with increased thirst, dehydration, increased pulse rate, breathlessness, a high temperature and collapse. Poisoning can be fatal. The patient should be removed from contamination, washed to remove the dinitro compound, given as much to drink as possible, and kept at rest; if the temperature rises it must be reduced by wet sheets and cold water. Breathlessness may require the use of oxygen. The dinitro compounds include DNOC and Dinoseb.

Dioxin: an organic chemical compound which may produce cancer and abnormality of the genes leading to congenital deformities.

Diphtheria: a severe infection most commonly affecting the upper respiratory passages, especially in the young, the infecting organism being *Corynebacterium diphtheriae*. This multiplies in the nose and throat and produces a powerful and dangerous toxin which poisons surrounding tissues and is carried by the bloodstream to other parts of the body. The toxin kills the mucous membrane lining the pharynx and upper air passages so that a grey membrane is formed and the surrounding tissues swell. The swelling and the membrane obstruct the larynx in cases where the infection is centred in that area and interfere with breathing, especially in young children, and it may be necessary to perform a tracheotomy to enable the child to breathe. In other cases the infection is centred on the tonsils, which become covered with a greyish-white membrane; it gradually turns black and sloughs off. The regional lymph glands are enlarged, and the child is ill for a week or so. Although there may be paralysis of the palate there are rarely any other complications if the infection remains confined to the tonsils. If, however, the infection extends to involve the uvula, the palate and the nasopharynx, the child becomes very ill, for the toxin passes freely into the blood. The membrane is dark and bloody, the lymph glands and the tissues of the neck swell, and the outlook is grave. Other forms of diphtheria are found in the nose, when the mucus discharged may be blood-stained and is highly infectious, and, in tropical areas, on the skin, where it may be hard to recognise; indolent ulcers form especially on the legs. The toxin formed by *C. diphtheriae* affects the heart and the nervous system; the pulse becomes weak, there are pains in the chest and the heart beats rapidly and often irregularly. Damage to the heart may be heralded by vomiting, which is a grave sign in diphtheria.

Towards the end of the illness, perhaps after some weeks, the nervous system may show signs of damage from which a complete recovery is possible; the palate may be paralysed, which alters the voice and allows food and drink to come up through the nose, the eye muscles may be affected so that vision is blurred and there may be a squint, and in severe cases the muscles of the pharynx may be affected making swallowing difficult. The paralysis may spread to the muscles of the larynx and even the muscles of respiration, but with expert care the child may be kept alive and will eventually recover. Treatment must at first be directed to neutralising the toxin, and for this purpose an antitoxin is available which must be given as soon as the disease is recognised. The organism is sensitive to penicillin in most cases, but the danger is not in the organism itself but in the toxin. Skilled nursing is essential.

Diphtheria is preventable. Routine immunisation of infants has made it a rare disease in Europe and the USA. Immunity to the disease may be tested by the Schick test, where a small amount of toxin is injected into the skin of the forearm; a red reaction shows susceptibility to infection. It is possible for people to carry the organism without showing signs of the disease, especially in the nose, or in sores on the legs which are not recognised; but penicillin will eradicate the bacteria. The incubation period of diphtheria is between two and six days, and the isolation period ten days subject to negative cultures.

Diphyllobothrium Latum: a very long tapeworm which lives in freshwater fish, and people who eat undercooked fish. It may be up to 25 m long, and is found in North America, the Baltic countries, in Japan, Switzerland and Northern Italy, and other places where there are freshwater lakes.

Diplopia: double vision, caused by interference with the movements of the eyes in relation to each other, usually because of weakness or incoordination of the muscles that move the eyeball. The image of the observed object does not fall upon corresponding parts of the two retinae. It may be transient and of no importance, but may be the sign of various diseases.

Dipsomania: *see* Alcoholism.

Disc: usually used to mean an intervertebral disc. *See* Spinal Column.

Disinfection: the destruction of bacteria by antiseptics (q.v.).

Disinfestation: the destruction of parasites and pests that can spread disease, for example lice.

Dislocation: displacement of a part from its normal position, used particularly when a bone is displaced from its normal relationship with another bone, as in disarticulation of a joint.

Disorientation: difficulty in locating oneself correctly in space and time.

Dissection: cutting apart; used both of separating the tissues during a surgical operation and of studying the structure of a dead body. A specimen that has been dissected to show some special feature is called a 'dis-section'.

Disseminated Sclerosis: *see* Multiple Sclerosis.

Disulfiram (Antabuse): a drug which interferes with the metabolism of alcohol and produces an excess of acetaldehyde in the blood. This leads to the development of disagreeable symptoms which include headache, nausea and vomiting, increase in pulse rate, and even low blood pressure which may lead to collapse. It is used in the treatment of alcoholism in selected cases and must only be taken under medical supervision; if it is prescribed, patients must not take any alcohol at all, for the reactions are to a certain extent unpredictable and variable, and may be produced by very small amounts of drink.

Diuretics: substances which increase the flow of urine. There are two main groups, those which act on the beginning of the distal convoluted tubule of the kidney (q.v.) and those which act on the ascending loop of Henle, and are called loop diuretics. The first group includes the thiazides; they stop the reabsorption of sodium, and are used in the treatment of high blood pressure, perhaps in combination with other drugs, and mild heart failure. Loop diuretics are more powerful, and include frusemide and bumetanide, they are used in heart failure and kidney failure. Both groups may cause loss of potassium in the blood, but spironolactone, besides being a weak diuretic, causes retention of potassium and potentiates the action of thiazide and loop diuretics. Amiloride and triamterene also cause retention of potassium, and can be given in combination with the other diuretics instead of giving potassium supplements.

Diverticulitis: inflammation of a diverticulum (*see below*) of the colon. There is pain in left lower side of the abdomen with diarrhoea or constipation. If the disease is severe the inflamed diverticulum may rupture and produce peritonitis, it may excite an area of inflammation which involves surrounding structures and form an abscess, or the area of inflammation may cause a fistula or opening to develop into the bladder or vagina or an adjacent loop of bowel. Treatment in these cases is surgical. If there is a considerable area of inflammation a lump may be felt in the abdomen, and only at operation is the diagnosis made between inflammation and a malignant tumour. If there is no abscess or suspicion of malignancy the patient may be treated conservatively in bed with the appropriate antibiotics which should include metronidazole.

Diverticulosis: a condition of the colon, usually involving the descending and pelvic parts, in which the circular muscle of the wall of the gut gives way and allows pouches of mucous membrane to protrude. These are the diverticula. It is usually found in middle age and later, and is of itself without significance; but in a number of people there is pain and a feeling of obstruction, probably caused by spasm of the colon, and alternate constipation and loose motions. The pain is relieved by passing a motion. The diagnosis is made by barium enema. Treatment is by altering the diet to include more fibrous material such as coarse wheat bran and apples and oranges. If inflammation occurs in the diverticula, the condition is called diverticulitis (*see above*).

Diverticulum: a sac protruding from a larger hollow organ, commonly the intestine, where diverticula are found in the duodenum, the jejunum and the ileum, but most commonly in the colon. They consist of pouches of mucous membrane lining the gut which protrude through a weak place in the circular muscle of the intestinal wall.

DNA: deoxyribonucleic acid, an extremely long molecule made up of two strands wound in a double helix found in chromosomes. It is the key to cellular reproduction, for it carries the information necessary to form proteins and enzymes and a duplicate copy of itself.

Doctor: a courtesy title accorded to qualified medical practitioners, except surgeons. The reason for this is that the physician's degree is Doctor of Medicine, but the surgeon's is Master of Surgery. Some say, however, that the usage commemorates the surgeon's descent from the barber surgeons of the sixteenth century. In the USA the courtesy title is extended to surgeons and dentists.

Dolichocephalic: long-headed; cf. Brachycephalic.

Douche: the treatment of any part of the body by a continuous flow of medicated water. The term is most commonly used in describing cleansing of the vagina; but this kind of douching is not recommended.

Dover's Powder: a remedy composed of saltpetre, powdered opium, liquorice, ipecacuanha and tartaric acid, once one of the most popular medicines to relieve various diseases and pains. It was devised by the privateer Captain Thomas Dover (1660–1742), who was a physician; his other claim to fame rests upon his rescue of Alexander Selkirk, the original Robinson Crusoe, from the desert island of Juan Fernandez.

Down's Syndrome or Disease: a congenital defect associated with mental deficiency and the well-known 'mongoloid' appearance. It has been found that instead of the normal 46 chromosomes there are 47 which gives the condition its other name, trisomy 21. It is the most frequent cause of mental retardation; about 1.5 per 1000 live births show this condition, but about two-thirds of foetuses with trisomy 21 fail to reach term. The incidence rises with the age of the mother, but amniocentesis (q.v.) will show if the foetus is abnormal and is therefore offered to older mothers. Parents in most cases show no genetic abnormality; although the adult female suffering from Down's syndrome can become pregnant, the male is sterile. About 40% of cases have associated congenital defects of the heart. Even with the most devoted attention few sufferers from Down's syndrome survive beyond the age of 50. (John Down, English physician, 1828–96)

Dracunculus: the Guinea worm. Found in Africa and parts of Asia where it is dry and hot, the infection is acquired by drinking water in which there are water-fleas carrying the larvae. The larvae penetrate the gut wall, pass into the tissues and there develop into adult worms, a process which takes up to a year. The adult worm makes its way through the tissues of the body and comes to lie under the skin, usually in the legs, where the skin gives way and the female worm lays the larvae. The worm may be removed by winding it onto a stick an inch or two a day, being careful not to break it. Metronidazole or niridazole by mouth helps to kill the worm and aid the extraction. Prevention of infection rests on making sure that drinking water does not contain water-fleas.

Dramamine: the proprietary name of dimenhydrinate, an antihistamine used to prevent travel sickness. It is important to realise that it may produce drowsiness, and it is not wise to drive after taking a dose.

Dressings: in general, dressings are applied to prevent organisms infecting a wound, to absorb blood and discharges, and to keep wounds from contact with the clothes. Many wounds do not need to be dressed after they have been treated, except for protection, and the dressings should be as light as possible. It is sensible to cover wounds that have just been inflicted; the dressing should be of sterile gauze if possible, but freshly laundered linen will do very well. Bind such dressings firmly in place, and if bleeding shows through do not disturb the first dressing but cover it with a further dressing. More dressings are used than is necessary, particularly those combined with adhesive tape. If a cut is at first covered, leave it open to the air as soon as possible; do not leave it covered until the skin goes soggy and white.

Dropsy: *see* Oedema.

Drug Addiction: *see* Addiction.

Drugs: any chemical substance used for medicinal purposes is a drug. The supply of drugs is regulated in the United Kingdom; certain drugs may be sold without prescription, others only on a doctor's prescription. Most drugs have two names: the generic name, which is its official name approved by the Pharmacopoeia Commission, and the proprietary name given by the manufacturer. The Misuse of Drugs Act of 1971 controls the manufacture, supply and possession of certain drugs named under Class A, B and C, listed according to their potential harmfulness if misused, and the Misuse of Drugs Regulations of 1985 lays down the classes of people who are authorised to possess and supply controlled drugs, while acting in their professional capacities, and lists controlled drugs under five schedules which specify the requirements for handling and prescribing the drugs.

Drugs, the Commercial Aspect: a great deal is said and implied about the conduct of manufacturers of what are described as 'ethical' preparations, i.e. those proprietary drugs which can only be obtained on prescription (in contrast to medicines which can be bought across the counter by anyone). Among the arguments brought against the drug firms are: *(1)* They make inordinate profits. *(2)* The cost of successful drugs is kept high. *(3)* Advertising to doctors is importunate, vulgar and meretricious. *(4)* The actions of drugs are misleadingly described. *(5)* There is confusing and unnecessary proliferation of names; a simple drug may be given as many names as there are drug firms selling it. *(6)* Drugs may be put on the market before they have been exhaustively tested. The firms in question deny that their profits are inordinate; they point out that successful drugs have to bear the cost of research which produces unsuccessful as well as successful preparations; advertising is in line with modern practice, and is if anything restrained; and claim that it is only fair that they should be able to use their own brand names. The last argument is answered by the fact that medicines cannot be offered on the market until they have met the requirements of the Medicines Commission set up under the Medicines Act of 1968 (in the USA the Food and Drug Administration).

Ductless Glands: *see* Endocrine Glands.

Dumbness: the primary cause of inability to speak is deafness from birth, for a child who cannot hear is unable to learn to speak. Some cases are due to defects in the mechanism of voice production or to mental deficiency and the inability to learn; cretins may be deaf and mute. Diagnosis and treatment are matters for the specialists.

Duodenal Ulcer: *see* Peptic Ulcer.

Duodenum: *see* Intestine.

Dupuytren's Contracture: named after Guillaume Depuytren (1777–1835), the French surgeon who described it in the nineteenth century, it is a condition in which the fibrous tissue of the palm of the hand contracts and gradually pulls the little and fourth fingers into flexion so that they cannot be straightened. The other fingers may be affected in time, so that the hand becomes crippled. It is found in older men, particularly diabetics. The treatment is surgical.

Dura: the dura mater, the outermost and toughest of the three meningeal membranes which surround the brain and spinal cord.

Dwarfism: there are two main types of dwarfism, one in which there is disproportion of the limbs, and the other where the limbs and body are in perfect proportion. The common example of the first group is achondroplasia, which is inherited. The skull is large, and the trunk of normal size, but the limbs are very short and thick. There is no mental abnormality. The cause of the disease is not yet known, and there is no cure. There are other rare conditions which lead to short-limbed dwarfism. Deficiency in the secretion of growth hormone by the anterior pituitary gland may be responsible for the perfectly proportioned type of dwarfism, in which case, after diagnosis, replacement therapy may be undertaken. Short stature of course also runs in families, but deficiency of the thyroid hormone or coeliac disease may stunt growth.

Dysarthria: difficulty in speech due to impairment of articulation, which may be caused by disease of the muscles, nerves or structures involved in the mechanism of speech, or a defect in the central nervous system.

Dyscrasia: a disorder brought about by lack of balance of essential factors. Once applied to states attributed to a 'bad condition of the humours', the term is now used only in connection with disease affecting the blood cells.

Dysentery: a condition in which there is diarrhoea with the passage of mucus and blood, and abdominal pain. Now used to describe two types of infection, one by bacilli of the *Shigella* genus, named after the Japanese bacteriologist Kiyoshi Shiga (1870–1957) who first isolated the dysentery bacillus, and the other infection by *Entamoeba histolytica*, amoebic dysentery.

Bacillary dysentery may be caused by *Shigella sonnei*, the least dangerous, *Sh. flexneri* or *Sh. boydi*, which are less mild, and *Sh. dysenteriae* which is the most dangerous. Most cases in the United Kingdom are caused by *Sh. sonnei*. The onset of dysentery is acute, about four days after infection with a margin of three days on either side, and in a moderate attack there is colicky pain in the abdomen, diarrhoea, nausea, vomiting and fever; the abdominal pain becomes worse, and there is tenesmus – straining to pass motions when there is nothing to pass. Mucus and blood constitute what motions there are. In severe cases there may be irregularity of the pulse, chest infection, neuritis, inflammation of the eyes and effusion into the joints of the legs. The chief danger is loss of fluids and salts, which must be replaced quickly especially in children and the elderly (*see* Dehydration). Most cases start to recover spontaneously in a week, but in more severe cases ampicillin, trimethoprim or ciprofloxacin may be given. It is possible to carry the infection in the bowel for some time, but it usually clears spontaneously.

Amoebic dysentery is found in tropical and subtropical countries and, rarely, in Europe and North America. The onset is less acute than that of bacillary dysentery, starting with watery diarrhoea and colicky abdominal pain and proceeding to the passage of blood and mucus. This may improve, and then relapse, and continue for some weeks. The diagnosis is made by microscopic identification of the cysts of *E. histolytica* in the motions or by serological tests. The dangers are the development of peritonitis in severe cases, and the formation of an abscess in the liver. Treatment as in all cases of dysentery is directed first to the correction of dehydration, and then metronidazole is the drug of choice; but if this is not successful diloxanide furoate may be used, which is active against chronic amoebiasis, or the older remedy emetine hydrochloride. People may carry and excrete the cysts of *E. histolytica* without being troubled by the disease, and in fact it is said that about one-tenth of the world's population is infected. However, infection commonly disappears after two or three years, although it may last for twenty. The disease takes more than three weeks to develop after infection, and may appear a long time after a traveller returns home after visiting a country where the amoeba is prevalent.

Dysentery is spread by poor standards of hygiene, for the infectious organisms are excreted in the motions and can be carried on the hands, by flies or in the dust. Carriers can be infective without being aware that they carry the disease.

Dyslexia: a defect in development in which there is an inability to read, not accompanied by intellectual impairment. In some cases a cause can be found, such as imperfect vision or hearing, but in others the reason is not understood. The condition usually comes to light in childhood, and if a dyslexic person does learn to read the spelling continues to be erratic.

Dysmenorrhoea: painful menstrual periods.

Dyspareunia: pain on sexual intercourse due either to physical or psychological causes.

Dyspepsia: discomfort in the process of digestion, which may be due to many reasons ranging from over-indulgence to disease of the stomach, for example peptic ulcer, intestinal disorder, or gall-bladder disease. If it persists it should be brought to the doctor's attention.

Dysphagia: difficulty in swallowing.

Dysphasia: impediment in speaking due to damage in the brain, in right-handed people on the left side and in left-handed people the right. There is difficulty in understanding speech and in writing and reading. *See* Speech Disorders.

Dysplasia: abnormality of development.

Dyspnoea: difficulty in breathing.

Dystrophy: wasting; condition brought about by defective nutrition.

Dysuria: pain or difficulty in passing urine.

E

Ear: the organ of hearing and of balance. It is divided into three parts: outer, middle and inner. The outer ear includes the visible ear, the skin-covered flap of cartilage called the pinna whose function is to collect sounds, and the canal through which sounds are conducted to the eardrum. The canal has an outer part of cartilage and an inner lining of skin which has hairs and glands which secrete wax in amounts that vary with the individual; it passes through bone to the middle ear, which is not visible because it lies behind the eardrum, a greyish thin membrane called the tympanic membrane which picks up sound vibrations.

The middle ear lies in a small cavity in the temporal bone which is continuous with the air cells in the mastoid bone; the cavity measures 15 mm × about 5 mm × about 5 mm. The width is variable and irregular, narrowing from 5 or 6 mm at the top to about 4 mm at the bottom; it is only about 2 mm opposite the middle of the eardrum, which is normally slightly drawn inwards, and set at an angle of 55° to the external canal. The important contents of the middle ear are the ossicles – a tiny chain of bones which transmits the movements of the drum to the organ of hearing in the inner ear. There are three bones in the chain: the malleus (hammer), incus (anvil) and stapes (stirrup). They are jointed together and are connected to the bone surrounding the middle ear by three ligaments, and are so arranged that there is a 22:1 increase in power and a 22:1 decrease in movement between the larger eardrum and the small oval window where the footplate of the stapes connects with the inner ear. There are two muscles in the middle ear, the tensor tympani which, as its name implies, keeps the eardrum drawn inwards, and the stapedius, which pulls the stapedius bone away from the oval window. These muscles, particularly the stapedius, damp the oscillation of the ossicles so that they prevent very loud noises from injuring the ear; if the stapedius is not functioning properly loud noises produce a very uncomfortable sensation. The Eustachian (auditory) tube runs from the upper part of the throat to the middle ear, so that the air pressure is kept equal on each side of the drum. If it becomes blocked, as it may in a common cold, the vibrations of the drum are dampened because the air in the middle ear is absorbed and atmospheric pressure becomes greater than the pressure in the middle ear. Hearing is then diminished and distorted.

The inner ear is made up of the organs of hearing and balance, which are systems of canals in the hardest part of the temporal bone, filled with fluid. There are two components of the system, the bony labyrinth and the membranous labyrinth lying inside; the fluid inside the membranous labyrinth is called endolymph, that between the bony and membranous labyrinths perilymph. The organ of hearing is called the cochlea, from its resemblance to a snail's shell. It contains a membrane called the basilar membrane which runs round inside the spiral and separates it into two spiral passages, upper and lower. The upper passage is again separated into two by another membrane, the vestibular membrane. Fluid filling the upper passage, the scala vestibuli, is set in motion by the movements of the stapes in the oval window, which is the lower termination of the scala vestibuli. The waves pass across the vestibular membrane into the cochlear duct, the middle spiral passage, and so reach the basilar membrane. Upon the basilar membrane is the organ of Corti (Alfonso Corti, 1822–76, Italian anatomist) which consists of rows of cells carrying fine hairs covered by the membrana tectoria like a soft roof. The hair cells are connected to the fibres of the acoustic nerve through the spiral ganglia. When the sound vibrations carried from the eardrum by the ossicles of the middle ear to the oval window disturb the fluid in the cochlea, and so move the basilar membrane, the hair cells move against the tectorial membrane and impulses are set up in the auditory nerve and carried to the brain. The sound waves are dissipated after they have set the basilar membrane in motion by the fluid in the scala tympani, the lowest spiral in the cochlea, which lies below the basilar membrane and opens into the middle ear cavity at the round window, covered by a membrane free to vibrate. The hair cells of the organ of Corti can be damaged by prolonged exposure to loud noise. The organ of balance is made up of three semicircular canals which lie in different planes of space. They arise from the central part of the labyrinthine system called the vestibule, from which on the other side the cochlea arises. They each have an ampulla, or dilated sac, in which there are hair cells, which sense the motion of the endolymphatic fluid in the semicircular canals and convey impulses to the brain through the vestibular part of the auditory nerve. In the vestibule lie two other structures, the saccule and the utricle, in which more hair cells detect gravitational forces. These hair cells carry on them otoliths, small deposits of calcium carbonate. The central connections of the organ of balance include nerve fibres running to the nerve cells controlling the muscles that move the eyeball, which assist the eye to remain fixed on a still object although the head and neck may move. Disturbance of the semicircular canals results in vertigo, nausea and vomiting (*see* Motion Sickness).

Earache: *see* Otitis.

ECG: *see* Electrocardiogram.

Echocardiography: the use of ultrasound to examine the heart; both the anatomy and function of the heart and its valves can be studied.

Eclampsia: fits or coma occurring in late pregnancy, associated with high blood pressure, oedema and the passage of protein in the urine. Pre-eclampsia is the state preceding this grave crisis, and may last for days or weeks, during which the blood pressure rises; if protein is found in the urine, the outlook is more serious. The treatment of pre-eclampsia is delivery of the child as soon as possible; the condition is dangerous both to mother and child, but signs that it is developing can be detected by regular antenatal examination, and eclampsia prevented.

Ectoderm: the embryo develops from three primary germinal layers, the outermost of which is the ectoderm, the middle the mesoderm and the inner the endoderm. The ectoderm gives rise to the skin, the nervous system and the organs of special sense.

Ectomorph: the type of bodily development in which ectodermal tissues predominate; there is a large surface area compared with the amount of muscle and bone, so that the figure is spare. Other types are endomorph and mesomorph (q.v.).

Ectopic Gestation: a condition in which the fertilised ovum becomes implanted outside the uterus, often in the Fallopian tube (q.v.) where the pregnancy may rupture and cause dangerous bleeding.

Ectropion: the eversion, or turning out, of the eyelid so that the conjunctiva is left exposed.

Eczema: a skin inflammation in which there is the formation of small vesicles with subsequent weeping, scaling and crusting. It is virtually synonymous with dermatitis (q.v.) but eczema is often used to describe inflammation of the skin when the cause is within the body. There is an hereditary form of eczema that is common, called atopic eczema, affecting up to 3% of children, which is recognised as a defect in the immunological system but is poorly understood. It is often accompanied by asthma or hay fever. The subjects are sensitive to a number of substances such as certain foods or house dust, but these are not the same as those usually found in allergic reactions. The condition usually shows itself by the time the child is six months old, and the symptom is itching, beginning on the face. As the child begins to move about, the skin of the knees and elbows becomes involved, together with the wrists and ankles. With increasing age the condition usually disappears, and is no longer apparent by the teens, although it may persist or show itself later in life by abnormal reactions to skin irritants. Treatment obviously starts with avoiding anything that is clearly setting up a reaction in the skin; emulsifying cream may be used instead of soap and to keep the skin moist. The condition varies from time to time, and in the more severe phase steroid creams may be used, but in a mild form, for example 1% hydrocortisone cream. It should be used for as short a time as possible. If the skin becomes infected the appropriate antibiotic should be used.

EEG: *see* Electro-encephalography.

Effusion: an outpouring of fluid into the tissues or a cavity in the body, for example into the knee or the pleural space.

Elastic Stockings: used in cases of varicose veins or oedema of the legs. They are made with various degrees of elasticity according to the support needed, and should be fitted by an expert.

Elbow: the joint formed by the bone of the upper arm, the humerus, and the two bones of the forearm, the radius and ulna. It is a hinge joint; rotation of the radius on the ulna takes place between these two bones and is not part of the movement at the elbow joint, which is formed mainly by the hook-shaped olecranon process of the ulna and the pulley-shaped trochlear groove on the humerus. The facet upon the head of the radius rests in contact with the round capitulum of the humerus, and the radius is bound more strongly to the ulna than to the humerus. The bony points that can be felt through the skin are the inner and outer, or medial and lateral, epicondyles of the humerus, and behind the joint the point of the elbow formed by the olecranon – the upper part of the ulna. The long axis of the upper arm is not in line with the long axis of the forearm when the elbow is extended and the palm of the hand open forwards because the transverse axis of the joint slopes downwards from outer to inner side, but the bones come to lie in the same line when the palm of the hand is turned round so that it faces backwards with the radius turned round the ulna. The angle between the long axis of the upper arm and that of the forearm with the elbow extended and the palm of the hand forwards is called the carrying angle, and differs in the male and female, in the male being about $173°$ and in the female $167°$. This is thought to account for the fact that women may have difficulty in throwing.

The elbow is bound together by powerful ligaments. The ulnar nerve passes behind the inner epicondyle of the humerus, and can be felt between the inner bony prominence and the point of the elbow; there is nothing between the nerve and the skin, and a blow here – on the funny-bone – produces pain and pins and needles all the way down the forearm and into the hand. There is a bursa overlying the olecranon which sometimes becomes inflamed and swollen, particularly if the arm is continually rested on the point of the elbow.

Fractures of the elbow are sustained as the result of direct injury, and as afterwards the elbow may remain stiff, or at least full movement be restricted, the fracture is immobilised so that the elbow is half bent, its most useful position. Dislocations can occur, the commonest being forwards and to the outer side, but the ligaments on the inner side of the joint are so strong that they may tear away part of the bone, and as the lower part of the humerus comes forward it may break the coronoid process, the upper end of the hooked part of the olecranon; dislocations are rarely simple. Tennis elbow is pain felt over the outer aspect of the elbow, where the extensor muscles of the forearm take origin from the lateral epicondyle of the humerus. It is the result of small tears in the muscle and over-use, and the treatment is rest. If a locally tender point can be found, injection with local anaesthetic may help, followed by injection of corticosteroids. Golfer's elbow is felt on the inner side, over the origin of the flexor muscles of the forearm. In both cases it may be worthwhile to review the player's technique which is often at fault.

Electric Shock: the amount of damage an electric shock produces depends on many factors, which are only partly dependent on the strength of the current. It is sadly true that the type of current most likely to injure people lies within the range that is best for transmission of electrical power and that cannot be avoided. But a current received through dry clothing is less dangerous than when the clothes are wet, or one received through the bare skin; if the body is earthed the shock is worse than if insulation is provided by rubber-soled shoes. The most dangerous room in the house is the bathroom, for if a shock is sustained through faulty wiring or faulty apparatus and the body is naked, wet and possibly earthed through the bath tub or the plumbing, the shock will be in many cases fatal. The effects of an electric current passing through the body fall into two classes: one, which can be called the shock effect, is not dependent on high or low voltage; the other is the effect of heating the body tissues, which produces burns and is more marked with high voltages. Shock leads to contraction of the muscles and interference with the rhythm of the heart and breathing, depending on the point of contact and the path followed by the current. The victim may be unable to let go of the object producing the shock if the current is alternating, and it is essential for the rescuer to switch off the current or, if this is impossible, to pad the hands with a dry cloth and stand on something dry. If the victim is in contact with high voltage, however, this will not help, and any touch is likely to result in two victims instead of one. If, after a shock, the heart and breathing appear to have stopped, external cardiac massage and artificial respiration are essential until skilled help arrives, for it is possible that the heart has gone into atrial fibrillation which is reversible or has stopped in asystole and can be started beating again. The same holds true of people who have been struck by lightning, which is direct current of high voltage: survival may depend on speedy application of cardiac massage and artificial respiration. Electrical burns are treated surgically, but may take a long time to heal; and it may be found that contraction of the muscles that lie around the spine has been violent enough to fracture vertebrae.

Electrocardiogram: an electrical record taken from the heart. When the heart muscle contracts and relaxes, changes in electrical potential are produced which may be picked up by electrodes placed on the surface of the body. The patient lies at rest and electrodes are applied to the skin; the recorder traces the changes of potential between the electrodes. The physician can change the leads in use as advisable, for various combinations are used to elucidate the diagnosis which is made from the shape of the tracing on the recorder. The record is commonly referred to as an ECG.

Electroconvulsant Therapy: a form of treatment in psychiatry introduced in the 1930s, in which an electric current is passed through the brain to produce loss of consciousness accompanied by convulsions. Being based on the (false) theory that epilepsy and schizophrenia were antagonistic conditions, and that one could not exist in the presence of the other, it was originally used in cases of schizophrenia; but later it was found to be effective in cases of depression, and continued in use until the range of modern antidepressant drugs were introduced, since when ECT has been confined to rare severe cases which do not respond to other treatment.

Electrode: the medium by which an electric current is passed between a conductor and the object to which the current is to be applied, or through which it is picked up. The anode is positive, the cathode negative.

Electro-encephalography: electrodes applied to the scalp pick up electrical currents arising from the activity of the brain. The precise processes underlying the production of these currents are not clear, except that they are a summation of the activity of perhaps millions of neurones. A basic rhythm is present when the eyes are closed in the occipital, that is the rear, part of the brain; this is the alpha rhythm with a period between 8 and 13 cycles a second. Beta rhythms are picked up from the vertex, the top of the head, and in front; they are faster than 13 a second. Delta rhythms are slow, less than 4 a second; they are normal in sleep and in children, but abnormal in conscious adults. Abnormal EEG records are useful in the diagnosis of many conditions, especially epilepsy, but unfortunately do not help in the localisation of tumours, where other techniques must be used.

Electrolyte: a substance that forms a solution through which an electric current can be passed, because the molecules break up into ions, that is atoms or groups of atoms with an electrical charge, those positively charged being cations and those negatively charged anions. If an electrical current is passed through the solution the cations are attracted to the negative electrode and the anions to the positive.

Electromyography: when a muscle contracts, changes of electrical potential are set up. These can be recorded through electrodes and the fluctuations inscribed on paper as an electromyogram or EMG.

Elephantiasis: gross swelling of the legs or genitalia caused by blockage of the lymphatic vessels by filariae, small worms about the size of a thread, transmitted by mosquitoes. There are a number of filariae, of which *Wuchereria bancrofti* and *Brugia malayi* cause elephantiasis. *See* Filariasis.

Elixir: a sweet liquid mixture containing a medicinal substance made up with alcohol or chloroform water.

Embolism: the blocking of an artery by material carried in the bloodstream from another part of the body. The material may be a fragment of blood clot, perhaps from a diseased valve in the heart or a clotted vein in the leg, a piece of tumour, a mass of bacteria, globules of fat or bubbles of air. The immediate result is that the blood supply to a segment of tissue is cut off, so that the tissue dies. If the part affected is not essential to life, a scar forms to replace the dead tissue. The process of tissue death following an embolism is called infarction, and the dead tissue an infarct. If the material blocking the artery contains bacteria an abscess will form, and if it contains cancer cells a secondary growth will develop. Fat embolism may occur after severe fractures, and air embolism can follow wounds of the head and neck.

Embolus: the material giving rise to an embolism. *See above*.

Embryo: the developing organism; in man the word is used of the growing organism between the second and eighth weeks of life, after which it is called the foetus.

Emetics: drugs which cause vomiting. The induction of vomiting after ingestion of a poison must only be tried if the patient is fully conscious and the poison is not corrosive or due to a distillate of petroleum. The only drug recommended is ipecacuanha, and it should be given within four hours. It may be useful in children, where the passage of a gastric tube to empty the stomach is impractical, and paediatric ipecacuanha emetic mixture is given in doses of 10 ml for children 6–18 months old, 15 ml for those older; the adult dose is 30 ml.

Emetine: one of the active principles of ipecacuanha, formerly used in the treatment of amoebic dysentery but now reserved for cases resistant to metronidazole or tinidazole.

Emphysema: the abnormal presence of air in the tissues. Used mainly of a condition of the lungs in which the alveolar air spaces are grossly enlarged, and found in conjunction with asthma and chronic bronchitis, being associated with cigarette smoking and air pollution. The main symptom is breathlessness, which, developing insidiously, may end with the patient unable to breathe adequately at rest, for the alveoli become so damaged that the exchange of gases between the blood and the air is barely adequate. Treatment is difficult, for the anatomical changes cannot be remedied. Obviously patients should not smoke, and infections of the lungs, which are likely to occur from time to time, must be treated. Drugs which dilate the air passages such as salbutamol may be useful, used in an inhaler, and in some cases corticosteroids may help. Physiotherapy and breathing exercises may assist, and in severe cases support may be found in the use of oxygen.

Empyema: an internal abscess, usually used of a collection of pus in the pleural cavity, consequent upon pneumonia, abscess or tumour of the lung, bronchiectasis, septic wounds of the chest, or (rarely now) tuberculosis. The treatment is aimed at draining the pus, getting rid of the infection and eliminating the space. Usually this can be achieved by the use of antibiotics and a drain inserted through the chest wall, but in difficult cases it may be necessary to undertake surgical operation.

Encephalitis: inflammation of the brain, usually the result of virus infection. Many viruses are known to produce this condition, and they vary in different countries. The most common in the United Kingdom is the mumps virus, followed by the echoviruses, Coxsackie viruses, measles virus, herpes simplex virus, which causes a dangerous encephalitis, the herpes zoster virus, the Epstein–Barr virus of infective mononucleosis, and adenoviruses. In some cases the illness does not show itself for a week or so after the infection has caused other signs: in measles or rubella, for example, one or two weeks after the rash. Encephalitis causes headache, neck stiffness, vomiting, and fever, just as in the case of meningitis, with confusion, clouded consciousness, and sometimes convulsions; various paralyses may develop. Treatment in many cases is difficult because of the lack of drugs working against viruses, but acyclovir and to a lesser extent vidarabine are active against herpes viruses.

Encephalography: making a radiological examination of the brain. It commonly referred to pneumo-encephalography, an outmoded method of X-ray examination of the brain, in which the ventricles were outlined by the injection of air or gas such as oxygen into the space occupied by the cerebrospinal fluid. The air was introduced by lumbar puncture.

Encephalopathy: a disease of the brain caused by degenerative process, or any condition except infection, for example high blood pressure, or repeated injury as in boxing.

Endemic: disease which is always present in the population, such as malaria in West Africa.

Endocarditis: inflammation of the membrane lining the heart, the endocardium. In an acute case, the organism may be *Staphylococcus aureus* or *Streptococcus pneumoniae*, and the infection may be fatal. There may be no previous history of heart trouble or defect in the heart. The subacute case is often due to *Streptococcus viridans* infection, and there is usually a history of trouble due to a heart defect such as congenital heart disease or aortic valvular disease. At one time rheumatic heart disease was the main underlying condition, but this has become comparatively uncommon, and while subacute endocarditis was a disease of younger people the age has now increased and patients are likely to be in their fifties. Other underlying causes of the infection may be cardiac valve surgery and drug addiction. Patients suffering from subacute endocarditis complain of ill-defined general malaise, a low-grade fever and various aches and pains. The diagnosis in most cases is made by a blood culture, for the infecting organisms are present in the bloodstream; when they have been identified the appropriate antibiotic can be given. Infection may be found to have occurred after dental treatment, or as a consequence of dental sepsis; it is therefore sensible to cover dental treatment in those susceptible to endocarditis by prophylactic antibiotics.

Endocrine Glands: those glands which do not have a duct but secrete their products directly into the bloodstream, as opposed to those glands which have a duct and can excrete their products directly to the place where they are to act, the exocrine glands. The secretions of the endocrine glands are called hormones, which through their actions play a fundamental part in the control of metabolism, growth, sexual development and function, and intellectual and emotional development; a proper balance of hormones is essential for life. The principal endocrine glands are the pituitary, hypothalamus, thyroid, parathyroid, adrenals, testes, ovaries, pancreas, kidneys, and certain parts of the intestinal tract and the brain. The function of the thymus gland in the neck is not fully understood, although it plays a part in the immunological process; Galen (AD 131–201) believed it was the seat of the soul. Descartes (1596–1650) thought that the pineal gland in the brain was the seat of the soul, but so far modern work has only shown that it influences sexual development in rats by secreting a hormone called melatonin. For fuller consideration of the ductless glands see under their separate headings.

Endoderm: the inner cell layer in the embryo from which are derived the digestive and urinary tracts and the lungs and airways.

Endometriosis: a condition in which the type of tissue that normally lines the uterus, the endometrium, is found in abnormal places in the abdomen. It is not certain how these deposits of endometrial tissue arise, but the common places where they occur include the surface of the ovaries, the peritoneum covering the bladder and pelvic colon, on the round ligaments of the uterus, at the umbilicus, on operation scars in the lower abdomen, and in the tissues between the vagina and the rectum. It causes dysmenorrhoea, pain in the lower abdomen, backache, dyspareunia, and if it involves the bowel, obstruction. Symptoms do not usually appear before the age of 30. The diagnosis is greatly helped by endoscopic examination of the lower abdomen through the laparoscope; treatment if needed may be by the use of a progestogen such as norethisterone, by the contraceptive pill, or by danazol, which stops the secretion of the gonadotrophic hormone by the pituitary gland.

Endometritis: inflammation of the lining of the uterus, which may follow abortion, criminal or otherwise, parturition, gonorrhoea, gynaecological operation, or may occur in old age. Treatment is by antibiotics according to the infecting organisms.

Endomorph: the type of development in which the endo-dermal tissues predominate – the body is round and soft. *See* Ectomorph, Mesomorph.

Endoscopy: the examination through an optical ins-trument of the interior of the body; the interior of the bladder is seen through the cystoscope, the lower part of the gut through the sigmoidoscope, the stomach through the gastroscope, the trachea and bronchi through the bronchoscope, the interior of the abdominal cavity through the laparoscope, and the interior of the knee joint is examined through the arthroscope. It is increasingly pos-sible to carry out surgical operations, through endoscopes, which now use fibre-optics, are internally illuminated and flexible, and such operations have earned the name 'keyhole surgery'.

Endothelium: a layer of cells derived from mesoderm which lines the blood vessels, lymphatic vessels, and the sinusoids of the bone marrow, liver and spleen, where it forms the reticulo-endothelial system. It also lines the peritoneum, and the abdominal cavity, being composed of simple squamous cells which slide easily over each other. *Cf.* Epithelium.

Endotoxin: a toxin found inside bacteria which is liberated into the tissues when the organism disintegrates, as opposed to exotoxins, which are secreted by the intact bacteria.

Endotracheal Tube: a tube passed into the trachea or windpipe through the vocal cords in order to establish a clear airway in an unconscious patient. It is used in the administration of anaesthetics, and can be introduced through the mouth or nose with the help of a laryngoscope. It commonly has an inflatable cuff round the end which seals off the trachea and prevents foreign matter such as blood or vomit reaching the lungs while the cough reflex is suppressed by the anaesthetic. The passage of an endotracheal tube is made easier by the use of a muscle-relaxing drug.

Enema: liquid injected into the lower bowel. Used to evacuate faeces from the rectum, or in radiography, when the enema contains barium, to outline the rectum and colon. Soft soap was formerly used for enemas, but it inflames the intestinal lining and is best avoided in favour of phosphate or sodium citrate. Retention enemas containing sulphasalazine or mesalazine are used in the treatment of ulcerative colitis.

Engagement: a term used in obstetrics. It means that the head of the foetus or, if it is not a head presentation, the presenting part has entered the brim of the pelvis.

ENT: abbreviation for ear, nose and throat.

Entamoeba Histolytica: an amoeba found in the large intestine in cases of amoebic dysentery. It is small, and when examined under the microscope usually contains red blood cells on which it has fed. It reproduces by splitting in two, and forms cysts if circumstances are unfavourable. The cysts remain alive for some weeks outside the body of the host, providing that the temperature is above 5°C and there is moisture in the environment. They are killed by temperatures above 50°C and by being dried. When they are eaten in contaminated food they pass through the stomach unchanged, but in the intestines the cyst wall disintegrates and the amoebae escape. The cysts contain four nuclei, and each nucleus splits into two, so that each cyst introduces eight amoebae into the host, which is usually human but may be monkey or ape. The amoebae are susceptible to the drugs metronidazole and tinidazole, and the cysts to diloxanide furoate. *See* Dysentery.

Enteric-Coated: the name for pills with a special coating to prevent their absorption until they reach the intestine.

Enteric Fever: typhoid and paratyphoid fever.

Enteritis: inflammation of the intestine, usually applied to the small intestine.

Enterobiasis: infection with threadworms (pinworms). *See* Worms.

Enterostomy: an artificial opening made into the intestine through the abdominal wall to link it with the exterior, or with another part of the alimentary tract as in gastro-enterostomy, a bypass made to short-circuit the duodenum in some cases of ulceration when a gastrectomy is not practicable. An enterostomy discharging onto the surface may be used as a temporary measure in cases of intestinal obstruction or permanently when the lower bowel has to be removed.

Enterotoxin: an exotoxin produced by staphylococci, which is comparatively heat stable. If eaten in food which has been colonised by staphylococci it produces violent vomiting and diarrhoea, which comes on suddenly and may last a day. The staphylococci themselves are not poisonous.

Enterovirus: one of a group of viruses which produce disease and enter by the alimentary tract. The group includes the Coxsackie viruses, echoviruses and the poliovirus.

Entropion: a condition in which the eyelid is turned in

towards the eyeball as the result of scarring or disease. *Cf*. Ectropion.

Enuresis: bed-wetting (q.v.).

Enzymes: biological catalysts responsible for most of the processes of metabolism both inside and outside the cells. (A catalyst is a substance in chemistry which accelerates the speed of a reaction without itself being part of the final product.) The enzymes are proteins, and are specific for one reaction or for a well-defined group of similar reactions. The speed of the reactions depends on the amount of enzyme present and the amount of the substance involved in the reaction, on temperature, the acid–base balance and a number of co-enzymes, inhibitors and activators. Many of the co-enzymes are related to vitamins, which explains why vitamin deficiencies alter metabolism so profoundly; but our knowledge of enzymes, although growing all the time, is far from complete.

Eosinophil: a white cell found in the blood which readily takes up the stain eosin when stained with Leishman's stain (Sir William Leishman, 1865–1926), a mixture of methylene blue and eosin. Eosinophil cells are increased in allergic states and in infestation with some worms, and the state of having an increased number of eosinophils in the blood is called eosinophilia.

Epanutin: the trade name for phenytoin sodium (q.v.).

Ephedrine: an alkaloid isolated from the plant *Ephedra equisetina*, or Ma Huang, used in Chinese medicine for many hundreds of years, but only known in the West since 1928. It is a sympathomimetic drug, that is to say it imitates the action of the sympathetic part of the autonomic nervous system. It increases the blood pressure, increases the heart rate, dilates the air passages and the pupil of the eye, constricts the mucous membranes of the nose and throat, and is active when taken by mouth. It is mainly used now in the form of nasal drops to relieve congestion of the nose, and in cold and cough cures, but must not be used by those who are taking MAOI (q.v.)

antidepressant drugs or men suffering from an enlarged prostate in whom it may cause acute retention of urine.

Epidemic: the occurrence of a number of cases of similar illness in excess of normal expectation.

Epidemiology: is concerned with the occurrence of disease in populations, and provides the scientific basis for the practice of public health and community medicine.

Epidermis: *see* Skin.

Epididymis: a structure lying on the rear aspect of each testis consisting of a head, body and tail. It is formed from a thin duct about 6 m long, coiled upon itself and connected to the back of the testis by 20 little ducts through which spermatozoa travel from the testis to be stored in the epididymis. From its tail emerges the ductus deferens through which the spermatozoa eventually reach the urethra and penis. It may be the site of infection, called epididymitis, which is often linked with infection of the testis (epididymo-orchitis). Cysts often form in the epididymis, especially in middle age. They are not dangerous.

Epigastrium: the upper part of the abdomen that lies within the angle of the ribs over the stomach.

Epiglottis: a leaf-shaped piece of cartilage covered with mucous membrane that lies at the back of the tongue over the opening of the larynx, the entrance to the air passages. In the larynx is the glottis, the vocal apparatus – the cords and the space between them. The epiglottis diverts food and drink from the back of the tongue towards the oesophagus, the food passage, and covers the entrance to the larynx during the act of swallowing. If a particle of food is inhaled, or there is anything wrong with the muscular co-ordination of the throat, the food 'goes down the wrong way', entering the glottis and irritating the vocal cords so that a paroxysm of coughing is set up, usually with a spasm of the cords and consequent difficulty in drawing a breath. *See* Choking.

Epilepsy: the 'falling sickness', in which there is an abnormality of brain function which shows itself as periodic paroxysmal activity resulting in a momentary loss of attention or consciousness in the minor form of the disease, 'petit mal', or prolonged loss of consciousness associated with generalised convulsions in major epilepsy or 'grand mal'. Psychomotor and autonomic equivalent attacks can occur. Recently a new classification has been drawn up, which describes petit mal attacks as absence seizures, grand mal as tonic-clonic seizures, and psychomotor or temporal lobe attacks as complex partial seizures. Petit mal attacks or absence seizures start during childhood, and it is rare for them to persist into adult life. The electro-encephalogram shows abnormality. Grand mal or tonic-clonic seizures begin with the tonic phase, during which the body becomes rigid and the patient falls. The tongue may be bitten and there may be incontinence, and the face becomes suffused with blood. This stage is followed by the clonic phase, when the body jerks with generalised convulsions. When this passes, the patient slowly wakes, at first confused, and then becoming fully conscious. The electro-encephalogram shows widespread electrical activity during an attack, and in many cases abnormal activity in between attacks. Partial epileptic attacks can occur, in which the abnormality is confined to one part of the brain, the normal function of which is mirrored in the attack, so that for example one side of the face twitches, or the thumb and index fingers move, and the movement spreads into the arm. Commonly the temporal lobe of the brain is involved, and although sometimes able to continue with simple activity the patient feels unreal and dizzy. There may be hallucinations; consciousness may be dimmed, and the face may twitch into grimaces. Often the attack will start with an uncomfortable feeling in the abdomen and chest, and indeed grand mal attacks in general may start after a premonitory feeling or aura which gives warning of an impending attack.

The only things that can be done for anyone having an epileptic fit are: remove anything nearby that could cause injury, turn the subject face down with the head to one side, and slap the back so that the tongue comes forward. There is no need to call an ambulance unless there is an injury, nor any need to try to force anything between the teeth.

In some cases there is an underlying cause for the development of epilepsy, but in most cases the reason is not understood. The onset of the condition will call for full investigation, and, unless there is some condition that can be set right, drugs are used to control the seizures. They are chosen according to the type of attack, and the dose is slowly adjusted upwards until the fits are controlled or until signs of overdosage appear. Carbamazepine is used for partial seizures and tonic-clonic attacks; phenytoin is also used, but has rather more unwanted effects; sodium valproate has recently been introduced but may have adverse effects on the liver and possibly the pancreas; primidone is converted to phenobarbitone in the body, and phenobarbitone itself, which has been used for years in the control of grand mal, is liable to produce drowsiness. Drugs used in absence attacks, or petit mal, are sodium valproate and ethosuximide. New drugs are being introduced, based on the finding of substances which, acting as transmitters of nervous impulses, excite or inhibit the activity of cells capable of developing spontaneous discharges. The inhibitory substances are gamma-aminobutyric acid and glycine, both amino-acids, and the exciting agents glutamate and aspartate. Drugs are being found to increase the effects of the inhibitory substances and reduce the effects of the excitatory ones. It should be noted that anticonvulsant drugs can interact with other drugs, possibly the most important interaction being between phenytoin and hormonal contraceptive pills, the action of which is impaired.

Many prominent men have suffered from epilepsy, but the social consequences of the condition can be grave; there may be difficulty in gaining employment, and the kinds of jobs that can be done may be restricted. Driving heavy goods vehicles is not permitted, although driving licences can be issued for motor cars if the subject has not had a grand mal attack for two years, or if the attacks have taken place asleep, the attacks have only been while asleep for a period of three years, and if driving a vehicle is not likely to be a source of danger to the public. Taking charge of moving machinery, working at heights or flying aircraft is obviously dangerous. If attacks have been controlled, the question may arise of stopping the drugs. Unfortunately no firm answer can be given, for there is at present no way of telling whether the attacks will recur. Epilepsy is inherited as an autosomal dominant characteristic, and children of those with grand mal may show abnormal electro-encephalograms although they do not necessarily show any signs of epilepsy. The marriage of two people with epilepsy should be undertaken only after the most careful thought.

Epinephrine: a hormone produced by the medulla of the suprarenal glands. *See* Adrenaline.

Epiphysis: the end of a long bone, separated from the shaft during growth by a plate of cartilage laying down new bone. When the individual is fully grown the cartilage disappears and the epiphysis fuses with the shaft.

Episiotomy: an incision made in the perineum during childbirth to prevent the mother being torn. An incision is under control, whereas a tear is not, and if it is necessary for the vaginal opening to be enlarged to allow the baby free passage, an episiotomy can be made under general or local anaesthetic. The incision is made starting in the midline and extending back to one or other side of the anus so that rectum, anus and the muscles controlling it are left intact. A tear sustained in childbirth may damage these structures and leave the mother incontinent. The episiotomy is repaired after birth.

Epispadias: a congenital deformity in which the urethra opens on the upper surface of the penis. In the worst form there is a gutter running the length of the penis. There may also be *ectopia vesicae*, where the bladder and front wall of the abdomen have failed to close. The treatment is surgical, the abnormal structures being reconstructed.

Epistaxis: nose bleeding. It may occur as the result of inflammation of the nose, injury, or – mainly in children – foreign bodies in the nose. Commonly, however, a small vessel just inside the nostril gives way for no apparent reason. Treatment therefore is to loosen the clothes round the neck, sit over a bowl or the sink and pinch the nostrils together below the bony part of the nose for five minutes by the clock. This may be repeated, and very often is successful. Blowing the nose will probably start the bleeding again. If bleeding persists, the doctor may pack the nose with gauze, and if this fails it may be necessary for the ENT surgeon to use diathermy to cauterise the bleeding point.

Epithelium: the sheet of cells that covers the body surface, both within and without. It develops from all three types of primordial germ cells: ectoderm, mesoderm and endoderm. The cells making up the epithelium lie on a basement membrane, and adhere firmly to each other. It is classified as simple when it is one cell thick, and stratified when there is more than one cell making up the layer. The shape may be squamous – like a scale – cubical or columnar; a professor of anatomy once said that they were like apples, pears and bricks. The layer may be of one type of cell, or mixed, in which case it is called transitional. Squamous epithelium allows diffusion, and lines the alveoli, the air sacs of the lungs. It lines moist surfaces where resistance to friction is necessary, such as the mouth, throat, oesophagus and vagina. When it is the outer layer of a stratified epithelium it can become full of keratin and forms the skin, hair and nails. Simple cubical or columnar epithelium is capable of absorption, and lines the small intestine. Cubical epithelial cells can have a 'brush border', or cilia, hairlike processes which vibrate, and are present in the air passages, where they are able to move sputum up from the lungs to the throat, and in the Fallopian tubes, where they move the egg from the ovary into the uterus. Transitional epithelium is able to resist the composition of urine, and lines the urinary system. Epithelial cells form secretory tissues, such as the sweat glands, and secrete substances into the gastro-intestinal tract as well as mucus. In some instances the secreting cells are grouped together as glands. Those which keep their connection with the surface and secrete onto it are called exocrine glands, while those which have lost the connection and secrete into the bloodstream are endocrine glands. Epithelial cells, because they line the body surfaces, are often damaged and lost. They are replaced by division of the remaining cells. An ulcer forms if the epithelium is destroyed, which heals by the proliferation of epithelial cells surrounding the damaged area. Epithelial cells can be transferred from another part of the body, as in skin grafting. If adhesion between the cells fails, and the cells proliferate to invade the basement membrane and surrounding tissues, a malignant tumour is formed, a carcinoma.

Epstein–Barr Virus: one of the group of herpes viruses, which is responsible for the disease infective mononucleosis, or glandular fever.

Ergometrine: an alkaloid isolated from ergot, which makes the muscle of the pregnant uterus contract, and is therefore used in the management of bleeding in an incomplete abortion, in the third stage of labour or in postpartum haemorrhage. It may be combined with oxytocin.

Ergosterol: originally isolated from ergot, this sterol is also found in yeast. If it is irradiated the substance calciferol is formed, which is vitamin D_2.

Ergot: a fungus, *Claviceps purpura*, which is parasitic on rye and wheat. At one time rye bread was a staple diet, and infested rye produced ergot poisoning, known as St Anthony's Fire: the limbs were afflicted with intolerable burning pain, became black and gangrenous and were eventually lost. Another form of ergot poisoning was called 'convulsive', as opposed to gangrenous: the skin itched, there were feelings as if insects were crawling on the skin (formication), and pins and needles. Convulsions ensued, and the victim might go blind or mad. During the last century ergot was used as a drug for its action on the muscle of the pregnant uterus, which was violently contracted, as midwives had known for years. Ergot proved to be the source of many alkaloids, all based on lysergic acid, which is not active unless combined with a base. The alkaloids used in medicine are ergometrine and ergotamine (q.v.).

In 1943, during an investigation of the action on the uterus of derivatives of lysergic acid, a scientist accidentally took a minute amount of lysergic acid diethylamide by mouth and became hallucinated. This led to the discovery that this derivative of ergot is one of the most powerful drugs known, for it acts in a dose of $1\mu g$ per kg body weight.

Ergotamine: an ergot derivative used in the treatment of acute migraine which does not respond to simple analgesics. It has the drawback that it may promote vomiting, and is therefore commonly used with an anti-emetic drug such as metoclopramide. Ergotamine may also give rise to muscular cramp and abdominal pain; It should be discontinued if any numbness or pins and needles develop in the toes or fingers Treatment should not be repeated within four days.

Erosion: appearance of the cervix uteri caused by re-placement of the normal squamous epithelium (q.v.) by columnar epithelium; the cervix is red rather than pink, and looks as if it has been inflamed or ulcerated. It is associated with an abnormally alkaline vaginal secretion, and may be found after pregnancy or on examination of patients complaining of vaginal discharge.

Erysipelas: infection of the skin and underlying tissues by group A streptococci. There is at first a fever, sometimes with vomiting and even confusion, and within 24 hours the skin at the site of infection, commonly the face or leg, becomes red and painful; the area has a raised edge. Blisters form, and may become crusted. The infection responds to penicillin and erythromycin.

Erysipeloid: a skin infection resembling erysipelas, but purple in colour rather than bright red. It is primarily an infection of animals, affecting meat, fish and poultry, and may be acquired through an abrasion or cut by those who work with the animals, particularly butchers. The infecting organism is *Erysipelothrix rhusiopathiae*, which is sensitive to penicillin. If left, the condition normally clears up spontaneously.

Erythema: reddening of the skin, caused by increased blood flow in the capillaries in response to many factors such as infection, slight burning, exposure to cold, or allergic response.

Erythema Multiforme: a skin disorder affecting the hands and feet rather than the trunk, showing round red patches which blister in the middle. They may occur on the eyes, the mouth and the genital organs; when the lesions are severe the condition is known as the Stevens–Johnson syndrome, and there may be a fever and other manifestations such as diarrhoea, arthritis, kidney failure and pneumonia. In half the cases the cause is obscure, but in others there is some infection such as herpes simplex; many drugs are known to excite the disease, among them sulphonamides, barbiturates and butazolidine. Treatment involves withdrawing the drug at fault, treating any concomitant disease, and the use of steroids in severe cases. The condition can recur.

Erythrocyte: a red blood cell. There are in health about 5×10^{12} red cells in each litre of blood. They contain haemoglobin, the substance which transports oxygen from the lungs to the tissues and returns to the lungs carbon dioxide, the product of cell metabolism. The normal content of haemoglobin in the blood is 145 g/100 ml, and each red cell is one-third haemoglobin. It is bi-concave, a shape which encourages the transfer of gases, measures about 7 μm in diameter and is 2 μm thick. The cells are made in the bone marrow, and have no nucleus except when they have just been made, when the remains of a nucleus can be seen. Such cells are called reticulocytes. Red blood cells last about 100 days.

Erythromycin: an antibiotic derived from the organism *Streptomyces erythreus*, with an action similar to that of penicillin. It is particularly useful in cases of whooping cough and legionnaires' disease, in campylobacter infection of the bowel and in chlamydia infections. It is often used in cases where the patient is sensitive to penicillin.

Erythropoietin: a hormone produced by the kidney which

promotes the production of red blood cells. The gene which regulates its structure has been identified, isolated and introduced into micro-organisms which have produced the hormone in quantities.

Eserine: also called physostigmine, an alkaloid extracted from the Calabar bean. It acts by inhibiting the enzymes which break down acetylcholine (q.v.). It was first known as a poison in West Africa, but is now used in opthalmology for the treatment of glaucoma; it contracts the pupil of the eye.

ESR: erythrocyte sedimentation rate. *See* Sedimentation Rate.

Essential Hypertension: high blood pressure which is not secondary to some other disease. *See* Hypertension.

Ethanol: ethyl alcohol, commonly referred to as alcohol.

Ether: diethyl ether, a volatile liquid used as an anaesthetic. After many years it is now falling into disuse, for it irritates the respiratory system and is highly inflammable. It causes nausea and vomiting, and has been superseded by more modern anaesthetic agents. It was first used in public by William Morton (1819–68) in 1846 at the Massachusetts General Hospital; this marked the introduction of general anaesthetics which made modern surgery possible.

Ethmoid: a small bone of irregular shape in the base of the skull. It helps to form the inner wall of the orbit, or eye socket, and the upper parts of the nose and nasal septum, the partition between the two sides of the nasal cavity. Parts of the bone are filled with air cells, the ethmoidal sinuses; the middle part of the bone which forms the roof of the nose is pierced by many holes through which pass branches of the olfactory nerve, the nerve of smell, as they travel from the nose into the skull and so to the brain.

Ethyl Alcohol: commonly called alcohol, used mostly for social purposes.

Ethyl Chloride: a volatile liquid which has been used as a local anaesthetic, for when sprayed onto the skin it evaporates rapidly and freezes the part. It was also once used as an agent for inducing general anaesthesia.

Ethylene Glycol: antifreeze, which has been used as a substitute for alcohol as an intoxicating liquor, with fatal results.

Eucalyptus: oil obtained from the eucalyptus tree, which is a popular remedy for coughs and colds applied externally as a rub or inhaled as a vapour. It is likely that when it is inhaled in steam it is the steam which has the relieving effect.

Eugenics: the study of means to improve the inherited qualities of human beings.

Eunuch: a castrated male.

Euphoria: a sense of bodily well-being and comfort, used in psychiatry to mean an exaggerated sense of well-being and cheerfulness regardless of circumstances, as seen for example in mania or those under the influence of drugs.

Eustachian Tube: the auditory tube, which connects the middle ear with the interior of the naso-pharynx in order to equalise pressures between the middle ear and the atmosphere. Named after Bartolemmeo Eustacio (1524–74), the Italian anatomist who described it in 1562.

Euthanasia: the recommendation that it should be legal to put to death those who are suffering from an incurable, painful and distressing disease by some painless method. It appeals mostly to laymen who have not seen much of death and have not been in a position to care for the dying. It is very rare to find that pain is so intolerable that it cannot be controlled by drugs; *in extremis*, if pain and distress can only be controlled at the risk of the patient's life, then that risk must be taken.

Exanthem: a skin eruption associated with some infectious fevers, such as measles and chicken-pox.

Exhibitionism: showing off the body in order to gain sexual attention; it sometimes extends to a display of the sexual parts in males.

Exophthalmos: forward protrusion of the eyeballs, which may be caused by a tumour in the orbit or thyrotoxicosis (q.v.)

Exostosis: an abnormal outgrowth of bone.

Exotoxin: toxic substance secreted by bacteria. Bacterial toxins can be modified into harmless toxoids and used to produce active immunity to the toxin, as in tetanus, where a course of toxoid by injection prevents the development of tetanus from a contaminated wound. If tetanus develops in a subject who has not been immunised, antitoxin contained in human immunoglobulin may be used. Similarly, toxoid is used in immunisation against diphtheria, and antitoxin is available. Besides the toxins of diphtheria and tetanus, very dangerous exotoxins are produced by the organisms of botulism and gas gangrene.

Expectorants: substances used in cough mixtures which are thought to have the action of liquifying sputum and making it easier for the patient to cough effectively. There is, however, no scientific foundation for their use.

Extradural Haemorrhage: the brain is covered by three membranes, the outer being the dura mater. It is closely applied to the inner surface of the skull, and in it run blood vessels, in particular the middle meningeal artery which is in the region of the temple. If the temple suffers a severe injury, or the skull is cracked and the fracture line runs across the temple, the middle meningeal artery may be torn so that blood escapes and forms an ever-increasing swelling between the dura and the skull. The classic story is that the patient regains consciousness after a blow on the head, and appears to have recovered; then after a time, which is variable, but may be a few hours, slips into a coma. This can mean that a patient is seen by a doctor after a head injury, is thought to have recovered, lapses into unconsciousness and dies. It is therefore very important that head injuries of any severity, particularly those which have caused loss of consciousness, should be admitted to hospital for at least 24 hours' observation. If the patient is not seen by a doctor after a head injury, and there is any change in consciousness in the hours following, medical aid should be sought at once. Drunkenness may be misleading, for there may be no clear history of a head injury, and the patient who starts to complain of a headache, becomes restless and confused, and has taken alcohol, may present difficulty in diagnosis. There is of course the possibility that the unconscious patient after a head injury never regains consciousness, and there is no lucid period, but the condition deteriorates. Diagnosis is made on the physical signs and brain scan, and the treatment is surgical evacuation of the collection of blood and arrest of the middle meningeal haemorrhage. *Cf.* Subdural Haemorrhage.

Extrapyramidal System: the nerves that control movements of the muscles, the motor system, run for the most part from the cortex of the brain into the spinal cord and along it in well-defined bundles of fibres called the corticospinal or pyramidal system, pyramidal because when they run through the medulla of the brain they raise the surface into a pyramidal shape. There are however other motor fibres running from the cortex to relay in the basal ganglia of the brain and brain stem and pass down to the muscles without passing through the pyramids, and they are, with the ganglia involved, called the extrapyramidal system. It is concerned with muscular posture and tone.

Extrasystole: normally the heartbeat follows a regular pattern: the pacemaker, called the sinuatrial node, which is a group of specialised cells in the right atrium, sets up an impulse which starts a wave of contraction passing through the atria. When this wave of contraction reaches the atrioventricular node, another group of specialised cells near the tricuspid valve, which lies between the right atrium and ventricle, it sets up an impulse in a bundle of specialised muscle fibres (the bundle of His) which passes into the interventricular septum, the partition between right and left ventricles, and makes the ventricles contract. A contraction of the heart arising from an impulse set up anywhere outside the sinu-atrial node is an extrasystole; it occurs commonly in healthy people.

Extravasation: an escape or discharge of fluid from a vessel into the tissues. For example an extravasation of blood occurs when a blood vessel has been injured, and if large forms a haematoma, if small a bruise. Injuries of the bladder or urethra may lead to extravasation of urine.

Exudate: matter composed of fluid, cells and debris which has, as the result of inflammation, escaped from the blood vessels to the surface or into the tissues.

Eye: the organ of vision. Just under an inch in diameter, the eyes are contained in bony sockets, the orbits, in the skull. They are moved in their sockets by the external ocular muscles – four straight muscles, the rectus muscles, running from the back of the orbit to cover the top, bottom and sides of the globe, and two oblique. The inferior oblique muscle runs from the inner forward part of the floor of the orbit obliquely backwards and is inserted into the upper outer back of the eyeball, but the superior oblique is more complicated. It starts at the back of the orbit from the inner part of the roof, runs forwards, and then hooks round a fibrous pulley called the trochlea to change direction completely, running obliquely backwards and outwards to be inserted into the upper outer part of the back of the eye near the inferior oblique. The muscles are supplied by cranial nerves; the rectus muscles by the oculomotor, except for the lateral muscle which is supplied by the abducent nerve, the inferior oblique by the oculomotor and the superior oblique by the trochlear. Co-ordination of eye movement takes place in the brain. When the muscles are incoordinated or paralysed the patient sees double.

The outer coat of the eyeball is called the sclera, an opaque layer of strong fibrous tissue which is continuous in front with the translucent cornea. The curve of the cornea is greater than the curve of the sclera, so that the cornea protrudes a little. Inside the sclera is a middle layer of pigmented tissue which forms the choroid at the back and the ciliary body and iris in front. In this layer run many blood vessels. The inner layer is the retina, which is thin and is the expanded end of the optic nerve. It is a complicated structure, but is essentially made up of nerve fibres, a plexus of their connections with the nerve cells of the retina and the rods and cones, the rods and cones themselves and blood vessels. The rods and cones are receptors sensitive to light, but in order to reach them the light has to pass through the other structures of the retina, which are almost transparent. The blood vessels are not seen because they remain still.

Filling the main part of the eyeball is the vitreous humour, a transparent jelly. At the front of the eyeball the lens, supported by the suspensory ligament from the ciliary body, shuts off the anterior chamber of the eye; in front of the lens is the pigmented iris, and then the transparent cornea. The anterior chamber of the eye is filled with aqueous humour which is like water. The rods and cones of the retina are light-sensitive cells, so named because of their shape. The rods contain rhodopsin, or visual purple, which is bleached by light. It is made from a protein and vitamin A. Rods are for monochrome vision, cones for colour vision (*see* Colour Blindness). There are two places in the retina where the structure differs from the rest: the fovea, where the retina is thinnest, so that light passes more directly to the colour-sensitive cones (there are no rods in the fovea), and the optic disc where the nerve leaves the eye and there are no rods or cones. The centre of an object focused by the lens normally lies at the fovea, and the optic disc forms the blind spot. Light entering the eye is first refracted by the cornea; the lens then focuses images sharply onto the retina, being transparent, bi-convex, with the curve at the back greater than that in front. It is normally held out by the suspensory ligament, so that when the muscle of the ciliary body contracts and the ligament slackens the lens, being elastic, becomes rounder, and as the distance from the front to the back surface becomes greater near objects are brought into focus. As we get older the lens loses its elasticity and it becomes more difficult to focus on things close at hand. The shape of the lens and of the eyeball itself can produce errors of refraction. If the surfaces of the lens are not spherical, astigmatism (q.v.) follows; if the lens brings the image to a focus in front of the retina, either because it refracts too sharply or the eyeball is too long from front to back, the result is short sight or myopia; if the opposite is true, and the lens cannot refract sharply enough or the eyeball is too short, the result is long sight or hypermetropia. These faults are corrected by lenses in spectacles, or contact lenses, or by altering the shape of the cornea (q.v.).

The amount of light entering the eye is controlled by the iris, which by contracting makes the pupil – the aperture in the centre of the iris – smaller. The muscle of the iris is supplied by the autonomic nervous system and is not under voluntary control. It works reflexly: the sympathetic system dilates the pupil, the parasympathetic constricts it. When a strong light falls on the retina the pupil at once contracts to cut down the illumination, but if the eye is in the dark the pupil opens widely. The response of the pupil to light depends on the central connections of the optic nerve in the brain stem and the integrity of the oculomotor nerve and ciliary ganglion. The fibres of the optic nerve carry impulses arising in the retina back through the optic chiasm, where half the fibres cross sides so that all the fibres 'seeing' the outside world on the right-hand side (those from the nasal side of the right retina and the outer, or temporal, side of the left retina) now go to the left-hand side of the brain and all the fibres sensitive to images on the left go to the right-hand side of the brain. The fibres relay in the midbrain and the impulses from the retina end in the visual cortex, which is at the back of the cerebral hemispheres, in the occipital pole. Information from the rods and cones is to a certain extent correlated in the ganglion cells of the retina which connect them to the fibres of the optic nerve, and further analysis is carried out in the cortex, but the processes by which we recognise what we see are by no means understood.

Injuries to the eye are of two kinds, penetrating and non-penetrating. Penetrating injuries call for immediate surgical attention; they have the added complication that inflammation of the iris, ciliary body or choroid (the uveal tract) which may follow injury may affect the sound eye and set up a sympathetic ophthalmia, which results in complete loss of sight. Non-penetrating injuries include abrasions of the cornea which are painful but heal well, displacement of the lens, and tears or detachment of the retina. Foreign bodies in the eye are a source of pain and inflammation; ordinary dust or grit may be dislodged by blinking, or sometimes by blowing the nose hard. It may be picked off the surface of the eye by the edge of a clean handkerchief, but care must be taken not to rub the eye. If the particle cannot be shifted easily medical aid is necessary.

Diseases of the eye are described under separate headings, e.g. Cataract, Conjunctivitis, Glaucoma, Trachoma. *Also see* Blindness, Colour Blindness, Perimetry, Steroscopic Vision.

Eyelids: the eyelids are composed of two folds of skin which cover the eyeball, lined on the inside by the thin conjunctival membrane and attached to a framework of fibrous tissue called the tarsal plates. They are surrounded by a thin muscle called the orbicularis oculi and the upper lid is raised by the levator palpebrae superioris. At the free margins are the eyelashes and modified sweat and sebaceous glands, the Meibomian glands, named after the German anatomist Heinrich Meibom (1638-1700); the secretions prevent the eyelids sticking together. Near the outer canthus, the angle of the eyelids, lies the lacrimal gland which secretes tears; the fluid passes across the surface of the eye to the inner angle, where it is picked up by the lacrimal puncti, small openings on the upper and lower eyelids, and passed into the lacrimal sac and so into the naso-lacrimal duct, which drains into the nose. The Meibomian glands may become infected and form a stye, or the duct may become blocked so that a cyst is formed in the eyelid, which is easily removed surgically. The lacrimal punctum may block, in which case tears overflow onto the cheeks, but this can be cleared by

233

the passage of a small instrument. Inflammation of the lacrimal sac, dacryocystitis, can occur and a swelling can be seen at the inner angle of the eyelid, and rarely concretions can block the sac or the naso-lacrimal duct. When eyedrops are used they should be introduced at the outer angle of the eyelids to be carried across the eye by the natural flow of the tears.

F

Facial Nerve: the seventh cranial nerve, supplying the muscles of the face and the stapedius muscle of the middle ear; sensation of the face is carried in the fifth cranial nerve.

Facies: in clinical medicine, the appearance of the face and expression which is characteristic of a particular disease, such as the mask-like face of Parkinson's disease, the stupid open-mouthed expression of children suffering from enlarged adenoids, the unmistakable appearance of Down's syndrome or the Hippocratic facies of approaching death – 'drawn, pinched and livid'.

Faeces: waste products from the intestines, consisting of food which has not been digested, mostly cellulose and fibre, dead cells from the lining of the intestine, water, mucus, and bacteria, the whole coloured by bile pigments.

Fainting: or syncope, transient loss of consciousness caused by temporary lack of blood supply to the brain. It can be caused by exposure to conditions which bring about pooling of blood in the trunk and limbs, such as lying in a hot bath, or lying in a warm bed, and then suddenly standing up, when the normal reflex compensating mechanism which constricts the arteries of the body and thus sends blood to the brain is not quick enough. This is particularly likely to happen in the elderly, who must stand up perhaps a little more slowly than they would like when getting out of bed or out of a chair. Standing in one position for a long time without moving, as on parade, or being in a hot atmosphere, may make one faint or feel faint; the face pales, the pulse becomes rapid and shallow, sweat breaks out and things seem far away and unsteady. Strong emotion may make the blood pressure fall enough to cause a faint. The blood which has pooled away from the brain is best returned by lying down, if possible with the legs raised, or sitting with the head bent forward between the knees. An isolated faint is not uncommon; but repeated attacks must call for medical advice, for they may be the sign of underlying illness.

Fallopian Tubes: named after the Italian anatomist Gabrielle Fallopius (1523–62), they are bilateral tubular structures which run from the ovaries on each side of the pelvis to the upper corners of the uterus, into which they open. At the ovarian end the tubes are open to the peritoneal cavity, but have fimbriated ends, that is, a fringe of processes, which lie close to the ovaries. They are lined with ciliated epithelium which collects the egg from the ovary and propels it down the tube into the uterus. Fertilisation, if it occurs, takes place in the Fallopian tube, and the fertilised ovum is normally carried into the uterus where it becomes implanted, but it can happen that the ovum becomes embedded in the wall of the tube and starts to develop as an ectopic pregnancy. As the ovum develops, the wall of the tube gives way and bleeds into the peritoneal cavity. If the bleeding is severe, the patient suffers pain in the lower abdomen, passes into shock and collapses; in less severe bleeding, she experiences recurrent attacks of pain and perhaps vaginal bleeding. Treatment is surgical, the abdomen is opened, the ectopic pregnancy removed and the bleeding stopped. An ectopic pregnancy does not mean that the woman is thereafter sterile.

Fallot's Tetralogy: the French physician Étienne Fallot (1850–1911) described in the last century a congenital condition of the heart that has four component defects: an opening in the interventricular septum, the partition between the right and left ventricles, a narrowing of the valve of the pulmonary artery, over development of the right ventricle and displacement of the aorta to the right. A child suffering from this condition is cyanosed, or blue, because the circulating blood cannot properly be oxygenated, and easily becomes breathless. The abnormality can be set right by surgery.

Farmer's Lung: a type of extrinsic allergic alveolitis, sometimes called hypersensitivity pneumonitis. It is due to the inhalation of dust from mouldy hay or straw containing an antigen which sets up an allergic reaction in the lungs. The dust has in it the spores of the organisms *Micropolyspora faeni* and *Thermoactinomyces vulgaris*, which infect the hay when it is damp and warm, and are released when it has dried out. In the summer, the patient develops an illness which produces headache, a fever, and various aches and pains, with a dry cough and shortness of breath. The disease may become chronic with continued exposure and result in fibrosis of the lung. It is recognised as an industrial disease. There are a considerable number of lung diseases of this type, affecting people from bird fanciers to woodworkers, which result from inhaling dust containing various antigens.

Fascia: fibrous tissue organised to form sheets which lie just under the skin, the superficial fascia, and round muscles, the deep fascia. The superficial fascia contains fat and the nerves and blood vessels running to the skin, while the deep fascia is densely fibrous; its strength varies from place to place, being very strong on the outside of the thigh but thin in the face. It forms sheaths for the muscles and compartments in which groups of muscles lie together.

Fasting: the length of time it is possible to exist without food varies with the circumstances. Without water it is only possible to live for a week or ten days, but given water and warm surroundings it is possible to live for a month or even two, especially if the drink contains fruit juice or glucose. Fasting as a health measure is recommended by some, but if the sedentary and perhaps overfed take to fasting and exercise too enthusiastically all they are likely to get is a peptic ulcer and coronary thrombosis.

Fat Embolism: in severe bone injuries fat globules may be released into the bloodstream and cause an embolism (q.v.).

Fatigue: there are two sorts of fatigue, one brought on by muscular exercise, and the other, psychological fatigue, by boredom. Muscular fatigue is due to the accumulation of the products of metabolism, in particular lactic acid, and

237

the onset can be delayed by training, which improves the metabolic capacity of muscle and encourages the growth of capillary blood vessels, so that the products of activity are removed more quickly. The fatigue of the long-distance runner is caused by the consumption by the muscles of glycogen; normally the muscles burn both glycogen and fatty acids, but in time the glycogen is used up leaving only the fatty acids available for use, and this cuts down the energy available. Training makes the conversion of fatty acids easier and alters the ratio between their use and the use of glycogen, so that less glucose is used and therefore lasts longer.

The fatigue that results from doing an uninteresting and boring job is different, for the reason is not lack of energy but lack of inclination. There remains fatigue brought about by physical disease such as anaemia, in which investigation will bring the cause to light and make treatment possible; it is not sensible to hope that self-treatment by advertised remedies can help.

Fat Necrosis: occasionally a hard lump appears in the breast, often after a blow, fixed to the skin and resembling a cancer but in fact composed of dead fat cells. The diagnosis is made by biopsy. Rarely the pancreas may be injured, or be the seat of severe inflammation, and pancreatic enzymes then escape into the abdominal cavity and kill fat cells in the omentum or mesentery. The enzymes may even cause necrosis in other parts of the body.

Fauces: the opening between the mouth and the throat, bounded above by the soft palate, below by the tongue, and on each side by the tonsils. The two folds of mucous membrane containing muscle fibres before and behind the tonsils are called the pillars of the fauces.

Favus: severe ringworm of the scalp found in tropical countries and the Middle East. It is chronic, and may lead to loss of hair.

Feeble-Mindedness: *see* Mental Defect.

Felon: an infection and abscess of the pulp of the finger.

Femur: the thigh-bone, the largest and strongest bone in the body. At the upper end its rounded head fits into the acetabulum of the pelvis to form a ball-and-socket joint, the hip joint, and its lower end forms a joint at the knee with the tibia, the weight-bearing bone of the leg, the joint being covered by the patella, the kneecap. The knee is a hinge joint, and rotation of the trunk on the foot takes place at the hip. The neck and the head of the femur are at an angle of 125° to the shaft, and rotation takes place round an axis joining the head of the bone to its lower end; it is along this axis that weight is borne. The part of the femur most likely to suffer a fracture is the neck, below the head or as it joins the shaft. This fracture is not common among adults in the prime of life, for the inside of the neck and shaft of the bone is buttressed by lines of dense bone formed along the lines of stress; but when in old age the bones lose their elasticity and become brittle, and are in elderly women perhaps affected by osteoporosis (q.v.), then a fracture of the neck of the femur is always a possibility even after a relatively trivial fall. This fracture is commonly treated by pinning or by the insertion of a prosthesis, an artificial hip such as is used in cases of osteoarthritis, and weight-bearing can begin very quickly. A fracture of the shaft of the femur is usually caused by direct violence, and takes longer to treat. First-aid treatment is to bind the legs together to stop the fracture moving.

Fenestration: an operation for otosclerosis which when it was introduced by the American surgeon Julius Lempert (1890–1962) was a great advance in the treatment of deafness, but which has become superseded by newer procedures.

Fetishism: a sexual abnormality, usually in men, in which erotic excitement is associated with inanimate objects such as women's shoes or underclothes.

Fever: a condition in which the body temperature is above normal, taken to be 37°C (98.4°F). In fact the body temperature varies throughout the day, being anything between 36.9°C and 37.5°C, at its highest in the late afternoon and evening and its lowest in the middle of the night. It is controlled by a centre in the brain which maintains a balance between heat production and its loss from the surface of the body. This mechanism is upset by infection by bacteria or viruses, which are thought to excite the macrophage cells of the reticulo-endothelial system to produce pyrogens, substances which make the temperature rise. A fever usually starts with shivering and a feeling of cold, although the body temperature is raised. When the shivering is pronounced it is called a rigor, a sign that the temperature has risen sharply. It is at this stage that convulsions may occur in young children; in older people a high temperature may be accompanied by confusion or even delirium. There is a headache, loss of appetite, sweating, and the muscles ache. The cause of the fever may be obvious; if it is not, it may be referred to as PUO, pyrexia of unknown, or uncertain, origin, and until the cause is known treatment must also be uncertain. A great number of conditions can produce fever, from obscure infections to allergies and drug reactions, and the course of a fever can be varied, from the common continuous fever to the intermittent fever of malaria – quotidian when the temperature rises every 24 hours, tertian when it rises every 48 hours, and quartan when the period is 72 hours. As the pattern of fever is important, one reading of the temperature is of limited significance, and periodic readings should be kept on a chart in doubtful or severe cases. Children tend to run a high temperature, and this may cause convulsions; but in the case of children under five these are not an indication of epilepsy. The temperature can be brought down by cooling the room, removing the bedclothes and sponging down with tepid water. Although aspirin is effective in reducing the temperature it should not be used for children under 12 years old. Paracetamol is recommended.

Fibrescope: an endoscope using glass or plastic fibres to carry images and light, which means that the instrument is flexible and more readily introduced into the body cavity that is being examined than the older endoscopes which were rigid.

Fibrillation: muscle fibres normally contract in an orderly and co-ordinated fashion. In fibrillation, the fibres contract independently and spontaneously.

Fibrin: a protein substance which forms the framework of blood clots. It is precipitated from the blood by the action of the enzyme thrombin or fibrinogen. *See* Coagulation of the Blood.

Fibrinogen: *see above.*

Fibro-adenoma: a benign tumour which is commonly found in the breast, consisting of glandular and fibrous tissue.

Fibroid: a benign tumour consisting of muscle and fibrous tissue enclosed within a capsule found in the uterus, usually in the body of the organ. It is commonest in childless women, and there is often more than one. Symptoms are menorrhagia (flooding at the periods) or bleeding between periods; there may be pain, and the size of the tumour may interfere with the bladder and cause difficulty in passing urine. If the fibroids are very large they can press on the veins running through the pelvis, which results in distended veins in the legs and swollen ankles. There is often sterility or miscarriage. The treatment is surgical removal, or in severe cases, or if the patient has passed childbearing age, removal of the uterus.

Fibroma: a benign tumour composed of fibrous tissue, usually small and unimportant.

Fibrosarcoma: a malignant tumour of fibrous tissue which grows relatively slowly, often in muscles near the surface of the body. It invades neighbouring tissues but is slow to spread to other parts; if it does so, it may metastasise to the lungs.

Fibrosis: the formation of fibrous or scar tissue in place of tissue which has been destroyed by injury, infection or deficient blood supply.

Fibrositis: a term used to describe muscular pain often associated with areas of particular tenderness in the back and neck, otherwise called muscular rheumatism. The cause is unknown, but it usually responds to physiotherapy or even the application of a counter-irritant liniment or cream to the overlying skin.

Fibrous Tissue: a great deal of the body consists of connective tissues, which are derived from mesoderm and form cartilage, bone, fibrous tissue, blood and lymph. Fibrous tissue is laid down by cells called fibroblasts, and may be loose or dense. It is composed of two proteins, collagen and elastin, and it may be unyielding or elastic, according to the proportions of these protein fibres present. Loose connective tissue, such as is found under the skin, contains fat cells and blood vessels, but dense connective tissue forming tendons contains only collagen fibres arranged in parallel, and is very strong. Similar strength is found in the ligaments of joints, but some have many elastic fibres in them, for example those joining the spines of the vertebrae of the neck and spinal column to form the ligamentum flavum, so called because elastic fibres are yellow. The sheets of dense fibrous tissue investing the muscles, the deep fascia, are made mostly of collagen fibres arranged randomly, while the tissue in the walls of the arteries has a preponderance of elastic fibres.

Fibula: the thin outer bone of the leg, which lies behind and to the outer side of the tibia, the shin-bone, and forms a joint with it at its upper end. The fibula plays no part in the knee joint, but its lower end articulates with the talus at the ankle. The bony projection on the outside of the ankle is the lower end of the fibula, and is called the external malleolus.

Filariasis: infection with nematode worms called filariae, which are the size of a heavy thread and vary in length. They are found in tropical and subtropical countries; those that infest man are *Wuchereria bancrofti*, *Brugia malayi*, and *Brugia timori*, which infest the lymphatic system and produce elephantiasis, *Onchocerca volvulus*, which produces skin disturbances and blindness, and *Loa loa*, which produces large swellings under the skin called Calabar swellings. The female worm when fertilised gives birth to microfilariae, which live in the blood or the skin until they are ingested by an insect biting the host. This acts as an intermediate host; in it the microfilariae develop into larvae, which when passed on by the insect biting another host become adult filariae. The process takes months to complete. One larva produces one worm, and the worms do not multiply in the host but only produce microfilariae. The intermediate host in Bancroftian and Brugian infestation is a mosquito, and that in *Onchocerca volvulus* the blackfly; *Loa loa*, which is found mainly in West Africa, is spread by redflies or mangrove-flies. The drug diethylcarbamazine is effective against all but *Onchocerca volvulus*, when the drug of choice is ivermectin.

Fingers: consist of three bones, the phalanges, joined together by hinge joints and strong ligaments; the thumb has only two phalanges. At their base, the first phalanges of the fingers make a saddle joint with the metacarpal bones of the palm at the knuckles. The movements of flexion (bending) and extension (straightening) are carried out by powerful muscles in the forearm whose tendons pass, two in front and two behind, to each finger; covered with synovial sheaths which contain fluid to enable them to move freely, they are inserted into the bases of the middle and terminal phalanges back and front, and the head of the first phalanx. Small muscles of the hand itself run from the palm to the fingers; the interosseous muscles move the fingers away and towards the middle finger – the thumb and little finger have their own named muscles to move them – and the lumbrical muscles of the palm assist in flexing the fingers at the knuckles and extending them at the phalangeal joints. Running along the sides of each finger are two small arteries and nerves which are of great importance in providing the particular sensitivity of the fingertips. The arteries come from the arterial arch in the palm formed by the radial and ulnar arteries, and the nerves are terminal branches of the median, ulnar and radial nerves of the forearm. On the front of the hand the ulnar nerve supplies only the little finger and the outer half of the fourth finger, the rest of the fingers being supplied by the median nerve, while on the back the ulnar nerve supplies the fifth, fourth and half of the third fingers, the median nerve the tips of the fingers and the radial nerve the rest of the back of the hand and the fingers as far as the tips. A point of practical importance is that the nerves of the fingers can be blocked by an injection of local anaesthetic at the sides of the base of the finger to provide anaesthesia of the whole finger. Injuries of the fingers are common, as are infections particularly of the pulp at the tips, and are important because so much depends on intact fingers. The blood supply can be affected by Raynaud's disease (q.v.), the joints by arthritis, and the skin by conditions brought about by the necessity for using the fingers to handle irritating, possibly dangerous substances. *Also see* Nails

Fissure: in anatomy, a cleft or groove in a structure. In disease, a crack or linear ulcer at the corner of the mouth or more importantly at the anus. In the mouth, small cracks in the skin become infected and as they are constantly moving and may be wet with saliva, they can be a long time healing, but attention to the infection and cleanliness will help. Fissures at the anus are very painful, and there may be a little blood and irritation. In children they may cause constipation because of the pain in passing a motion, which sets up a vicious circle because the motions become hard and tear the fissure. Mild cases may respond to treatment aimed at keeping the motions soft; the use of a local anaesthetic ointment may help, but it should not be used for more than a couple of weeks for it may make the skin sensitive. The skin round the anus should be washed after passing a motion. In more severe cases the surgeon may dilate the anus under anaesthetic, which often relieves the condition, but it may be necessary to remove the fissure and the surrounding tissue.

Fistula: an abnormal communication between an internal structure and the surface of the body, or between two internal organs. It may arise from developmental error, as in the neck when a branchial arch fails to fuse and leaves a channel running from the region of the tonsil to the outside of the neck; from a blocked duct from a gland as when a salivary duct is blocked and saliva discharges through the cheek or under the chin; from injury, as when the urethra is torn and urine passes through the damaged tissues and skin; and because of disease, as when a fistula is formed between the bowel and the bladder as the result of a malignant tumour. A fistula may be found between an artery and a vein, formed in the course of development or as the result of injury. One of the commonest examples of fistula is that occurring between the interior of the rectum and the skin by the anus, the ano-rectal fistula, caused by an abscess in the region. The treatment in all cases is surgical.

Fits: *see* Epilepsy.

Flat Foot: fallen arch, or pes planus. A condition normal in infants and many children, and in people who have never worn shoes. The foot has an arch on the inner side, between the two areas which bear weight, the heel-bone or calcaneus and the heads of the bones of the foot, the metatarsals. This arch is supported by strong ligaments which bind the bones together, and by the muscles of the foot. If they fail, the arch flattens; the foot becomes painful. This can occur because of general debility or overweight, long hours of standing, arthritis of the feet, after illness and confinement to bed, or after a fracture of a bone in the foot. Treatment is exercise designed to strengthen the muscles of the sole and attention to general health; supports for the arch may relieve discomfort, but they do not restore the strength of the muscles and ligaments. It may be noted that many people have flat feet which do not cause any trouble.

Flatulence: gas in the stomach or intestines which may become evident in noises or borborygmi in the abdomen, and discomfort relieved by belching or the passage of wind from the anus. Many cases of frequent belching are due to the unconscious swallowing of air, a habit which is not uncommon; others are associated with a hiatus hernia (q.v.). At the other end of the digestive tract the gas is a mixture of that swallowed and the products of fermentation in the colon, mostly methane and hydrogen sulphide, and the amount depends in part on the type of food that has been eaten.

Fleas: the common flea producing an irritating bite is *Pulex irritans*, but dog and cat fleas can also be a nuisance. There are over 200 species of this insect, but only 20 are found to bite man; of these the most annoying is *Tunga penetrans*, the jigger flea found in Africa and Central America, which burrows into the skin usually of the feet and sets up irritation, infection and ulceration. It has to be removed surgically. Other fleas are the vectors of disease, notably plague. The flea is infected with *Yersinia pestis*, the organism of plague, by biting an infected rat; the plague organisms then multiply in the flea's oesophagus, blocking it. When it bites another creature it cannot draw blood, but regurgitates the mass of bacilli into the bloodstream of the victim. Rats infected with plague die, and the flea, whose life is threatened by starvation and dehydration because its oesophagus is blocked, in its search for a warm-blooded host may light on a human being and so spread the disease.

Fleming, Sir Alexander (1881–1955): English bacteriologist who discovered penicillin, and with Lord Florey (1898–1968) and Sir Ernst Chain (1906–79) was awarded the Nobel Prize in 1945.

Flexibilitas Cerea: an abnormal condition found in advanced schizophrenia in which the subject's limbs remain in whatever position they are placed by the observer.

Flooding: the common name for excessive bleeding in women whether during the menstrual period, when it is called menorrhagia, or between periods, when it is described as metrorrhagia.

Fluid Balance: the average output of urine is between 1200 and 1500 ml a day, and the loss of fluid from perspiration and in the breath up to 1000 ml, so that on average the intake of fluid has to be two or three litres. The commonest way for sick people to lose fluid is by vomiting or diarrhoea, and not only fluid is lost but also essential electrolytes. If left to themselves the sick, especially the elderly, tend to drink too little, and must be encouraged to take as much fluid as possible. *See* Dehydration.

Flukes (trematodes): leaf-shaped parasitic flatworms which can infest the intestines, liver, lungs and the blood. They have at least two hosts in their lifetime, one usually a mollusc. When the eggs are discharged from the host they can only survive in the wet, and if they fall into freshwater they develop as free-swimming miracidia. If they find a suitable mollusc as intermediate host they continue their development into cercariae, which are free-swimming. Some then find another intermediate host, such as a freshwater fish or crustacean, before they reach their final destination, and develop into adult flukes. The most important trematode is *Schistosoma*, which causes bilharzia (q.v.). Praziquantel is the drug used in treating most cases of trematode infestation.

Fluorescein: the dark orange-red dye resorcenolphthalein. If dissolved in alkaline solution it emits green fluorescence, and is used in medicine in various applications.

Fluorinated Hydrocarbons (freons): used widely as aerosols, they have proved fatal to 'sniffers' particularly if they undertake violent exercise, such as running, directly afterwards. The heart is affected; if there is additional lack of oxygen it may stop beating. The ventricles may take on a fast rhythm as a result of the action of the aerosols and even go into fibrillation.

Fluorine: a halogen element which is one of the normal constituents of bones and teeth. Taken in excess it is poisonous, but one part per million in the water supply is not only harmless but will keep 60% of children free of dental caries.

Fluoroacetic Acid: derivatives of this acid are used to kill rats in sewers, but they are very poisonous, and if as little as 30 mg is taken by mouth it may prove fatal. The subject becomes apprehensive, nauseated, develops an irregular pulse, and may have convulsions. There is no antidote.

Flying: *see* Air Travel.

Foetus: in viviparous creatures, the unborn offspring developing in the uterus. Before eight weeks after conception, the child in man is called the embryo, and after that time the foetus. The ovum is fertilised in the Fallopian tube, and in the first week passes into the uterus where it becomes implanted. In two weeks it has grown to be about half an inch long, and by the fourth week the embryo has become curved like a comma and buds appear which will be the ears and the limbs; in the following week the eyes appear and the segments of the limbs are defined. At the end of two months the embryo has taken on a human appearance with a nose and separate fingers, and the tail which has hitherto been prominent is reduced to a rudiment; the embryo is now just over an inch long. In the third month the limbs are clearly human, the finger and toe nails appear, and sex can be distinguished. In the fourth month the foetus is between four and six inches long, hair has appeared and the legs are proportionately longer. In the sixth month the foetus is about twelve inches long, eyelashes and eyebrows appear, and a month later the eyes open and the foetus is capable of being born alive. During the final two months the foetus becomes plumper and the skin develops its final colour. At birth the infant should weigh about six and a half to seven and a half pounds and be about 20 inches long. Before birth the foetus is dependent on the mother's blood for its food and oxygen, exchange takes place through the placenta, attached to the wall of the uterus, although there is no direct connection between the blood supply of the foetus and mother. The umbilical cord connects the foetus with the placenta and it contains two arteries and two veins; after birth it becomes atrophied and withers away.

Folic Acid (pteroylglutamic acid): part of the vitamin B complex found in green leaves, particularly spinach; also found in yeast. It is essential for the formation of normal red cells, and without it the red cells are fewer and larger than they should be, a state called megaloblastic anaemia. Lack of sufficient folic acid in the diet or impaired absorption because of intestinal disease leads to deficiency of the vitamin, which is also found in chronic alcoholism and as the result of taking certain drugs such as phenytoin. In pregnancy the mother needs twice as much folic acid in the diet as she did before, and it is often given as a routine to pregnant women, along with iron.

Follicle: a very small secreting gland, or cyst. In the ovary the ovum develops in a small cystic space filled with fluid, called a Graafian follicle after Regner de Graaf (1641–73), the Dutch physician who first described it.

Follicle Stimulating Hormone: one of the hormones of the anterior pituitary gland which stimulates the formation of the ovum in the ovary and spermatozoa in the testis. Commonly abbreviated to FSH.

Fomentation: the application of a hot sometimes wet dressing to a part to produce counter-irritation, or to encourage the flow of blood to the area and so help boils and superficial infections to localise and drain. Also the poultice itself.

Fomites: articles that have been in contact with an infected person such as clothes, bedding, toys, books, etc., that might be capable of spreading the infection.

Fontanelle: when it is born the baby's skull-bones have not completely come together, and there are six places where the gaps are closed by membrane. The largest is on top of the head where the frontal bone in front and the two parietal bones at the sides leave a gap of a square inch called the anterior fontanelle through which can be felt the pulsation of the brain; the level sinks if the infant is dehydrated. The gap is normally closed by 18 months.

Food Poisoning: can be due to toxic chemicals contaminating the food, to eating poisonous plants or, in most cases, to bacterial infection. The commonest organisms are *Salmonella, Staphylococcus aureus,* and *Clostridium perfringens*;

very rarely *Clostridium botulinum*. Occasionally *Bacillus cereus* is at fault: it may be found in boiled or fried rice kept at a high temperature, as well as in other sorts of food. *See* Diarrhoea.

Foot: the foot is very similar in structure to the hand (q.v.). Each toe has three phalanges, except the great toe, which like the thumb has only two, and they articulate with the metatarsal bones which correspond to the metacarpal bones of the hand. The metatarsal bones articulate with seven tarsal bones at the ankle, as opposed to eight carpal bones in the wrist, but the joint forms a weight-bearing right angle unlike the wrist. The arrangement of blood vessels and nerves is similar to that of the hand and fingers. The weight of the body is borne on three main points: the heel, the head of the first metatarsal bone, and the head of the fifth metatarsal, with the heads of the intervening metatarsals taking a share. There are two arches in the foot, one longitudinal and the other transverse, which are maintained by the shape of the bones of the ankle and the strong ligaments of the sole of the foot aided by the pull of the tendons of the long muscles running from the leg into the foot and toes and the short muscles of the foot itself. In addition there is a strong layer of deep fascia running along the sole of the foot from the ankle to the toes, called the plantar aponeurosis. The bones of the ankle are the talus, which makes a saddle joint with the bones of the leg the tibia and fibula, below it the calcaneus, the heel-bone, and in front the navicular and cuboid and three cuneiform bones. The bones are bound together by strong ligaments, and the talus, navicular and calcaneus are joined to the fibula and tibia by the powerful lateral and medial ligaments of the ankle. The foot is drawn down by the muscles of the calf, acting through the Achilles tendon, and upwards by the muscles passing to the foot in front of the joint.

Foramen: a natural opening especially into or through bone for the passage of blood vessels or nerves. The largest is the foramen magnum at the base of the skull through which the spinal cord passes into the vertebral column. The foramen ovale is an opening between the two sides of the heart in the foetus, which closes normally at birth. If it persists it can be closed surgically.

Forceps: an instrument with two blades and handles for taking hold of objects, pulling, or cutting. Some are used to take hold of tissues, usually called dissecting forceps; some to compress, such as the Spencer–Wells artery forceps with fine blades and ratchet handles to catch and hold bleeding arteries; some to cut, such as bone forceps strong enough to cut through bone; and some to assist in the delivery of the baby in childbirth, the first of which was invented by the man midwife Peter Chamberlen (1560–1631).

Foreign Bodies: anything found in the body which is not naturally there. Examples are objects found in the digestive tract of children who have swallowed them, such as coins, which normally pass naturally, or safety-pins which may not. Beads may be found in the nostrils or ears; and the eyes are not infrequently irritated or injured by foreign matter. Foreign bodies are of prime importance in military medicine, for if they are not removed they can cause chronic infection and prevent wounds healing. But few objects can have been so thoroughly foreign as that encountered by an English surgeon who is alleged to have removed from a patient's rectum a bust of Napoleon.

Forensic Medicine: that part of medicine concerned with the law.

Formalin: a 40% solution of the gas formaldehyde, used for fixing and preserving tissues, and in dilution as an antiseptic.

Formic Acid: a substance found in the stings of certain insects such as ants, bees and wasps.

Fossa: used in anatomy to mean a depressed or hollow area.

Fractures: in theory fractures of bone can occur in any part of the skeleton, but in practice they are most commonly found in certain well-defined areas: for example, the most common fracture of the forearm is Colles' fracture at the wrist, and the most common in the leg Pott's fracture at the ankle. This is partly due to the varying strength or weakness of bones in different areas, and partly to the similar ways in which people tend to have accidents, for example falling on the outstretched hand in the former and 'turning the ankle over' in the latter. Several different types of fracture are described: the simple fracture, in which the bones are broken cleanly with little laceration of the surrounding tissues and no break in the skin surface; the greenstick fracture, characteristic of injuries in children, when the bones, being still soft and not fully calcified, bend rather than break right through; open or compound fracture, when the fracture is associated with a break in the skin surface; complete and incomplete fracture, when the bone ends are separated or together; comminuted fracture, when the bone is splintered into pieces; and impacted fracture, where one part of the bone is driven into the other.

In early life bones contain a good deal of fibrous tissue and are more likely to bend than break, but with increasing age they come to contain an increasing amount of calcium and become more brittle. Bones are broken often by indirect violence; the force is applied at some place other than where the break occurs, and is transmitted to the point of fracture as when a fall on the shoulder results in a broken collar-bone. Direct violence is usually associated with injury to the surrounding tissues, and the bone is broken at the point of impact; the fracture therefore is often compound. If a bone is weakened by cysts, tumours or certain diseases associated with decalcification it may break spontaneously or as the result of minor stress; such fractures are called pathological.

When a bone is broken, bleeding at the site from vessels within the bone and in its surrounding membrane, the periosteum, forms a clot round the fracture, within which cells derived from the periosteum start to lay down new bone. The swelling round the fracture is called a callus, which is at first soft, and then as calcium is deposited becomes hard. As the new bone is formed the shape of the callus is refined to form the definitive callus which knits the two broken ends of the bone together and restores its original strength.

Signs of a fracture are pain, which may not be great; swelling; bruising which takes time to develop, and in some cases shows at a site removed from the fracture as in the case of a fracture of the upper humerus, the bone of the upper arm, where the blood may track down and appear as a bruise above the elbow; deformity, which may not be obvious; abnormal movement; grating or crepitus when the broken ends move on each other; loss of function; and tenderness.

First aid is directed to covering an open fracture with a clean dressing – a freshly laundered handkerchief will do in the absence of sterile dressings – and immobilising the broken bone. Splints must be long enough; adequate splints can be made from rolled-up magazines for the arm or a walking stick or broom handle for the leg. Fractures of the upper arm can be bound to the side, and legs can be bound together. No attempt should be made to remove clothes from simple fractures of the limbs. The patient will be shocked, and must be kept warm; movement must be reduced to a minimum, as it may be very painful and may displace the fracture. The best rule is 'splint them where they lie'. Fractures of the collarbone and arm are more comfortable in a sling, with the hand high and supported in the sling. If there is any suspicion that the spine is broken the patient is left undisturbed; do not move him or her without skilled help.

Fragilitas Ossium: also called osteogenesis imperfecta, a rare inherited disease in which the bones are abnormally fragile.

Framboesia: *see* Yaws.

Freud: *see* Psychoanalysis.

Friar's Balsam: balsams are substances exuded from the trunk of certain trees, which contain resins and oils. Friar's balsam, otherwise compound tincture of benzoin, is used in hot water to form a vapour to be inhaled in chest infections.

It is the moist hot air rather than the balsam which is helpful.

Frostbite: exposure to cold interferes with the vitality of the tissues largely but not entirely by affecting the circulation. In response to severe cold the arteries and arterioles contract so that the part, usually the fingers, hands, toes or feet show areas of hard white skin. The affected part should be kept warm and dry, and when possible the circulation restored by warming gently, using water comfortably hot; sometimes the skin may subsequently go black, but when it sloughs off the tissue left is substantially normal. In more severe cases surgery may eventually be needed when the full extent of the damage is apparent.

Frozen Section: when operating for a growth the surgeon may not be able to tell whether it is malignant or not, and this may make a great difference to the operation. It is possible for a biopsy to be taken, frozen and cut into sections for the pathologist to examine under the microscope and provide a quick answer.

Frozen Shoulder: a condition in which the shoulder is painful and movement is lost. It may follow an injury, or there may be no history of damage; but the shoulder joint is so complicated and so often used and abused that it is no wonder that it may become painful spontaneously. There are a number of names for the condition reflecting the number of structures in the shoulder, ranging from capsulitis to subacromial and subdeltoid bursitis; but from a practical point of view it remains poorly understood and difficult to treat. Local injections of corticosteroids are used, and physiotherapy designed to mobilise the joint; but in many cases the condition is slow to respond, and it takes up to two years for full recovery. It is important that after any injury to the arm or shoulder the shoulder joint is actively exercised and not allowed to stiffen, for full movement may never be regained.

Fructose: fruit sugar, also called laevulose.

Fruit: most fruit contains at least 80% water, the amount being less in starchy fruit such as bananas and greatest in melons. The pulp consists mainly of starch and sugar, the other constituents being acids such as citric, malic and tartaric, and essential oils or volatile substances which give the characteristic flavour. Most fruit contains vitamin C and vitamins of the B complex as well as carotene, the precursor of vitamin A, and various minerals including potassium, iron and calcium. Fruit also provides a good deal of dietary fibre, but little energy or protein.

Frusemide: a powerful diuretic acting on the loop of the renal tubule. *See* Diuretics, Kidney.

Fugue: a patient may suffer from a change of consciousness in which acts are carried out apparently with a purpose, but of which there is no recollection afterwards. This is a state of fugue; it may occur in epilepsy, and in transient global amnesia.

Fulguration: the destruction of tissue by means of sparks; but also applied to the burning of tumours in the bladder by diathermy through the cystoscope, which takes place under water.

Fumigation: the process of burning or volatilising substances in order to produce vapours which destroy infective organisms and vermin. Formerly used after infectious fevers, it is now rarely employed.

Functional Disease: a term used to describe symptoms that have no discoverable basis in physical disorder, and are therefore assumed to have a psychological origin.

Fungus: a plant with no chlorophyll, living on other plants or animals as a parasite or saprophyte. Fungi range from the one-celled yeasts to the many-celled moulds and mushrooms. They are the source of many antibiotics including penicillin and the tetracyclines; but some of them are poisonous. They also cause a number of diseases, either by producing spores which give rise to allergic lung diseases, or by invading the body, usually superficially as in ringworm. The diseases they produce are called mycoses.

Funny-bone: *see* Humerus.

Furuncle: a boil (q.v.).

G

Gait: the way in which people walk often gives important information about the medical condition from which they suffer. Typical are the gait of severe flat foot with the toes turned out and the feet placed flat on the ground, the dragging leg of hemiplegia following a stroke, and the hesitating shuffle of Parkinson's disease.

Galactocoele: a cyst in the breast containing milk, caused by obstruction to a milk duct.

Galactogogue: a substance which increases the flow of milk. There are a number of drugs which may produce galactorrhoea, an excessive or abnormal production of milk, including those used to combat nausea and vomiting such as metoclopramide and the phenothiazines and the drug methyldopa used in high blood pressure.

Galenical: originally a prescription made up by Galen (AD ?131–201), physician to the Roman emperor Marcus Aurelius, the term is now applied to preparations which contain vegetable as opposed to chemical substances.

Gall-bladder: a pear-shaped receptacle with muscular walls, lying attached to the under-surface of the liver. It is part of the biliary system which receives bile from the liver, stores and concentrates it, and discharges it to the intestine. The bile is collected in the liver by small ducts which join until two large ducts are formed; these, the hepatic ducts, leave the liver in a deep fissure called the porta hepatis, which also admits to the liver the portal artery and vein with nerve plexuses and small lymphatic vessels. After they leave the porta hepatis the right and left bile ducts unite to form a common duct which runs down to the duodenum, the first part of the small intestine. It is joined by the duct which comes from the gall-bladder, the cystic duct, and below this the name changes to the bile duct.

This receives the pancreatic duct before it reaches the duodenum.

The gall-bladder is a cul-de-sac, and the only way in and out is through the cystic duct. After it has emptied, bile coming down the hepatic duct from the liver is held up by the closing of the biliary sphincter, a muscle which surrounds the end of the bile duct at the duodenum, and it finds its way up the cystic duct through a spiral valve made up of a fold of mucous membrane into the gall-bladder. Here the mucosal lining withdraws fluid from the bile and concentrates it, while the muscle of the wall of the gall-bladder relaxes to accommodate the increasing volume until the signal comes for it to contract and expel the concentrated bile into the duodenum through the now relaxed sphincter. This signal is given about half an hour after the beginning of a meal, and comes both from the brain via the vagus nerve and from the intestine, for a hormone called cholecystokinin (CCK) is released from the mucosa of the duodenum in response to the presence of food. The function of the gall-bladder can be observed by X-rays; a fat-soluble iodine compound given by mouth is excreted by the liver in the bile and concentrated in the gall-bladder, where it is radio-opaque and outlines the organ. The examination is called cholangiography. *See* Cholangitis, Cholecystitis, Cholelithiasis.

Galls: enlargements produced in plants and trees by the puncture and laying within of eggs by insects. One produced on the oak *Quercus infectoria* by the insect *Cynips gallae tinctoriae* contains tannic and gallic acids, and was once used as an astringent application with or without opium in cases of bleeding haemorrhoids.

Gallstone: *see* Cholelithiasis.

Galvanism: named after Luigi Galvani (1737–98), the Italian physician who noted the effect of electricity on frogs' legs, galvanism is the use of direct current to stimulate the contraction of muscles which otherwise would waste from disuse. It was at one time believed that the passage of direct current through the tissues was generally beneficial, and it was used in a number of diseases, but there is no scientific justification for the belief.

Gamma Globulin: globulins are proteins which are soluble in salt solution but not in plain water, and they can be divided into three groups by their electrophoretic mobility – alpha globulins have the greatest, beta intermediate, and gamma the least. Gamma globulins are rich in antibodies (see Allergy), and the term was used to denote globulins with antibody reactions; but not all such globulins show electrophoretic gamma behaviour, and the term now used is immunoglobulins (q.v.).

Ganglion: (1) A collection of nerve cells in the course of a nerve or a network of nerve fibres outside the central nervous system. (2) A cystic swelling found in relation to a tendon. Often found on the wrist, the swelling is composed of a material like jelly enclosed in a fibrous capsule; there may be more than one. They are not in any way dangerous, but may be inconvenient, and the traditional way of treating them is to burst the cyst with a sharp blow from the family Bible. They can of course be burst by steady pressure, but are liable to recur, and it may be best to have them removed surgically.

Gangrene: death of tissue, as the result of an inadequate blood supply, which may be followed by bacterial infection and putrefaction. Dry gangrene is the result of arterial blockage, wet gangrene of arterial and venous insufficiency and bacterial infection. In dry gangrene the part, possibly a finger or toe, becomes black and shrivelled; a zone of demarcation develops between the dead and living tissue, and in time the dead tissue separates and falls off. Gangrene, especially of the foot, is a complication of diabetes mellitus, and special attention must be paid to the feet in this disease. It may also follow wounds, burns, frostbite, the action of drugs such as ergot, adrenaline used with a local anaesthetic for injection, and exposure to strong acids or alkalis; in the past, dressings of phenol have been at fault. The treatment of gangrene may have to be surgical removal of the affected parts. Gas gangrene follows the infection of dead muscle by *Clostridia*, particularly *Clostridium perfringens*. As the organism multiplies in the dead tissue it produces toxins which kill surrounding healthy tissue, and so the infection spreads rapidly, to a fatal outcome unless treatment is rapid and thorough. All infected tissue must be removed; antisera are available, and oxygen under 3 atmospheres pressure may be given to the patient at intervals, for it kills the organisms which are anaerobic. Penicillin may be used in large doses.

Gargles: although gargles have no effect on infections of the throat, they do clean the mouth and can relieve irritation. In cases of mild sore throat it may be useful to gargle with a solution of two soluble aspirin tablets in water; the local anaesthetic effect of the aspirin helps, and when swallowed the gargle relieves any headache and keeps the temperature down.

Gas Poisoning: since natural gas replaced manufactured (town) gas, there has been a great reduction in the number of cases of carbon monoxide poisoning. Nevertheless, the possibility still exists of carbon monoxide being formed in the home by the incomplete burning of natural gas, which with poor flues and ventilation can result in chronic tiredness and ill health, possibly with headaches and nausea. Severe cases can be fatal. It is important to be sure, if you use a gas appliance, that it is in good order and properly installed, for the symptoms of carbon monoxide poisoning are insidious and can be difficult to diagnose. *See* Carbon Monoxide.

Gastrectomy: a surgical operation for the removal of the stomach, partial or total.

Gastric: relating to the stomach.

Gastric Ulcer: *see* Peptic Ulcer.

Gastritis: inflammation of the stomach.

Gastro-enteritis: inflammation of the stomach and intestines, usually due to bacterial or viral infection, producing diarrhoea and vomiting, but often self-limiting. *See* Diarrhoea, Dysentery.

Gastro-enterology: the study of the digestive system, i.e. the stomach, intestines, liver and pancreas.

Gastro-enterostomy: an opening made surgically between the stomach and the small intestine.

Gastroscope: an endoscope for viewing the interior of the stomach. No anaesthetic is needed for the examination, which is perhaps uncomfortable but safe.

Gastrostomy: an operation on the stomach in which an opening is made between the stomach and the overlying abdominal wall, used in cases in which the oesophagus is blocked or the patient is unable to swallow. A self-retaining catheter or tube is introduced into the opening through which the patient is fed.

Gel: a colloid which has the consistency of jelly.

Gelatin: a colourless and transparent substance made from the collagen of the connective tissue of animals, used in medicine for capsules and suppositories.

Gelsemium: the root of the yellow jasmine, containing gelsamine, a poisonous alkaloid. It has been used in the treatment of migraine and neuralgia, but is unreliable in its effects and poisonous except in very small doses.

Gene: a factor which controls the inheritance of a specific characteristic. Deoxyribonucleic acid (DNA) is the substance through which the composition of proteins and the structure of cells in the organism are passed from parents to offspring, and the gene can be regarded as a region of the very long spiral DNA molecule.

Generic: the official name of a drug is the generic name, as opposed to the brand name given it by the manufacturer.

General Paralysis of the Insane: also known as GPI and dementia paralytica, this disease is a manifestation of the third stage of syphilis (q.v.). It has become very rare since the advent of penicillin, which has made syphilis almost the easiest of the sexually transmitted diseases to cure if treated early, but used to produce progressive mental deterioration, sometimes with delusions of grandeur, until the dementia proved eventually fatal.

Genetics: the study of heredity (q.v.). Since the discovery by Watson and Crick in 1953 of the way in which deoxyribonucleic acid (DNA) present in the chromosomes is able to carry the messages for the formation of protein and is also able to undergo replication and mutation, it has recently become possible to break into DNA molecules and insert nucleic acid molecules from elsewhere. This is genetic engineering, and it has become feasible to form various new hereditable characteristics in organisms. It may even be that hereditary diseases carried by an identified gene can in the future be cured by altering the gene in the developing embryo.

Gentian: the root of the yellow gentian can be used as a bitter to stimulate appetite, and is an ingredient of various aperitifs.

Gentian Violet: an aniline dye used by microscopists as a stain. As crystal violet it may be used on unbroken skin as an antiseptic, but stains clothes and skin a deep violet which is hard to remove. Used sometimes before operations to mark the skin at the site of the proposed operation.

Genu Valgum: knock-knee.

Genu Varum: bow-legs.

Geriatrician: a physician specialising in the care of those over 65 years old.

Geriatrics: the branch of medicine that deals with the diseases of age and studies the problems of growing old.

The term was first used by the American physician Ignaz L. Nascher in 1909 and between the wars in England Dr Marjorie Warren took a lead in organising a department for the care of the aged in London, but little was done until after the Second World War when, with an increasing number of older people in the population and the inception of the NHS, geriatrics was first recognised as a specialty. The problem of the old is essentially one of industrial society in which families tend to become small and the old, being unproductive, are regarded as financial liabilities. Improved medical knowledge, better living and working conditions, and the absence of great wars have altered the expectation of life so that the fastest-growing section of the population is over 60 years old. In the world as a whole, the proportion of elderly people in 1950 was 8.5%; in 2025 the proportion is expected to be 13.7%. Age overtakes people in different ways, and, while some are incapacitated at 60, many are able to function much longer. Nevertheless age brings its own difficulties, many of them due to social conditions; those who have to lead solitary lives may lose interest in themselves and their general attitude changes for the worse. While the work of the geriatrician is concerned to a large extent with chronic medical conditions – although obviously the elderly suffer from acute conditions too – the social, economic and general circumstances in which the patient lives are part of the physician's interest perhaps to a greater extent than in the case of younger people, and to this end a team of health and social workers of various disciplines is needed. The aim is to support the elderly in their wish to be self-sufficient by co-ordinating the services available. While it remains true that many elderly people are cared for by their relatives or friends, an increasing number will come to depend on professional care as the age of the population rises, and the specialty of geriatrics will be more in demand. Research on an international scale into ageing is on the increase, encompassing economic and social matters as well as medical.

German Measles: *see* Rubella.

Gestation: the period between conception and birth in viviparous animals. Gestation in women, calculated from the beginning of the last menstrual period, lasts about 40 weeks.

Giardiasis: a protozoan infection with *Giardia lamblia*, a parasite with flagellae found in the small intestine. It produces cysts, which are passed in the faeces and spread by contaminated food and water. The organism is found all over the world, but is most common in the hotter countries; it causes acute or chronic diarrhoea, and is a cause of traveller's diarrhoea in some cases. It is also liable to infect those with immune deficiency syndromes. The condition is treated with metronidazole or tinidazole; cases of cyst carriers who have no symptoms may also be treated with these drugs.

Gibbus: a deformity of the spine, as in a hunchback; a hump. The medical name is kyphos.

Giddiness: *see* Vertigo.

Ginger: prepared from the root of *Zingiber officinale*, which comes from East India and the Caribbean, it can be used in medicine as a carminative to stimulate the gastric juices and relieve flatulence.

Gingivitis: inflammation of the gums.

Glanders: a disease of horses, donkeys and mules, which is due to infection by *Pseudomonas mallei*, which has virtually been eliminated in the Western world. It could be passed on to man, and the disease was almost invariably fatal.

Glands: a specialised group of cells which secrete or excrete substances which are not the same as those needed for their own metabolism, and which act on other tissues and in places other than the gland itself. Glands are exocrine, when the secretion is removed through a duct, or endocrine, when it passes into the bloodstream. The word is also used to mean a lymph node (q.v.).

Glandular Fever: *see* Infective Mononucleosis.

Glauber's Salt: sodium sulphate, named after the German physician Rudolf Glauber (1604–68) who discovered it. He called it *sal mirabile*; it is a laxative.

Glaucoma: a disease of the eye occurring usually after middle age, in which the pressure of the fluid inside the eye rises and damages the optic nerve and the retina because the normal drainage passages at the margin of the iris are blocked and the aqueous humour cannot escape. Glaucoma can be acute or chronic; in acute glaucoma the eye becomes red and very painful and the sight is lost. A light shone into the eye shows up a greenish-grey colour, and the eyeball feels hard. Immediate medical attention is necessary if the sight is to be preserved, and consists of the use of drugs to reduce the pressure in the eye and surgical removal of part of the iris. In chronic glaucoma the pressure builds up over a matter of years. Vision at the edges of the visual fields is gradually lost, perhaps without it being noticed, and eventually acuity goes. The appearance of the interior of the eye undergoes typical changes, and these can be picked up by the optician at routine examination; it is important that they should be, because the earlier treatment begins the more likely it is to be successful. Eye-drops containing a beta-blocker such as timolol are often used because they reduce the production of aqueous humour, but operation may be required.

Gleet: a slight watery penile discharge typical of chronic gonorrhoea.

Glioma: a tumour of the brain or spinal cord arising from neuroglial tissue, which is the supporting tissue of the nervous system. Although regarded as malignant, these tumours do not spread outside the nervous system, but invade the tissue in which they lie so that there is no clear line between normal tissue and the new growth. This means that it is not possible to remove the tumour with any degree of certainty; moreover, it is in most cases not possible for the surgeon to try to remove it without damaging the brain or spinal cord so badly as to leave the patient severely disabled. Some gliomas are cystic, and it may be practical to drain the cyst, and a few are confined to areas of the brain which can be removed without an entirely crippling effect, but the outlook in this type of tumour is bleak.

Globulin: a class of protein found extensively in animals and plants, soluble in weak salt solutions but not in water. Globulins exhibit electrophoretic activity according to which they can be classified into alpha, beta and gamma groups; those in the blood are divided into immunoglobulins (q.v.) and non-immunoglobulins, which have many functions.

Globus Hystericus: the feeling that there is a lump in the throat preventing swallowing or producing choking, characteristic of certain neuroses and caused by anxiety.

Glomerulonephritis: a disease of the kidneys affecting the glomeruli, formerly known as Bright's disease. *See* Kidney.

Glomus Tumour: there are normally in the fingertips, and other parts of the body such as the ears and the face, communications between small arteries and veins which when open allow the blood to bypass the capillary vessels. These are called glomus bodies and are concerned with the regulation of skin temperature. Occasionally they form very small pink tumours, which are extremely tender and painful; they may occur under the nail, and only respond to surgical removal.

Glossina: the tsetse fly, a biting fly which transmits the trypanosomes of African sleeping sickness.

Glossitis: inflammation of the tongue.

Glossopharyngeal Nerve: the ninth cranial nerve, which contains both motor and sensory fibres, supplying motor impulses to the stylopharyngeus muscle in the throat, the secretory nerve to the parotid salivary gland, and relaying sensation from the throat, the tonsil and the back third of the tongue, including the sensation of taste. It also carries sensation from the middle ear, from the carotid body, which is concerned with the chemical composition of the blood, and the carotid sinus which monitors the blood pressure.

Glottis: that part of the larynx in which the voice is produced, i.e. the vocal folds or cords and the opening between them, the *rima glottidis*.

Glucagon: a hormone secreted by the pancreas which causes a rise in circulating blood sugar by increasing the release of glucose from the liver; its action is the opposite to that of insulin. It is used by injection in the treatment of low blood sugar occurring in the diabetic patient; it can safely be injected below the skin or into muscle, and can therefore be used by a layman and left with diabetic patients or their relatives to use if a dose of insulin is not balanced properly by an adequate intake of food and hypoglycaemic coma results.

Glucose: also called dextrose, a simple sugar, is the substance into which all higher carbohydrates are converted in the body; it is the main source of energy when it is broken down into water and carbon dioxide. It is absorbed without having to be digested. It is not advisable, however, to take glucose just before an endurance sport, for it decreases the use of fatty acids in the muscles and so leads to exhaustion of the muscle glycogen (*see* Fatigue). Leave at least three hours between taking glucose and starting the event; once it has started, glucose can be taken towards the end in small quantities of a dilute solution.

Glue Ear: secretory otitis media, found in children between six months and 10 years old. A factor in the development of this condition is chronic blockage of the Eustachian tube (q.v.), and another is infection of the middle ear, which may have been successfully treated. The symptom is deafness, for the middle ear becomes full of a sticky thick material which interferes with the movement of the ear-drum and the ossicles. Many mild cases resolve spontaneously, but it may be necessary to insert a small hollow plastic tube called a grommet into the ear-drum to allow ventilation of the middle ear. This small operation may be accompanied by removal of the adenoids (q.v.).

Glue Sniffing: solvent abuse. A practice among children and adolescents, usually between 12 and 16 years old, which involves inhaling the vapour of solvents, often those used in glue making, for example the glue used for model aeroplanes. A number of solvents have been implicated, among them toluene, trichlorethane, trichlorethylene, tetrachlorethylene and carbon tetrachloride, contained in such common domestic items as nail polish remover, dry cleaning fluid, paint thinners and hair lacquer; all kinds of aerosols have been used. The object is to become intoxicated; the effects are quick, and the sniffer becomes euphoric and excited, then confused. In many cases there are hallucinations. Recovery takes place inside an hour, often leaving the subject feeling ill and giddy. In some cases damage has occurred to the liver and kidneys, which may not be related to the amount of solvent inhaled; deaths have resulted from intoxication, from consequent accidents or loss of consciousness and inhalation of vomit. The effect of the inhalation of freons used in aerosols has already been noted (*see* Fluorinated Hydrocarbons). Petrol vapour has an intoxicating effect, which is quickly produced, but if inhaled in excess unconsciousness and coma may follow. Prolonged exposure to petrol fumes has resulted in acute leukaemia. Solvent abuse is rarely a solitary habit, and most children are led into it by curiosity or because 'their friends do it', and it is usually a passing fad; but there are those who become habituated and need psychiatric help.

Gluteal: pertaining to the region of the buttocks.

Gluten: protein of wheat and other grain. It becomes sticky on the addition of water, and can be separated from the starchy carbohydrate part of flour and used to make bread and rolls for diabetics and in reducing diets. It can cause a gluten-sensitive enteropathy called coeliac disease, in which the intestinal mucosa is damaged, probably by an immunological reaction, the tendency to which runs in families. It may be recognised at any age, but often infants show signs of it after they have been weaned. The motions are large, pale and offensive and loose; there is abdominal discomfort and loss of weight. If it is allowed to continue, signs of malnutrition may develop. The condition is treated by banning gluten from the diet, and gluten-free flour is readily available. In some patients the condition does not show itself until later in life, and some who have hardly any symptoms are discovered through an abnormal blood count or a family survey.

Glycerin: glycerol, an alcohol used infrequently as a purgative, but often added to various medicines because of its sweet taste. With gelatin, it forms the basis of many pastilles, and is used as a suppository in cases of constipation.

Glyceryl Trinitrate: also known as nitroglycerine, it is used in the relief of angina; taken in tablets under the tongue, it relaxes smooth muscle and so dilates the blood vessels, including the coronary arteries. It also reduces the venous return to the heart, thus diminishing its load. It may cause low blood pressure, headaches and flushing, but tolerance develops to these unwanted effects. It should be noted that the tablets do not last for more than eight weeks. The drug is also available in long-acting preparations and in plasters to be applied to the skin. *See* Angina Pectoris.

Glycogen: a substance comprising a large number of molecules of glucose. It is stored in the liver and muscles, and from it glucose can be derived as needed in the body for the production of energy.

Glycosuria: the presence of glucose in the urine. *See* Diabetes Mellitus.

Goitre: a swelling of the thyroid gland in the neck. Simple goitres, that is those not associated with under or overactivity of the gland, are attributable to a deficiency of iodine in the diet, and they are found in many mountainous parts of the world such as the Alps, the Andes and the Himalayas, as well as other places where there is little iodine in the water or soil. They can be prevented by the inclusion of iodine in the diet, and this also reduces the number of cretinous children. Iodine can also be administered by the injection of iodine in oil, which releases the iodine slowly over a period of years, and the size of the goitres can be diminished by the use of thyroxine, the thyroid hormone. The thyroid can be the site of malignant growth, which in younger patients may show as a hard nodule, and in older people as a more diffuse hard enlargement. The treatment is surgical removal. Goitres associated with myxoedema, deficiency of thyroid hormone, and thyrotoxicosis, overactivity of the gland, are dealt with under those headings.

Gold: in the form of sodium aurothiamolate or auranofin, it is given by injection and by mouth respectively in cases of rheumatoid arthritis which have failed to benefit from NSAIDs (q.v.). It has to be used cautiously, for it may cause damage to the kidneys or blood disorders, as well as skin rashes. The effect is not immediate, and may take as long as three months to show; the mode of action is not fully understood.

Golfer's Elbow: *see* Elbow.

Golgi Apparatus: part of the endoplasmic reticulum of cells which lies near the nucleus, a complex of membranes and vesicles forming an organelle, the function of which is not understood. First described by Camillo Golgi (1843–1926), the Italian pathologist.

Gonadotrophin: human chorionic gonadotrophin, abbreviated to HCG. Secreted by the trophoblast, a layer of cells on the outside of the blastoderm, the mass of cells produced by reduplication of the fertilised ovum, it is concerned with the suppression of menstruation and the embedding of the developing embryo in the uterus. It is present from the earliest days of pregnancy, and can be detected in the urine about two weeks after a missed period and so provides an early test for pregnancy.

Gonads: the organs that produce spermatozoa and ova: the testis and ovary.

Gonorrhoea: a common sexually transmitted disease, caused by the gonococcus *Neisseria gonorrhoeae*. In the male, a discharge from the penis with pain on passing water begins between two and ten days after infection. The discharge is thick and yellow. If it is left untreated, the discharge turns clear and sticky; the epididymis of the testicle may become inflamed, and lymphatic glands draining the area are enlarged and painful. Most importantly a stricture may develop in the urethra, causing later difficulty in passing water. In women there is a discharge from the urethra and vagina, but these are not infrequently unnoticed; in children, usually the victims of sexual assault, the external genitalia may show signs of inflammation. The most important complication in women is pelvic inflammation involving the Fallopian tubes, for this leads to pain, possibly an abscess, chronic inflammation and infertility. Because the symptoms of the original infection may be overlooked it is important that the slightest suspicion of exposure should call for medical attention. It is uncommon now for newborn infants to acquire infection of the eyes from the mother, but once this was a cause of blindness. Treatment has been revolutionised by antibiotics: ampicillin or amoxycillin, in one large dose of 3.5 g together with probenecid, which reduces the excretion of penicillin, is effective except in cases where the organism is penicillin-resistant, when spectinomycin or cefuroxime may be used. Prophylactic eye-drops are used on newborn babies.

Gout: a disease associated with a high level of uric acid in the blood, causing painful inflammation usually of one joint, the first joint of the great toe, which suddenly becomes red, swollen and acutely painful. The disease is commonest in men, the first attack occurring between the ages of 30 and 60; it is not found in boys before the age of puberty, nor in women until after the menopause. Other joints may be affected such as the knee, the elbow, ankle and wrist, but only one at a time. It may be associated with stones in the kidney, and sufferers are usually overweight. Attacks may occur at any time; some people have only one attack of pain, or it may recur at intervals of months or even years. In severe cases deposits of urate crystals may form, called gouty tophi, at the joints and sometimes on the ear, and the kidneys may be damaged. Treatment is by NSAIDs (q.v.) or colchicine in the acute attack, and

271

the pain commonly starts to go in one or two days. In severe cases it is possible to lower the level of uric acid in the blood by using allopurinol, which decreases the production of uric acid, probenecid, which increases its excretion, or sulphinpyrazone, which does the same, but these drugs must not be given during an acute attack; indeed, they may when first administered precipitate an attack.

Graft: a term applied to tissue removed from a person, animal or plant and implanted in another or the same organism to make good a defect or, in the case of a plant, to build a composite individual plant. In human beings skin, bone, and blood vessels are used in grafting within the same subject; it is also possible to graft from one person to another, a technique called transplant surgery (q v)

Gram's Stain: a method of staining bacteria introduced in 1884 by the Danish physician Hans Gram (1853–1938). The staining method is to use crystal violet, then iodine solution, then ethanol or ethanol-acetone, and then counter-stain. The bacteria which are stained purple are called Gram-positive, those which have been decolourised and have taken up the counter-stain Gram-negative. This method of staining separates bacteria into two large groups, Gram-positive and Gram-negative.

Grand Mal: *see* Epilepsy.

Granulation Tissue: the tissue formed by fibroblasts and endothelial cells which grows over a raw surface in the process of healing. It looks like red velvet and is very resistant to infection. As healing proceeds it is covered by epithelial cells, which on the surface form skin; the endothelial cells form small blood vessels and lymphatics, and the fibroblasts lay down fibrous tissue which contracts to form a scar. Formation and contraction of fibrous tissue is increased by the presence of infection, so that scarring is worse when the wound has been infected. The process of the formation and development of granulation tissue is called organisation. A mass of granulation tissue is called a granuloma.

Granulocytes: white blood cells containing granules, divided into neutrophils, eosinophils and basophils according to their staining reaction. They are otherwise called polymorphonuclear leucocytes.

Graves' Disease: *see* Thyrotoxicosis.

Gravid: pregnant; primigravida, one who is in her first pregnancy.

Greenstick Fracture: a type of fracture found in the long bones of children, usually due to indirect violence, where the bone does not break completely; one side of the bone breaks while the other bends. This is due to the preponderance of connective tissue over calcium apatite in the structure of growing bone, which makes it to a certain degree flexible.

Gregory's Mixture: a mixture of compound rhubarb tincture, light magnesium carbonate, sodium bicarbonate and strong ginger tincture used as an antacid and purgative for digestive upsets. It is now known as compound rhubarb mixture, but remains just as disagreeable. (James Gregory, 1753–1821)

Grey Powder: containing mercury and chalk, this was once used as a 'teething powder' for infants. Not for nearly half a century after the description of a disease in infants called acrodynia or pink disease was it realised that it was due to mercury poisoning, and after the use of grey powder and similar mercury-containing compounds in infancy had been abandoned the disease almost disappeared.

Grinder's Disease: a disease of the lungs once seen in knife-grinders, caused by inhaling particles of steel.

Grippe: influenza.

Griseofulvin: an antibiotic active against fungus infection when given by mouth. It is concentrated in keratin, and is therefore useful for infections involving the skin and nails. It is used in intractable or widespread infections, and treatment has to be continued for a month or more. It should not be taken during pregnancy.

Groin: the area which includes the upper thigh and lower abdomen, in which hernias and enlarged lymphatic glands may occur. Also used as a non-medical euphemism for genitalia, as in 'a kick in the groin'.

Grommet: a small plastic tube used to ventilate the middle ear in cases of glue ear (q.v.).

Growing Pains: pains occurring in children during the course of development, usually felt in the legs and back. They are due to a variety of causes, none of which is to do with growing, and although such pains are unlikely to be serious skilled advice should be sought.

Gubernaculum: a cord of tissue formed during the development of the testis which connects the testis with the scrotum while it is still inside the abdominal cavity. When the testis descends during the seventh and eighth month of intrauterine life the gubernaculum guides the way.

Guinea Worm: *see* Dracunculus.

Gullet: the oesophagus (q.v.), a long muscular tube connecting the throat to the stomach.

Gumboil: an abscess at the root of a decayed tooth which produces pain and swelling in the face. In its early stages pain may be relieved by hot mouthwashes and aspirin, but penicillin and a visit to the dentist are usually prescribed by the doctor.

Gumma: a hard granulomatous swelling occurring in the third stage of syphilis anywhere in the body. It develops anything between one and ten years after the primary infection.

Gynaecology: that branch of medicine dealing with the diseases of women.

Gynaecomastia: abnormal enlargement of the male breast. This may happen about the time of puberty, and is due to hormonal imbalance. It is not of consequence, and almost always subsides. Gynaecomastia may be produced by hormonal imbalance later in life; it may be associated with overaction of the thyroid in thyrotoxicosis (q.v.), liver disease, and with the use of oestrogens in the treatment of carcinoma of the prostate.

Gyrus: one of the convolutions on the surface of the brain.

H

Haem: an iron compound present in the respiratory pigments of many animals and plants. In combination with the protein globin it forms haemoglobin, and enables the molecule to carry oxygen.

Haemangioma: a tumour composed of blood vessels. *See* Angioma.

Haematemesis: the vomiting of blood. This can occur from the bleeding of peptic ulcers (q.v.) and needs urgent medical attention if the blood is fresh; if the bleeding has been slow, the appearance of the blood is altered by partial digestion, and it then resembles coffee grounds.

Haematocoele: a cavity containing blood, caused for example by an injury when blood escapes into a natural cavity or into loose connective tissue.

Haematocolpos: retention of menstrual blood in the vagina by an imperforate hymen.

Haematology: the branch of medicine which deals with the blood and its disorders.

Haematoma: a swelling containing blood effused into the tissues, usually as the result of injury.

Haematomyelia: bleeding into the spinal cord.

Haematuria: the presence of blood in the urine; it may come from any part of the urinary tract, and be of serious or relatively little consequence. Some indication of the site of the bleeding may come from the appearance of the urine, which may be dull brown or smoky when the blood comes from the kidneys and brighter if it comes from the bladder. If the blood comes from the bladder or the urethra it will appear at the beginning of the stream. Bleeding from the kidneys may be a sign of various diseases, among them stones and tumours, and bleeding from the bladder may be a sign of a tumour or may accompany severe cystitis. In the urethra bleeding may be a sign accompanying a fractured pelvis or other injury, or an enlarged prostate gland. Other causes of haematuria are scurvy, purpura or other blood disease, or in the tropics bilharzia (q.v.); in some cases no cause is found.

Haemochromotosis: bronzed diabetes, a hereditary disease in which there is an abnormality in the metabolism of iron which results in the deposition of iron in the tissues, especially the heart, liver and endocrine glands. The skin is discoloured, and the damage to the pancreas causes diabetes. Men are affected more than women. Treatment includes the control of the diabetes by insulin and the removal of iron from the body by taking quantities of blood from the circulation at regular intervals.

Haemocytometer: apparatus for counting blood cells.

Haemodialysis: *see* Renal Dialysis.

Haemoglobin: about one-third of the substance of red blood cells is made up of haemoglobin, a pigment containing four haem groups and the protein globin. Its function is the carriage of oxygen to the tissues, when it is bright red, and the removal of carbon dioxide, the waste product of cell metabolism, when the colour is darker.

Haemoglobinuria: free haemoglobin will pass through the kidneys and colour the urine dark red. This may happen after running or walking on a hard surface, and appears to be caused by damage to the red cells in the vessels of the sole of the foot; the condition is called march haemoglobinuria and is not of significance. Haemoglobinuria may occur during sleep, when urine passed in the morning is discoloured; there may be abdominal pain. It is due to a deficiency in the production of red cells in the bone marrow and may lead to iron deficiency anaemia. Other possible causes of haemoglobinuria are poisoning by arsine, potassium chlorate or quinine, and some infections, for example yellow fever and malignant malaria (blackwater fever). It may be a consequence of extensive burning or crushing injuries.

Haemolysis: the breakdown of red blood cells and the liberation of blood pigment into the bloodstream. It may occur in a number of conditions, including haemolytic disease of the newborn, after heart valve surgery, and after the bite of certain venomous snakes.

Haemolytic Disease of the Newborn: a condition brought about by the interaction of an antibody present in the blood of the mother with the blood of the foetus. The incompatibility nearly always involves the Rh or the ABO systems, most commonly the Rh system (*see* Blood Groups), and results in the destruction of the red cells of the foetus, with consequent anaemia and jaundice. Sensitisation of an Rh-negative mother occurs if she has an Rh-positive baby, cells from whose blood pass into the mother's circulation usually during delivery. Sensitisation can also occur from a blood transfusion. It is in a subsequent pregnancy with another Rh-positive baby that the trouble arises. All mothers should have their ABO and Rh groups identified early in pregnancy, and those who are Rh(D)-negative followed during pregnancy to see if they develop anti-Rh(D) antibodies, although they are unlikely to do so during their first pregnancy. If the baby is found to be at risk, amniocentesis may be carried out to assess the degree of jaundice, measures taken to counteract the disease range from interuterine transfusion to exchange transfusion after birth, which after 36 weeks may be induced early. Recently the whole outlook on the disease has been altered by the discovery that sensitisation of Rh-negative mothers can be prevented by an intramuscular injection of anti-D(Rh$_0$) immunoglobulin immediately after the birth of an Rh-positive infant.

Haemophilia: a disease of the blood in which there is a deficiency in the blood-clotting mechanism (deficiency of factor VIII) which leads to repeated haemorrhages, spontaneous or as the result of minor injuries. It is hereditary, and passed down in the female line, although only males suffer from it (X-linked recessive characteristic). Sometimes known as the royal disease, it has in the past run in royal families: Queen Victoria carried haemophilia, passing it on to her grand-daughter the Tzarina of Russia whose son Alexis had the disease. It also passed into the Spanish royal family through Queen Victoria's daughter Beatrice. The Hapsburgs, too, are said to have suffered from haemophilia. Bleeding in haemophilia commonly occurs in the muscles and joints of the legs, which may lead to muscle wasting and damage and deformity of the joints. Bleeding may occur elsewhere, and accidents and operations are always potentially dangerous. Treatment is the intravenous infusion of factor VIII; in milder cases the analogue of the posterior pituitary hormone vasopressin, desmopressin, may be used for its action in increasing the concentration of factor VIII. Cases are usually referred to special centres for advice and treatment.

Haemoptysis: the spitting of blood. It may be a sign of disease or may mean nothing at all; it may be produced by bleeding from the gums or from the nose, or more seriously from the lungs. If its origin is not obvious, blood in the sputum should be regarded as warranting medical advice.

Haemorrhage: bleeding, which may be internal or external, arterial, venous or capillary. In arterial bleeding the blood is bright red, and may spurt out with the beat of the heart; venous blood is darker and escapes in a steady stream; capillary blood oozes from the damaged tissues. Most bleeding can be controlled by pressure over the wound; severe arterial bleeding may need pressure above the bleeding-point where the artery can be compressed against bone. The use of tourniquets is dangerous, but if they have to be used on a limb they must be loosened frequently, must be visible and must be pointed out to others if the care of the patient is transferred. Venous bleeding, for example in the case of an injured varicose vein, can be stopped by elevating the limb as well as using pressure on the bleeding-point. If blood shows through a first dressing it is better to put another dressing over it than to take the first dressing off. If internal bleeding is suspected the patient must be kept still and warm; it is not sensible to give anything by mouth if internal injuries are present, but dryness in the mouth may be helped by sucking ice.

Haemorrhoids (piles): varicose enlargement of the rectal or anal haemorrhoidal plexuses of veins. External haemorrhoids are dilatations of the inferior or anal veins, and lie covered by skin at the anus, while internal piles are dilatations of the superior or rectal veins, lie at the junction of the rectum and anal canal, and are covered by mucous membrane. They are common, and can cause bleeding on passing motions, discomfort and irritation, and pain. External haemorrhoids are often not noticed unless they become thrombosed, when the clot is very painful. Internal haemorrhoids may be unnoticed until they cause bleeding, but they may become prolapsed and protrude from the anus; in some cases they can be replaced easily, but in others they cannot, and may become thrombosed and infected, when they are painful and very distressing. There may be a combination of external and internal haemorrhoids. Treatment of mild cases, where occasional bleeding and irritation are the only symptoms, is to keep the bowel motions regular and soft, and wash round the anus with cold water after passing a motion. In more severe cases various treatments are used, ranging from injection of the haemorrhoids with a sclerosing solution, to induce them to shrivel, to surgical removal.

Haemostasis: the arrest of bleeding.

Haemostatics: substances which help in the arrest of bleeding. Those that have been used for local application include adrenaline, fibrin foam, perchloride of iron, cobwebs and witch-hazel, but they are only effective against slight bleeding or oozing. A more powerful agent is tranexamic acid, which inhibits fibrinolysis and the activation of plasminogen (*see* Coagulation of the Blood), and is given by mouth or by injection.

Haemothorax: blood in the pleural cavity, the space between the chest wall and the lung. It may be the result of a penetrating wound or injury, or the presence of a malignant tumour. Occasionally it may accompany an infarct of the lung. It may be suspected after a chest injury if the pain, shock and shortness of breath are greater than might be expected from the outward appearance of the injury. Treatment is surgical.

Hair: grows from hair follicles, small pits in the skin containing a sebaceous gland. In the wall of the follicle is a muscle, the arrector pili. The hair grows from a hair papilla at the bottom of the follicle, which forms the hair bulb; this is continuous with the hair shaft, which is composed of dense keratinised epithelial cells containing pigment. It has an outer cortex in which the cells are tightly bound together and an inner medulla, where the cells are larger and looser, separated in part by air spaces. Growth is at a rate of about 1 cm a month, and takes place over three years. There is then a resting phase, and then after three months the old hair is pushed out by a new one. In the human, hair follicles are all at a different stage in the cycle, as opposed to other hairy mammals where the cycle is synchronous and shorter and leads to moulting; but illness or an emotional disturbance can disturb the cycle so that hairs fall out before they are due. The distribution of the hair, the pattern and the colour are hereditary; the growth of body hair is largely determined by the sex hormones. *See* Baldness, Hirsutism.

Halitosis: bad breath, common in all people sometimes and in some people all the time. It is often imaginary, but may be caused by bad teeth, inflammation of the gums, severe tonsillitis, or bronchiectasis, a disease of the lungs. A very uncommon disease of the nose, ozaena, may be at fault; but many people believe they have bad breath when it is not true.

Hallucinations: false perceptions of things that are not there. They may involve any of the senses – vision, hearing, taste, smell or touch; they may be induced by drugs, including alcohol, brain disease, the trances of mediums and witch-doctors, religious ecstasy, and psychosis. The classic instance of hallucination of hearing occurs in schizophrenia. The significance of hallucinations must be judged in the context of the individual's ordinary beliefs and cultural level, and in relation to the rest of the subject's behaviour and history.

Hallucinogen: any substance that induces hallucinations, for example cannabis, lysergic acid diethylamide (LSD), and mescaline.

Hallux: the great toe.

Haloperidol: a drug of the butyrophenone group used in the treatment of schizophrenia and mania. It has the drawback that it is liable to produce disorders of the extrapyramidal system (q.v.), but it may be used in emergencies to contain uncontrollable behaviour or relieve severe anxiety. It has also been used in cases of stuttering and hiccups. In the form of haloperidol decanoate it is used as a depot injection, with an action that lasts for four weeks.

Halothane: an anaesthetic agent given by inhalation, commonly used with oxygen or nitrous oxide and oxygen mixture for induction and maintenance of general anaesthesia, because it is not unpleasant to take, does not irritate the air passages and is not generally followed by post-anaesthetic vomiting. It has, however, the disadvantage that repeated administration can cause severe damage to the liver. The commonly used trade name is Fluothane.

Hammer Toe: the toe in this deformity is drawn up and bent like an inverted V, and is liable to become painful because it rubs on the shoe. The treatment is surgical.

Hamstrings: the tendons that lie behind the knee and flex that joint.

Hand: the ability of man to oppose the thumb to the other fingers so that small objects can be grasped and manipulated is one of the distinguishing features of the human race, and makes the hand a most delicate, flexible and intricate instrument. It possesses 27 bones: 8 carpals in the wrist, roughly arranged in two rows of four each, 5 metacarpals in the palm, and 14 phalanges in the fingers, the thumb having two and the fingers three. From the muscles of the forearm 9 tendons run in front of the wrist, passing under a retaining ligament, and enclosed in complex synovial sheaths, to be attached to the fingers and thumb where they bring about flexion, and 6 run behind the wrist to extend the fingers and thumb and to move the thumb outwards. Six muscles act on the wrist. The turning of the hand palm downwards is termed pronation and upwards supination, and these movements are brought about by pronator and supinator muscles of the forearm and the biceps. Because supination is the more powerful movement this determines the direction of the thread in such objects as corkscrews and wood screws. Forming the ball of the thumb and little finger and filling the spaces between the metacarpal bones in the palm are the short muscles whose function is to separate and bring the fingers together and bend the hand at the knuckles. The blood supply to the hand comes from the radial and ulnar arteries, the former passing down the inner side of the forearm, the latter down the outer side. They join to form two arches, deep and superficial, in the palm, from which branches run to the digits. The ulnar nerve supplies the skin with sensation over the little finger and half the fourth finger on the front of the hand, and on the back the little, fourth and half the third fingers. The median nerve supplies the other digits on the front of the hand and the back of the tips of the fingers, while the radial nerve supplies the remainder of the back of the hand. *See* Fingers.

Hangover: most of the symptoms of hangover (apart from those caused by drinking impure alcohol of dubious ancestry) are brought about by the diuretic and irritant powers of alcohol; more fluid is lost than is taken in, and the stomach develops gastritis. It is instructive to pour a little whisky or gin onto a cut. The remedy for dehydration and gastritis is to drink two pints of water before retiring for the night; two pints – four tumblers – is a lot of water, and it may take some determination to drink it down; but the result may be thought worth the effort. The remaining gastritis and headache may be reduced by taking an alkaline stomach powder and an aspirin the next day.

Hapten: chemical group which is capable of exciting an immune response when combined with a protein molecule.

Hare Lip: *see* Cleft Palate.

Harvey, William: English physician born in Folkestone in 1578. In 1628 he published the work *De Motu Cordis*, which for the first time described the circulation of the blood. He died in 1657.

Hashimoto's Disease: a familial auto-immune disease of the thyroid gland, producing a goitre with an increase of fibrous tissue and infiltration of lymphocytes. Antibodies to thyroglobulin are found in the patient, who may suffer from other auto-immune disease. In time the condition may produce myxoedema; the treatment is the administration of thyroxine. *See* Auto-immune Disease. (Hakuru Hashimoto, 1881–1934)

Hashish: the dried stalks and leaves of *Cannabis indica*.

Hay Fever: seasonal allergic rhinitis and conjunctivitis. A reaction is set up in the mucous membrane of the nose, and often the conjunctiva of the eye, by the pollen of various grasses and plants; these can to a certain extent be identified by skin tests, and desensitising injections prepared, but the results are disappointing and the course of injections may precipitate dangerous anaphylactic reactions. However, a range of antihistamine drugs is available, from which one can be selected to suit the individual patient, and the regular use of sodium cromoglycate as a nasal spray or drops, and as eye-drops, in many cases prevents the development of the allergic reactions. In severe cases corticosteroids can be used as a nasal spray, or in extremely disabling conditions they can be taken by mouth.

Hazeline: hamamelis, or witch-hazel, prepared from the leaves and bark of *Hamamelis virginiana*, and used as an astringent extract or ointment for the skin or in suppositories for the treatment of haemorrhoids. It is sometimes used in a lotion for rubbing over strained muscles or sprained joints.

Headache: one of the commonest complaints seen by a doctor. Headaches may be due to fever or an infection, but most can be described as 'tension' headaches, consequent upon tension of the scalp and neck muscles associated with anxiety, depression or overwork. The headache may last for a short time, and be relieved by a simple analgesic; but may be chronic, coming on every day for months, in which case treatment is difficult and often depends on the identification of an underlying depression or chronic anxiety. These headaches are different from migraine (q.v.) in that the patient does not suffer from vomiting, usually has the pain all over the head, often described as a pressure or a band round the skull, does not have any visual disturbance and can carry on at work. Cluster headache is a condition that usually affects men. There is a one-sided very severe headache coming on every day for about an hour or two for a period of a month or longer. It may happen at night, and the pain is felt centring on the eye, which may be bloodshot and watering. After a series of attacks the pain disappears, but may recur after a year of two. Treatment during the period of attacks is the use of ergotamine by mouth or in a suppository, taken before the time at which the attacks usually occur. Headache can be referred from the eye, as in glaucoma, from infected sinuses, from the teeth, or from the upper cervical vertebrae, which when affected by arthritic change can irritate the upper cervical nerves which run up to the scalp at the back of the head. Serious conditions that produce headache are temporal arteritis, meningitis, subarachnoid haemorrhage or subdural haemorrhage, and cerebral tumours, which are dealt with under separate headings. It may be noted that a high blood pressure is rarely a cause of headache.

Head Injuries: may be closed or open, and involve any degree of interference with consciousness from a momentary dizziness to coma and death. The scalp, skull, the membranes covering the brain and the blood vessels associated with them, and the brain itself can all be injured. The scalp is commonly bruised or lacerated and, because the blood supply is so free, any laceration bleeds profusely and generally looks far worse than it is. Bleeding is controlled by pressing the scalp against the bone round the bleeding area so that the vessels supplying it are cut off, when the worst of the bleeding has stopped a pressure dressing can be applied. Hair quickly becomes matted with blood, and this makes many injuries look worse than they are; there should be no hesitation in cutting hair off in order to see the extent of the wound and make the control of bleeding easier. Open injuries that involve the skull and underlying brain should be covered with a clean dressing or freshly laundered cloth, and no attempt made to apply disinfectants or any other medication. The skull can be fractured by a serious blow while the scalp is apparently undamaged, but a fracture of the skull is not by itself important (except that it gives an indication of the force encountered) unless it runs across the temple, the ear or the nose, or the bone is depressed. It is not usually possible to tell if the skull has been fractured without X-rays. Apart from direct violence or open fractures where the injury is obvious, the brain may be severely damaged by the sudden shear strains imposed by acceleration and deceleration caused by a blow on the head. These disrupt the white matter of the brain, and at the same time the cortex may be bruised on the under-surface of the temporal and frontal lobes by contact with the ridges of the base of the skull. It is the extent and severity of the damage to the white matter that determines the degree of loss of consciousness; the injury to the cortex may show itself by loss of function if it is in an area where the function is localised, and later may be in part responsible for the changes that can follow a severe head injury. These include epilepsy, change of personality and loss of function. The most important thing in helping an unconscious person is to make sure that the airway (q.v.) is clear, for complications can follow if there has been any degree of asphyxia. All cases of injury causing unconsciousness should be observed for 24 hours in hospital, for there is a possibility that haemorrhage may occur inside the skull as a result of damage to the middle meningeal artery; in such a case consciousness may be regained, only to be lost again as the extent of the haemorrhage increases. *See* Concussion, Extradural Haemorrhage.

Hearing Aids: basically miniature amplifiers small enough to be worn behind the ear, with a plastic insert for the ear itself. Their response can be varied to suit the patient's hearing loss, which is measured on the audiometer, and both the investigation of the deafness and prescription of a suitable aid are carried out in specialised hearing aid clinics. Because they are only amplifiers they are more satisfactory for those with conductive rather than nerve deafness. *See* Deafness.

Heart: the heart is essentially two pumps lying side by side, one to pump blood from the lungs out into the body, the other to pump blood from the body into the lungs. Each pump has two chambers: in the first, the atrium, blood collects from veins. When the atrium contracts, the blood passes through a non-return valve into the second chamber, the ventricle; when the ventricle contracts blood is prevented from returning into the atrium and is pumped out through another non-return valve into the arteries. When the ventricle relaxes and the cycle begins again the arterial valves close. The pump which circulates blood from the veins of the body into the lungs is the right side of the heart, and that which pumps blood returning from the lungs out into the body is the left side of the heart. The two pumps, which in function are separate, do not in fact lie side by side, for the anatomy is such that the right side spirals and partially encircles the left. Seen from in front, the right atrium and right ventricle lie in front of the left; all four chambers lie in about the same horizontal plane. The heart lies obliquely in the chest between the lungs with its base in the midline behind the breast bone, and its left border is about three and a half inches to the left of the midline. When it contracts it turns and the apex, which is part of the right ventricle in front and the left ventricle behind, can be felt to beat in the fifth space between the ribs; it turns because the left ventricle has a thicker wall than the right, for it has more work to do. It pumps the blood at a pressure of some 120 mm Hg, while the pressure in the right ventricle is far less. The veins supplying the right heart are the superior and inferior venae cavae, which form part of the wall of the atrium, and the right ventricle therefore pumps venous blood through the pulmonary artery into the lungs. When the blood has circulated through the lungs and is full of oxygen it returns to the left atrium through four pulmonary veins, two on each side. This arterial blood is then pumped out through the left ventricle into the aorta, the great artery of the body, and so through the arteries and arterioles into the capillaries, where it gives up its oxygen for carbon dioxide and returns through the venous system to the right side of the heart again.

The non-return valve between the right atrium and right ventricle is called the tricuspid valve; the outlet from the right ventricle is the pulmonary valve. The outlet valve from the left ventricle is the aortic valve, and that between the left atrium and ventricle the mitral valve, which is the only valve to have two cusps; the other valves have three. The tricuspid and mitral valves have cords and muscles like guy-ropes running between them and the inner walls of the ventricles to support them, but the pulmonary and aortic valves have no such support. All the valves are set in fibrous rings. The valves open silently, but when they close they set up vibrations in the bloodstream which can be heard through the chest wall as sounds. These sounds are traditionally represented by the words 'lubb-dup'. The first sound is the almost simultaneous closure of the mitral and tricuspid valves, the second is made up of two sounds, the aortic valve closing fractionally earlier than the pulmonary. Another sound sometimes heard in healthy young people is low and soft and occurs during ventricular filling. If the valves are diseased and cannot open or shut properly, eddies are formed in the bloodstream and 'murmurs' are heard.

Contraction of the heart begins in the atria, and is excited by a pacemaker, an island of specialised tissue called the sinu-atrial or SA node, situated in the right atrium. The wave of contraction spreads quickly through the muscle of the right and left atria, and reaches another island of specialised tissue low in the right atrium called the atrioventricular or AV node. From the AV node a bundle of fast conducting fibres called the bundle of His runs into the upper part of the partition between the ventricles, the interventricular septum, and branches into right and left divisions which ramify in the walls of the ventricles and spread the impulse to contract. (Wilhelm His, 1863–1934)

The heart is contained within an outer fibrous sac and two layers of membrane which can slide over each other called the pericardium. The layers are separated by a thin film of fluid, and the heart can move in relation to the structures round about. It has its own blood supply through the coronary arteries. Heart muscle is specialised, and consists of short irregular branched fibres which adhere to each other and form a network. The muscle is striated, like voluntary muscle, and each cell has its own spontaneous rhythm, but the cell with the fastest rhythm drives the others; these cells are in the SA node.

Diseases of the heart are dealt with under their own separate headings.

Heart Block: When one of the conducting channels in the heart, the atrioventricular (AV) or the bundle of His, is interrupted the rhythm of the heartbeat changes. In complete AV block the pulse rate may drop to below 40/min., and the patient is subject to fainting attacks. The condition is usually due to fibrosis, most often in elderly people, and the treatment is the insertion of a pacemaker. *See* Heart, Pacemakers.

Heartburn: a burning pain felt behind the breastbone extending into the throat. It is associated with conditions that allow reflux of the acid contents of the stomach into the lower oesophagus, such as hiatus hernia (q.v.). It is relieved by alkalis, for example aluminium hydroxide or magnesium carbonate.

Heart Failure: the heart may fail to carry out its function properly because of congenital or acquired disease, and the failure may be mainly of the right or left side (*see* Heart). The commonest type of failure is left-sided, following disease of the mitral or aortic valves, coronary insufficiency or high blood pressure. The exact mechanism of heart failure is complex, and the diagnosis is a clinical one. Patients complain of breathlessness on exertion, and as the condition progresses the amount of exercise possible diminishes. In time it becomes difficult to take breath, and patients often find that it is easier to breathe sitting up than lying down. Attacks of severe breathlessness may take place in the night. In addition the patient feels tired and unwilling to make much effort to do anything. Swelling of the legs, beginning at the ankles, develops and the collection of fluid in the tissues may extend to the abdomen. The lungs may become waterlogged, adding to the difficulty in breathing. Simple measures to relieve the breathlessness and oedema are rest in bed, and avoidance of food containing sodium, such as salt. More severe cases need treatment with diuretics (q.v.) and in some cases digitalis is useful, especially where there is atrial fibrillation. Drugs may be used to reduce the resistance of the arteries, for in response to the decreased output of a failing heart the arteries tend to contract to maintain the blood pressure and so increase the burden on the heart. It is also of benefit to reduce the tone in the veins. There are a number of drugs available which include nitroglycerin and nitroprusside, both having a direct action on the smooth muscle of the blood vessels, others which block the action of adrenaline, some which prevent the formation of the hormone angiotensin, and yet others with different actions, from which the appropriate choice can be made in each case.

Heart-Lung Machine: in cardiac surgery the heart and the lungs can be bypassed, with the blood pumped and oxygenated outside the body by this apparatus. Operations can then be carried out on the heart while it is empty and still.

Heat Stroke: heat is lost from the body by dilation of the blood vessels in the skin and convection and conduction in the surrounding air, and also by the evaporation of sweat from the body surface. As long as the temperature of the skin is about 1°C less than the temperature in the interior of the body, and the temperature of the air less than 32°C, the skin vessels can keep the temperature regulated except during exercise, when the additional evaporation of sweat is required. In a hot dry climate the body becomes acclimatised and produces more sweat with a lower content of salt, but unacclimatised people can become overheated fairly easily on taking exercise, particularly if they are dry. Many hours spent in a hot humid atmosphere can also lead to overheating. If the mechanisms are not adequate the interior temperature rises, and the subject begins to pant, suffers from headache, and becomes irritable, fatigued and even confused; if overheating persists the heart and circulation grow weak and sweating stops, with ultimate collapse. Treatment is aimed at bringing the temperature down, for example by sponging down with lukewarm water. Heat exhaustion may occur after exposure to heat for some days, and involves lack of water and salt lost in the sweat. There is fatigue and giddiness, and perhaps cramp in the muscles. The intake of salt has to be raised in hot climates, particularly by those performing heavy work, but salt tablets are liable to irritate the stomach, and the extra salt is best taken with the meals. A drink to replace water and salt loss quickly can be made up of eight level teaspoons of sugar and one level teaspoon of salt in one litre of water.

Hebephrenia: one of the subdivisions of schizophrenia, occurring soon after puberty, consisting of rapid deterioration in the mind, with lack of social interest, self-centred delusions, hallucinations and absurd behaviour.

Heberden's Nodes: small hard swellings on the finger joints in some cases of arthritis. (William Heberden, English physician, 1767–1845)

Heliotherapy: treatment by the sun's rays, once popular but now confined to cases of psoriasis, who benefit greatly by exposure to natural sunlight.

Helminths: parasitic worms. *See* Worms.

Hemianopia: loss of one half of the visual field.

Hemiballismus: uncontrolled movement of the limbs on one side of the body.

Hemiplegia: paralysis of one side of the body, usually caused by a stroke.

Hemlock: *Conium maculatum*, a plant containing the poisonous alkaloid coniine, a woodland flower found in damp places. Socrates was put to death by a draught of hemlock.

Heparin: a substance found in many tissues of the body, but mostly in the liver, which prevents the clotting of blood by interfering with the formation of thrombin from prothrombin (*see* Coagulation of the Blood). It is used in medicine to prevent clotting, and acts quickly; but the action is shortlived, and it has to be given by injection, either into the veins or under the skin. It is particularly useful in cardiac surgery and renal dialysis. If haemorrhage should be provoked, the antidote is protamine sulphate.

Hepatitis: inflammation of the liver, caused by virus infection, many drugs, and various chemicals including alcohol. Viruses causing hepatitis are described as A, B, D, non-A and non-B (NANB); a virus C has recently been found to be responsible for many cases of NANB, and another virus, hepatitis E, has also been found. The Epstein–Barr virus of infectious mononucleosis can cause hepatitis, as can the viruses of yellow fever and herpes simplex, and the cytomegalus virus, which may infect people with immunosuppressive disease.

In hepatitis A the incubation period is about a month, and infection shows itself by a period of malaise rather like flu; this is followed in ten days or so by jaundice. The disease is self-limiting and recovery takes place without treatment, although it may be weeks before the patient feels fully recovered. The virus is excreted in the faeces, and transmitted by the contamination of food or by contact with an infected person. It is very common in some tropical and subtropical countries.

NANB hepatitis is most likely to be transmitted by blood transfusion, or dirty needles used by drug addicts, and the illness is usually mild, although some cases progress to chronic hepatitis.

Hepatitis B is found in the blood and body fluids, and is transmitted by personal contact, by sexual congress, and by contaminated syringes, needles, and other sharp objects. The incubation period may be as long as six months. Those infected may subsequently suffer from chronic liver disease, and may remain carriers for many months or even years. It is said that there are in the world more than 200 million carriers of hepatitis B, but it is particularly likely to be found in institutions for the mentally handicapped.

The virus of hepatitis D is only found in association with the B virus, on which it depends for its multiplication. If it infects a carrier of hepatitis B it may increase the severity of the liver condition.

Hepatitis E is associated with contaminated water supplies, and occurs in developing countries.

Prevention of infection with the virus of hepatitis A rests on passive immunisation with immunoglobulin, which is given by intramuscular injection; protection lasts for about three months, and can be given to travellers to countries where the disease is known to be common just before they leave, and to close contacts of known cases. It is however possible to produce active immunity to hepatitis B by a course of three injections of a vaccine made either from the plasma of human carriers of the disease, or, increasingly, by biosynthetic techniques. This should be given to all those who may come into contact with the disease, including babies born to mothers who are carriers. Immunity takes up to six months to develop, and lasts between three and five years. Recent work suggests that treatment with interferon (q.v.) may help in cases of hepatitis.

Heredity: this vast subject which forms the theme for the science of genetics can be only summarily dealt with here. The scientific study of heredity was initiated by the Austrian monk Gregor Johann Mendel (1822–84) who, although one of the greatest scientific geniuses, died virtually unknown. He published his work *Versuche über Pflanzen-Hybriden* in 1866 but it was not until 1900 that it was recognised for what it was. Mendel's most important experiments were carried out on the common garden pea, in which it is a relatively simple matter to distinguish several inherited characteristics and to cross-fertilise one plant with another. Thus some seeds are round, others wrinkled; some are green, others yellow; some plants are tall, others dwarf. By deliberately fertilising one plant with another, Mendel was able to show how such characteristics are handed on. It might be supposed that traits of this type mingle to produce others which are a compromise between the two, for example that the offspring of a tall and a dwarf parent would be medium-sized, and so it sometimes turns out in nature where few characteristics occur in pure form. But Mendel was able to show that when pure tall and dwarf lines are crossed the offspring are hybrid talls, because the characteristic of tallness is dominant, and when these are interbred the third generation is in the proportion of one pure tall to one pure dwarf and two hybrid talls. The pure lines when mated with each other breed true, only producing talls or dwarfs; but when the hybrids (who all appear tall) breed, the above proportions are found. The underlying reason for these proportions, although unknown to Mendel, is apparent when we consider the process of cell division and reproduction. Every living cell (with rare exceptions such as the human red blood cell) contains a central nucleus which is responsible for cell metabolism and also carries the material which is the agent of heredity in the form of the chromosomes; ordinarily these are in a confused network which resembles a roughly crumpled skein of wool, but when cell division is about to occur this breaks up into numbers of separate chromosomes. These are rod, comma or globular-shaped paired bodies along which are strung the genes which are the actual carriers of the units of heredity. The cell in dividing narrows at the middle, and the chromosomes divide equally down the centre of each one so that when the narrowing becomes a distinct waist, and then a dumb-bell shape just before the two new cells separate, each part will contain the same genes as the other. This process is called mitosis and obviously there is little possibility of variation, for the two cells which have separated in this way contain the same hereditary material. But the mechanism of evolution is divergence, and this factor is introduced by sexual reproduction when two cells unite, each with a different hereditary content. Before this can happen the number of chromosomes must be halved in the sex cells, or gametes; the paired chromosomes instead of dividing down the middle, go half to one cell and half to another; thus in the human the cells of the body contain 46 chromosomes, but spermatozoa and ova contain 23; when fertilisation takes place the full number is again present.

Consider again Mendel's tall and short pea plants. Each pure-bred tall pea and each pure-bred dwarf contains in every cell two units (or genes) for tallness or dwarfism, so that when the sex cells are formed they will contain only factors for tallness or dwarfism. The hybrids, on the other hand, have cells which contain one gene for tallness and one for dwarfism, and when they divide to form sex cells some will carry only tall characteristics and others only dwarf ones. When the two hybrids are crossed the possibilities for the offspring are: tall unites with tall, tall unites with dwarf, dwarf unites with tall, and dwarf unites with dwarf. There will be one pure-bred tall, one pure-bred dwarf, and two hybrids which appear tall but are not pure-bred. The gene which imposes its appearance on the hybrids is the dominant gene, the other the recessive.

According to commonly accepted theory the genes are totally unaffected by any events in the life of the individual who carries them, and changes in the genetic constitution of a species are brought about by natural selection, which weeds out useless traits by causing those who carry them to die out earlier than those with useful variations. To take an example, in a wood near London a certain moth had a wing colour which perfectly fitted in with the light grey bark of the trees on which it usually rested. It was invisible to hungry birds. But gradually the smoke of the growing city blackened the trunks of the trees, and the light-coloured moths were easily seen and picked off by predators. Some, however, had chance variations of wing colour which were nearer in tint to the blackened trunks, and they not only survived but increased since they naturally produced a higher proportion of dark-winged offspring. Today no light-winged moths survive. This is natural selection; another mechanism of evolution is mutation, in which the genes are changed by factors which are not fully understood; it can, however, be caused by ionising radiation such as X-rays or atomic radiation. *See* Cell, Genetics.

Hermaphrodite: a rare condition in which both male and female sex organs are present, due to developmental abnormality.

Hernia: the abnormal protrusion of one structure through another. The commonest type is protrusion of part of the abdominal contents through the abdominal wall, which in men may occur in the inguinal region, or groin, above the inguinal ligament, which runs obliquely from the bony protuberance of the pelvis felt in the outer part of the lower abdominal wall called the anterior superior iliac spine, to the pubic bone near the midline. There is a weakness of the abdominal wall where the spermatic cord and blood vessels run from the testis into the abdomen in the inguinal canal, and a pouch of peritoneum protrudes and comes to lie along the spermatic cord. It may extend all the way into the scrotum, or be confined to the canal, and may contain small intestine or omentum (q.v.). This is called an indirect hernia; in a direct hernia there is a bulge and weakness of the muscles behind the inguinal canal, through which the peritoneum protrudes.

Indirect hernias may be congenital, that is present at birth, or may show themselves later in life, and are not dangerous as long as they can be replaced easily in the abdomen; they usually disappear when the man lies down. It is however possible for them to become irreducible and incarcerated, with the contents still supplied with blood, or strangulated, when the blood supply is cut off and the condition becomes very dangerous. The treatment of simple reducible inguinal hernias should always if possible be surgical repair; an irreducible or strangulated hernia is a surgical emergency. The use of a truss, a pad placed over the inguinal canal and kept in place by a steel spring, is only to be recommended if the patient is unfit for operation. In the female, the hernia in this region is usually below the inguinal ligament, and the protrusion expands through the femoral canal where the artery and vein run over the brim of the pelvis into the thigh. These hernias are likely to become strangulated, and if they contain small bowel the condition becomes dangerous. Again the treatment is surgical.

Other types of abdominal hernia are umbilical, found in infants when the umbilicus does not close off properly, which can confidently be left to close itself; para-umbilical, due to separation of the muscles in the midline just above the umbilicus; and ventral, where the separation is in the midline above or below the umbilicus. These may need surgical closure. Incisional hernias occur when muscles involved in surgical incisions later weaken and give way, and they too may have to be surgically repaired. There are other places where the abdominal contents may protrude, but they are rare, except in the upper abdomen where a knuckle of stomach may slip through the diaphragm and form a hiatus hernia (q.v.).

Heroin: diamorphine, a powerful derivative of morphine, which is easily soluble and produces less nausea than morphine. Used in medicine as a narcotic analgesic, especially in terminal illness, it has been greatly abused by addicts to the extent that the World Health Organization wishes its manufacture to be discontinued, and it is not possible to use it medically in the USA and other countries.

Herpes Simplex: caused by the herpes simplex virus, HSV, which may be acquired at any age, but commonly at first gives rise to no symptoms, although antibodies and immunity develop; the virus persists in the nerve ganglions and may give rise to recurrent manifestations of disease later. HSV has two types, type 1 which gives rise to most infections and type 2 which is found in genital disease. Type 1 causes cold sores round the mouth and nose; it may also cause a mild form of meningitis, or a much more dangerous encephalitis which follows a first infection, and is not likely to affect those with cold sores or other types of herpes. Type 2 is transmitted by sexual contact, and the herpetic blisters appear on the genital organs and may be very painful, especially in the female; it is very liable to recur. Herpes infection is dangerous to patients who have immune deficiency conditions, for example AIDS. Treatment of herpes on the skin and genitals is the administration of acyclovir by mouth or locally as a cream, or the local application of idoxuridine solution.

Herpes Zoster: the virus responsible for this disease is the same as that responsible for varicella, or chicken-pox: the varicella-zoster or V-Z virus. The original infection produces chicken-pox, which is a very infectious disease, being spread by droplets from the mouth and nose. It is a common, and usually mild, disease of childhood. An immune reaction is set up by the virus, which as in herpes simplex persists in the nerve cells of ganglions. Later in life, when the immunity is lost after about 40 years, it may reappear in the skin and produces herpes zoster. The attack is usually preceded by pain in the area affected, which is commonly on the trunk, on one side, and confined to the area of skin supplied by one nerve root. Vesicles then appear and scab over in about a week, although the pain may persist and later be troublesome, and the skin in the area may become very sensitive to the touch. The most dangerous area for the disease to appear is in the face and forehead, for the eye may be involved and this may lead to complications. Treatment for the skin of the trunk involves early local application of idoxuridine solution to the vesicles for four days following their appearance, and this usually relieves the pain and lessens the discomfort which may follow; when the disease affects the eye, injections of vidarabine or acyclovir may be given, but they must be used early in the infection. The pain of neuralgia following herpes zoster is unfortunately often difficult to treat. While chicken-pox may be caught from a patient with herpes zoster, the converse is not true.

Hexachlorophane: a skin disinfectant which may be used as a dusting powder in newborn infants to prevent infection of the severed umbilical cord, or as a cream to disinfect the hands.

Hiatus Hernia: protrusion of the upper part of the stomach through the diaphragm, which may lead to an escape of gastric acid into the oesophagus and consequent pain behind the breastbone, 'heartburn', and regurgitation of the stomach juices as 'water-brash'. The symptoms are worse after a heavy meal, and on lying down, so that they commonly appear on going to bed; they are relieved by standing up. Stooping over may produce symptoms, and should be avoided. The head of the bed can be raised on blocks. Sufferers are usually overweight, and an effective reducing diet often relieves the condition; much discomfort can be avoided by taking antacid mixtures.

Hiccup: spasmodic contraction of the diaphragm and muscles of respiration followed by closure of the vocal cords. What function could be served by this is not clear, but a bout of hiccups can be stopped by a shock, drinking iced water, rebreathing air from a bag and thus increasing the concentration of carbon dioxide in the blood, or by sniffing pepper to provoke sneezing. Intractable hiccup may occur in disease of the nervous system, for example encephalitis, or metabolic disturbance such as uraemia.

High Blood Pressure: *see* Hypertension.

Hip Joint: the ball-and-socket joint between the ball-shaped head of the femur, the thigh-bone, and the acetabulum, a cup-shaped hollow in the side of the pelvis. Because it has a very strong fibrous capsule with powerful ligaments it is rarely dislocated in adults, but some children are born with an ill-formed joint which is easily dislocated, a condition called congenital dislocation of the hip. If it is diagnosed early in life it can be corrected by the use of special splints; the test for the condition is easy, and routinely carried out in infant welfare clinics. If it is left the individual walks with a waddling gait. Because the hip joint transmits considerable weight and is in constant movement it is in later life liable to become the seat of osteoarthritic disease, which causes increasing pain and difficulty in walking. One of the great advances in surgery has been the introduction of the artificial hip joint, which consists of a metal head to replace the femoral head and a plastic socket for the acetabulum. About 95% of patients experience freedom from pain after the operation, and 75% of artificial hips are expected to last for 20 years.

Hippocratic Oath: Hippocrates was a Greek physician who lived in Cos from about 460 to 370 BC and is universally recognised in the West as the 'Father of Medicine'. He and his school left many writings, among which is the Hippocratic oath, which has been accepted as the foundation for codes of medical conduct ever since:

I swear by Apollo Physician, by Asclepius, by Health, by Heal-all, and by all the gods and goddesses, making them witnesses, that I will carry out, according to my ability and judgement, this oath and this indenture: To regard my teacher in this art as equal to my parents; to make him partner in my livelihood, and when he is in need of money to share mine with him; to consider his offspring equal to my brothers; to teach them this art, if they require to learn it, without fee or indenture; and to impart precept, oral instruction, and all the other learning, to my sons, to the sons of my teacher, and to pupils who have signed the indenture and sworn obedience to the physicians' Law, but to none other. I will use treatment to help the sick according to my ability and judgement, but I will never use it to injure or wrong them. I will not give poison to anyone though asked to do so, nor will I suggest such a plan. Similarly I will not give a pessary to a woman to cause abortion. But in purity and holiness I will guard my life and my art. I will not use the knife either on sufferers from stone, but will give place to such as are craftsmen therein. Into whatsoever houses I enter, I will do so to help the sick, keeping myself free from all intentional wrong-doing and harm, especially from fornication with woman or man, bond or free. Whatsoever in the course of my practice I see or hear (or even outside my practice in social intercourse) that ought never to be published abroad, I will not divulge, but consider such things to be holy secrets. Now if I keep this oath and break it not, may I enjoy honour, in my life and art, among all men for all time; but if I transgress and forswear myself, may the opposite befall me. (*The Doctor's Oath*, by W.H.S. Jones, Cambridge University Press.)

Hippus: normally the pupil of the eye contracts and dilates rhythmically but imperceptibly – hippus is a condition in which the movement is exaggerated and obvious. It continues all the time and is not stopped by changes in the level of light nor by accommodation.

Hirschsprung's Disease: *see* Megacolon.

Hirsutism: the growth of superfluous hair, especially in women. It is due to androgenic hormones, and commonly starts soon after the onset of the menses. If the periods are normal, there is very little likelihood of underlying disease, but if they cease or are very irregular there may be some cause such as a polycystic ovary. Treatment is of the underlying cause, if there is one, but in the common case where none is evident removal of the offending hair, for example by electrolysis, may be sufficient; in more severe cases, drugs which antagonise the action of androgens may be used, for example cyproterone. In some cases the contraceptive pill has the desired effect, for it decreases the activity of the ovaries, which normally secrete weak androgens.

Histamine: a substance found throughout the body. It is of considerable importance, and has a number of actions on the tissues. Secreted by basophilic cells and mast cells, as a hormone it causes smooth muscle to contract, both that surrounding the airways of the lungs, and that surrounding the gut, dilates arteries and capillaries and stimulates the secretion in the stomach of gastric acid and pepsin. It is released in the antibody–antigen reaction of allergy (q.v.) and is responsible for many of the symptoms, and is also concerned in the process of inflammation. It has been found that there are two types of receptors through which histamine produces its effects, H_1 and H_2. Antihistamine drugs of the conventional kind used in treating allergic reactions act upon H_1 receptors; comparatively recently drugs have been introduced which act upon H_2 receptors. These are used in the treatment of peptic ulcers, for they decrease the secretion of gastric acid. The first of these drugs was cimetidine, which was followed by ranitidine; other drugs have followed, namely famotidine and nizatidine.

Histology: the study of the microscopic structure of tissues.

Histoplasmosis: a fungus infection by the organism *Histoplasma capsulatum*, found mostly in the USA. The fungus is found in the soil where bird excreta are present, and if it is inhaled affects the lungs, but may spread throughout the body.

Hives: nettle rash or urticaria (q.v.).

HLA (Human Leucocyte Antigen): this antigen, which is present in all cells with nuclei, was first identified in work on human white blood cells. It plays a most important part in determining whether transplanted tissues will be rejected by the recipient.

Hoarseness: commonly due to infection of the throat and larynx, when the treatment is that of the underlying condition and resting the voice. It may be caused by irritation of the vocal cords by misuse; this results in swelling and thickening, and possibly the development of polypi – small excrescences of the membrane covering the cords. The treatment is to give up shouting; polypi can be removed surgically. If however hoarseness develops in the absence of infection or misuse of the voice, it is important to seek medical advice, for it may be due to a tumour of the larynx, in which case early treatment is essential.

Hobnail Liver: *see* Cirrhosis.

Hodgkin's Disease: a disease of the reticular and lymphatic tissues of the body, twice as common in young men as young women, first described by the English physician Thomas Hodgkin (1798–1866). It causes painless enlargement of the lymph glands, commonly in the neck or axillae, and may be accompanied by a fever and night sweats. As the disease spreads other lymph glands become enlarged, and the skin may itch; the spleen may become enlarged, and later the liver, and groups of glands may interfere with the function of neighbouring structures. The diagnosis is made by biopsy of an enlarged gland. The treatment of this formerly incurable disease has been revolutionised by advances in deep X-ray therapy and chemotherapy, and now the majority of cases can look forward to a cure.

Holistic Medicine: an emphasis on the concept of the patient as a whole, rather than a case suffering from a particular disease regardless of background and individual characteristics, marks this medical philosophy. There is in fact nothing new about this approach to medicine, which has always been adopted by any good medical practitioner.

Homatropine: an alkaloid derived from atropine, used to dilate the pupil of the eye.

Homoeopathy: a system of medicine founded by C.F.S. Hahnemann (1755–1843), a physician of Leipzig. Being dissatisfied with the state of medicine, he put forward in 1796 his new principle of the 'law of similars', to the effect that diseases should be treated by substances which produce symptoms similar to them in healthy people (*similia similibus curantur*). Four years later he produced his other principle, that drugs should be given in almost infinitesimal doses, believing that the smaller the dose, the greater the effect. Hahnemann's views caused great antagonism in Leipzig, and he had to leave, ending up in Paris where he ran a successful practice based on his principles; they were in retrospect an advance on most orthodox medicine of the time, for they delivered his patients from the over-prescription of many spurious remedies. Homeopathic medicine is practised today more in European countries than in the USA, and some practitioners allow drugs to be used in certain cases in more orthodox doses: but without scientific evidence to support its tenets homoeopathy remains difficult for most doctors to accept.

Homograft: a graft taken from another individual of the same species. Also called allograft.

Homosexuality: *see* Sex.

Hookworm: *Ankylostoma duodenale* and *Necator americanus* are hookworms which infest man. The worms are found in tropical and subtropical countries; they live in the upper part of the small intestine and lay eggs which pass out of the gut, but cannot develop into larvae unless they fall into damp and moist places. The larvae are able to burrow into the skin, so that anyone coming into contact with water or mud where the larval worms are present runs the risk of infection. The same risk is present if drinking water becomes contaminated, but simple sanitation will prevent this. When the hookworm has entered the skin it makes its way in the case of *N. americanus* into the lungs, and in *A. duodenale* into muscle, where the larvae develop further. They then migrate into the duodenum. When the larvae enter the skin they cause small pustules, often referred to as 'ground itch', and the dermatitis can last for a number of days. In the lungs they cause a cough, but the main symptoms are caused by the worms sucking blood from the walls of the duodenum. In a heavy infestation there is anaemia, discomfort in the upper abdomen, malnutrition and oedema. *A. duodenale* may live for fifteen years, but *N. americanus* only for three. Treatment is with the drugs bephenium, pyrantel or mebendazole; iron is given for the anaemia, with folic acid.

Hordoleum: a stye, inflammation of a sebaceous gland in the eyelid.

Horehound: a group of perennial herbs found throughout Europe, although not very common in Britain where the white or common horehound is infrequently found and the black horehound only occurs south of the Forth and Clyde. The dried leaves of the former, *Marrubium vulgare*, are used to relieve coughs; they are either mixed with sugar or prescribed in a fluid extract – more often nowadays by herbalists than physicians.

Hormones: substances secreted by cells which, passing into the body fluids, influence other cells in tissues or organs in other parts of the body.

Horner's Syndrome: a group of signs and symptoms resulting from paralysis of the sympathetic nerves in the neck. They are: drooping of the upper eyelid; sinking-in of the eyeball; constriction of the pupil; and loss of the power of sweating on the affected side. (Johann Horner, Swiss ophthalmologist, 1831–86)

Hospice: during the last 20 years or so, increasing attention has been given to the needs of the incurable and dying; the Hospice movement, devoted to the care of patients in the terminal stages of illness, has grown from the special homes established and maintained usually by religious organisations since the end of the last century. The mediaeval hospice was a place of rest for travellers; the modern hospice is not only a place of rest, but extends its work into the community, using its knowledge to ameliorate the suffering associated with impending death and helping the general practitioner caring for the dying.

Hospital: from the Latin *hospitium*, a place for guests and those needing shelter. There were hospitals of a sort for the sick attached to temples in ancient Egypt from about 4000 BC, where patients slept in the hope that the gods would cure them; the temple of Asclepius at Cos in Greece, associated with Hippocrates, the 'Father of Medicine' (460–370 BC), was originally based on the same hopes, but became more scientific as under his influence diseases became better understood. In the East, the Indian Emperor Asoka founded a hospital at Surat, and the famous Sultan Harun al Rashid who died in AD 809 built numerous hospitals in Baghdad. Constantinople under the Byzantine empire had the Pancrator, which was far in advance of anything contemporary in Europe, with specialists in various branches of medicine, women doctors for childbirth, a pharmacy and an almoner's department, disinfection of the patients' clothes on admission, and issue of clean clothing and bedding while under treatment.

In the Middle Ages there were infirmaries in monasteries, and lazar-houses for those who suffered from leprosy. In England, following the dissolution of the monasteries, infirmaries fell into lay hands, and in 1601 the Poor Law put the care of the poor in the public domain. Up to 1700 there were four voluntary hospitals in the kingdom; in 1800, sixty-one; and during the nineteenth century the number rose into the hundreds. The important events which made hospitals as we know them possible and needed were the discovery of anaesthetics, which completely transformed the practice of surgery, the increasing understanding and knowledge of bacteriology, which reduced the dangers of sepsis and infection, and the improvements in the standard of nursing initiated by Florence Nightingale as the result of her experiences in the Crimean War, which she introduced to St Thomas's School of Nursing in London. As a result it became clear that a hospital rather than home was the best place to care for the sick

Hourglass Stomach: the appearance seen in an X ray of a stomach constricted in the middle as the result of spasm or more commonly the scarring of old ulceration.

Housemaid's Knee: a swelling of the bursa in front of the kneecap due, as the name suggests, to excessive kneeling.

Humerus: the bone of the upper arm, articulating with the shoulder-blade (scapula) at the upper end in a ball-and-socket joint, and with the radius and ulna, the two bones of the forearm, at the elbow in a hinge joint. The inner prominence of the humerus at the elbow is called the funny bone; behind it directly under the skin runs the ulnar nerve, and a blow upon it is extremely painful

Humours: a term now used only for the aqueous and vitreous humours of the eyeball, but formerly associated with a theory of the nature of disease originating with the Pythagorean philosophers in the sixth century BC, but accepted by Hippocrates, Aristotle and Galen and in one form or another by most physicians well into the eighteenth century. The theory ascribed temperaments and diseases to excess or deficiency of the four humours, which were fluids contained in the body: blood, which made a man sanguine and cheerful; phlegm, a dull-watery humour which made a man calm and phlegmatic; choler, which was yellow bile and made a man bad-tempered and choleric; and melancholy, or black bile, which made a man sad. Although as a theory to account for disease this view is long outdated, the terms persist to describe basic types of personality.

Hunterian Chancre: the primary sore of syphilis, which has an ulcerated hard base. The discharge is thin and watery. It derives its name from the London surgeon John Hunter (1728–93), who inoculated himself with syphilitic matter in order to demonstrate how the disease was passed on and how it developed.

Huntington's Chorea: a rare familial neurological disease, inherited as a Mendelian dominant. It shows itself between the ages of 30 and 40 and is characterised by involuntary movements of the limbs and mental deterioration leading to complete dementia. No treatment is possible. It is however becoming possible to identify the gene defect, and the disease may in the future therefore become identifiable very early in foetal life by chorionic villus sampling. *See* Chorea.

Hutchinson's Teeth: narrowed and notched incisor teeth typical of congenital syphilis, named after Sir Jonathan Hutchinson (1828–1913), the surgeon who first described them.

Hyaluronidase: a naturally occurring enzyme which has the property of breaking down hyaluronic acid, the cement substance, or ground substance, of tissues so that the tissue planes are opened up. It is found in the venom of snakes and spiders, and in leeches; it also occurs in mammalian testes. It is sometimes used to speed up the absorption of injected drugs and fluids.

Hydatid Disease: infection with the dog tapeworm, *Echinococcus granulosus*. The natural cycle for this worm is from dogs to sheep, or other herbivores, who form the intermediate host; they eat the eggs which have been shed from an infected dog, and the developing worm passes into the liver, lungs or other parts of the animal, where

307

it forms cysts containing other developing worms. When a dog eats the offal from an infected sheep the worms reach full growth and come to infest the jejunum, whence eggs are shed in the dog's faeces onto grass where sheep may graze. Humans become the intermediate host accidentally by infection from dogs, and cysts may be formed in the lungs, liver, muscles, and other parts including the brain. These may burst or become infected, or in the brain interfere with function or cause symptoms of increased pressure within the skull. If the cyst bursts, it may set off a fatal anaphylactic reaction (see Anaphylaxis), or in the lungs cause coughing and blood-stained sputum, and daughter cysts with developing worms are seeded in the neighbouring tissues. Surgical removal of cysts may be necessary, but the operation is difficult for the cysts are fragile. Spread of the disease has been controlled in many countries by preventing dogs from eating offal, and by worming them regularly.

Hydatidiform Mole: a disease of the superficial layer of the chorion, the outer of the two membranous layers covering the foetus in the uterus, in which the uterus becomes full of vesicles like grapes; it results from abnormal development of the fertilised ovum. The patient progresses normally for the first months of pregnancy, but after about four months there is a certain amount of bleeding, sometimes a watery discharge, and occasionally the escape of vesicles from the mole. There may be pain in the back and loins, and the uterus is bigger than expected for the date. The mole must be removed, for in one in ten cases it may undergo malignant change. If the patient is content to have no more children, the uterus and mole may be removed together; otherwise she must attend the clinic for regular reviews after the mole has been taken away.

Hydrargyrum: mercury.

Hydrocarbon: an organic compound consisting entirely of hydrogen and carbon atoms; according to the arrangement of the atoms and the properties of the compound, hydrocarbons are classified as alicyclic, aliphatic and aromatic. Alicyclic compounds have a cyclic structure but no benzene ring; aliphatic have no carbon ring; and aromatic hydrocarbons have a ring structure with double bonds, the benzene ring.

Hydrocephalus: an abnormal amount of fluid in the head. The brain contains cavities called ventricles which are normally full of cerebrospinal fluid, which is formed in the ventricles by the blood vessels of the choroid plexuses. The ventricles communicate with the outside surface at the base of the brain, and the fluid runs upwards to be absorbed through special structures called arachnoid villi into the blood in the venous sinuses contained in the dura mater, the outermost of the three membranes surrounding the brain. If the channels through which the fluid passes are obstructed, so that it cannot be absorbed, hydrocephalus follows, with dilation of the ventricles. If the obstruction is in the ventricular system, it is called a non-communicating hydrocephalus; if outside, communicating. Hydrocephalus in infants is very often of unknown origin, but may be due to narrowing of the aqueduct, a passage between the third and fourth ventricles, as a result of bleeding into the ventricles or infection. It is also associated with spina bifida. It is manifested by enlargement of the head, especially the forehead, because the bones of the skull have not fused. The child may suffer from headache, difficulty in movement and squint. If investigation fails to identify any underlying treatable cause, and the child has impairment of mental capacity or movement, a shunt may be placed between the ventricles and the peritoneal cavity to drain the surplus fluid. Acquired hydrocephalus is usually the result of a tumour blocking the passage of the cerebrospinal fluid, and is non-communicating; a block may follow inflammation or, rarely, bleeding after an injury.

Hydrochloric Acid: a solution of the gas hydrogen chloride in water. It is contained in normal stomach juices in a diluted form.

Hydrocoele: a common condition of men in which there is a collection of fluid in the tunica vaginalis, the sac which surrounds the testicle. It may occur at any age, but is more common as age advances. There is usually no obvious cause, but in some cases there is underlying disease. A painless, smooth, elastic swelling of the scrotum develops, which is full of straw-coloured fluid that can be drawn off through a wide-bore needle. As the swelling usually recurs after this has been done, it is advisable to have an operation if possible, when the sac containing the fluid can be removed. Hydrocoele in infants usually disappears by itself.

Hydrocortisone: a corticosteroid with glucocorticoid action, used commonly in 1% creams and ointments for skin conditions, as well as for replacement therapy and the suppression of allergic and inflammatory reactions. *See* Corticosteroids.

Hydrocyanic Acid: a poison contained in the seed kernels of cherries, apricots, almonds and peaches. There is a small amount in cassava flour. *See* Cyanides.

Hydrogen Peroxide: being decomposed into water and oxygen when brought into contact with the tissues, especially in the presence of dead cells and pus, hydrogen peroxide exercises its action as a cleanser by virtue of its freed oxygen. It is used in a concentration of 6% (20 vols) and is mild, safe, and ordinarily non-irritant; it is useful in removing dressings that stick, in cleaning wounds and ulcers, in disinfecting small amounts of drinking water, as a mouthwash, in treating inflammation of the gums, in removing wax from the ears, and in stopping bleeding from capillary oozing.

Hydronephrosis: distension of the pelvis of the kidney with greater or lesser destruction of kidney tissue and loss of function. The cause is obstruction to the flow of urine, which may be brought about by various conditions inside and outside the urinary system. A stone lodged in the ureter, or a tumour, may cause obstruction, as may malfunction of the neuro-muscular control of the pelvis of the kidney or of the ureter, which may be congenital. Stricture or narrowing of the ureter may follow tuberculosis or the removal of a stone, and congenital stricture may be present at the junction between ureter and bladder. Beyond the bladder strictures may form in the urethra after gonorrhoea or the removal of a stone. Tumours outside the ureters may block them, or lower in the urinary tract an enlarged prostate can block the urethra. The symptoms depend on the site of the obstruction, and range from pain in the loin and renal colic to difficulty in passing water. Symptoms associated with infection may dominate the picture, and bring the disease to notice, for all these conditions are likely to be accompanied by infection. Treatment of hydronephrosis is treatment of the underlying condition, but if the kidney is so badly affected that function has been lost it may be advisable to remove it. The aim in treatment is to preserve as much kidney function as possible.

Hydrophobia: *see* Rabies.

Hydrotherapy: the use of water in treatment externally or internally, once so popular that the fortunes of whole towns were founded on their waters. Taking the waters has now lost its wide appeal, but spas still exist on the Continent, and the waters of mineral springs, now bottled, command a wide market.

Hydroxycobalamin: a form of vitamin B_{12} used in the treatment of pernicious anaemia.

Hygiene: the science of the preservation of health.

Hymen: the membrane at the external opening of the vagina, usually present in virgins. It may be without perforation in young girls, causing retention of the products of menstruation when it starts and accumulation of blood in the vagina, a haematocolpos.

Hyoid Bone: a small U-shaped bone at the base of the tongue, which can be felt in the neck about an inch above the Adam's apple. It is usually broken during strangulation, a fact which may prove very important in the investigation of a death.

Hyoscyamus: from this plant is prepared hyoscine, or scopolamine, an alkaloid useful in the prevention of motion sickness, vertigo and nausea; it counteracts the action of the parasympathetic nervous system, like atropine, and relaxes spasm of smooth muscle, both in the gastro-intestinal tract and in the ureters. It may be used as premedication before a general anaesthetic to diminish the secretions of the bronchi. In overdose it may produce hallucinations, excitement and confusion.

Hyperactivity: *see* Hyperkinesis.

Hyperacusis: abnormal sensitivity to sounds, or abnormally acute sense of hearing.

Hyperaemia: congestion of a part with blood.

Hyperaesthesia: increased sensitivity to touch, or to pain in the skin, or abnormally increased sensitivity in one of the organs of special sense.

Hyperchlorhydria: excess of hydrochloric acid in the stomach.

Hyperemesis: excessive vomiting, which when it occurs in pregnancy is called hyperemesis gravidarum. It begins in the early months of pregnancy, and is commonest with the first child. It is treated psychologically, but may require the removal of the patient to hospital, the use of drugs and the replacement of fluid and salts lost.

Hyperglycaemia: excessive sugar in the blood. *See* Diabetes Mellitus.

Hyperhidrosis: excessive sweating. Apart from obvious causes, such as a hot room or taking exercise, this may be caused by a high temperature, by excessive secretion of thyroid hormone in thyrotoxicosis, by taking alcohol, by diabetes, or by the emotions of fear or anxiety, particularly in young people. Obviously keeping cool and calm is important; sweating is inhibited by 20% aluminium chloride hexahydrate in alcohol applied to a dry skin.

Hyperkinesis: excessive activity of the motor system. Certain children show excessive activity, allied to impulsive restlessness and aggression. They tend to do badly at school. It has been described as a syndrome with a basis in a bodily disease, but the state is not well understood, and various remedies have been suggested including the exclusion from the diet of tartrazine, a red, yellow or orange food-colouring agent. Some have recommended the use of amphetamines in treatment. However, the children appear to grow out of the condition in time.

Hypermetropia: long sight, caused by the eye being too short from lens to retina or having a lens without sufficient refractive power. The ability to focus on objects near at hand is restored by a convex spectacle lens. The sight tends to grow longer with age.

Hypernephroma: a malignant tumour of the kidney, commoner in men than women and commonest in those over 50. It usually causes the passage of blood in the urine, and a dull ache in the loin. The tumour may be removed surgically with a good hope of complete success, but sometimes solitary secondary deposits are found in the lungs, or in bone; these too may successfully be removed.

Hyperpiesis: another word for high blood pressure or hypertension.

Hyperplasia: an abnormal increase in the number of cells in a tissue, and consequent increase in size of the organ or structure.

Hyperpyrexia: an abnormally high temperature, usually defined as a fever reaching 41°C (106°F).

Hypertension: high blood pressure. The importance of this condition lies in the fact that many people who die of disease of the cardiovascular system are found to have had a blood pressure higher than normal. The normal blood pressure for a healthy young adult is accepted as being 120 mm of mercury when the heart pump contracts (systole) and 80 mm mercury when it relaxes (diastole). It is measured by inflating a cuff placed round the upper arm, which is connected to an instrument containing a column of mercury; the pressure in the cuff raises the level of the column of mercury, and is expressed as the number of millimetres of mercury supported in the column. The pressure in the artery of the upper arm is estimated by listening with a stethoscope over the artery in front of the elbow; when the pressure obliterates the artery, no sound is heard; when blood begins to flow as the force of the heartbeat overcomes the pressure in the cuff, eddies are set up in the blood and a beat is heard. The height of the column of mercury when the sound is first heard is taken as the systolic pressure, that is, the pressure exerted by the force of the heart when it contracts. As air is allowed to escape from the cuff at a rate of about 3 mm at a time, the sound continues until suddenly it dies away, at first becoming muffled and then disappearing altogether. The height of the column of mercury is noted at both these points, and the disappearance of the sound is usually taken as the sign that the artery is fully open and the heart is relaxed in diastole. Other means of taking the blood pressure may be used, but the results are still expressed in millimetres of mercury. The difficulty comes in recognising a reading which is significantly high, for the pressure varies from time to time according to circumstances. The experience of having the blood pressure taken is enough to send it up in some people; relaxation is important in getting a true reading, and if necessary the subject should lie down for a quarter of an hour, although the best readings are taken with the patient sitting down, the arm being on a level with the heart. A series of three readings at intervals can be taken in doubtful cases. Opinions vary on figures which should be taken to warrant treatment, some believing that the diastolic figure is most important, others placing more reliance on the systolic figure; however, a reading greater than 140/90 merits further attention, and one of 160/100 calls for treatment. Even so, factors such as the age of the patient must be taken into consideration. A high blood pressure by itself causes no symptoms, and is usually discovered on routine examination. A high blood pressure may in time however cause breathlessness, heart failure, coronary artery disease, stroke and disturbances of vision. Headache is not a symptom, but may lead the doctor to take the blood pressure and discover that it is raised. Treatment, in the great majority of cases where there is no underlying cause for the high blood pressure, is first directed to weight control and advice to avoid smoking. In many cases loss of surplus weight is sufficient to bring the pressure down to reasonable levels. In others, it is necessary to use a thiazide diuretic or a beta-blocker (q.v.), or a combination of both. If these fail, other drugs may be added or substituted such as nifedipine or prazosin, but there is such a range of possibilities that each physician will be able to select what is best for each individual patient. It is essential that whatever is prescribed should be taken regularly, and that patients should be followed up at regular intervals.

Hyperthermia: the treatment of certain diseases by the artificial production of a high temperature, a process that has largely fallen into disuse. The word may also be used to mean hyperpyrexia (q.v.).

Hyperthyroidism: overaction of the thyroid gland. *See* Thyrotoxicosis.

Hypertrophy: an increase in size of an organ or tissue as a result of increased work or stress imposed, for example the increased size of the breasts during pregnancy and lactation.

Hypnosis: an artificially induced state of passivity in which there is an increased inclination to believe and follow suggestions. Induced trances have been part of the stock-in-trade of medicine men, witch-doctors, religious devotees and others for centuries, but hypnotism was first used in Europe as a therapeutic tool by Anton Mesmer (1734–1815) who from 1774 onwards was the rage first of Vienna and then Paris. Physicians such as Charcot subsequently used hypnotism, as did Freud, at one time, and before the advent of anaesthetics it was tried during surgical operations. Hypnotism requires a willing subject and a confident hypnotist; suggestions made will not be carried out if they conflict to any great extent with the subject's own wishes.

Hypnotics: drugs which induce sleep.

Hypocalcaemia: a low level of calcium in the blood. The normal level is 2.3–2.8 mmol/l. An abnormally low level may be the result of deficiency in the secretions of the parathyroid gland, sometimes damaged in operations on the thyroid; deficiency in vitamin D; or may be induced by over-breathing. A possible consequence of hypocalcaemia is tetany, in which the neuro-muscular system is over-excitable; there are tingling sensations in the face and hands, and the muscles of the legs and feet, hands and arms may go into spasm so that the hands and feet are stiff and distorted. Spasm of the muscles of the face may produce a caricature of a grin called *risus sardonicus*. Tetany should not be confused with tetanus.

Hypochlorhydria: a deficiency of hydrochloric acid in the stomach. Complete absence of the acid is called achlorhydria. Neither of these conditions by themselves cause symptoms, but they may be found in association with cancer of the stomach, pernicious anaemia, or chronic gastritis.

Hypochondria: the upper lateral parts of the abdomen, lying to right and left of the epigastric region.

Hypochondriasis: morbid preoccupation with the health, often extending to a fixed belief in the existence of a physical disease although there is no evidence of it. The hypochondriac may be suffering from a mental illness such as depression, anxiety neurosis or even schizophrenia, but a large number of sufferers do not fit into these categories, being men often with a family history of preoccupation with bodily functions. Complaints usually centre around the abdominal organs, but may include the head, heart and lower back; nothing that is said or demonstrated by special investigations will convince the patient more than briefly that nothing is wrong. Treatment of any underlying psychological cause will help, but cases in which none are found are very difficult to deal with, especially when it is remembered that sooner or later the complaint will be well-founded.

Hypodermic: hypodermic injections are those given under the skin, as opposed to intramuscular or intravenous injections. The word has by extension come to mean the syringe and needle used.

Hypogastrium: the lowest part of the abdomen.

Hypoglossal Nerve: the twelfth cranial nerve, which supplies the muscles of the tongue. *See* Cranial Nerves.

Hypoglycaemia: a low level of glucose in the blood. Normal values range between about 5.0 to 3.5 mmol/l, and symptoms are likely to appear if the level falls below 2.5 mmol/l. By far the most common cause of this is failure in a diabetic to cover the dose of insulin or similar drug with food, although there are a number of rare conditions that can lower the blood sugar. The patient experiences sweating, palpitations, tremor of the hands, hunger and excitability, and goes pale. The onset is sudden, and there may be confusion and clumsiness, sleepiness and unconsciousness. Often the patient recognises the first signs of trouble and can take sugar, which aborts the attack, but if it is unforeseen and progresses the treatment is to give sugar by mouth if possible; if not, intravenous glucose is required, or an intramuscular injection of 1 mg glucagon which may revive the patient enough for glucose to be taken by mouth. *See* Diabetes Mellitus.

Hypokalaemia: a level of potassium in the blood lower than the normal range, which is 3.8–5.5 mmol/l. It may be caused by excessive vomiting or diarrhoea, or by diuretics.

Hypomania: a state of mental excitement less in degree than that of mania.

Hyponatraemia: a low level of sodium in the blood; normal range is 135–150 mmol/l. As with hypokalaemia, may be caused by excessive diarrhoea and vomiting. In salt deficiency due to heat exhaustion the blood sodium levels are found to be normal.

Hypophysis: the pituitary gland.

Hypopituitarism: deficiency of the secretions of the pituitary gland (q.v.).

Hypoplasia: underdevelopment of a tissue or organ.

Hypopyon: collection of pus in the anterior chamber of the eye.

Hypospadias: a congenital malformation of the penis, in which the genital folds fail to unite normally in the midline, and the orifice of the urethra may lie anywhere along the under-surface of the organ or in the perineum. Treatment is by plastic surgery.

Hypostasis: the pooling of blood in the vessels and fluid in the tissue spaces of the dependent parts of the body when a poor circulation is unable to overcome the effects of gravity. Hypostatic congestion of the feet and ankles occurs in heart failure, and those who are old, enfeebled and bedridden may develop hypostatic congestion of the lungs leading to pneumonia.

Hypotension: abnormally low blood pressure. Apart from that caused by excessive blood loss and shock, and severe disease, low blood pressure may be postural, especially in the elderly, when getting out of bed or a chair and standing up may result in giddiness or even fainting. The same may happen after being confined to bed in illness, or in treatment by some drugs for high blood pressure. It means that sudden standing must be avoided: sit on the side of the bed for a while on getting up, and remember that it is likely to happen when getting up from a chair in a warm room. Wearing elastic stockings to prevent the blood pooling in the legs may help. The blood pressure may also fall on standing up for a long time in one position, but this may be prevented by moving the legs or by standing on tiptoe from time to time to pump the blood out of the legs.

Hypothalamus: that part of the brain that lies at the base, below the third ventricle and below the thalamus (*see* Nervous System). Its integrity is essential for life, for it controls the 'vegetative' functions: body temperature, the appetite, blood pressure and fluid balance, and sleep; it can be said to be the physical basis of the emotions.

Hypothermia: abnormally low body temperature. Accidental exposure to cold of infants or the elderly can result in serious illness. Infants kept in a room temperature below 18°C (64°F) may become too cold, and although all infants are liable to be affected, premature and weakly babies are more likely to be harmed. The affected infant becomes quiet, shows little sign of hunger, and feels cold to the touch. The skin is red, and the limbs may be swollen. At first the pulse is quick, but as the temperature falls it slows down. Rewarming must be slow, and if possible carried out in hospital in an incubator. The aged, who may be solitary, sick with unrecognised disease and undernourished, may be found to be suffering from the effects of cold in the winter, although they may not complain of it; the signs are confusion or semi-consciousness and slow breathing and pulse rate. The body temperature taken rectally falls below 35°C (96°F), and the blood pressure is low. The effects of cold are often complicated by other disease which may not at first be apparent, and sometimes the patient may have been taking sleeping pills or alcohol. Warming must be slow and careful, beginning with covering the patient with a blanket but no more, and the patient should be admitted to hospital. It is perhaps worth noting that fit adults exposed to extreme cold, as may happen if people out walking become lost or cut off, render themselves more likely to become hypothermic if they take alcohol without food, for it disturbs the normal reflexes which keep the body warm.

Hypothyroidism: deficiency of the hormone secreted by the thyroid gland. *See* Myxoedema.

Hysterectomy: the surgical removal of the womb, or uterus. Subtotal hysterectomy removes the body of the uterus but not the cervix (i.e. the portion protruding into the vagina); total hysterectomy may be carried out for a number of conditions, and may involve removal of the ovaries as well as the Fallopian tubes, but in women under the age of menopause every effort is made to preserve at least one ovary to ensure subsequent hormonal balance. If the ovaries have to be removed, hormonal balance can be achieved by giving the hormones by mouth. When the uterus is small and the condition for which the operation is carried out warrants it, the organ may be removed through the vagina, thus obviating the necessity for an abdominal incision. Contrary to general belief, hysterectomy does not lead to a loss of sexual desire.

Hysteria: a mental disorder characterised by dissociation, that is, the apparent cutting-off of one part of the mind from the other; a high degree of suggestibility both from the self and others; and a great variety of phenomena which may at first give the impression of organic disease, although the condition is wholly psychological in origin. *See* Neurosis.

I

Iatrogenic Disease: disease unwittingly produced by the doctor: for example, the mere fact of taking the blood pressure, especially if done repeatedly, can produce anxiety in the patient even when this is objectively unnecessary. On the whole it is only those who have a fund of anxiety waiting for an apparently rational hook on which it may be hung who respond in this way, but the doctor has to be aware that an apparently innocuous word or unguarded gesture may be interpreted wrongly. Apart from psychological difficulties, a good deal of iatrogenic illness is produced by the unwary use of drugs, for unwanted side-effects and the complexity of drug interactions can trap the most skilled prescriber.

Ichthammol: a dark brown viscous fluid with a distinctive fishy odour derived from certain bituminous schists, which has some antiseptic action and is mildly irritating to the skin. It is used, often in combination with zinc, in an ointment or cream for treating chronic eczema, having a milder action than coal tar.

Ichthyosis: a disorder in which the skin is coarse, cracked and scaly, resembling the skin of a fish. It may be inherited and present at birth, the appearance being worse over the shins and the backs of the elbows; there is very little disability apart from the scaly appearance, and it does not predispose to other skin diseases. It may develop in old age, when a scaly skin is not uncommon, but it differs from the congenital type in that it itches.

Icterus: jaundice.

Icterus Gravis Neonatorum: jaundice of the newborn. *See* Haemolytic Disease of the Newborn.

Idiocy: a term no longer used for the lowest grade of mental deficiency.

Idioglossia: the continued utterance of meaningless sounds, as in some mental defectives or demented schizophrenics. In certain religious sects it is regarded as a sign of peculiar holiness.

Idiopathic: a term applied to diseases when their cause is unknown, or of spontaneous origin.

Idiosyncrasy: response to drugs or other substances which is particular to an individual.

Ileitis: inflammation of the ileum. It occurs in a localised area in the last part of the ileum, which forms the last three-fifths of the small intestine, and may extend into the colon; described by the American surgeon B. B. Crohn (1874–1983) in 1932, it is often called Crohn's disease. The cause is not known, but recent research suggests that small blood clots obstruct the arteries supplying the lining of the gut. The consequence is that the wall of the bowel becomes swollen and red, and the mucosal lining ulcerated. Loops of the bowel may become adherent to neighbouring structures, such as other parts of the bowel or the bladder, and fistulae may form between them. Symptoms are diarrhoea and abdominal pain, and sometimes this mimics an acute appendicitis. The diagnosis is clear on X-ray examination of the bowel with barium contrast, which outlines the narrowing of the bowel and may show ulceration or a fistula if one is present. Medical treatment includes attention to the anaemia which may be present and the use of corticosteroids; surgical treatment may prove necessary if the narrowing of the bowel has caused obstruction, or if a fistula has formed.

Ileo-caecal Valve: the lower end of the small gut, called the ileum, opens into the large gut at the place where the colon joins the caecum, the blind end of the large bowel that lies in the right lower part of the abdomen, and from which the appendix arises. At the junction of the small and large gut there is a valve consisting of two 'lips' surrounded by a thickening of the circular muscle of the intestine. The function of this valve is not clear, but it may prevent the contents of the ileum from running too quickly into the colon.

Ileostomy: an artificial opening between the ileum and the exterior, made surgically in the right lower abdominal wall when the colon has been removed, usually for ulcerative colitis. Although the idea seems disagreeable, patients with an ileostomy are a good deal better off than they were with ulcerative colitis, and can lead a perfectly normal life.

Ileum: the last three-fifths of the small intestine, continuous with the jejunum above and the colon below. The differences between the jejunum and the ileum develop slowly and progressively so that the separation of the small intestine into two-fifths jejunum and three-fifths ileum is to some extent arbitrary. Although after death the small intestine can be stretched out to seven or eight metres, in life when the muscle is active it measures only about three metres.

Ileus: an obstruction of the intestine, which may be due to a number of causes including obliteration of the lumen by a tumour, strangulation in a hernia, twisting of the intestine round an adhesion or round itself, or paralysis of the wall of the gut. This can often accompany an 'acute abdomen', peritonitis or an abdominal injury. In obstruction the abdomen becomes distended and the patient vomits, no motions or flatus are passed, and the sounds which the bowels normally make are sparse or absent. There may be little pain, unless the obstruction sets up a colic or spasm of the bowel muscle. The treatment is gastric suction through a tube passed into the stomach, and intravenous fluids and electrolytes until the diagnosis is made, when it may be possible to remove the obstruction by operation. Paralytic ileus may be expected to recover spontaneously.

Illusion: a false mental interpretation of a real sensory stimulus, as when the conjuror produces a rabbit out of an empty hat. Also an idea which is unreal and has no basis in fact.

Imbecility: formerly defined as the second most severe degree of mental defect after idiocy, the term is now outdated.

Imhotep: the first physician whose name has come down to us, Imhotep was an Egyptian who lived during the third dynasty, about 2980 BC. As time went on he became worshipped as the god of healing.

IMI: intramuscular injection.

Imipramine: a drug used in the treatment of depression, one of a group called tricyclic antidepressants (q.v.).

Immune System: consists of the cells and organs of the body concerned with the processes of ensuring immunity. Foreign matter entering the body as micro-organisms of disease, or proteins which are capable of setting up immune reactions, carry characteristic antigens which the body recognises as not belonging to itself. The antigens excite certain cells in the body to produce antibodies, which are responsible for neutralising and killing the foreign invaders. Cells producing immunoglobulins which carry the antibodies are the lymphocytes, which are small white cells circulating in the blood and lymphatic fluid, and contained in the lymphatic glands, the spleen, bone marrow and thymus gland, the tonsils and the patches of lymphoid tissue in the intestine. In the main the immune system is silent and efficient in operation, but there are some reactions which are not helpful, for example allergies (q.v.) and the rejection of grafts (*see* Transplant Surgery).

Immunisation: the process of developing resistance in the body to the invasion of organisms and foreign matter. It may be naturally acquired by infection with a disease, be artificially produced by inoculation against a disease or a toxin elaborated by a particular organism, or be conferred passively by the injection of immunoglobulins. Active immunisation was first used against smallpox by injecting people with pus from a person suffering from the disease, but it was dangerous. In 1796 Edward Jenner, a Gloucestershire doctor who had noticed that patients who caught cowpox from infected cows did not subsequently catch smallpox, injected a boy with matter from a patient with cowpox and after a time injected him with matter from a victim of smallpox; he did not develop the disease. Jenner's invention was called vaccination, from the Latin *vacca*, a cow, and from it sprang the modern science of immunology, and the names vaccine and vaccination. As a result of worldwide vaccination against smallpox the disease has finally disappeared. The discovery that diseases were caused by micro-organisms came in the nineteenth century, and the way was open for the recognition of the antigen–antibody reaction and the elaboration of vaccines against other infective diseases. *See* Allergy, Vaccination.

Immunity: the process in the body of identifying and getting rid of invading organisms and foreign matter.

Immunoglobulins: globulins which are active as antibodies. Those derived from animals have been almost abandoned, as they were liable to cause dangerous anaphylactic reactions, in favour of those derived from human blood. These are divided into two classes, normal immunoglobulins and specific immunoglobulins, and they are used to provide passive immunity. Normal immunoglobulin is prepared from human blood plasma and, given by intramuscular injection, confers temporary immunity from hepatitis A, measles, and to a certain extent rubella. The usual dose, 2 ml, gives protection for about three months, but pregnant women exposed to rubella need a bigger dose. Specific immunoglobulins are prepared from the blood of patients who are recovering from the disease in question, or of actively immunised donors. They are available for hepatitis B, tetanus, and rabies, but active immunisation by inoculation is to be preferred if possible. Immunoglobulins are prepared against other diseases, but may be scarce. Anti-D (Rh_0) immunoglobulin is used in cases where rhesus-negative mothers have rhesus-positive babies, to prevent the formation of antibodies in the mother's blood to rhesus positive blood cells which may be transferred during childbirth (*see* Haemolytic Disease of the Newborn). The immunoglobulin must be given within 72 hours of the birth.

325

Immunology: the study of the immune system, which includes not only the reactions in disease but also those concerned in the rejection or acceptance of grafts.

Impaction: the wedging of two objects together so that separation is difficult; for example, a tooth may be impacted by a neighbouring tooth, or be so firmly locked in its socket that removal is troublesome. An impacted fracture is one where the broken ends of the bone are pushed into each other; faeces in chronic constipation may become impacted, that is, so hard and dry that they cannot be passed out of the rectum without special measures being taken.

Impetigo: an infection of the skin, particularly of the face, with streptococci or staphylococci, which is found in children and is very contagious. It starts as a small pustule; when this breaks, a yellow scab forms and spreads. It is treated by an antibacterial ointment, of which there are several including chlortetracycline, mupirocin and fusidic acid preparations. It should be remembered that infection can be carried by face-flannels and towels.

Impotence: inability in the male to achieve or maintain an erection. It can be the result of disease; diabetes is a well-known cause, and some diseases of the nervous system can be at fault. Endocrine disease affecting the testicles and the secretion of androgens is rarely present; more commonly impotence is the result of drugs used in the treatment of high blood pressure, depression and anxiety. The majority of cases, however, are psychological in origin, and result from feelings of guilt, anxiety, distaste for the sexual act either in general or in a particular case, latent homosexual tendencies or sheer ignorance. The ability in men to have sexual intercourse satisfactorily is dependent on many factors, among which are self-confidence and self-regard, and it happens that failure on one occasion perpetuates itself, owing to the fear on each subsequent occasion that all will not be well. Since erection is almost impossible in the presence of the conflicting emotions of anxiety and desire, love and fear, impotence results in such circumstances. Treatment, in the absence of organic factors, is psychological, and directed towards removing anxiety and depression. Aphrodisiacs are useless, and in the case of cantharides, 'Spanish fly', dangerous. Nearly all men are at some time impotent, but if a single occasion is regarded anxiously as indicating the possibility of future failure the condition is likely to persist. Desire and introspection cannot exist together, and anxiety is the most potent anaphrodisiac. Excess of alcohol can induce impotence.

Inanition: the state resulting from starvation.

Incisions: there are a great number of named surgical incisions particularly in the abdominal region, perhaps the most famous of which is McBurney's incision, made in the right lower part of the abdomen for the removal of the appendix, in which the muscles are split rather than cut (Charles McBurney, 1845–1913). Another named incision commonly used is that of Hermann Pfannenstiel (1862–1909), which is made transversely just above the pubic bone so that when it heals it is covered by the pubic hair. It is used for pelvic operations in women. The standard surgical incisions in the abdomen are the median, in the middle line above or below the umbilicus, the paramedian which is to one side of the midline, the transverse and the oblique, which may in the case of operations on the kidneys run round under the lowest ribs in the flank. In making an incision the surgeon's aim is to weaken the muscles as little as possible, splitting them rather than cutting through them.

Incisors: the front four teeth of the upper and lower jaws; their function is cutting, as opposed to molars which grind.

Incompetence: when applied to the valves of the heart, this refers to conditions in which they will not close completely, and so allow the blood to flow back into the chamber from which it has been pumped. The non-return valves in the veins of the leg may become incompetent; this leads to the development of varicose veins (q.v.).

Incontinence: inability to control bladder or bowels; when control of both is lost the condition is called double incontinence. It occurs in infancy and the second childhood of old age, in diseases of the nervous system, and weakness of the muscles of the pelvic floor in women (stress incontinence).

Incoordination: inability to co-ordinate movements, caused by damage to the sensory nerves which inform the brain about the position of the limbs and trunk, defects in the brain itself, or disorder of the motor nerves or the muscles.

Incubation Period: the time elapsing between infection with the organisms of a disease and the appearance of symptoms. In any given disease it is relatively constant. People who have been exposed to an infectious disease and may be incubating it are known as contacts, and should be watched, for they may become highly infectious as soon as the first signs of disease appear. Roughly speaking, incubation periods may be divided into short, intermediate and long; the incubation periods for common infectious diseases are:

Short (up to seven days): diphtheria, scarlet fever, bacillary dysentery, influenza, plague, cholera, meningitis.

Intermediate (one to two weeks): measles, chicken-pox (may be up to three weeks), glandular fever, typhoid fever, whooping cough.

Long (more than two weeks): rubella (up to three weeks), mumps (up to three weeks), hepatitis A (up to four weeks), hepatitis B (a matter of months).

The quarantine period is the maximum incubation period plus two days added, but for the usual childhood infections quarantine is not practical. Cases should be kept as far as possible at home after they develop symptoms; contacts of diphtheria and close contacts of typhoid and paratyphoid fever can have specimens taken for culture to make sure that they are not carrying the disease. Those who have been in contact with meningococcal meningitis can be given prophylactic rifampicin. The periods of infectivity of common fevers are: *chicken-pox*: from five days before the rash appears until the vesicles have all scabbed over, and the scabs are disappearing;

Measles: from the time symptoms appear until five days after the rash has appeared;

Rubella: from a week before the appearance of the rash until the fifth day after;

Mumps: from seven days before symptoms appear until they have gone;

Whooping cough: from one week after exposure to infection until three weeks after the start of the cough.

Indian Hemp: *see* Cannabis Indica.

Indigestion: *see* Dyspepsia.

Indole: one of the compounds normally found in faeces which is in part responsible for the characteristic smell.

Indomethacin: one of the group of non-steroidal anti-inflammatory drugs, NSAIDs (q.v.).

Induction: setting in motion or beginning, used mostly of anaesthesia or labour.

Induration: the hardening of a tissue or organ.

Industrial Disease: *see* Occupational Disease.

Infantile Paralysis: *see* Poliomyelitis.

Infants and Infant Welfare: it is important to realise that the term 'normal infant' simply means the average; this may be quite misleading in an individual case (for example as far as weight is concerned infants who are quite healthy may fall considerably short of, or exceed, the average weight). The figures given here are only rough guides and no anxiety should be felt if one's own child does not conform, unless there are other signs that its condition is not satisfactory.

Weight At birth the average baby weighs 7–7½ lb (3.2–3.4 kg). The weight is approximately doubled by the fifth month, trebled by the end of the first year, and at the end

329

of the second year the child should weigh about 28 lb
(12.7 kg). After the first week, when there is a slight initial
loss, the weight increases by about 6–8 oz (170–226 g) a
week, but minor variations are of little significance and
small infants (for infants vary in size within normal limits
as much as their parents) may do quite satisfactorily with
a weekly gain of 4–6 oz (113–170 g).

Height This again varies as greatly as does the height of
the parents, but broadly speaking the hereditary factor
in height does not make its influence felt until about the
fifth year; before that time height is largely dependent
on nutrition. At birth the average baby is about 20 in
(508 mm) long, and at the end of the year about 28 in
(701 mm); the height increases about 3½ in (90 mm) a
year thereafter until the fifth year.

Sleep During the first month the baby sleeps nearly all the
time except for feeding, washing and dressing, but by the
sixth month this has gradually altered to about 12 hours
at night, 2 hours in the morning, and 2 or 3 hours in the
afternoon. At 1 year the period of sleep is 12 hours at
night, 1 or 2 in the morning and 1 in the afternoon; at
18 months the afternoon sleep may be omitted for it may
result in loss of sleep at night. Bedclothes should be warm
but light, and the room darkened and well ventilated but
without draughts.

The cot For the first two or three months the most
convenient is the Moses basket. When the baby grows
bigger, it needs a cot which has a solid head to keep off
draughts, and bars sufficiently close together to prevent the
head passing through and becoming stuck.

Movements and walking Newly born babies can grasp
objects, suck and swallow, but movements of the arms
and legs are not co-ordinated; by the end of the third
month the baby can usually lift up its head. By six months
it begins to sit up, by the ninth month to crawl and by ten
months to stand up. Walking begins about the twelfth or
fourteenth month.

Speech Single words may be spoken by the end of the first
year, but what can reasonably be described as speech does
not make its appearance until the end of the second.

General management The mother should be free from anxiety, relaxed and not given to fussing. Feeding difficulties

may arise from the infant's awareness of the mother's tension, and in later life there is no surer way to make a child neurotic than to fuss over it and give the impression that the world is a dangerous place. Neurosis is one of the most infectious diseases known.

Feeding Should be under the advice of the health visitor, the welfare centre, or the paediatrician, but it must be said that if at all possible the infant should be breast-fed. The idea that a schedule of feeding must rigidly be observed regardless of the child's cries of hunger is not sensible; it will be found that if the infant is at first fed on demand it will develop a regularity suited to its own needs.

Clothing Should be light and loose and preferably made of wool, silk and wool, or cotton; it must not be easily inflammable. The body should be able to get a reasonable amount of fresh air and sunshine and be free to move. New clothes should be washed before they are worn for the first time, for they are often dressed with substances that can irritate the baby's skin; and if a washing machine is used, make sure always that it is rinsing thoroughly.

Bathing After birth the baby is thoroughly washed in water a little above blood heat (37.8°C, 100°F) and the stump of the umbilical cord dried by swabbing, dusted with antiseptic powder and covered with a dressing. Daily sponging is carried out thereafter while keeping the cord dry until it separates on or about the tenth day. In a month or so the temperature of the bath should be lowered to tepid and after the daily bath the baby should be allowed to lie naked and kick freely.

Teeth The lower central incisors appear from the fifth to the eighth month, and the other incisors follow, first in the upper jaw and then in the lower. The 20 milk teeth should all be present at the end of the second year, and the permanent teeth begin to erupt from about the fourth.

Weaning This should be a natural process, and from the fourth month, or as advised, the feed can be supplemented by fruit or vegetables which can be reduced to a puree or mash, or a bland cereal such as rice. Most foods are suitable for a young baby as long as they are prepared without salt, added sugar or strong spices. Foods high in fat like hard cheeses are best left till later in the first year, and soft cheeses except those made with pasteurised milk avoided altogether. Egg is best left until after six months, and it should be hard boiled. Egg in prepared baby foods has been treated to kill bacteria. Begin by offering solids once a day, and gradually increase over six weeks; the baby should by then be having three small solid feeds a day.

General health   Symptoms and signs of ill health include fever, restlessness and irritability, lethargy and persistent crying (crying itself is not necessarily anything to worry about and the mother will soon learn to recognise the cry of pain or discomfort). Colds which block the nose are extremely distressing to babies and coughs should call for advice from the health visitor or the welfare clinic. Vomiting small amounts is not necessarily serious; the normal child brings up small amounts of fluid, especially if it is overfed, but violent vomiting with or without diarrhoea should receive medical attention. Diarrhoea is an indication for asking for professional help, but constipation is rarely a cause for worry and many babies who are perfectly healthy tend to be constipated. It is only worth considering if it is persistent or accompanied by other signs of ill health. Here it should be pointed out that the habit of 'potting' regularly when the infant is unable for anatomical reasons to control its bowels is to be avoided; the child's bowel functions should be allowed to develop control in their own good time.

Infarction: when an artery is suddenly blocked by thrombosis or by an embolus and there is no collateral (alternative) circulation to keep the tissues nourished, a wedge-shaped area will die, the apex of the dead tissue being at the point where the blocked vessel begins to be solely responsible for the supply of oxygen and nourishment. The area of dead tissue is called an infarct, and the process whereby the blood supply is cut off and necrosis ensues is called infarction.

Infection: infectious diseases are those caused by invasion of the body by organisms from outside; they are characterised by the fact that they can be passed on from one person to another or from an animal to a person. The organisms concerned are called pathogens, and include bacteria, viruses, protozoa, worms, and fungi. In general, the symptoms of an infection are fever, sweating, sometimes chills and shivering, headache, pain in the muscles, malaise, sometimes skin rashes, and various manifestations depending on the system affected, such as cough, diarrhoea, vomiting, or localised swelling and pain when the infection is confined to one area, as it might be in the case of a boil or a carbuncle. It was not until the last century that the discovery of the micro-organisms of disease made it possible to explain infectious diseases; until then all sorts of explanations had been put forward, ranging from climatic conditions to the relative positions of the stars. Since the work of Pasteur (1822–95) in France and Koch (1843–1910) in Germany the micro-organisms of most infective diseases have been found and identified, and in recent years the advent of electron microscopy has made it possible to study viruses in detail. The discovery of sulphonamides in 1935 and the subsequent discovery of penicillin, first used in 1941, which started the proliferation of modern antibiotics, have revolutionized the treatment of infections to the extent that medical practice has changed considerably for the better and the average expectation of life has increased. So far, however, viruses have proved for the most part immune to treatment by drugs; but the development of immunology and the discoveries of vaccines active against viruses have resulted in the extirpation of smallpox and greatly diminished the incidence of poliomyelitis. Immunisation can also limit the prevalence of mumps, rubella, measles, hepatitis B, yellow fever and rabies, all virus infections against which other treatment is ineffective.

Infectious Mononucleosis: otherwise called glandular fever, is caused by infection with a herpes virus, the Epstein–Barr virus. It is a disease of young adults, especially common in universities and colleges. The mode of transmission is not certain, but may be by droplet infection. Many cases infected do not show any signs of the disease, but those who do develop a sore throat, with enlargement of the glands of the neck and depression and malaise. Often there is also a streptococcal infection of the throat. In a few cases there is a rash like measles, but more often a rash is caused by giving the patient ampicillin for the sore throat;

this or a related penicillin must be avoided. A reaction to ampicillin in infectious mononucleosis does not mean that the patient is thereafter sensitive to penicillin. The spleen is enlarged in half the cases, and therefore patients must not take part in violent games for a couple of months. The disease in most cases runs its course in a month or so; some suffer for longer, but this is exceptional. Complications are not common, but they include jaundice, rarely a benign meningitis, and very rarely encephalitis. In these cases steroids are used, but the majority of cases recover without treatment.

Infective Endocarditis: infection of the lining of the heart, which may be acute or subacute. It may be found in those who have a pre-existing congenital heart condition or valvular disease, but may occur without any obvious heart abnormality. It may affect patients after heart surgery for valvular disease, and is liable to develop in drug addicts who use drugs intravenously. Infecting organisms vary, but often streptococci or staphylococci are responsible. The patient complains of fever, aches and pains and feels ill. Bacteria are found in the blood on culture in the majority of cases, and the appropriate antibiotic is used, usually by intravenous injection. Prevention of the disease in those who are known to be susceptible, that is those with congenital heart conditions, those who have had surgery for valve defects, and those who have a valvular disease of the heart, involves taking appropriate antibiotics before any surgical procedure likely to result in the introduction of bacteria into the bloodstream. The most common surgery of this sort is that involved in dental treatment.

Infestation: the presence on or in the body of parasites such as ticks, mites and fleas, or other multicellular organisms.

Inflammation: the local reaction of the body to damage caused by infection or injury. The characteristics of inflammation were described by Celsus in the first century AD as *rubor*, *tumor*, *calor* and *dolor*: redness, swelling, heat and pain. To this Galen added, in the second century AD, *functio laesa*, impairment of function. Inflammation starts at the point of damage with dilation of the blood vessels, so that the blood suffuses the part and the skin becomes red and hot. Soon the circulation at the centre of the affected area slows down, white blood cells stick to the walls of the smallest vessels and begin to make their way through them into the damaged tissues, and fluid passes from the blood into the tissue spaces causing swelling. The white blood cells destroy and remove invading organisms, remove dead tissue, and then aid in the process of repair. Antibodies pass out of the blood vessels in the fluid escaping into the tissues, as well as fibrin, which helps to contain the infection. A thick cellular barrier is formed as a fence round the infected area, but bacteria may escape into the lymphatic vessels and travel up to the lymph glands which drain the part, and set up inflammation elsewhere. As the cells and bacteria in the centre of the inflammatory process die, with the extravasated tissue fluid they may form pus, which is eventually discharged.

Influenza: acute infection with the respiratory virus influenza A, B or C. The incidence of the disease is seasonal: in the United Kingdom it is usually at its worst between December and May. The infection is spread by droplets in the breath of infected people, who are infective from a day before symptoms show themselves until about a week afterwards. The incubation period is between one and four days. The onset is sudden, with a high temperature, shivering, headache, aching pain in the bones and muscles and a cough, loss of appetite and severe malaise. In children and the elderly the disease can be dangerous, but in most cases recovery begins after about four days, often leaving the patient depressed. Treatment consists of rest in bed with plenty to drink and aspirin or paracetamol for the headache and fever. Antibiotics are useless, except in those cases where there is a secondary infection of the lungs. Prevention by immunisation is difficult, because the surfaces of the viruses carry haemagglutinins (H) and neuroaminidases (N) which may change, especially in the A type, and when they do the infection becomes more widely spread and more dangerous. The World Health Organization system for identifying strains names the type, the place where it was isolated, the number, and the year, and each year the WHO recommends which strains should be used to prepare vaccines. B and C types are more stable than A, and change less, but the illness they cause is less severe. Influenza vaccines are recommended for the elderly, especially those suffering from chronic lung, heart, or kidney disease, or diabetes. The vaccines are grown in chick embryos and are therefore not to be given to those who are sensitive to eggs. The best control of the disease would be the isolation of influenza victims, but it is not the sort of disease which keeps people away from work if they can walk.

Infra-red: electromagnetic radiation beyond the red end of the spectrum with a wavelength shorter than radio waves It may be used to heat the tissues in physiotherapy; in medical photography, the use of infra-red sensitive film shows up the patterns of blood vessels in the skin.

Infusion: a watery preparation of a vegetable drug made by steeping the appropriate part of the plant in water and straining. One of the weaknesses of such preparations is difficulty in standardisation, for the amount of drug present in different preparations varies. Senna, digitalis, quassia, gentian and cinchona have been prepared in this way, as well as tea and coffee. Another meaning is the intravenous administration of fluids under the influence of gravity.

Inguinal Region: the groin.

Inhalation: a method of introducing drugs into the body by way of the lungs. Some anaesthetics are given this way; often drugs in inhalers are used in obstructive diseases of the air passages, such as salbutamol and terbutaline in asthma. The drugs may be in aerosol form or prepared as a dry powder, for some people find it easier to use a powder inhaler than an aerosol, where inspiration must be synchronised with the release of the aerosol, and the breath then held for ten seconds. Spacing devices increase the space between the aerosol container and the mouth, and make breathing technique easier. Aqueous aerosols may be used in a nebuliser, driven by an oxygen cylinder or an electric compressor, and are very useful in acute asthmatic attacks. In bronchitis and respiratory infections, traditional inhalations of aromatic substances such as benzoin tincture or menthol and eucalyptus in hot water are useful because they encourage the inhalation of hot moist air; the same effect can be achieved by keeping a kettle steaming in the room.

Inhibition: the prevention or deactivation of a process. In the popular sense people are said to be inhibited or to have inhibitions when they are shy, unsociable or afraid of expressing undue emotion.

Injection: the act of forcing liquid into a part of the body, usually by means of a needle and syringe. Most commonly injections are made under the skin (subcutaneous), into muscle (intramuscular) or into veins (intravenous). The most rapid way of getting a drug into the circulation is by intravenous injection; intramuscular injection takes longer to act, but is the way to make an injection in an emergency if you are uncertain how to do it. Clean the skin, and thrust the needle into the fleshy upper outer part of the arm about three inches below the point of the shoulder; let the needle go straight into the arm for at least an inch and make the injection. Another place to use is the upper outer part of the buttock, where the needle can be allowed to penetrate further into the muscle. An injection into the arm is absorbed more quickly than one into the rump. Before you make the injection, first pull the plunger of the syringe back a little to make sure the point of the needle is not in a blood vessel, and then make the injection slowly and firmly. If you are using soft ampoules with the needle attached you will not be able to do this, but no harm is likely to be done if you make the injection into the upper outer part of the arm or the buttock.

Innocent: sometimes used of benign as opposed to malignant tumours.

Inoculation: accidental or intentional introduction of foreign matter into a living organism or culture medium. Used of the injection of vaccines to prevent disease.

Inquest: inquiry into the circumstances and cause of a death, held before a coroner.

Insanity: *see* Mental Illness.

Insecticides: substances lethal to insects. The older chlorinated hydrocarbons such as DDT, aldrin and dieldrin proved to be very stable and therefore persistent in the food chain. They have been succeeded by organophosphorus compounds, carbamates and sometimes dinitro compounds; if used properly these are not harmful, but if misused they can be poisonous. Organophosphorus compounds, being derived originally from nerve gases, inhibit the action of cholinesterase and increase the amount of acetylcholine (q.v.) in the body. Carbamates have a similar action. Dinitro compounds turn the skin yellow, and speed up the metabolic processes in the body. producing sweating, a racing pulse, dryness and thirst and over-breathing. Treatment is directed towards lowering the temperature and replacing fluids.

Insemination: the transfer of semen into the vagina naturally or artificially.

Insomnia: inability to sleep is one of the most common complaints encountered by doctors. It is clear that people vary greatly in the amount of sleep they need, some being content with eight hours, others with six or less; others need ten hours' sleep. Many great men have slept very little, and at odd times. There have even been claims from some saying that they never slept at all, for example one Dr Pavoni in Northern Italy, who died in his eighties. He did not sleep to any significant degree for over sixty years, but instead amassed a comfortable fortune by doing other doctors' night calls. The most frequent cause of sleeplessness is anxiety. Obviously there are other causes of insomnia, for example pain, and some sleep so lightly that they may be woken by cold feet, or slight noises in the night; age may bring with it broken sleep. Nevertheless, worry is the most common cause of insomnia. and as things appear at their blackest at three in the morning sleeplessness is liable to feed upon itself. The best aid to sleep is a quiet mind, and treatment of insomnia must be directed to that end. Sleeping pills, usually one of the benzodiazepines, can be useful in the short term, but the danger of taking sleeping pills is that they can become a habit which is difficult to break, although common sense says that once they have served their purpose they should be abandoned. Unfortunately among the effects of withdrawing benzodiazepines may be anxiety and insomnia, so that a vicious circle can be set up. If three weeks' treatment with sleeping pills is not successful, it is best for the doctor to search for the underlying anxiety or depression and treat that.

Insufflation: the blowing of air, gas or a powder into a cavity; for example blowing into the lungs in artificial respiration, or blowing a suitable powder into the ear to cure local disease.

Insulin: the pancreas has two types of secreting cells, those which elaborate digestive enzymes carried to the duodenum through the pancreatic duct, and others which form isolated groups called the islets of Langerhans and secrete the hormones insulin and glucagon. The existence of insulin had been postulated in 1909, but it was not isolated until 1921 when the Canadian workers Macleod (1876–1935), Banting (1891–1941) and Best (1899–1978), working in Toronto, finally succeeded and gained a Nobel Prize. The function of insulin is, roughly speaking, to enable the body to use sugar. When the level of sugar in the blood rises, the secretion of insulin is stimulated; it has two main actions, the first being to increase the rate at which sugar is withdrawn from the blood into the tissue cells, and the second to decrease the rate at which sugar is passed into the blood by the liver. Besides increasing the storage of glycogen, the forerunner of glucose, in the muscles and increasing the rate at which glucose is used in the tissues, insulin stimulates the formation of protein in muscle, stimulates the formation of fat, and prevents its breakdown. Lack of insulin causes the disease diabetes mellitus (q.v.) and the great importance of the Toronto work was that it made the treatment of diabetes possible by the injection of insulin. The insulin used in treatment has been mainly derived from pork or beef pancreas, but recently it has been possible to make human insulin by recombinant DNA technology or modifying pork insulin by enzymes.

Intensive Care: with recent advances in knowledge and the proliferation of machines and apparatus capable of sustaining and measuring vital processes, it has become necessary to concentrate both the skill needed to employ the apparatus and the apparatus itself in special wards in hospitals which supplement the general medical and surgical wards. These special wards have succeeded the recovery units which were formerly maintained in conjunction with operating theatres, and are called intensive care units; into them are admitted patients after serious operations, accident victims, and medical patients suffering from poisoning or other conditions that threaten their lives but retain a hope of recovery. In the intensive care unit may be found ventilating machines, renal dialysis machines, apparatus for recording the heart rate and its electrical activity, the temperature and breathing rate and function, and the blood pressure, as well as apparatus for carrying out biochemical and possibly X-ray investigations. The unit is often under the care of an anaesthetist, whose specialised knowledge is most suitable for the duty, and staffed by specially trained nurses.

Intercostal: used to describe the blood vessels, nerves and muscles lying between the ribs.

Intercurrent: applied to a second disease or infection occurring during the course of the original disease.

Interferons: proteins, first described in 1957, produced by lymphocytes and fibroblasts which render cells resistant to infection by viruses, and also have an action against certain tumours. They are specific to each different species, and human interferon has until recently been difficult to extract, so that with very limited supplies investigative work has been restricted. It is now possible, however, to use recombinant DNA technology to increase the supply, and it may be that this group of substances, now being used in the treatment of certain leukaemias, may prove useful against malignant tumours and in the treatment of virus infections. It has recently been reported that interferon has been used successfully in the treatment of hepatitis.

Intermittent Claudication: painful cramp in the muscles of the calf which comes on after exercise, caused by arterial disease in the arteries of the leg. It appears after a constant degree of exercise, and patients know how far they can walk before the legs become painful; after a rest the pain goes. The reason for the pain is similar to that in angina pectoris; the muscles are starved of oxygen by the poor blood supply, and are unable to get rid of the waste products produced during contraction. If the case is suitable, reconstructive arterial surgery may be considered.

Interstitial: interstitial tissue is 'background' tissue, which supports the active tissue of an organ. It is usually fibrous.

Intertrigo: chafing between two contiguous skin surfaces, for example, below pendulous breasts; also the resulting dermatitis.

Intervertebral Disc: *see* Spinal Column.

Intestine: the alimentary canal after it leaves the stomach. It is divided into small and large intestine; the small intestine is the longer, and is continuous with the stomach at the gastro-duodenal junction. The duodenum is the first part of the small intestine, a short section of gut; it derives its name from the fact that it is about 12 finger-breadths long – some 25 cm. It is divided for the purpose of description into four parts which form a C with the concavity to the left, surrounding the head of the pancreas. The first part of the duodenum is continuous with the stomach at the pylorus and is susceptible to the formation of ulcers; the bile duct and the main duct of the pancreas enter the second part, having joined just before they open into the duodenum. The third and fourth parts complete the sweep of the C, and are continuous at the duodeno-jejunal flexure with the jejunum, the first two-fifths of the small intestine; the remaining three-fifths is called the ileum. The jejunum and the ileum are together about three metres long in life, but after death when the muscle has lost its tone can be stretched out for about eight metres; they are attached to the back wall of the abdominal cavity by the mesentery, a membrane only 15 cm long at the base but as long as the small intestine at its intestinal edge. It fans out in many convolutions, and carries the blood vessels which supply the small intestine. The duodenum has no mesentery, but is applied to the back wall of the abdominal cavity, and the same is true of the ascending colon, the first part of the large intestine. The terminal part of the ileum joins the ascending colon in the right lower part of the abdomen just above the caecum and appendix. The circumference of the colon is greater than that of the small intestine, and instead of being surrounded completely by smooth muscle the colon has three bands of muscle running longitudinally, starting at the appendix and running as far as the rectum. These bands are called the taeniae coli and they pucker the gut lengthways; it is divided into sacculations by circular muscles. On the surface of the large intestine are small bags of fat called the appendices epiploicae. The ascending colon runs up the right side of the abdomen to the hepatic flexure near the liver, where it is continuous with the transverse colon. This part of the colon is suspended by a mesentery, and from it hangs the back fold of the omentum (q.v.). The transverse colon turns downward near the spleen on the left of the abdomen at the splenic flexure, where it is once more adherent to the back wall of the abdominal cavity. At the brim of the pelvis the descending colon again acquires a mesentery and becomes the sigmoid colon, which is continuous with the rectum; this passes downwards out of the peritoneal cavity and joins the anal canal 3 cm above the anus. The functions of the intestines are described under the heading Digestive System, and its diseases under separate headings.

Intoxication: the state caused by poison; in particular applied to the state of being poisoned by alcohol.

Intracranial: inside the skull.

Intradermal: in the skin.

Intramedullary: within the spinal cord or the medulla oblongata; within the marrow cavity inside bones.

Intramuscular: inside a muscle.

Intrathecal: within a sheath; an intrathecal injection in the spine is made into the space lying between the arachnoid and pia mater, the membranes covering the spinal cord, where the cerebrospinal fluid lies.

Intrauterine Device (IUD): a device usually of copper wire wound round a plastic or silver core, fitted inside the uterus for the purpose of contraception. The device can stay in position for between three and five years, and is most suitable for older women who have borne children.

Intravenous: within a vein.

Intubation: the introduction of a tube into the body, used mostly of the process of inserting a tube into the trachea to maintain an airway during the administration of an anaesthetic, or for the purpose of artificial respiration by a breathing machine.

Intussusception: a condition in which a part of the intestine telescopes into the next segment. The large intestine can prolapse into itself, the last part of the ileum can prolapse into the caecum, or be drawn into the ascending colon, and the small intestine can telescope into itself. Most cases occur in infants between the ages of four to nine months, but it may be seen in adults, usually complicating the presence of a tumour or polyp of the intestine. An intussusception causes intestinal obstruction with colic and vomiting, and the motions may contain mucus mixed with blood, called a 'redcurrant jelly' stool. The condition may relieve itself, but recur, and the treatment is surgical.

Inunction: the act of rubbing into the skin an ointment or oil.

343

In Vitro: literally 'in glass', a term used to describe a biological reaction which takes place under laboratory conditions rather than 'in vivo', in the living animal or human being. The fact that a certain drug has an action in vitro does not mean that it has the same action in vivo.

Involution: the return to normal size of the uterus after childbirth, or the shrinking of tissues or organs which may occur in old age.

Iodine: an element essential for the secretion of the thyroid hormones thyroxine and tri-iodothyronine, usually present in sufficient quantities in normal diets. There are certain mountainous areas in the world where this is not so, and the population is liable to suffer from goitre, but this can be prevented by using iodised salt. Iodine is used as a skin antiseptic, but is liable to cause sensitivity reactions, as it may when used in radio-opaque preparations for radiological investigations. It is used regularly in medicine in its radioactive form, ^{131}I, in the diagnosis and treatment of disease of the thyroid gland; it has a half-life of eight days.

Iodoform: tri-iodomethane. Although it has been used a great deal on wounds, especially in the Latin countries, iodoform has only a weak antiseptic action.

Iodophthalein: a compound excreted quickly by the liver into the bile ducts and gall-bladder. It is radio-opaque, and has therefore been used to show up the biliary apparatus on X-ray plates and give an indication of the efficiency of secretion and concentration of bile.

Ipecacuanha: derived from the South American plant *Cephaelis ipecacuanha*, it contains the alkaloid emetine, and may be used as an emetic in cases of poisoning if the patient is fully conscious and the poison is neither derived from petrol nor corrosive. It has been for years included in expectorant mixtures in small quantities, but there is no evidence that it has any influence in loosening a cough.

Iridectomy: the operation of removing part of the iris, usually performed for glaucoma.

Iris: that part of the pigmented coat of the eye which lies behind the cornea. It has a central aperture, the pupil, through which light enters the eyeball to fall on the retina. The amount of light admitted is controlled by the size of the pupil, which is varied by the contraction or relaxation of the muscle fibres of the iris. The brighter the light, the smaller the pupil.

Iritis: inflammation of the iris. The iris, ciliary body and choroid (*see* Eye) make up the uveal tract, and they have the same blood supply, so that infection can easily spread from one to the other. According to the extent of the inflammation, it is called iritis, iridocyclitis, or iridocyclo-choroiditis; in the last the whole pigmented part of the eye is affected. There are a number of causes, including herpes, syphilis and toxoplasmosis. The uveal tract is also involved in sympathetic ophthalmia, a condition which develops in an intact eye after a penetrating wound of the other eye; it may require the removal of the injured eye to save the good one.

Iron: this element is essential for the formation of haemoglobin, the pigment in the red blood cells which carries oxygen. Deficiency of iron leads to anaemia, but a normal diet supplies sufficient iron, except in pregnancy where the requirement is much greater and extra iron may be needed. Although there is a popular belief that iron is a tonic, it does no good except in cases of anaemia, which are easily recognised by a simple blood test. The belief is very old: Hippocrates knew that iron salts improved many patients but did not know why, and in the Middle Ages when diets were poor, and for various reasons anaemia must have been common, some people felt better for drinking water in which a sword had stood. Confusion between the effects of iron in unrecognised anaemia and the semi-magical properties of a warlike metal is not unnatural.

Irradiation: treatment by exposure to radiation of any kind, but usually refers to treatment by ionising radiation. *See* Radiation.

Irrigation: the washing-out of a cavity or wound by a stream of water or other liquid.

Irritable Bowel Syndrome: an obscure but common condition in which the patient complains of disturbance of bowel function with ill-defined abdominal discomfort. The motions are frequent, with the passage of a small amount of faeces which may be mixed with mucus; this alternates with periods of constipation. The complaint is chronic, with periods of remission, and appears to be brought on by anxiety. No abnormality of the bowel is found on investigation, and treatment is difficult because drugs aimed at relieving anxiety and depression have little effect. The use of bran in the diet, or other 'bulking' agents, may prove beneficial. The condition is also known as irritable or spastic colon, but there is a suggestion that the small intestine is involved as well as the colon.

Ischaemia: inadequate blood supply to a part of the body, caused by spasm or disease of the blood vessels or failure of the general circulation; if it is prolonged and severe, the tissue dies. Different tissues resist ischaemia for varying periods; the brain is very sensitive to lack of oxygen, and cannot survive intact for more than five minutes, but the skin can survive for hours – if it did not, it would be impossible to sit down for long. The survival times of some organs such as the kidneys, liver and heart are very important in transplant surgery, and the resistance of tissues to ischaemia can be increased by lowering the temperature, but too low a temperature may itself prove dangerous. Partial ischaemia of muscle is painful, and lack of oxygen together with the accumulation of the products of metabolism is the cause of the pain of angina pectoris, intermittent claudication and some sorts of cramp.

Ischiorectal Abscess: an abscess occurring between the rectum and the ischium, part of the pelvis (see below). This type of abscess may be associated with a *fistula in ano*, a communication between the rectum and the skin at the anus. The treatment is surgical.

Ischium: the lower posterior part of the pelvis upon which one sits. The actual part that bears the weight of the sitting body is the tuberosity of the ischium, and it can be felt under the skin as a large bony prominence. It has a bursa over it which may become inflamed and painful, a condition sometimes known as weaver's bottom. The ischium develops as a separate bone in early life, but fuses with the ilium to form the os coxae, the hip-bone, before adult life. The lines of fusion run through the acetabulum, the socket of the hip joint.

Ishihara Test: test for colour blindness devised by Shinobu Ishihara, Japanese ophthalmologist (1879–1963), which consists of several coloured cards printed with coloured spots arranged in patterns, some of which cannot be perceived by the colour blind, while other patterns appear only to the colour blind and not to those with normal vision.

Iso-immunisation: the development of antibodies against an antigen from another individual of the same species, as in haemolytic disease of the newborn (q.v.).

Isolation: the separation of an infective patient from others, so that the infecting organism is not spread. It is also required to protect those with a deficient immune system, such as patients after transplant operations or suffering from an immune deficiency disease, from infections normally trivial but to them potentially dangerous. The technique in the first case is called barrier nursing, in the second reverse barrier nursing.

Isoniazid: a powerful drug used in the treatment of tuberculosis. It is given in combination with other drugs, usually rifampicin and pyrazinamide, for the first three months of treatment, and subsequently in combination with rifampicin for the six to nine months needed to eradicate the disease. It may be used in the prophylactic treatment of susceptible close contacts of tuberculosis.

Isotonic: solutions which have the same osmotic pressure, i.e. which will not bring about diffusion one into the other through an intervening membrane, are isotonic. A 'normal' solution, for example 0.9% sodium chloride, will not draw fluid from human tissues nor be absorbed into them; but hypertonic solutions will withdraw fluid from the tissues and hypotonic solutions will be drawn into them.

Isotope: a chemical element which has the same atomic number as another, but a different atomic mass. It has the same number of protons in the nucleus, but a different number of neutrons. Radioactive isotopes change into another element over the course of time, the change being accompanied by the emission of electromagnetic radiations, and they are used in medicine because they can be traced and because some of them become concentrated in one place in the body and can then influence the surrounding tissues by their radiation. An example is the use of ^{131}I in the treatment of thyrotoxicosis. Other isotopes can be used to irradiate the body from the outside, or can be implanted surgically into the part to be irradiated. Most elements are in nature a mixture of several isotopes.

Itch: *see* Pruritus.

IVP: intravenous pyelogram. Radiological technique for demonstrating the outline and function of the kidneys, ureters and bladder. An intravenous injection of a radio-opaque substance selectively excreted by the kidneys is given, and radiographs taken subsequently show the degree of concentration achieved by the kidneys, the outline of the pelvis of the kidney and the ureters, and the outline of the bladder. Radiographs taken after emptying the bladder show whether there is any malfunction of the bladder or obstruction to the passage of urine.

J

Jaborandi: *Pilocarpus microphyllus*, a South American plant, the leaves of which contain pilocarpine (q.v.).

Jacksonian Epilepsy: focal epilepsy, named after John Hughlings Jackson (1835–1911) who first described it. Usually the result of a localised area of disease or injury in the motor cortex of the brain, but sometimes occurring in idiopathic epilepsy, the attack starts in the index finger and thumb, the toes or round the mouth; the muscles start recurrent contractions which spread to involve neighbouring muscles to a greater or lesser extent. Consciousness is not lost unless the attack spreads so far that it becomes a grand mal attack, and attacks may be confined to one limb or the face. The essentials of a Jacksonian attack are that it begins in a definite place and spreads from there in a definite progression.

Jalap: a powerful purgative obtained from the root of the Mexican plant *Exogonium purga*. It is now rarely used. (Sometimes mis-spelt jolop.)

Jaundice: a yellow discoloration of the skin, whites of the eyes, and mucous membranes, caused by the deposition of the bile pigment bilirubin in the tissues. Bilirubin is the product of the breakdown of haemoglobin from spent red blood cells, and it is excreted normally by the liver in the bile. Jaundice can be caused by excessive production of bilirubin, by obstruction of the biliary apparatus through which the bile is passed into the intestines, or by disease of the liver preventing the excretion of bilirubin. Excessive production of bilirubin occurs in haemolytic anaemias, such as haemolytic disease of the newborn, in which red cells are destroyed in large numbers; in this type of anaemia the urine is not discoloured nor the motions pale. In obstructive jaundice, where the bile passages are blocked, as for example when a gallstone is impacted in the biliary duct and the bile cannot be excreted into the intestines, the motions become pale; the bile is absorbed into the bloodstream and is excreted by the kidneys, turning the urine dark. The skin may itch. In hepatitis the liver cells are damaged and cannot excrete bilirubin; moreover the swelling blocks the small bile channels within the liver. The condition may be the result of infection (*see* Hepatitis) or poisoning by such substances as phosphorus, carbon tetrachloride or various drugs. Again, the urine becomes dark and the motions pale.

Jaw: the upper jaw is formed by the two maxillary or cheekbones, and the lower jaw by the mandible. There are 16 permanent teeth in each jaw, and the teeth of the upper jaw slightly overlap the teeth of the lower jaw. The upper jaw is fixed to the base of the skull, the lower jaw forms a hinge with the temporal bone just in front of the ear. A finger in the ear will feel the head of the mandible moving to and fro. In addition to the simple hinge movement, the head of the mandible can slide backwards and forwards so that the point of the lower jaw can be moved from side to side and a grinding motion imparted to the teeth. The muscles that act on the lower jaw are the two temporal muscles, which can be felt to harden in the temples when the teeth are clenched, and the pterygoid and masseter muscles which help to close the jaws and move the mandible from side to side. A number of weaker muscles aided by gravity drop the lower jaw. In the joint between the head of the mandible and the temporal bone there is a cartilage to facilitate movement, which sometimes clicks and can get out of place and lock the jaw. Dislocation of the lower jaw can only take place forwards, and it can happen in over-enthusiastic yawning. The remedy is to stand in front of the patient and place the thumbs on the back teeth, while the fingers are put under the point of the jaw. Press the thumbs down and the fingers up, and the muscles will pull the head of the mandible back into its socket. A fractured mandible can be supported by a bandage passing under the jaw and over the top of the head.

Jejunum: the second part of the small intestine. *See* Intestines.

Jerks: the reflex jerks elicited by the doctor on striking the tendons at the knee, ankle and elbows are the response of the muscles to sudden stretching. If a normal response is present it shows that the muscle stretch receptors are working, and that the sensory nerves which carry the impulses from the stretch receptors to the spinal cord and the motor nerves which carry the reflex impulse to the muscles are in order; it also shows the state of that segment of the spinal cord where the reflex path lies. Abnormal responses involve absent or exaggerated jerks.

Jigger: *Tunga penetrans:* a flea which burrows into the skin of the feet, causing intense irritation and ulceration. Scrub mites, *Trombiculidae*, which can spread scrub typhus, are also called jiggers.

Jogger's Nipple: irritation and inflammation of the nipple caused by the friction of the clothes over the chest during jogging.

Joints: are formed where one bone meets another. They may be immovable, as in sutures where the bones of the skull join, or where the bones are united by fibrous tissue, or where the bones are separated by cartilage but bound together by fibrous tissue as in the symphysis pubis. Movable joints are synovial joints, in which the joint surfaces are covered by cartilage, and bound together by a joint capsule of fibrous tissue. The joint is lined by the synovial membrane, which is a slippery membrane secreting synovial fluid to lubricate the joint and sustain the cartilage. The fibrous capsule has thickenings which are the intrinsic ligaments of the joint. There may also be gaps in the capsule through which the synovial membrane protrudes to form bursae which help the muscles and tendons to move easily over the joint; bursae may also be associated with muscle movements but not connected directly with the joint. Some joints have within them, between the cartilaginous bone ends, separate plates of cartilage, the menisci, which act as shock absorbers and adapt to the movements of the joint, adding to its stability. The shape of the joint obviously determines the movement possible, and the common shapes are ball and socket, as in the hip; hinge, as in the knee; saddle-shaped, as in the thumb; pivot, which allows rotation as happens when the head of the radius moves in relation to the ulna in pronating and supinating the forearm; and plane, as in the wrist. Joints are in many instances combinations of these shapes. The stability of a joint depends greatly on the muscles acting upon it, on the shape of the joint and the ligaments of the capsule.

Jugular: the external and internal jugular veins of the neck drain blood from the brain and the rest of the head into the great veins of the chest.

Jurisprudence: medical jurisprudence, or forensic medicine, is concerned with any aspect of medicine which relates to the law. There is a mass of legislation which regulates a great deal of medical practice, questions of neglect and malpractice may come before the courts, and many insurance cases rely on medical evidence. There is no one specialty to deal with these matters of civil law, but there are specialists concerned with criminal law. The police surgeon is a general practitioner who has a contract with the local police force to give medical help in criminal cases, and there are pathologists designated by the Home Office to handle suspicious and criminal deaths. Forensic science has grown out of forensic medicine, and now many branches of science which are not primarily medical have become involved in the detection of crime.

K

Kahn Test: a serological test formerly used in the diagnosis of syphilis, now superseded by the Venereal Disease Research Laboratories test (VDRL test). (Reuben Kahn, American bacteriologist, 1887–1979)

Kala-azar: a disease caused by infection with a parasite of the genus *Leishmania*, and spread by sandflies. Leishmania can infect the skin, causing disfiguring ulceration, or the internal organs, causing the disease kala-azar, also known as black fever or dumdum fever. It is found in many hot parts of the world, including the shores of the Mediterranean, the Middle East, India, China, Kenya and the Sudan, and Central and South America, particularly Brazil. The hosts for the parasite may be human beings, foxes, dogs, gerbils and various rodents. The onset of the disease may be a month to some years after infection; the parasite multiplies in the reticulo-endothelial system (q.v.), and causes fever, painful enlargement of the spleen, wasting, and anaemia. The patient develops a distended abdomen, and looks like the victim of famine. Treatment is the administration of antimony in the form of sodium stibogluconate, and prevention the avoidance of sandflies and their bites, and the control of dogs, rodents and other hosts.

Kaolin: aluminium silicate, or china clay. It is used in the treatment of mild diarrhoea, sometimes in a mixture with morphine; it is mixed with other ingredients in the preparation of poultices, when it is put between layers of gauze, and can be warmed under a grill before application.

Kaposi's Sarcoma: a malignant growth formerly known to affect African children and Mediterranean men over the age of 50, who developed the tumour on the legs. In 1981 it became apparent that the tumour was affecting a different section of the world's population, and it was found to be associated with the immunodeficiency disease AIDS. Now about a quarter of those suffering with AIDS present with the tumour, which is thought to be due to a virus infection.

Keloid: an overgrowth of scar tissue at the site of a cut or burn. The scar, instead of disappearing, spreads and sends out offshoots like claws which pucker the surrounding skin, often over three months after the injury. The skin may be affected on the chin, neck, chest or shoulders, particularly if it is stretched. Treatment is difficult, because attempts to remove one keloid may well result in the formation of another. Radiotherapy after excision may help.

Keratin: a fibrous protein containing sulphur, the substance of which horn, hair, the outer layer of the skin, and the nails are composed. It is also part of the structure of the enamel of the teeth.

Keratitis: inflammation of the cornea of the eye, the result of infection or injury. Keratitis is one of the complications of herpes zoster affecting the fifth cranial nerve, which supplies the face, or of foreign bodies in the eye. The danger is ulceration of the cornea and the formation of opaque scars which interfere with vision and which may require a subsequent corneal graft. At one time keratitis was often caused by congenital syphilis.

Kernicterus: the staining with bilirubin of the basal ganglia of the brain in infants suffering from haemolytic disease of the newborn (q.v.). It may cause toxic degeneration of the nerve cells with resulting disabilities including spasticity and mental defect.

Kernig's Sign: characteristic of irritation of the meninges, and therefore of meningitis. With the patient lying flat, the hip is flexed until it is at right angles to the body; the leg cannot then be extended at the knee, and any attempt to straighten it produces pain. The same sign is present to a lesser degree in cases of sciatica caused by irritation of the nerve roots by a prolapsed intervertebral disc. (Vladimir Kernig, 1846–1917)

Kerosene: paraffin oil. Room heaters using paraffin in badly ventilated surroundings can give off enough carbon monoxide to be poisonous, but the inhalation of paraffin fumes is unlikely in normal conditions to be dangerous. If it is swallowed, however, it may set up an irritation of the lungs which produces fever and interference with breathing, and irritation of the gut with abdominal pain, diarrhoea and vomiting.

Ketones: substances produced in the body by the imperfect breakdown of stored fats in severe diabetes mellitus and starvation.

Khellin: a substance derived from the fruit of an Eastern Mediterranean plant, *Ammi visnaga*, which has for centuries had the reputation of curing renal colic. It is also used for the relief of asthma and angina pectoris, for it is an antispasmodic.

Kibe: an alternative word for chilblain.

Kidney: the two kidneys lie one on each side of the spinal column behind the peritoneum on the back wall of the abdominal cavity at the level of the second lumbar vertebra, the left kidney lying slightly higher than the right. They lie in fat, and can move with the breathing; applied to their upper poles are the suprarenal glands, and leading from their inner borders are the ureters, the tubes through which urine is conveyed to the bladder. Human kidneys are about four inches long, weigh about 150 g, and are covered by a layer of tough fibrous tissue which forms a capsule. The arteries, veins and nerves enter and leave the substance of the kidneys at the inner border, like the ureter; this point is called the hilum. If kidneys are cut in half lengthways, it can be seen that their substance is divided into cortex, the paler part near the surface, and medulla, much darker tissue which forms pyramids pointing towards the pelvis of the kidney, the cavity in the hilum into which the urine drains and from which run the ureters. The kidney is made up of about a million microscopic structures called nephrons, which are the functioning units of the organ. Each nephron starts as a small bunch of capillary blood vessels, called a glomerulus, surrounded by a membrane enclosing a space. The combined glomerulus and surrounding membrane is called a Malpighian body, after the Italian physician Marcello Malpighi (1628–94) who first described it. From the Malpighian body runs the tubule, a prolongation of the membrane surrounding the capillary tuft, which is about 30–40 mm long; the first part, being twisted, is called the proximal convoluted tubule. After the convolutions the tubule runs straight towards the medulla, and bends back onto itself like a hairpin at the loop of Henle, first described by the German anatomist Friedrich Henle (1809–85). It becomes twisted again to form the distal convoluted tubule, and eventually ends in a collecting duct which drains about 10 nephrons and joins other ducts to open into the pelvis of the kidney.

The blood supply to the kidneys is through the right and left renal arteries, which branch directly from the abdominal aorta; venous blood drains through the renal veins into the inferior vena cava. The lymphatic vessels follow the course of the blood vessels, running to the glands which lie beside the aorta. The kidneys are responsible for keeping the acid–base balance of the blood constant, keeping the electrolyte content of the body balanced, and for eliminating waste matter containing nitrogen. These functions are essential for life, and a human being can only survive without kidneys for two or three weeks. In health a large amount of blood filters through the Malpighian bodies, where fluid is filtered off into the tubules at an overall rate of about 125 ml a minute. This is far greater than the amount of urine eventually lost. In the proximal convoluted tubule salt and water are reabsorbed and waste products left with enough water to keep them in solution; the processes of adjusting the amounts of water and electrolytes absorbed, and the regulation of the acid–base balance of the blood, are carried out to fine limits in the rest of the tubule.

Three main factors influence the activity of the kidneys: the blood pressure in the capillaries; the rate of circulation of the blood; and the state of the cells lining the tubules. The hormones acting upon the kidneys are the suprarenal hormones aldosterone and cortisol, which influence the excretion of sodium; vasopressin or antidiuretic hormone, secreted by the pituitary gland, which regulates the amount of water lost; the growth hormone, also secreted by the pituitary, which regulates sodium excretion; the parathyroid hormones which influence the excretion of phosphates; and the hormones secreted by the gonads, which have some effect on the regulation of water and sodium balance. The kidneys themselves secrete two hormones, renin and erythropoietin. Renin acts on a globulin called angiotensinogen, which is formed in the liver and present in the blood, to produce angiotensin, which has a powerful effect in raising the blood pressure. Damage to the kidney caused by an insufficient blood supply can increase the amount of renin secreted and so raise the blood pressure; but a raised blood pressure can itself lead to a poor blood supply, thus setting up a vicious circle. Erythropoietin is the hormone which regulates the formation of red blood cells; it is not clear whether it is itself formed in the kidney, or whether the kidney produces a substance which acts upon another in the blood, as in the case of renin, to form the hormone.

Disease of the kidney may be accompanied by anaemia, and some tumours of the kidney produce too much erythropoietin with a consequent excess of red blood cells. Diseases of the kidney are discussed under their own headings: *see* Hypernephroma, Nephritis, Pyelitis, Renal Calculus; *also see* Renal Dialysis.

Kinaesthetic Sensation: sensory impulses generated in the muscles and joints to indicate to the central nervous system their position and degree of tension, so that the brain can control and correlate the complicated motor signals that must be sent to the muscles to produce smooth motion or maintain the posture. Kinaesthetic sensations do not appear in consciousness all the time, but the position of the limbs is normally accurately known as the end result of a number of different sensory impulses. A breakdown in the system is disabling, for it is not then possible to generate fine movements nor relate the position of the limbs to the body with the eyes shut. Various everyday movements, such as walking, become difficult. One of the ways in which patients can become aware of a deficiency in kinaesthetic sensation is that they totter when bending over at the washbasin with the eyes closed to wash the face.

King's Evil: scrofula, tuberculosis of the lymph glands, with cold abscesses and chronic discharge, which, it was once believed, could be cured by a touch of the royal hand. This power was claimed by (or imposed upon) the royal houses of England and France and maintained in England until the time of the Stuarts; it died out under the Hanoverians, although the Stuart claimants practised it during their exile and even during their invasions of the country. This does not necessarily imply that they believed in the power Charles II, for one, certainly did not.

Kino: obtained from the dried trunk of the Indian tree *Pterocarpus marsupium*, this is an astringent, and is (or was) used internally for diarrhoea, and also as a gargle for oedema of the larynx and vocal cords arising from misuse of the voice.

Kleptomania: the uncontrollable pathological urge to steal objects which are not really wanted. Those who steal compulsively in this way, usually from shops, are commonly middle-aged women, often about the time of the menopause, of impeccable character, well able to pay for the trivial and useless things they steal. The compulsion may persist in the face of discovery and even prosecution; in most cases no clear psychiatric reason can be found, but in general it appears to be a symptom of unhappiness, and may even lead to suicide. When the condition afflicts men, usually over 60, it appears to be confined to stealing books. Kleptomania has nothing to do with the common offence of shop-lifting, for which excuses are sometimes made along these lines.

Knee: although the knee is the largest and one of the strongest joints in the body, it is a complicated joint, and it transmits so much weight and is liable to so much stress that it often operates at the limit of its strength and in the case of athletes, especially footballers, it not uncommonly becomes the site of injury and the cause of disability. It is a hinge joint between the femur, the thigh-bone, and the tibia, the weight-bearing bone of the lower leg, the two condyles of the lower end of the femur articulating with two corresponding condyles on the upper surface of the tibia; it is stabilised by the action of the great muscles of the thigh and strong ligaments. Neither the patella, the kneecap, nor the fibula, the subsidiary bone of the lower leg, take part in forming the weight-bearing joint. Two semilunar cartilages divide the joint, lying between the femur and the tibia on the inner and outer sides. The joint is covered by a fibrous capsule, indistinguishable in places from the expansions of the tendons closely applied to it. The strongest parts of the capsule are at the sides, where it forms the medial and lateral ligaments. At the front, the capsule is lacking behind the tendon of the quadriceps muscle, and the synovial membrane lining the joint bulges upwards to form the suprapatellar bursa. There is a well-defined ligament running from the femur to the tibia on the inner side of the joint, adherent in its upper part to the edge of the medial semilunar cartilage: it is called the tibial collateral ligament. On the outer side of the joint there runs the fibular collateral ligament, which is more like a cord, and is not attached to the lateral meniscus but attached above to the femur and below to the fibula. Inside the joint there are two very important ligaments, the anterior and posterior cruciate ligaments, which cross each other, running from the tibia below to the internal surfaces of the two condyles, the weight-bearing surfaces of the femur. The anterior cruciate ligament runs from the inner side of the intercondylar eminence of the tibia near the front end of the internal semilunar cartilage upwards, backwards and outwards to the femur, and the posterior cruciate ligament runs from the outer part of the intercondylar eminence near the back end of the internal semilunar cartilage upwards, forwards and inwards to the inner condyle of the femur. The cruciate ligaments are very strong and prevent the knee from being dislocated forwards or backwards. They are tightened when the knee is fully extended. The patellar ligament, which passes across the front of the knee, is the tendon of the quadriceps muscle of the front of the thigh, and the patella, the kneecap, is a sesamoid bone in the tendon, which is inserted into the tibia just below the joint. It covers and strengthens the front of the knee, and the action of the muscle is to extend, or straighten, the joint. The two cartilages in the knee, the menisci or semilunar cartilages, are there to allow smooth movement between the weight-bearing surfaces of the femur and tibia and to act as shock-absorbers. The lateral meniscus is nearly a complete circle, thicker on its outer edge, and it is attached to the intercondylar eminence of the tibia at its ends as well as being attached by its outer edge to the edge of the tibia by a coronary ligament. The medial meniscus is similarly attached, but it is less extensive than the lateral meniscus, forming a C, and it is attached to the joint capsule as well as the tibia. It is therefore less able to move, and is more liable to injury. Both the cartilages are vulnerable, they are liable to be torn if the knee is twisted while the weight is borne upon it.

Knock-knee (genu valgum): may be caused in children by rickets, but sometimes occurs with no known cause. The condition is more common in girls than boys, but unless the deformity is gross it corrects itself as the child grows up. It may be associated with other minor deformities, particularly of the backbone.

Koch's Postulates: a statement devised by Robert Koch, German bacteriologist (1843–1910, Nobel Prize winner 1905), of the evidence necessary to prove that a given disease is caused by a particular micro-organism: *(1)* The organism must be found in every case of the disease. *(2)* It must be isolated and grown in pure culture. *(3)* The pure culture must reproduce the disease when inoculated into a suitable animal. *(4)* The organism must be found in, and recovered from, the experimental animal.

Koilonychia: spoon-shaped fingernails, sometimes found in chronic anaemia. Such nails may be brittle.

Koplik's Spots: small white spots appearing on the inside of the mouth in cases of measles about three days before the rash develops. (Henry Koplik, 1858–1927)

Korsakoff's Syndrome: a mental disorder occurring in toxic states resulting from both inorganic and organic poisons, and frequently associated with polyneuritis. It was first described in 1887 by the Russian neurologist Sergei Korsakoff (1854–1900) in connection with alcoholic poisoning. Its typical features are a poor memory for recent events and a tendency to invent tales of non-existent happenings, although the patient is apparently fully conscious and aware. For example, the patient may not remember who the doctor is, the time of day, the date or what he was doing the day before, but will make up for the loss by addressing the doctor by another name and giving a long and circumstantial account of a fictitious visit home that very morning, although he has been in the hospital for weeks. The commonest cause of the syndrome is chronic alcoholism and consequent deficiency of thiamine (vitamin B_1). After treatment recovery may take a long time, and in many cases there remains a varying degree of memory defect and emotional deterioration.

Krameria: or rhatany, is the root of a South American plant, *Krameria triandra* from Peru or *K. argentea* from Brazil, which has much the same astringent action as kino (q.v.).

Kupffer Cells: star-shaped endothelial cells in the sinusoids of the liver which are part of the reticulo-endothelial system (q.v.). (Karl W. Kuppfer, 1829–1902)

Kuru: a disease of the brain caused by a transmissible slow virus, found in Papua New Guinea in 1957. It is fatal, and affects the cerebellum and other parts of the brain, resulting in progressive unsteadiness and inability to control movements. The disease was passed on by the practice of cannibalism: the brains of dead relatives were eaten by the women and children, who, it is said, took to cannibalism because they were denied meat by the men. At post-mortem examination, the underlying change in the brain was a diffuse spongiform encephalitis, similar to that found in scrapie in sheep and bovine spongiform encephalitis in cattle. The disease has disappeared with the disappearance of cannibalism.

Kwashiorkor: malignant malnutrition, found in children from very poor homes and in famine throughout the world. The cause is extreme deficiency of protein in the diet, and the disease develops when the child is weaned from the breast. The children suffer from chronic diarrhoea, oedematous swelling of the body, including the face, patches of peeling skin which may ulcerate, apathy, loss of appetite and failure of growth. They may also be suffering from tuberculosis or malaria, or be harbouring intestinal worms. Treatment is the identification and treatment of accompanying disease, and the introduction of nourishment by cautious steps. Many cases respond well to dried skimmed milk, which can be mixed with bananas, or flour and butter, with supplements of vitamins, and attention to potassium and magnesium requirements. As the children have a poor appetite, they must be fed little and often; when the appetite returns, feeding should be increased only slowly and carefully.

Kyphosis: pathological curvature of the spine in which the concavity of the curve is directed forwards, giving rise to the deformity of the hunchback.

L

Labium: part of the vulva, the female external genitals (q.v.).

Labour: parturition, the process of giving birth. When pregnancy in the human has lasted for more or less 280 days the contractions of the uterus known as labour pains begin. Labour is divided into three stages: dilation of the cervix, the neck of the womb; delivery of the child; and expulsion of the placenta, the afterbirth. At the beginning of labour the child is normally lying head downwards in the womb, surrounded by the amniotic fluid and enclosed in the membranes. As the contractions proceed the opening of the cervix begins to dilate, and part of the membranes thrusts forward like the finger of a rubber glove to help the process. The pressure within the uterus and the stretching cause the membranes to rupture and the amniotic fluid breaks out – the breaking of the waters. At the end of the first stage the cervix is fully dilated, and the birth canal clear. The head of the baby is driven down by the contracting uterus through the cervix into the vagina, the contractions become stronger, more frequent and prolonged, and the abdominal muscles help as the head moves down and is born. The baby's body follows, and after a resting period of 20 or 30 minutes contractions begin again and the placenta is expelled. In most cases any abnormalities, such as a breech presentation where the baby is the wrong way round, will have been found during the antenatal period, and the obstetrician will be prepared, but if labour is difficult it may be necessary to help by using instruments to grasp and guide the baby's head during the second stage. Most labours would terminate successfully without skilled help, but the birth is much easier and safer with the help of the obstetrician and midwife.

Labyrinth: the inner ear (q.v.). Labyrinthitis is inflammation of the inner ear, and causes vertigo, nausea and vomiting.

Lacrimal Apparatus: the parts concerned with the secretion and drainage of tears.

Lactation: the period during which the infant is suckled at the breast. During pregnancy the milk-secreting tissue of the breast proliferates under the influence of the hormones oestrogen, prolactin and progesterone. Towards the end of pregnancy the ducts are full of colostrum, a pale yellow fluid rich in protein and containing antibodies. Milk is secreted by the mother between one and three days after the birth, and continues while suckling reflexly stimulates prolactin secretion by the anterior part of the pituitary gland. Suckling also stimulates secretion of oxytocin from the posterior pituitary, which causes the muscle cells in the walls of the minute ducts in the breast to contract and expel milk. Prolactin secretion inhibits ovulation, thus preventing conception, until about six weeks after the child is weaned, when menstruation returns.

Lactic Acid: made by the fermentation of milk sugar, or lactose, by lactobacilli, as in the souring of milk. It is also produced in the muscles by the breakdown of glucose without oxygen to provide energy. If it is allowed to accumulate in the muscles, for example by an inadequate circulation of blood, muscular fatigue follows with pain. At one time, sour milk in the form of koumiss or yoghourt was thought to prolong life, but unfortunately statistics do not bear out this claim.

Lactose: milk sugar.

Laevulose: fruit sugar, also called fructose.

Lamblia Giardia: *see* Giardiasis.

Lamella: a thin plate of bone; or small discs of gelatin and glycerin impregnated with various drugs which can be placed below the lower eyelid, where they dissolve.

Laminectomy: when operating on the spinal cord or lumbar intervertebral discs it is necessary first to remove the overlying vertebral arches or laminae. This operation is called laminectomy.

Lancet: a small two-edged pointed surgical knife formerly used for opening abscesses and letting blood.

Lanolin: fat obtained from sheep's wool, used as a base for ointments because it does not go rancid and can penetrate the skin. It is capable of absorbing and mixing with water; but it may cause sensitisation of the skin and subsequently provoke a reaction.

Laparoscopy: the examination of the interior of the abdominal cavity through an endoscope, called a laparoscope; a small incision is made into the abdominal wall, and gas is introduced to make the examination possible. The procedure can be carried out under local anaesthesia, and is also called peritoneoscopy.

Laparotomy: a surgical operation to open the abdominal cavity, either to make an inspection of the contents or as a preliminary to further surgery. To be quite correct, laparotomy means an incision through the flank, but the word is hardly ever used in this sense now.

Laryngectomy: the removal of the larynx, an operation carried out for malignant growths. Patients without a larynx can be taught to speak by using various techniques.

Laryngitis: inflammation of the larynx, usually caused by a virus infection as in the common cold; it can be caused by harmful dust or vapour. At one time it could be part of an infection by diphtheria, syphilis or tuberculosis, but such cases are now rarely seen. In infants laryngitis causes croup; adults lose their voice or become hoarse.

Laryngoscope: an instrument for looking into the larynx. It is possible to see the interior of the larynx through a mirror, reflecting light from a mirror on the observer's forehead, or the laryngoscope may carry its own light. In an anaesthetised patient it is possible to use an instrument with a blade which depresses the tongue, so that the interior of the larynx can be seen directly.

Larynx: a fairly rigid framework of cartilages, held together by ligaments and moved by attached muscles, at the upper end of the trachea. It is lined with mucous membrane continuous above with that of the throat, and below with the lining of the trachea. It forms the lump visible in the neck as the Adam's apple, and its chief function is the production of the voice, for it contains the vocal cords.

Laser (Light Amplification by Stimulated Emission of Radiation): the powerful beam of light energy produced is increasingly used in surgery, and has proved particularly useful in ophthalmic operations because the eye is largely devoid of significant optical scatter, unlike other tissues, so that an optical beam can be focused on tissue deep inside the eye; coagulation and cutting is then possible without the risk of infection and in many cases without the need for anaesthesia.

Lassa Fever: first seen in a town called Lassa in northern Nigeria in 1969, Lassa fever is a virus infection carried by the rat *Mastomys natalensis* found in sub-Saharan Africa. The infection is thought to be spread to humans by contamination of food by rat's urine, and from person to person by contact with blood or other body fluids and by airborne infection. In outbreaks of the disease in Nigeria and Sierra Leone upwards of 30% of patients have died, although it is probable that some cases are mild and go undiagnosed. The disease causes sore throat, headache and fever, and proceeds to diarrhoea and vomiting, pains in the chest and abdomen, and swelling of the eyelids and face. The patient becomes increasingly ill and weak and may go into coma. Those who survive begin to improve after two or three weeks. The drug tribavirin has been used in treatment.

Lathyrism: a disease of the nervous system found in certain parts of the world, particularly central India, caused by eating the pea *Lathyrus sativa*. It is marked by progressive paralysis of the legs and pain in the loins.

Laudanum: tincture of opium, until modern times a popular remedy for deadening pain and bringing sleep.

Laughing Gas: nitrous oxide, a general anaesthetic used in dental and other short operations by itself, and in combination with volatile anaesthetics in longer procedures.

Lavage: irrigation, usually used in referring to gastric lavage, the washing out of the stomach through a stomach tube for severe alcoholic intoxication or poisoning.

Laxatives: *see* Constipation.

Lazarette: a hospital for the poor and diseased, particularly those suffering from the plague or other foul diseases.

Lead: a poisonous metal, once used widely in paints and water pipes and giving rise not infrequently to poisoning. It was also used a great deal in industry without particular precautions. Acute lead poisoning causes severe abdominal colic, with constipation, or may cause epileptic fits. Chronic lead poisoning may cause abdominal pain, anaemia, kidney damage and damage to the nervous system. This may result in difficulty in walking due to foot-drop, and in using the hands because of wrist-drop. It is also thought that chronic mild lead poisoning may impair the intelligence in children. Few paints now contain lead, and the composition of water pipes is carefully supervised, but in the United States children living in slum areas have contracted lead poisoning from flaking paint and old plaster, and from burning car batteries for warmth. Recently the emission of lead from car exhausts, derived from tetraethyl lead added to petrol for its anti-knock properties, has been thought to be dangerous. The treatment of lead poisoning is by penicillamine by mouth or sodium calciumedetate by intravenous injection.

Leaders: the popular name for tendons.

Lecithin: a complex fat found in large amounts in the brain and nerves as well as semen and the yolk of eggs.

Leeches: the medicinal leech, *Hirudo medicinalis*, was once used to draw blood from 'congested areas', for example from the temples in the case of headache – although the thought of leeches on the temples might persuade the patient that the headache was not so bad after all. The leech is shaped like a worm and has a mouth like a sucker at one end which contains three teeth; it also has a sucker at the other end by which it attaches itself. They secrete a substance, hirudin, which prevents the blood clotting. Land leeches, *Haemadipsa* and *Phyrobdella*, infest tropical swamps and wet places; they attach themselves to the ankles and lower legs, being able to find their way through clothes and into boots. Their bite is painless, and their presence may not be suspected until it is found that the wounds are bleeding. It may need a firm dressing to stop this, because of the action of hirudin. Water leeches are most unpleasant, for they are liable to enter the body through the natural orifices, and set up bleeding. Leeches may be persuaded to drop off by the application of salt or alcohol, but those water leeches that find their way into the body may have to be removed by endoscopy. It is possible that leeches may again be used in surgery, for they can help in the technique of skin grafting by reducing swelling in the grafted skin.

Left-handedness: mancinism, or sinistrality, may be accompanied by a left master eye, a tendency to read from right to left, and mirror-writing – Leonardo da Vinci was left-handed. In right-handed people the left side of the brain is dominant; the speech centre is on the left. In 40% of left-handed people the right hemisphere is dominant, the speech centre being on the right, but contrary to what was once believed the speech centre is still on the left in 60% of cases. It is more likely to be on the right when left-handedness runs in families. About 10% of people are naturally left-handed, but there has been a tendency to try to make children right-handed because so many things are arranged for a right-hander. It is far more sensible to encourage them to be ambidextrous.

Leg: although in common speech the whole of the lower limb is referred to as the leg, anatomically the leg is that part which lies between the knee and the foot. It has two bones, the tibia and the fibula, the tibia being the large weight-bearing bone which articulates with the femur, the thigh-bone, at the knee, and with the talus at the ankle. The fibula is a smaller bone; it bears no weight, but lies on the outer side of the tibia, and affords origin to a number of muscles, as well as taking part in the ankle joint. The tibia and fibula are bound together by a strong membrane, the interosseous membrane, and by strong ligaments where they form the ankle joint with the talus. Although the fibula bears no weight, it is very important in maintaining the stability of the ankle. The lower end of the tibia forms the medial malleolus, the bone felt on the inner side of the ankle, and the lower end of the fibula the lateral malleolus, felt on the outer side. The muscles of the front of the leg raise the foot at the ankle, and in doing so raise the inner border of the foot; they also extend the toes. Two muscles arising from the fibula, peroneus longus and brevis, at the outer side of the leg, pull the foot down at the ankle and tend to turn the foot out. The tendon of peroneus longus helps maintain the arch of the foot. The muscles of the calf, at the back of the leg, are in two groups, superficial and deep. The superficial muscles are the gastrocnemius, soleus and plantaris, the last being very much smaller than the other two, which are large and strong, pulling the foot down through the Achilles tendon at the back of the heel. The deep group includes the flexor muscles of the toes, which help in extending the ankle. The muscles are supplied by branches of the sciatic nerve, named the common peroneal and the tibial nerves. The principal arteries of the leg are the anterior and posterior tibial arteries, branches of the popliteal artery, which is a continuation of the femoral artery of the thigh. The veins are divided into superficial and deep groups, which communicate with each other through communicating veins which have valves allowing the passage of blood from superficial to deep veins. It is incompetence of these valves which allows the superficial veins to become enlarged and form varicosities.

Legionnaires' Disease: named after an outbreak of pneumonia which occurred in Philadelphia in 1976 at a convention of the American Legion, in which 29 people died. As a result of this a new organism was identified and called *Legionella pneumophila*; since then several other *Legionella* species have been found. The organism flourishes in water, particularly if it is at about 30°C, the temperature in most cooling towers and condensers in air-conditioning systems, which can give off air infected with the bacteria in fine drops of water. The disease cannot be spread from person to person, but only in infected drops of water which are inhaled. It develops a week after infection, with a fever, headache, and pains in the muscles, progressing to pneumonia. In some cases symptoms such as diarrhoea and vomiting, with abdominal pain, occur. The antibiotic used in treatment is erythromycin, with rifampicin in resistant cases.

Leiomyoma: a tumour of the unstriped or involuntary muscle in an internal organ.

Leishmaniasis: infection with a protozoon of the genus *Leishmania*, which is found in dogs and rodents and transmitted by sandflies. The infection may be of the skin, where it produces indolent sores, or it may be in the internal organs (*see* Kala-azar). Leishmaniasis is found in hot and dry countries both in the Old World and the New, and is treated by sodium stibogluconate. The skin sores may have to be treated surgically. (Sir William Leishman, English bacteriologist, 1865–1926)

Leishman's Stain: used principally to stain blood films, the stain is a combination of methylene blue and eosin.

Lemon: a source of vitamin C, its juice containing 60 mg ascorbic acid per 100 g. It has been recommended as an aid to slimming, but of itself has no effect; however, a diet of unsweetened lemon juice might lead to a loss of weight by destroying the appetite.

Lens: light entering the eye is first refracted in the cornea; it then passes through the lens, which is capable of changing its shape and so bringing images into sharp focus on the retina. The lens is held out at its edge by the suspensory ligament, so that it assumes its greatest diameter and least thickness. When the ciliary muscle contracts, it slackens the suspensory ligament and allows the lens to become more globular; its refractive power is increased and images of near objects are brought into focus on the retina at the back of the eye. The lens is bi-convex, the front less curved than the back, with a firm central part, the nucleus, surrounded by softer tissue. It is normally translucent, but becomes slightly yellow, flatter and less resilient with age. If cataracts form, the lens becomes opaque, but it can be removed to restore sight. *See* Cataract.

Leontiasis: overgrowth of the bones of the face and forehead which eventually produces the appearance of a lion. A similar appearance may be produced by leprosy.

Leprosy: also known as Hansen's disease (Gerhard Hansen, Norwegian physician, 1841–1912), now occurs in many tropical and subtropical countries, but has disappeared from Northern Europe. It is caused by *Mycobacterium leprae*, which in many ways resembles the organism of tuberculosis. There are two main types of leprosy: the lepromatous and the tuberculoid, the differentiation being made on the nature of the tissue reactions to the infection seen on microscopy. The disease is one of overcrowding, and it is thought that infection is spread by the nasal secretions of patients, but the exact way in which it happens is not known. Certain nerves are affected, becoming thickened and easily felt through the skin, which leads to anaesthesia and paralysis of the hands and feet. The skin is the site of change, large flat discoloured areas developing in tuberculoid leprosy and nodules with thickening of the skin in the lepromatous form. These nodules and thickened areas may affect the nose, the face, the palate, and the larynx, affecting the voice. The eyes may become inflamed. In time the cartilage and bones of the nose may be eaten away. The sensations of pain and temperature are lost as the nerves are affected, so that the fingers and toes are repeatedly injured and infected, eventually becoming shortened and useless. The disease may take years to develop after infection; the greatest incidence of leprosy is among those aged between 20 and 35. The drug dapsone is used in treatment, combined with rifampicin and clofazimine, according to recommendations from the World Health Organization. Treatment of the lepromatous type of disease must continue for at least two years, and of the tuberculoid type for upwards of six months. There are more than 10 million people suffering from leprosy in the world, but there is little danger of contracting the disease, even in a leper colony, provided that intimate personal contact is avoided.

Leptospira: micro-organisms like very fine corkscrews which are in constant motion. *Leptospira interrogans* is divided into many serogroups; the organism is carried by a number of creatures, the most important being rats, although cattle and dogs are included in the list. Infection is passed on in the urine, blood or tissues of infected animals through small abrasions in the skin or through intact mucous membranes, for example in the nose and throat. It may also be acquired by drinking infected water. The incubation period is a week or two, and infection shows itself by fever, severe headache, and pains in the muscles. There may be abdominal pain with nausea and vomiting. The kidneys and liver are affected, and in the form known as Weil's disease there is jaundice and possibly kidney failure. The organism is sensitive to penicillin, tetracycline and other antibiotics.

Lesbianism: female homosexuality. *See* Sex.

Lesion: a non-specific term meaning the damage done to the tissues of the body by injury or a disease process, e.g. a wound in the case of injury, or a boil in the case of infection. (Latin *laesio* from *laedere*, to hurt.)

Leucocyte: the leucocytes are the white cells in the blood. They are classified as polymorphonuclear leucocytes or polymorphs, lymphocytes and monocytes. Granulocytes are further divided into neutrophils, basophils or eosinophils, according to their staining characteristics. Polymorphs are 10–12 μm in diameter, small lymphocytes 7–10 μm, large lymphocytes up to 20 μm, and monocytes between 16–22 μm. The proportions in which they are present in the blood in health are: neutrophils 60–70%, eosinophils 1–4%, basophils 0–1%, lymphocytes 25–30%, and monocytes 5–10%. The total number is $4–11 \times 10^9$/l. This is raised in inflammatory conditions and abnormally low in other conditions, such as poisoning of the bone marrow by drugs. The state in which the count is increased is called leucocytosis, and that in which it is decreased leucopenia.

Leucoderma: a condition of the skin in which patches of white appear. It may be caused by diseases such as pityriasis versicolor or leprosy, or by vitiligo, an auto-immune condition which is common. The only harm it causes is the social embarrassment of the patient; but the blemish may often be camouflaged by make-up. It may affect coloured people; about one in three patients are cured spontaneously.

Leucoplakia: a condition in which the patient develops thickened white patches on the tongue, cheeks or gums which cannot be scraped off. In many cases no cause is found, but some may be put down to infection with *Candida*, smoking or syphilis. The treatment is the treatment of the infection if present, or the cessation of smoking. A number of cases develop malignant change, but this can be diagnosed and dealt with if patients attend regularly for follow-up.

Leucotomy: an operation now rarely performed. First introduced by the Portuguese neurologist Antonio Moniz (1874–1955) in 1935, it had as its object the severance to a greater or lesser degree of the white matter of the frontal lobes of the brain. It was intended for the treatment of intractable mental illnesses, such as depression, obsessional neurosis and chronic schizophrenia. Progress in drug therapy overtook the operation, and now it can only be justified in very rare cases where all else has failed and in which there is otherwise no hope of improvement.

Leukaemia: a malignant disease involving overproduction of white blood cells. Leukaemia may be acute or chronic, and according to the type of cell involved can be divided into myeloid or lymphatic. Acute lymphatic leukamia is mostly a disease of children, and acute myeloid leukaemia a disease of those over 55; the chronic leukaemias occur in people over 40. There is no clear cause for the disease, but it has been found in association with exposure to radiation; the dose of radiation likely to be harmful is not at present known. Radiation causes acute lymphatic leukaemia or chronic myeloid disease. Exposure to benzene has also been known to result in leukaemia. In acute disease, there is failure of the normal function of the bone marrow, leading to a lack of red blood cells, platelets necessary for blood clotting, and white cells necessary to fight disease, so that the patient becomes anaemic, and liable to develop infections and haemorrhages. In addition the liver and spleen are enlarged, as are the lymph glands These changes are to a greater or lesser extent common to all types of leukaemia, but enlarged lymph glands in the chest are particularly liable to cause trouble in acute lymphatic disease.

In all leukaemias, the diagnosis is made by examination of the blood. Remarkable progress has been made in the treatment of acute lymphatic disease, and there is now a range of drugs available which may be used. There is a very reasonable hope of recovery, but treatment has to continue for a long time. Special attention has to be paid to the possibility of the disease affecting the central nervous system. Acute myeloid leukaemia is also treated with various drugs, and radiotherapy may be employed, as well as bone marrow transplantation.

Chronic myeloid leukaemia is a rare disease, and patients suffer from anaemia, which is reflected in the complaint of tiredness, and enlargement of the spleen which may be painful. Busulphan is the chemotherapeutic agent used; radiotherapy may be employed, with bone marrow transplantation to follow. Chronic lymphatic leukaemia may produce enlargement of the lymph glands, and generalised ill health, but quite a number of cases have no symptoms, and the disease is only diagnosed when a blood count is done. Treatment may not be needed for a time, but if the symptoms of enlarged glands, anaemia, or ill health demand it, the drug chlorambucil is commonly used, or in some cases prednisolone followed by chlorambucil. Radiotherapy may be used on the enlarged glands or spleen. Patients are particularly likely to develop intercurrent infections, which are treated as they arise.

Leukorrhoea: an abnormal white discharge from the vagina.

Levodopa: a drug used in the treatment of Parkinson's disease (q.v.).

Libido: the sexual impulse.

Lichen Planus: a skin disease which is characterised by shiny smooth-topped papules with a violet tinge which may start on the ankles or wrists, or the palms of the hands or soles of the feet, or the back. The papules may spread, and when they heal leave behind dark patches. In the mouth, where they may cause ulcers, they leave a white pattern like lace. They may be very irritating, and need cortisone skin ointments or creams to allay the itching. The condition slowly resolves, perhaps taking as long as a year to disappear.

Ligaments: strong bands of fibrous tissue which hold the bones together and stabilise the joints.

Ligature: a piece of material, e.g. thread or catgut, used to tie off blood vessels or other structures.

Lightening: occurs after the 36th week of pregnancy when the head of the foetus engages in the brim of the pelvis. The uterus and its contents descend a little in the abdomen and relieve the feeling of distension.

Lightning: those struck by lightning suffer the passage of a direct electrical current of very high amperage and voltage, and are likely to stop breathing; the heart may also stop, and artificial respiration and external heart massage is essential. It may be successful if started up to a quarter of an hour after the injury, and is therefore always worth trying.

Lignocaine: a commonly used local anaesthetic with a

swift action, which can be injected in concentrations of ½-1% or applied to mucous membranes at a strength of 2-4%. It can also be used in inducing epidural or spinal anaesthesia, and has an action in restoring the normal rhythm of the heart after it has been disturbed by myocardial infarction (q.v.), when 100 mg can be given intravenously followed by 4 mg a minute over 30 minutes.

Linctus: any syrupy medicine, often a cough mixture.

Linea Alba: a whitish line running down the middle of the muscular wall of the abdomen, formed by the junction of the flat tendons of the external oblique, internal oblique and transverse muscles after they have split to enclose the two longitudinal rectus muscles.

Liniments or Embrocations: liquid preparations designed to be rubbed into the skin for muscular or joint pains. They act by counter-irritation, for anything which produces irritation of the overlying skin tends to relieve pain in deeper structures. They should be applied by gentle massage, which is in itself beneficial. Traditional liniments are made of methyl salicylate (oil of wintergreen), turpentine and camphor, but there are a number of creams on the market which are perhaps more convenient to use. Some claim to penetrate the skin, introducing remedies into the affected area, but there is little evidence that this is so.

Lip: sometimes the site of uncomfortable cracks and fissures appearing in cold weather, which respond to simple ointment or lip salves, except when they become infected when an anti-bacterial ointment is needed. Cold sores, usually caused by the virus of herpes simplex (q.v.), may need to be treated with acyclovir cream. Boils forming on the lips, especially the upper one, must be treated seriously, for the infection is liable to spread. Ulcers may form inside the lips, and can be treated with corticosteroids in tablets or ointment kept in contact with the ulcers. The primary sore of syphilis may be found on the lip; it appears between two and four weeks after infection as a small nodule, which is painless. This breaks down to form an ulcer, and is very infectious. Cancer of the lip is rare; it was at one time associated with smoking clay pipes.

Lipaemia: the presence in the blood of abnormally large amounts of fats or fatty substances, including cholesterol.

Lipoma: a tumour often occurring just below the skin, composed of fat cells. It is harmless, and if necessary can be removed easily.

Liquorice: prepared from the dried roots and underground stem of the plant *Glycyrrhiza glabra*, it has been used in medicines for centuries. Carbenoxolone, a derivative of glycyrrhizinic acid, an active principle of liquorice, is used in the treatment of peptic ulcers, as is liquorice with the glycyrrhizin removed.

Listeria: *Listeria monocytogenes* is a micro-organism which can survive at low temperatures and multiply despite refrigeration. It is found in the earth and vegetation, and in many wild and domestic animals, birds and fish, being able to infect human beings through contaminated food and especially dairy products; it may be found in cheese, particularly soft cheese, and in milk, and as it can survive refrigeration and in some cases pasteurisation and is only killed by adequate cooking, cold prepared food may be infective. It is liable to produce disease in the very young and the elderly, and in those with immunosuppressive conditions. Most importantly it can affect pregnant mothers, who develop a mild attack of fever, with diarrhoea, sore throat, headache, and pain in the abdomen or back, which may be so mild that it is disregarded. The infection is passed on to the foetus, and may result in the premature birth of an infant with chest infection and a rash. Unfortunately some of the infants are born dead, and some develop inflammation of the brain and its coverings, a meningo-encephalitis. The organism may persist in the genital tract, and in some cases the infection is passed on to the infant in this way at birth; persistent infection may also be the cause of habitual abortion. After a birth the mother may suffer from a recurrence of symptoms, developing up to three weeks after labour. The treatment is with penicillin, erythromycin or tetracycline, ampicillin or amoxycillin being the preferred penicillins. In 1989 there were 291 cases reported in Britain, with the deaths of 26 unborn or newborn babies.

Lithiasis: a condition in which stones or concretions are present.

Lithium: a metallic element. As lithium carbonate, it is used in the treatment of mania and manic-depressive illness. It has recently been introduced in the form of lithium succinate ointment as a treatment for seborrhoeic dermatitis.

Lithotomy: the operation of cutting for a stone. Cutting for bladder stones is one of the most ancient operations in surgery, dating back at least to the time of Hippocrates, who considered it so dangerous that it should be left strictly to specialists (*see* Hippocratic Oath). The operation continued to be carried out by lithotomists for centuries, demanding great fortitude on the part of both patient and surgeon, for there was no anaesthesia and the results could be catastrophic; nevertheless there must have been successes, for the operation persisted until the discovery of anaesthetics, which made things a great deal less traumatic. At the turn of the last century the discovery of X-rays made diagnosis much more certain, and stones could then be seen in the kidney and ureters and removed. Using endoscopic instruments, it has for many years been possible to break up and remove stones from the bladder and ureters without opening the abdomen, but recently great advances have been made in the removal of stones from the kidneys; using X-ray guidance, instruments can be passed into the pelvis of the kidney through a small incision in the flank, and stones, if necessary broken up by ultrasonic probes or the shock waves produced by the spark gap of an electrohydraulic lithotriptor, can be removed or the fragments passed in the urine. Stones can also be broken up by extracorporeal lithotripsy (*see* below).

Lithotripsy: recently a technique has been introduced

which avoids any kind of surgical incision for the removal of stones from the kidney or gall-bladder, called extracorporeal shock-wave lithotripsy. The lithotripsy machines rely on a shock wave produced in one of three ways: spark gap, electromagnetic or piezo-electric. The stones are localised by X-rays or ultrasound, and the shock waves focused on them reduce them to fragments. In the case of kidney stones, the fragments are passed in the urine; gallstones, however, are not washed out in the same way, and passage relies on strong contractions of the gall-bladder, which in many cases is diseased and may be incapable of contraction. The place of lithotripsy in the treatment of gallstones is not yet clear, but it is the treatment of choice in many cases of kidney stones, for no anaesthetic, or at the most a short intravenous injection of an analgesic, is needed, and the patient does not have to stay in hospital.

Liver: the largest gland in the body, the liver lies in the right upper part of the abdominal cavity, under the diaphragm and covered by the lower ribs. It extends upwards to the level of the sixth rib. It weighs about 1500 g and is soft. For the purposes of description it is divided into four lobes, but to all intents it is a single organ shaped rather like a wedge. It is supplied with blood by the hepatic artery, a branch of the abdominal aorta, and by the portal vein which brings blood from the intestines; about one-fifth of the blood coming to the liver arrives through the hepatic artery, the remaining four-fifths coming from the portal vein. Blood leaves the liver through the hepatic vein, which joins the inferior vena cava. Branches of the hepatic artery and the portal vein run in company to sinusoids within the liver, small blood spaces which take the place of capillaries. The sinusoids are lined by liver cells across which the blood passes before it is collected in veins which join to form the hepatic vein. The liver cells form bile, which is carried away in ducts running in company with the branches of the artery and portal vein. The hepatic ducts carrying bile join together to form right and left bile ducts which leave the liver at the porta hepatis, where the hepatic artery and portal vein enter the liver, and join to form the hepatic bile duct.

The liver is essential; without it life is not possible. It has many functions, some concerned with the formation and breakdown of proteins, carbohydrates and fats, and their storage. Others are concerned with the metabolism of hormones and drugs, the secretion of bile, and the conversion of toxic products of nitrogen metabolism into urea. The liver oxidises alcohol, and stores the vitamins A, D, E, and K. The chemical processes take place in the cells of the sinusoids, the 'raw materials' being brought from the intestines by the portal vein and the rest of the body by the hepatic artery; a number of poisons and diseases can attack the cells, but fortunately they have great powers of regeneration.

Liver Fluke. *Clonorchis*, *Fasciola* and *Opisthorcis* are genera of flukes which infect the liver of humans. They live in the biliary tract, and their intermediate hosts are snails. *Clonorchis* and *Opisthorcis* find a further secondary host in freshwater fish, and the infection occurs where people eat raw fish, particularly in the Far East. Flukes may infect fish-eating mammals other than man, such as cats and dogs. *Fasciola* is the sheep liver fluke, and the snail infects vegetation and water; in sheep and cattle raising countries the infection spreads to humans through infected water. *See* Flukes.

Loa Loa: a filarial worm of West Africa, which infests the subcutaneous tissues, causes transient swellings (Calabar swellings) and intense itching, and is sometimes seen crossing the eye beneath the conjunctiva. It is spread by the mango fly, and treated with diethylcarbamazine citrate. *See* Filariasis.

Lobe: a well-defined part of an organ; the brain, lungs, liver and thyroid gland are for example made up of lobes, which are defined by their shape, by partitions of connective tissue, or by fissures in the organ.

Local Anaesthesia: anaesthesia of a localised area of the body, as opposed to general anaesthesia, when the whole body is rendered insensitive to pain. The first local anaesthetic, introduced in 1884, was cocaine, which was applied to the surface of the eye and throat. It was, however, liable to be poisonous and addictive, and was replaced by procaine which is much safer and can be injected into the skin or into nerves to block the area they supply. There are now a number of local anaesthetics, but the most commonly used is lignocaine, which can be used as a surface anaesthetic, injected into the skin or nerves, or used in inducing spinal or epidural anaesthesia when injected into the spinal subdural or extradural spaces. Bupivacaine may be used when a longer duration of anaesthesia is required, for its effect in nerve blocks can last for up to eight hours. It is, however, slower in action than lignocaine, and may take up to half an hour to be fully effective.

Lochia: the normal discharge from the womb after child-birth. It may last for one or two weeks.

Lockjaw: *see* Tetanus.

Locomotor Ataxia (tabes dorsalis): a manifestation of the third stage of syphilis, much less common now than once it was. Appearing up to 20 years after the original infection, the disease involves the posterior root ganglia of the spinal nerves, with degeneration of the posterior columns of the spinal cord in which sensory fibres ascend to the brain. The patient complains of sudden pains in the legs, known as lightning pains, and a feeling when walking as if being on cotton wool. There may also be impotence, difficulty in passing water, attacks of double vision and unsteadiness in the dark. As the disease progresses there is increasing ataxia (incoordination of movement), and inability to sense where the body and limbs are in space, which causes the tabetic to sway and fall in the dark, or if the eyes are closed. There may also be a profound disorder of the nerves supplying the abdomen, so that the patient feels acute severe abdominal pain with vomiting and even rigidity of the abdominal wall simulating an 'acute abdomen'. The knee joint may become disorganised as the result of repeated small injuries, and ulcers may develop in the soles of the feet. Blindness may follow atrophy of the optic disc. Since the advent of penicillin in the treatment of syphilis, the disease is rarely now seen in this advanced stage.

Lordosis: exaggerated forward curvature of the spine in the lumbar region; the lower back is abnormally hollow.

Lotions: solutions or suspensions in water which when applied leave a thin amount of the contained drug spread on the skin, and cool it by evaporation; alcohol may be added to assist this action. Shake lotions contain an insoluble powder, and when they evaporate leave a coating of the powder on the skin, e.g. calamine lotion.

Louse: a parasitic insect which has been with man since pre-history; although there are many varieties of lice, there are only two which breed on man, *Pediculus* and *Pthirus*. *Pediculus humanus capitis* lives on the head, and is common in schools, where it is spread by direct contact and by combs and hairbrushes. It is not caught because of any kind of dirtiness. The eggs are laid on the hair, where they leave empty white egg containers or 'nits' about a centimetre from the scalp. They make the head itch, but are of no great consequence and are treated by malathion or carbaryl lotion. *Pediculus humanus humanus* is the body louse, bigger than the head louse and capable of spreading typhus, relapsing fever and trench fever. It lives in the clothes rather than on the body. *Pthirus pubis* is the crab louse, found in the pubic hair and usually spread by sexual intercourse. These lice are also treated with malathion or carbaryl; lindane may be used, but some lice are resistant to it.

LSD: lysergic acid diethylamide, derived from ergot, one of the most potent drugs known – 1 µg/kg is enough to produce symptoms of poisoning, which start with a period of vague apprehension. This is followed by a disturbance of the autonomic nervous system, producing hot and cold sensations, and then there develop visual and spatial hallucinations and feelings of anxiety, persecution, depression and hostility with considerable confusion. The symptoms of intoxication arise about 30 minutes after the drug has been taken and last for a few hours, but the effect of the drug does not wear off completely for a day. Treatment may include the use of a minor tranquilliser such as diazepam, but it may not be easy to control the effects of LSD; it has been known for people under the influence of the drug to become criminally violent. Although an unbiased observer is in little doubt that the effects of LSD are quite disagreeable in many cases, and not an unmixed pleasure in many others, the attraction of the drug as a means to the titillation of the senses has proved irresistible to some and it has become accepted as part of the drug taker's armamentarium. It seems likely that it can produce long-term damage to the mentality particularly in those who were not entirely normal when they started taking the drug.

Lucid Interval: the interval of consciousness which may follow a period of unconsciousness and precede a lapse into coma in cases where a head injury has started extradural bleeding from the middle meningeal artery or one of its branches.

Lues: syphilis.

Lugol's Iodine: a solution of iodine 5% and potassium iodide 10% in water which may be used in the pre-operative treatment of thyrotoxicosis.

Lumbago: pain in the lower back, commonly caused by a strained ligament in the spine. The treatment is rest and heat.

Lumbar Puncture: the introduction of a hollow needle into the spinal canal in order to draw off a specimen of cerebrospinal fluid for laboratory examination, or to introduce drugs, spinal anaesthetics or radio-opaque substances for X-ray investigations. The puncture is made between the third and fourth or fourth and fifth lumbar vertebrae, where the point of the needle cannot harm the spinal cord, for it ends at the level of the second spinal vertebra. The puncture is usually made under local anaesthesia.

Lunar Caustic: silver nitrate.

Lunatic: one who is moonstruck, a mentally deranged person. *See* Mental Illness.

Lungs: the organs in which exchange of gases and vapours takes place between the air, or whatever gas is being inspired, and the blood. The respiratory system consists of the lungs, air passages, the muscles that control breathing, and the pleural cavities. The right and left lungs are divided into lobes; the right lung has three, upper, lower and middle, and the left two, upper and lower. Each lung has an apex which reaches up to the level of the collar-bone, and a base which rests on the diaphragm, which is roughly at the level of the tenth rib, although it reaches the level of the twelfth rib behind and is as high as the eighth rib in front. The bronchi (the air passages) and the blood vessels enter the lungs at the root or hilum on the inner surface. Right and left lungs are separated by the structures of the mediastinum which contains the heart and great blood vessels, the oesophagus and, in its upper part, the trachea. Although it is not apparent from superficial examination, each lobe of the lungs is separated by sheets of fibrous tissue into segments, each with its own bronchus and blood supply; the number varies from five in the right lower lobe to two in the middle lobe. Inspired air enters the mouth and nose, passes into the pharynx, and enters the trachea through the larynx. The trachea is a tube prevented from collapsing by about 20 rings of cartilage; it is about 10 cm long, and at its lower end branches into right and left bronchi. The right bronchus divides into branches for the upper and lower lobes, the branch for the middle lobe coming from the lower main bronchus. The left bronchus divides into two branches. The lobar bronchi divide in turn, the two branches together having a greater area in cross-section than the bronchus from which they derive. The branches continue to divide into two until the smallest air passages, the bronchioles, are only some 0.2 mm in diameter.

Branches of the pulmonary artery and vein accompany the branches of the bronchi. When the bronchioles reach their terminal branches, small ducts protrude from them which open into air sacs, the alveolar sacs, which are lined by alveoli, one cell thick, surrounded by a meshwork of capillary vessels, also with walls one cell thick, the barrier between blood and air being less than 1 μm. This is where the exchange of gases takes place; the total area available for the exchange is over 50 square metres. Blood containing carbon dioxide exchanges the gas for oxygen contained in the alveoli.

Air is drawn into the lungs by the movements of the chest wall and the diaphragm. The inner surface of the chest cavity and the outer surfaces of the lungs are lined by the pleural membranes which are slippery and slide freely over each other. The lungs themselves have very little muscle in them, and that only to control the size of the bronchi and bronchioles; they cannot move themselves, but can respond to changes of pressure in the chest because they are elastic. When the chest wall is raised and the diaphragm held still or lowered by contraction of its muscle, the capacity of the chest is increased and the pressure lowered; air under atmospheric pressure then passes into the lungs. When the pressure in the chest is increased by lowering the chest wall, and the dome of the diaphragm rises, the air leaves the lungs. The process depends on the chest being airtight and the air entering only through the mouth and nose.

As air enters the respiratory system it is warmed and moistened, and dust and other particles of matter are caught in the mucus secreted by the cells lining the air passages. The cells have cilia, processes like hairs, which beat upwards and propel the debris out until it is removed by coughing. The nervous control of breathing is automatic, but while it can to a certain extent be over-ridden there comes a time when the breath can voluntarily be held no longer, and automatic control comes into action again, because there is a rising concentration of carbon dioxide in the blood and the respiratory centre in the brain is extremely sensitive to the presence of carbon dioxide.

Lupus: *Lupus vulgaris* is tuberculosis of the skin, now increasingly rare; it occurs mostly on the face and nose, taking the form of small nodules which leave scars behind. It responds to the anti-tubercular drugs. *Systemic lupus erythematosus* is a disease which has a multitude of symptoms; it is more common in women than men, and is characterised by the presence of a large number of autoantibodies in the blood, which react with the patient's own cells. It may affect the skin, when red scaly patches or papules appear on the bridge of the nose and the cheeks, the ears, the backs of the hands and the upper trunk. The rash may take some time to appear, or the onset may be acute, often after exposure to the sun; the red patches may run into each other, and the centres heal up and scar while the edges extend. The skin rashes may take a number of forms, not always easy to recognise. The disease may affect the central nervous system, and cause severe headaches and depression as well as other manifestations; it may affect the kidneys, lungs, and the heart, as well as causing anaemia. It is a chronic disease, and patients suffer remissions and exacerbations. The treatment varies according to the patient's needs, and may be simple or may involve the use of chloroquine, an antimalarial drug, and corticosteroids; as the disease is one of the immune system, immunosuppressive drugs may have to be used such as azathioprine.

Luxation: dislocation.

Lycanthropy: the delusion that a man has changed into a wolf, the werewolf of legend. *See* Zoomorphism.

Lye: a mixture of sodium hydroxide and sodium carbonate, once but no longer used in the household. It was an extremely corrosive poison.

Lyme Disease: first described as the result of cases occurring in Lyme in the USA in 1977, the disease is caused by the micro-organism *Borrelia bergdorferi*, and spread by ticks, mosquitoes and biting flies. The tick bite develops as a small red pimple that spreads out on the skin as a red, itching and possibly painful area; the centre clears, leaving an expanding circle of affected skin. This condition is called erythema migrans, and may be accompanied by a headache, pains in the muscles and joints, and a fever. Red areas of skin may develop in places unconnected with the original bite, and these manifestations may persist for some weeks. The disease may continue, some months after the original infection, to involve the joints, especially the knee; the heart, with irregular pulse, shortness of breath and pain in the chest; and the central and peripheral nervous system, with encephalitis and neuritis. Similar illnesses have occurred in Europe where the tick *Ixodes ricinus* is found to carry the disease, possibly from dogs, who can suffer from arthritis caused by *B. bergdorferi*. The organism is sensitive to antibiotics, including tetracyclines, penicillin and erythromycin.

Lymph: the fluid found in the lymph vessels; it is clear and slightly yellow, containing lymph cells and, if it derives from intestinal vessels, particles of fat. It originates in the tissue spaces, being derived from the fluid which filters through the walls of the capillary blood vessels. It may contain particles as big as bacteria if it is draining from an infected area.

Lymphadenitis: inflammation of lymph glands, or nodes.

Lymphangitis: inflammation of the lymph vessels, which may be seen as thin red lines running up the forearm in some cases of infection of the fingers or hand.

Lymphatic Leukaemia: *see* Leukaemia.

Lymphatic System: the tissue fluid which moves out of the capillary blood vessels into the tissue spaces is for the most part taken up in the capillaries again, but some is carried away in the lymphatic system, which has small capillary vessels which join to form larger vessels, usually as a plexus round the blood vessels. The lymph vessels run from all parts of the body into groups of lymph nodes; a number of small vessels run into a node, and leave it as one larger vessel. Like veins, they have valves which direct the lymph centrally: vessels join to form trunks, which eventually come together to form the thoracic duct, the right broncho-mediastinal trunk, and trunks running from the arms and head and neck on each side. These run into the great veins at the root of the neck. The lymphatics draining the intestine are particularly important, for they take up fat absorbed in the intestine and carry it through the thoracic duct into the bloodstream.

Lymph Nodes: also known as lymph glands. Small collections of lymphoid tissue lying in the course of the lymph vessels; several small vessels come together at the nodes, leaving as one larger vessel. Lymphocytes are formed in the lymph nodes, as are antibodies, and they form filters to intercept foreign matter and bacteria, consequently often becoming the seat of infection themselves, when they become enlarged and painful. If the infection is overwhelming they may break down and suppurate, as can happen in the groin in consequence of an infection in the leg, or in the armpit in a severe infection of the hand or arm. The lymph nodes draining the tonsils often become enlarged in a throat infection. Collections of lymph nodes are found at junctional areas of the body, i.e. at the knee, groin, elbow and armpit, as well as in the neck, at the roots of the main bronchi in the lungs, and along the aorta in the abdomen. Generalised enlargement of the lymph nodes may develop in various systemic diseases, and localised enlargement may be found in cases of malignant disease where the nodes have intercepted malignant cells breaking away from the primary growth.

Lymphocyte: a round white blood cell, concerned mainly with the immune system and formed in the lymph nodes and elsewhere in the reticulo-endothelial system. Lymphocytes play a most important part in the immune system, and are divided into two classes, B and T cells, the latter being formed in the thymus gland. B cells produce antibodies, which become more specific as the cell matures into a plasma cell. T cells have four types: helper (Th), suppressor (Ts), cytotoxic (Tc) and delayed hypersensitivity (Td). The Th cells play a part in the development of antibodies by the B cells; the Ts cells check this activity, and form with the Th cells a regulating system for the immune response. Tc cells kill infected cells in the tissues, in particular those infected with viruses, and are dependent on Th cells for their action, as are the Td cells which also take part in the cellular response. Tc and Td cells are involved in the process of graft rejection. *See* Allergy, Immune System, Leucocytes.

Lymphogranuloma: lymphogranuloma venereum is a venereal disease caused by infection with the organism *Chlamydia trachomatis*. The infection is found in Africa, the Caribbean, South America and South-East Asia. A small blister, which may ulcerate, appears at the site of infection on the genitalia up to three weeks after infection, and then painful swelling of the lymph glands in the groin develops. The enlarged lymph glands may break down and suppurate. Tetracycline or sulphonamides are used in the treatment. Lymphogranuloma has been used as a name for Hodgkin's disease (q.v.), especially on the Continent.

Lymphoma: a number of conditions that involve swelling of the lymph nodes which is not caused by inflammation, metastatic malignant disease or Hodgkin's disease, have been called lymphomas. They are rare, and the diagnosis is made on microscopical examination of lymph nodes removed at biopsy. Treatment is by radiotherapy or chemotherapy, according to the particular needs of each case.

Lymphosarcoma: a malignant disease of the lymphoid tissue, not including Hodgkin's disease. It is not common, but occurs mainly in middle-aged men. There is painless swelling of lymphatic nodes, particularly in the neck, and sometimes enlargement of the tonsil; sometimes a group of nodes presses on neighbouring structures and so produces symptoms. Treatment is by cytotoxic drugs, possibly by radiotherapy.

Lysol: a soapy solution of cresol once used as a household disinfectant; it was not infrequently used in suicide attempts, being caustic and highly irritant.

Lysozyme: an antibacterial enzyme found in tears, saliva, bronchial secretions and egg-white.

M

McBurney's Point: named after the New York surgeon McBurney (1845–1913), this is the point at which the maximum tenderness is felt in the abdomen in a case of acute appendicitis. It lies on a line drawn between the umbilicus and the right anterior superior iliac spine – the bony point felt at the outer end of the fold in the groin – two-thirds of the way from the umbilicus in the right lower abdomen. It is quite possible to have acute appendicitis without having great tenderness at this point, but it is not common. McBurney also developed an incision used in taking out the appendix which involves splitting rather than cutting the muscles of the abdominal wall.

Maceration: the softening of a solid by fluid. In medicine, the softening and damaging of the tissues by water, as in the case of a corpse many hours drowned.

McNaghten Rules: drawn up by the House of Lords in the last century after an attempt to assassinate Sir Robert Peel which resulted in the death of his private secretary. The rules state that for a defence of insanity to be successful the defendant must prove that he was at the time of the crime suffering from such a defect of reason because of his mental condition that he did not know what he was doing; or, if he did know, he did not know that what he was doing was wrong.

Macrophages: large cells present in connective tissue and in the walls of blood vessels, also called phagocytic cells, or histiocytes. They can be fixed, or can move about to pick up foreign particles or fragments of disintegrated cells. They form part of the reticulo-endothelial system (q.v.).

Macula: a stain or spot, used in anatomy to mean an area distinguishable from its surroundings by its colour or other peculiarity. The macula of the retina is a yellow spot at the back of the retina, which has in it a central depression called the fovea. Here the retina is thinnest and the vision most acute.

Macule: a flat discoloured spot in the skin, as distinct from a papule, which is a raised spot. Rashes are often maculopapular, having raised areas of discoloration surrounded by flat areas.

Madura Foot: a tropical disease in which the foot swells and its tissues and bones become riddled with sinuses caused by infection with a fungus. It is one of a group of chronic infections called mycetomas, caused by fungi or actinomycetes, and the legs and feet are most commonly affected, although the disease may be found in the arms, the chest and elsewhere. Treatment with dapsone, rifampicin or sulphonamides is long and may only be partially effective; surgery may be needed.

Magnesium: a metallic element used in medicine in the form of its salts: magnesium carbonate, hydroxide and trisilicate are used as antacids in the treatment of peptic ulcers and gastritis. Magnesium hydroxide mixture (milk of magnesia) has a slight laxative action, and magnesium sulphate (Epsom salts) a more powerful one. The element is a constituent of chlorophyll, and so an essential part of life; it is essential for human beings, playing a part in the functioning of nerves and muscles, and in energy metabolism. A normal diet supplies the requirements.

Magnetic Resonance Imaging (MRI): *see* Nuclear Magnetic Resonance Imaging.

Mal: sickness, disease; *see* Epilepsy.

Malaise: a vague feeling of general discomfort.

Malaria: a disease caused by infection with the malaria parasite, a protozoan organism of the genus *Plasmodium*. Four species of the genus infect man, and they are all carried by female anopheline mosquitoes (q.v.), which flourish in tropical and subtropical countries. The mosquito bites a human being, and introduces into the blood sporozoites, small fusiform cells with one nucleus. They have to find their way to the liver within an hour or they die; but if they do find their way there, they grow and reproduce. After a week, the parasites leave the liver as merozoites, which pass into the blood and invade the red blood corpuscles, where they start cycles of growth and reproduction. When the merozoite enters the red blood corpuscle, it takes the form of a ring and within a few hours fills the cell completely. Fission of the parasite takes place, and each one gives origin to 16 daughter cells. While the merozoite is growing it is called a trophozoite, and when fission starts a schizont. The 16 new merozoites are liberated into the bloodstream from the red blood cells in which they developed, and the asexual reproduction cycle starts again as they invade new red blood cells. The attacks of periodic fever characteristic of malaria coincide with the liberation of the daughter merozoites into the bloodstream. While the asexual merozoites start their reproductive cycle in the red cells, sexual forms of the parasite called microgametes (males) and macrogametes (females) begin to appear in the blood. These can only survive and reproduce in a mosquito, and if one comes along and bites the human they pass into the stomach of the mosquito where microgametes and macrogametes join to produce a zygote, which pushes its way out of the stomach. On the outside of the stomach there is formed an oocyst within which many sporozoites develop. When fully grown the asexual sporozoites travel into the mosquito's salivary glands and wait until the mosquito bites another human being.

Malaria manifests itself in four ways, according to which species of plasmodium is responsible for the infection. All four produce headache and shivering, sweating and pains in the limbs. In infections with *P. falciparum*, known as malignant tertian malaria, which takes from five to ten days to develop, the patient suddenly feels cold, starts to shiver, and may vomit. This coincides with the merozoites leaving the red blood cells and entering the bloodstream; because the maturation of the parasites in falciparum malaria is not well synchronised, the fever is not regular, and paroxysms may occur every day (quotidian) or irregularly. Falciparum malaria is called malignant malaria because clumps of the organism may block capillaries in vital organs; the parasites adhere to the vessel walls and damage them, and this may happen in the brain, kidneys, liver, spleen, bone marrow and lungs. The patient becomes anaemic, perhaps jaundiced, may develop convulsions and coma, and may pass blood in the urine (blackwater fever). Involvement of the brain is most dangerous to life; involvement of the kidneys may lead to kidney failure. Infection with *P. vivax* takes about two weeks to produce symptoms, *P. ovale* takes a day or two longer, and *P. malariae* a few days more. Some infections with *P. vivax* may take between a month and a year to show themselves. The parasites in *P. vivax* and *P. ovale* are liberated from the red cells every 48 hours, producing a tertian fever, while in *P. malariae* the cycle takes place every 72 hours, producing a quartan fever. These types of malaria are relatively benign, although unpleasant, and rarely cause death. However, the spleen commonly becomes enlarged in infections with *P. vivax*, and is consequently prone to rupture.

Chloroquine is the drug used in cases of benign malaria, but unfortunately *P. falciparum* has in many places become resistant to it and therefore quinine, sulphonamide-pyrimethamine combinations (Fansidar) or mefloquine, a drug which has recently been introduced, must be used. Travellers to areas where malaria is prevalent should start prophylactic drugs a week before travelling, and continue for four weeks after their return. For North Africa and the Middle East, chloroquine 300 mg weekly or proguanil 200 mg daily are recommended; for India and China, the rest of Africa and Central and South America, proguanil daily and chloroquine weekly; and for South-East Asia and the rest of the world where malaria occurs advice should be sought from the doctor or the travel agent. Mefloquine can be used prophylactically once a week. Anopheline mosquitoes are most likely to bite in the evening, when it is sensible to wear long sleeves and trousers or other covering for the legs; bites are most likely to occur in sub-Saharan Africa. Great efforts have been made in many parts of the world to control mosquitoes by using insecticides, but there are places such as the Niger delta where the task appears to be impossible.

Malignant: when used of a tumour it means cancerous; the term is also applied to dangerous conditions which progress rapidly such as malignant malaria or malignant hypertension.

Malingering: the feigning of illness in order to gain some advantage.

Malleolus: the bony projection at the ankle, formed by the lower end of the tibia on the inside and the lower end of the fibula on the outside.

Mallet Finger: if the extensor tendon which normally straightens the end of the finger is torn away from the base of the bone at the last finger joint, or cut through, the fingertip is left permanently half-flexed and is called a mallet finger. It may be treated surgically by repair of the tendon.

Malleus: a small bone in the middle ear. *See* Ear.

Malnutrition: a condition arising from deficiency in the diet or deficiency in the absorption or metabolism of food.

Malta Fever: *see* Brucellosis.

Mammary Gland: the breast (q.v.).

Mammogram: a radiological examination of the breast to identify or exclude tumours. It is simple, and recommended as a three-yearly routine in women between the ages of 50 and 65.

Mandible: the lower jawbone.

Mandragora: *Mandragora officinarum*, the oriental mandrake, contains hyoscine, and was once used as a sedative and narcotic. *Cf. Othello*, III, iii, 331.

Mandrake: a forked root with magical properties, the mandrake shrieked when pulled out of the ground in such a way as to send men mad, so that it had to be rooted up by dogs. It was thought to be an aphrodisiac and promoter of fertility in women, but the poet Donne believed differently: 'His apples kindle, his leaves, force of conception kill' ('The Progress of the Soul'). *See also* Genesis 30: 14–18.

Manganese: a metallic element essential for life, but only minute quantities are needed; no cases of manganese deficiency have been recorded. It may be used in medicine in the form of potassium permanganate as an antiseptic. If manganese fumes or dust are inhaled to excess, patients develop a condition very like Parkinson's disease.

Mania: a mental state characterised by elevated mood, exaggerated activity and rapid speech, with ideas of self-importance. Subjects are inclined to alternate manic periods with periods of depression, a condition called manic-depressive disorder.

MAOIs (monoamine-oxydase inhibitors): drugs sometimes used in cases of depression. They take about three weeks to become effective, and have the disadvantage that they interact with certain substances to stimulate the release of noradrenaline at the nerve endings; this results in a sudden dangerous elevation of the blood pressure. The main substance liable to produce this effect is tyramine, which is found in many foods, for example cheese, or meat or yeast extracts such as Bovril and Marmite. Substances used in proprietary cough medicines and cold cures may have the same effect. A patient prescribed an MAOI is given a card carrying a warning and setting out the precautions that must be taken. The principal MAOIs are phenelzine and isocarboxazid.

Mantoux Test: a test devised by Charles Mantoux (French physician, 1877–1947) for infection with tuberculosis. An injection of a solution of purified protein derivative of tuberculin (PPD) is made into the skin, and a positive reaction of inflammation in the skin over 10 mm in size is likely to indicate an infection. The Heaf test is a variation of the Mantoux test.

Marasmus: progressive wasting away, particularly in infants.

Marburg Disease: a virus infection first described in 1967 when it affected laboratory workers in Marburg who had been in contact with a group of vervet monkeys from Uganda. In 1976 there was an outbreak of severe haemorrhagic fever in the Sudan and Zaire which was found to be caused by a virus identical with the Marburg virus, but carrying a different antigen. This was called the Ebola virus. Both infections are now referred to as African haemorrhagic fever, and a number of cases have occurred. Although the cases at Marburg were connected with monkeys, it has not been proved that monkeys are the carriers of the disease. Infection from monkey to man was by contact with infected body fluids, and the same is true of infection from man to man.

Marfan's Syndrome: named after the French physician Bernard Marfan (1858–1942) who described the condition in 1896, the syndrome is characterised by long thin fingers, toes, arms and legs, increased height, deformity of the spine and breastbone, and abnormality of the heart and eyes. The aortic valve in the heart is incompetent, and the lens of the eye is dislocated. The syndrome is inherited as a dominant trait.

Marihuana: *see* Cannabis Indica.

Marrow: the marrow of the bones in an adult is red or yellow. Red marrow is found in the skull, ribs, pelvis, breastbone, the bodies of the vertebrae and the ends of the long bones. It is actively engaged in making the cells of the blood. Yellow marrow is full of fat; in early life, it is active and red, but by the end of the period of growth it has become inactive. In times of crisis it is still capable of regaining activity, and it then becomes red again.

Masochism: a sexual perversion in which satisfaction is gained from being cruelly treated. It takes its name from the stories of the nineteenth-century Austrian novelist von Sacher Masoch.

Massage: a manipulative treatment used in physiotherapy. The masseur or masseuse uses passive movements of the muscles, limbs and joints, and by stroking, pinching, pressing and kneading stimulates the tissues. The various movements are described as effleurage, stroking towards the heart; stroking, which is away from the heart; pétrissage or kneading; frictions or circular movements; and tapotement or beating the tissues with the edge of the hand.

Mast Cells: large cells found in many places in the body, particularly in connective tissues and the mucosal surfaces. If they are damaged, or activated by an antibody–antigen reaction, they release histamine and other substances which increase the passage of fluid from the blood vessels, lower the blood pressure, increase secretion from the mucous membranes, and contract smooth muscles. They also attract white blood cells. Massive activation of the mast cells results in anaphylactic shock (q.v.).

Mastectomy: the removal of the breast. Simple mastectomy is the removal of the breast alone; radical mastectomy, which may be carried out for cancer, involves removal of the breast together with the muscles on which it lies and the lymph nodes in the armpit. This severe operation is intended to remove all the tissue into which the cancer might spread, but it is not carried out as often as it once was, for it has been found that a simple mastectomy, or even the removal only of the cancerous lump in the breast, followed by hormone therapy, and possibly chemotherapy and radiotherapy, may give equally good results and is far less disfiguring.

Mastic: a resin derived from the tree *Pistacia lentiscus*, used in microscopy and dentistry.

Mastitis: acute mastitis is an inflammation of the breast which most commonly occurs in nursing mothers in association with cracked or depressed nipples. Treatment is by penicillin; feeding from the normal breast may not have to be stopped, although the milk should be expressed manually from the infected breast while it is inflamed. Chronic mastitis is not an infection, but a name used for changes which produce benign lumps in the breast, possibly in association with cysts; the changes are probably dependent on hormonal imbalance, for it is found that the condition is improved by the contraceptive pill.

Mastoiditis: inflammation of the air cells in the mastoid process of the temporal bone, once not uncommon in association with middle ear disease, but since the advent of antibiotics rarely seen.

Masturbation: self-stimulation of the sexual organs is almost universal and is in fact a normal stage in sexual development. It is found in nearly all boys and most girls, although the sexual impulse in women tends to be less conscious than in men until it is awakened. Masturbation produces no ill effects physically and the only harm that can follow to the mind is when feelings of guilt are attached to the act. It is abnormal if carried out to excess, when it indicates severe anxiety rather than immoderate sexuality; if it is practised in preference to normal sexual relations, it indicates that there is something seriously wrong with the individual's personal relationships.

Maxilla: the bone of the upper jaw, which also takes part in the formation of the orbit or eye-socket, the nose and the hard palate. It contains the maxillary antrum or sinus, a hollow cavity which communicates with the nose and is liable to become inflamed in sinusitis.

Measles: an acute virus infection which appears in epidemics, often in the winter and spring. It commonly affects children between the ages of three and six; up to a year old, children are protected by the antibodies passed to them by their mother. The infecting organism is a paramyxovirus, which is spread in droplets by coughing or sneezing. The incubation period is from 10 to 12 days, and then the patient develops a fever, a cough and a runny nose, and shows Koplik's spots inside the mouth – small bright red spots with a white centre. The eyes may be red. About two weeks after infection the rash appears on the forehead and neck, spreading to cover the trunk and then the limbs. Usually patients recover in about a week. Measles can have unpleasant complications, which include pneumonia, middle ear infection and, rarely, encephalitis. In the developing world these complications are more frequent, and measles can be a dangerous disease. Active immunisation is strongly advised, ideally between 14 and 16 months in the West but earlier in developing countries, where infection tends to affect children in their first year. One attack of measles confers immunity for life.

Meatus: an opening to a natural passage in the body, for example external auditory meatus, the opening to the ear.

Meckel's Diverticulum: a hollow blind appendage sometimes found growing from the small intestine about 50 cm from the ileo-caecal junction. It varies in size, the average length being about 5 cm. It is the remains of a structure in the embryo called the vitello-intestinal duct, which in the early stages of development connects the yolk sac to the midgut. It may be connected to the umbilicus by a fibrous cord. In later life it may be the seat of infection, or ulceration, because in some cases it contains gastric cells. It is possible for the gut to become twisted round a persisting connection to the umbilicus, causing an obstruction. The diverticulum was first described by the German anatomist J.F. Meckel (1781–1833).

Meconium: a dark green semi-fluid material consisting of bile and debris discharged from the infant's bowels at birth or immediately afterwards.

Median Nerve: one of the nerves of the arm. It originates in the brachial plexus of nerves in the root of the neck, runs down the upper arm, passes in front of the elbow, down the forearm and ends in the palm of the hand. It has no branches in the upper arm, but in the forearm it supplies most of the muscles which flex the fingers and wrist, and in the hand the short flexor and opponens muscles of the thumb and the first two lumbrical muscles of the palm. It also supplies the skin over the front of the palm, thumb, index, middle and half the fourth fingers, and the backs of the tips of the thumb and second, third and fourth fingers. It may be injured by compression in the carpal tunnel as it passes over the wrist into the palm, giving rise to the carpal tunnel syndrome (q.v.).

Mediastinum: the space in the chest between the two lungs. It contains the heart and great vessels, the oesophagus, the lower end of the trachea, the thoracic duct, various nerves, the thymus gland and lymph nodes.

Mediterranean Fever: *see* Brucellosis.

Medulla: the inner part of a structure or organ. Also used to mean the marrow of a bone, the spinal cord (medulla spinalis), and that part of the hind-brain continuous with the upper end of the spinal cord, the medulla oblongata.

Megacolon: abnormal enlargement of the colon, which may happen in consequence of prolonged use of certain laxatives such as senna and cascara. It may be congenital: in Hirschsprung's disease (aganglionic megacolon) there are no nerve ganglion cells in the wall of the rectum; the absence of nerve cells may extend upwards into the colon. The affected part of the gut cannot move, and therefore forms an obstruction, above which the colon becomes loaded with faeces and grossly distended. The baby is constipated, its abdomen becomes distended, and it may vomit. The symptoms may take some time to develop, in some cases only becoming apparent after a year or longer. The treatment is surgical removal of the affected part of the bowel, with functional continuity being restored. Harold Hirschsprung was a Danish physician (1830–1916).

Megaloblastic Anaemia: due to deficiency of vitamin B_{12} or folic acid, in this type of anaemia the red cells are immature and larger than normal. *See* Pernicious Anaemia.

Megalomania: delusions of grandeur.

Megrim: another term for headache; migraine.

Meibomian Cyst: a cyst on the inside of the eyelid caused by blockage of the duct from one of the Meibomian glands which normally open at the edge of the eyelid. It is treated by a simple incision made under local anaesthetic. (Heinrich Meibom, German anatomist, 1638–1700)

Meiosis: the type of cell division in which each daughter cell ends up with half the number of chromosomes that were in the original cell. This kind of division occurs in the formation of the sex cells, so that while the cells of the human body each have 46 chromosomes, the spermatozoa and ova have only 23. If this were not so, the new individual formed by the fusion of spermatozoon and ovum would have double the number of normal chromosomes.

Melaena: black motions, caused by altered blood originating from haemorrhage in the stomach or intestines, by iron taken as a medicine, or by some red wines.

Melancholia: a state of mental depression and wretchedness.

Melanin: the dark pigment of the skin, the choroid layer of the eye, and the hair.

Melanoma: a tumour of cells containing melanin. The tumour is malignant, and produces secondary deposits. It occurs most often on the legs in women, and on the neck, head and trunk in men. The darker the skin, the less likely it is to develop a melanoma; the incidence varies according to the amount of ultraviolet light to which the skin is exposed, but it is not more common in outdoor than indoor workers, being related more to sunbathing. Ultraviolet light is not the only factor concerned in the development of the tumour, for it may develop in those who never expose the skin to the sun. Malignant melanomas may arise in previously existing moles, and if one starts to grow, bleed or change in any way, medical advice is necessary.

Melanuria: dark-coloured urine, or urine which turns dark if left standing, found in cases of jaundice, certain melanotic tumours, altered blood from haemorrhage into the urinary tract, and the rare conditions of alcaptonuria and porphyria.

Memory: defects in memory may result from faulty perception during preoccupation with other matters and paying little attention to what is going on or being said; but a deficient memory may be an early sign of cerebral disease such as Alzheimer's disease (q.v.). *Also see* Amnesia, Korsakoff's Syndrome.

Menarche: the first appearance of the menstrual periods.

Mendelism: *see* Heredity.

Ménière's Disease: a disorder of the inner ear, causing recurrent acute vertigo, deafness and tinnitus. As time goes by, the deafness becomes worse but the attacks of giddiness improve. The noises in the ear are usually present all the time, but are worse during the attacks of giddiness, which are bad enough to make the patient vomit and collapse. Attacks last about a day, but are liable to come in groups, with intervals of a few weeks or months. Those affected are usually 40 or 50 years old. The cause is thought to be excessive fluid in the inner ear; various drugs have been used, among them hyoscine, beta-histine and cinnarizine. Prochlorperazine is useful in treating the vomiting. Surgical decompression of the fluid in the inner ear has been carried out, with varying results. *See* Ear. (Prosper Ménière, 1799–1862)

Meninges: the membranes surrounding the brain and spinal cord. The outer membrane, the dura mater, is a firm fibrous sheet adherent to the inner periosteal membrane of the skull, which splits to enclose various large blood spaces into which flow the cerebral veins. These blood spaces are called the intracranial venous sinuses, and they cannot either collapse or dilate. The dura also forms three large folds which project into the cranial cavity; they are called the falx cerebri, the tentorium cerebelli and the falx cerebelli. The falx cerebri separates the two cerebral hemispheres, and the tentorium is a shelf which separates the inside of the skull into two compartments – the upper or supratentorial space, containing the cerebral hemispheres, and the lower or infratentorial space, containing the cerebellum and brain stem. The two spaces are connected by the tentorial notch, which is occupied by the midbrain. The falx cerebelli is a small midline fold beneath the tentorium. The biggest venous sinus, the transverse, runs in the edge of the tentorium where it is attached to the skull, and the other large sinus, the superior sagittal sinus, runs in the attached edge of the falx cerebri. The whole arrangement of the dural folds looks very much like the folds inside a walnut shell. Arteries, notably the middle meningeal, run in the substance of the dura. The membrane is not attached to the vertebra in the spinal column as it is to the skull, and movements of the vertebrae can take place independently of the dura covering the spinal cord. The arachnoid mater lies below the dura, and is separated from it by a potential space, containing in health only a little tissue fluid. Beneath the arachnoid is the pia mater, a soft thin membrane intimately adherent to the surface of the brain. Between the arachnoid and the pia run many thin fibres – from which the arachnoid is named, for the fibres look like a spider's web – and between the two membranes is a space occupied by the cerebrospinal fluid and the arteries and veins running to the brain. Arachnoid granulations or valves project into the venous sinuses through which the cerebrospinal fluid is returned to the bloodstream. Between the pia and arachnoid are a number of collections of cerebrospinal fluid, for the pia dips down into the sulci of the cortex while the arachnoid does not. In some places the spaces are large, and are called cisterns, the largest being at the base of the brain over the medulla oblongata.

Meningioma: a fibrous tumour arising from the meninges; it is not malignant unless it penetrates the skull, when the portion that breaks through may give rise to secondary tumours, but removal may prove difficult and dangerous when the tumour grows about the base of the brain. It produces symptoms according to its position by direct pressure on the brain, and it also competes with the brain for the limited space within the skull, thus producing symptoms of increased intracranial pressure such as severe headache, deterioration of vision, and in extreme cases vomiting and disturbance of consciousness. The treatment is surgical removal; the operation for removal of a meningioma on the upper surface of the brain is one of the most satisfactory in neurosurgery.

Meningitis: inflammation of the meninges. It is possible for the meninges to become infected as a result of injury to the skull, or infection of the middle ear, but in general meningitis is caused by a variety of bacteria, viruses and sometimes fungi. The symptoms of meningitis are in general headache, fever, nausea, vomiting, backache, and dislike of light (photophobia). There is stiffness of the neck, and in children there may be convulsions. There may be a history of respiratory infection. Often the meningeal irritation is due to a virus infection, the commonest being mumps; measles can be responsible, as can a variety of other viruses, including the herpes virus, but they do not usually cause accompanying infection of the brain (encephalitis) and recovery is the rule. Infection due to the poliomyelitis virus is now rarely seen because of the success of the immunisation programme, and mumps and measles will for the same reason become increasingly rare. Bacterial meningitis is usually caused by *Neisseria meningitidis*, *Streptococcus pneumoniae* or *Haemophilus influenzae*. Infection is spread by droplets from the nose and is encouraged by crowded conditions. In meningococcal infections (spotted fever) patients, who are often under five years old, may develop a rash. The diagnosis is confirmed by lumbar puncture, and the drug of choice in cases of infection with *N. meningitidis* and *Str. pneumoniae* is benzylpenicillin; in cases of haemophilus infection it is chloramphenicol, although this drug has to be used with care in infants, for it is dangerous. Since the introduction of antibiotics the mortality of bacterial meningitis has decreased from about 75% to less than 5%. Vaccines are now available against *N. meningitidis* and *Str. pneumoniae*, and the drug rifampicin can be used prophylactically against infection with meningococci and *H. influenzae*. Tuberculous meningitis has become rare in the West, but is still to be found in developing countries where it is a serious disease. The treatment is by the anti-tubercular drugs isoniazid and rifampicin.

Meniscus: a semicircular or crescentic cartilage in a joint, usually used to refer to the semilunar cartilages in the knee (q.v.). Also the surface of a column of liquid.

Menopause: the capacity for reproduction in women begins to decrease at about the age of 40 to 45, and the periods cease at about 50, either abruptly or more frequently gradually, with increasing intervals between. There is a gradual change in the function of the ovaries, and there is a decrease in the level of oestrogens in the blood. These hormonal disturbances at the cessation of menstruation may cause hot flushes, atrophy of the breasts, possibly atrophy and dryness of the vagina, reduction of the size of the uterus, a tendency to weakness of the muscles of the pelvic floor, and rarefaction of the bones (osteoporosis). Associated with these changes there may be insomnia, depression, lack of concentration and fatigue, although there is no unanimity of opinion on whether such symptoms can truly be attributed to hormonal change; the menopause occurs at a time of life when other changes are common, for children leave home, parents become older and may need more support, friends and relatives are older and more liable to illness. Nevertheless, the physical discomforts can and should be helped by hormone replacement therapy. Oestrogen alone carries a risk of carcinoma of the uterus, which is avoided by giving oestrogen combined with progesterone in cyclical doses. If the patient has had a hysterectomy, the progesterone need not be given. The length of treatment depends on the individual and on the beliefs of the doctor, for views differ, but the dosage can be reduced when the symptoms have been controlled, and then withdrawn altogether.

Menorrhagia: excessive blood loss at the monthly period. It may be due to a number of factors: nervous and emotional causes are not uncommon, or there may be a defect in the clotting mechanism of the blood. It is found in some girls after puberty, but is usually then due to hormonal factors and irregular ovulation. The trouble in most cases rights itself. Hormonal imbalance may be caused by administration of the combined contraceptive pill, or in older women by hormone replacement therapy at the time of the menopause. Bleeding before or after the periods may occur (metrorrhagia) and in general it is true to say that any bleeding which occurs between periods needs investigation. Any bleeding which happens after the menopause is also a sign that investigation is needed.

Menstruation: the monthly loss of blood and mucous membrane occurring throughout the reproductive life of women and females of the higher apes. The lining of the womb, the endometrium, is a soft velvety covering in which the fertilised ovum embeds itself, and it is grown monthly in the expectation of pregnancy. If this does not occur, the endometrium is discharged with a varying amount of blood. This cycle is controlled by hormones secreted by the ovaries, which are in turn controlled by the pituitary gland, which has a connection with the hypothalamus in the brain. The hypothalamus releases a gonadotrophin-releasing hormone (GnRH), which stimulates the release of follicle stimulating hormone (FSH) and luteinising hormone (LH) by the pituitary body. The ovaries secrete oestrogens and progesterone. The cycle begins after menstruation when the endometrium is repaired under the influence of oestrogens, while the follicle in the ovary containing the ovum develops under the influence of FSH. Release of the ovum from the ovary follows a mid-cycle surge of LH, brought about by a feedback effect of oestrogens from the follicle developing under the influence of FSH; there is then secretion of progesterone as well as oestrogen. After a period of quiescence, the endometrium under the influence of LH and progesterone proliferates. If no pregnancy develops, the oestrogen and progesterone levels fall, and the endometrium is discarded. The endometrium is then repaired under the influence of oestrogens, the follicle in the ovary under the influence of FSH again makes ready to shed its ovum, and the cycle repeats. Of the usual 28 days of the cycle about 5 are taken up by premenstrual congestion, 4 by the menstrual flow, 7 by the period of repair and 12 are spent in a state of quiescence. Ovulation occurs about the mid-period, usually in a 28-day cycle on the 14th day before the beginning of the next period.

In such a complicated cycle, there are various things that may interfere and give rise to irregularities; they range from the effects of illness to minor psychological upsets. In the case of the latter, the cycle normally returns in a couple of months. The pursuit of athletics and strenuous exercise may result in irregularity or even in loss of the periods (amenorrhoea) for reasons which are not fully understood, but no lasting harm is done, except that in the long run it is possible that low oestrogen levels may lead to osteoporosis. The periods return to normal if training is less demanding. In general investigation of amenorrhoea in people who are otherwise healthy is called for if the condition lasts for more than a few months; obviously the first test will be for pregnancy. Dysmenorrhoea, or pain at the time of the period, is a condition that may develop in the late teens or early twenties. As it is associated with an increased production of prostaglandin synthetase, NSAIs such as indomethacin or ketoprofen may be useful in treatment; another approach is the use of the contraceptive pill. If no improvement is obtained in about six months, further investigation may be necessary. It usually disappears with the birth of the first child.

A considerable number of women are troubled by symptoms which begin about a week before the period is due, including irritability, depression, headache, a feeling of tension, sometimes accompanied by swelling of the fingers and legs and a feeling that the abdomen is bloated, and perhaps dizziness or palpitations. This has been called premenstrual syndrome, or PMS. It is not fully understood, but fluctuations in hormone levels must be to some extent concerned. Because the condition is not properly understood, treatment is varied and not always successful. However, the first essential is a firm diagnosis that this condition is responsible for the symptoms, a diagnosis that is not always easy to make. Vitamin B_6, piridoxine, may be recommended, or a multi-vitamin preparation, together with dietary advice. Reduction of sugar and salt intake, eating regularly, with plenty of green vegetables, and cutting down the fat intake will help. It is important to keep the weight within bounds, and to avoid excessive smoking, drinking, or consumption of coffee and tea. In many cases these simple measures help a great deal. Thiazide diuretics, or spironolactone, may also be used. It is sensible to relax as much as possible, put off difficult decisions until after the period, get a good night's sleep, and take regular exercise. In cases where simple measures do not help, other treatments are possible under expert advice. Progestogens have been used, but results have been conflicting.

Mental Defect: terms formerly used to categorise mental deficiency such as idiocy, imbecility and feeble-mindedness are now obsolete, and cases are referred to as being mentally retarded or handicapped. The laws which relate to such cases and to mentally disordered people were consolidated by the Mental Health Act of 1983. Mental retardation, or subnormality, is a state of arrested or incomplete mental development, and it means that the subject needs special training and care; severely subnormal people are unable to take care of themselves and are not capable of independent life. Children are classified as educationally subnormal (ESN) to a moderate or severe degree, or profoundly retarded when the Intelligence Quotient is below 30. There is usually an identifiable disease in severely subnormal children, the most common being Down's syndrome (trisomy 21). Others include congenital infection with rubella, cytomegalovirus, or toxoplasma. Alcoholism during pregnancy may lead to the child being mentally subnormal.

Mental Illness: mental illnesses are not illnesses in the usually accepted sense of the word, being forms of social maladaptation predisposed to in a greater or lesser degree by heredity, and influenced by such factors as upbringing and religious belief. Insanity is in many ways a legal rather than medical concept, and in many ways a social and cultural concept; nevertheless, there is always something that is inconsistent about psychotic or insane beliefs. Mental disorders may be separated into various groups, but they tend to run into each other. The neuroses include anxiety, hysteria, phobias, hypochondria and obsessions. The affective disorders include depression and mania, and manic-depressive conditions where the mood changes. Schizophrenia may be acute or chronic; there are many symptoms. The patient suffers from delusions, often of persecution, hallucinations of hearing, abnormal emotional responses, and disordered thought. The behaviour is strange, withdrawn or intrusive and possibly violent. The chronic schizophrenic is likely to be withdrawn, perhaps listening to the voices, and depressed. Memory and consciousness are unaltered. In paranoia, there are hallucinations and delusions, often, but not necessarily, of persecution. The state may be acute, when recovery is the rule, or chronic, when the delusions may lead to violent behaviour. Great advances have been made in the treatment of mental illnesses, which have led to active and optimistic attitudes with patients no longer cooped up in asylums but encouraged to live in the community, and as far as possible to live a normal life. Admissions to psychiatric wards and hospitals are if possible made informally; if this is not possible, the patient's civil rights are most carefully safeguarded. In England and Wales, the Mental Health Act of 1983 allows compulsory emergency admission at the request of the nearest relative or an approved social worker who has seen the patient in the last 24 hours, with a medical recommendation by a doctor who knows the patient, or one (usually a psychiatrist) who is recognised for this purpose, or failing that by any other medical practitioner. A compulsory admission order lasts for 72 hours; the patient must be admitted within 24 hours. In Scotland and Northern Ireland the details differ a little. In England and Wales detention for assessment (28 days) and treatment (six months renewable for six months and then yearly) on the grounds of mental disorder of a degree to warrant compulsion in the interest of the patient's health or to protect other people can be undertaken on application from the nearest relative and an approved social worker, with two independent medical recommendations; discharge can be ordered by the doctor in charge, the hospital managers or the nearest relative, but the latter can be over-ruled if the patient is declared by the doctor to be dangerous. Appeal is to the Mental Health Review Tribunal. In Scotland, long-term detention requires the approval of the Sheriff, and appeal is to him.

Menthol: an alcohol derived from peppermint oil, or made synthetically. It is mildly antiseptic, and has a slight effect as a local anaesthetic. It is customarily used in inhalations, often with benzoin or eucalyptus, and in various lotions and ointments.

Meprobamate: a tranquilliser used in the short-term treatment of anxiety; it is not as effective as the benzodiazepines, and is more likely to produce unwanted effects and dependence.

Mercaptopurine: a drug that prevents the division of cells, used in the treatment of leukaemia.

Mercury: once used in medicine, but now abandoned because of its toxic properties. Metallic mercury is not absorbed, but mercury vapour can be inhaled, and because of the high vapour pressure at room temperature metallic mercury must be handled with care. Mercury salts are poisonous, and if swallowed produce severe inflammation of the stomach and intestines, with vomiting and diarrhoea, abdominal pain and collapse, followed by kidney damage and perhaps failure. The treatment of acute poisoning is the administration of dimercaprol, which may have to be followed by renal dialysis. Chronic poisoning may occur in industry among people handling inorganic and organic mercury salts, and shows itself by insomnia, loss of appetite, and disturbances of behaviour. Mercuric nitrate was once used in making felt, and hat-makers would inhale the vapour from hot felt; hence the expression 'mad as a hatter'. Other manifestations are inflammation of the gums, shaky hands and eventual kidney damage. Dimercaprol or an analogue, DMPS, is used in treatment, possibly with penicillamine, as in the treatment of poisoning with other heavy metals.

Merozoite: *see* Malaria.

Mescaline: an alkaloid present in the cactus *Lophophora williamsii*; it is a psychomimetic drug which produces various symptoms of madness in those who take it. The perceptions are changed so that the drugged subject suffers from hallucinations, illusions and changes of time sense, feelings of unspecified anxiety and perhaps persecution. The drugs mescal and peyotl were used in religious ceremonies among the Mexican Indians, in which, it was said, communal hallucinations occurred, and mescaline has been used like LSD (q.v.) to 'enlarge the bounds of experience' – at least, that is the excuse given for taking psychomimetic drugs and inducing temporary madness.

Mesencephalon: the midbrain.

Mesentery: a double layer of peritoneum which attaches the intestine to the posterior abdominal wall, and carries the blood vessels, lymphatic vessels and nerves that supply the gut.

Mesmerism: hypnosis, named after Anton Mesmer (1734–1815), who practised hypnotism and invented the concept of animal magnetism. *See* Hypnosis.

Mesoderm: the middle of the three primary germinal cells in the embryo, from which are derived the bones, muscles, blood, blood vessels, kidneys, gonads and connective tissues.

Mesomorph: a type of bodily build in which there is a preponderance of tissues derived from mesoderm, i.e. muscle and bone. *See also* Ectomorph, Endomorph.

Mesothelioma: a malignant tumour of the mesothelium of the pleura, pericardium or peritoneum. In the case of the pleura the tumour is in the majority of cases caused by inhaling asbestos fibres.

Metabolism: the total sum of all the chemical processes by which the substance of the body is produced and maintained (anabolism); the production of energy in the body (catabolism). The basal metabolic rate is the minimum energy taken up by the body for the vital processes, measured by the oxygen consumption at rest.

Metacarpals: the five bones of the hand which articulate with the bones of the wrist and the phalanges, the bones of the fingers and thumb. The heads of the metacarpals form the knuckles of the clenched fist.

Metastasis: a cancerous or malignant growth spreads both by direct extension and by the separation of cells which make their way through the lymphatic vessels or blood vessels to other parts of the body, where they grow and form secondary tumours. The process is called metastasis, and the new tumours secondaries or metastases.

Metatarsals: the five bones of the foot which run between the ankle and the toes.

Metatarsalgia: pain in the region of the metatarsal bones, sometimes caused by flat feet or by arthritis. It is often due to excessive weight falling on the heads of the second, third and fourth metatarsal bones, and can be helped by pads placed behind the heads of these bones.

Meteorism: excessive gas in the intestines.

Methadone: an opioid analgesic drug used in the treatment of addiction to morphine and heroin, for which it can be substituted and gradually withdrawn. It is itself a drug of addiction, but in small amounts may be used in cough mixtures.

Methanol: methyl alcohol, used as a solvent in industry. It has an intoxicating action, but is much more poisonous than ethyl alcohol, and has an action on the optic nerve which produces blindness. A fatal dose of methanol may be as little as 30 ml, and blindness may follow a dose of 10 ml. Methyl alcohol may contaminate improperly distilled alcoholic drinks. Methylated spirits is a mixture of 5% methanol and 95% ethyl alcohol. First aid treatment for methanol poisoning is a stomach wash-out; further treatment is carried out in hospital, but no treatment for the blindness is known.

Methicillin: a penicillin which is active against penicillin-resistant *Staphylococcus aureus*; it can only be given by injection, and is not often used.

Methotrexate: a drug which prevents the normal division of cells, used in the treatment of lymphatic leukaemia and a number of solid tumours. It is also used in the treatment of severe arthritic psoriasis, and is an immunosuppressive agent.

Methylene Blue: a blue dye used in staining material for microscopy. It is also used intravenously in the treatment of acute toxic methaemoglobinaemia, a condition in which the iron in haemoglobin is changed by one of a number of substances into the ferric form, when haemoglobin is no longer capable of giving up its oxygen to the tissues. Such substances are chlorates, nitrites, and others including the drugs phenacetin and the sulphonamides. There is a rare form of methaemoglobinaemia which is hereditary.

Methysergide: a drug sometimes used in the treatment of migraine. It may have the dangerous unwanted effect of inducing fibrosis of the heart valves, pleural membranes and the tissues that lie behind the peritoneum in the abdominal cavity.

Metritis: inflammation of the womb.

Metropathia Haemorrhagica: a condition in which there is thickening of the lining of the uterus and irregular bleeding. The bleeding may be heavy and painless, and preceded by missed periods. It is caused by prolonged unopposed action of oestrogens, for the ovary does not shed an ovum and no progesterone is secreted. The diagnosis is made by microscopic examination of the material obtained from curettage; the treatment is the administration of progesterone, or in cases over the age of 40 removal of the uterus may be considered.

Metrorrhagia: bleeding from the uterus occurring outside the normal period. *See* Menorrhagia.

Microbe: a micro-organism, especially one capable of causing disease.

Microbiology: the study of micro-organisms; often used as a synonym for bacteriology.

Micturition: the act of passing urine.

Middle Ear: that part of the ear which separates the ear-drum from the inner ear; it contains the ossicles, three small bones which transmit sound vibrations from the ear-drum to the nerve mechanisms of the inner ear. Because it has a communication to the nose through the auditory tube, it is liable to become infected. *See* Ear.

Migraine: a severe headache, often confined to one side, which recurs at intervals; it may run in families. Some patients experience attacks before the age of 10, and in most cases the first attack occurs before the age of 30. Attacks, which in many cases are preceded by an aura, usually of flashing lights before the eyes or zig-zag figures, recur several times a year in most cases, although the frequency varies. There may be premonitory pins and needles in the hands and arms, or tingling round the mouth. The headache follows the aura, and the patient may vomit. Often felt only on one side, the pain may spread, and is made worse by noise, light, and any kind of exercise; it builds to a climax in a few hours, and may last for a day. In a severe attack the patient has to go to bed and sleep. Aspirin or paracetamol may help, and are best taken in dispersible form in water. Ergotamine is often prescribed, and may be taken as a suppository or can be breathed in from an inhaler. However it is taken, the prescribed dose of ergotamine should not be exceeded, and treatment should not be repeated within four days. The vomiting may be eased by metoclopramide taken at the beginning of an attack. A number of drugs have been recommended for use in preventing attacks, among them pizotifen, beta-blockers such as propranolol, and the antidepressive amitriptyline. The calcium channel-blocker nifedipine may also be used. Methysergide (q.v.) is sometimes used, but has dangerous unwanted effects. The diet should be considered, for alcohol, chocolate, cheese, and other kinds of food may be found to be precipitating factors; fatigue, lack of sleep, and anxiety can cause an attack. Women may find attacks worse before or during menstruation. The basis for the disease is thought to be in the cerebral circulation, with spasm and following dilatation of the arteries, but it is imperfectly understood.

Miliary: like a millet seed; used of multiple small lesions, for example those that can occur in the lungs in widespread tuberculosis.

Millions Fish: *Lebistes reticulatus*, which have been cultivated in some parts of the world to live in areas of standing water, where they eat mosquito larvae and so help in the control of malaria.

Miosis: the contraction of the pupil of the eye. Miotics are drugs which cause contraction of the pupil.

Miscarriage: the expulsion of the foetus before it is capable of sustaining independent life, which is taken to be about the 28th week. Later expulsion is described as premature labour. A considerable number of pregnancies end in a miscarriage, usually before the fourth month. The miscarriage may threaten; there is painless bleeding. The patient should go to bed and rest, and if the miscarriage proceeds, bleeding becomes more profuse and is accompanied by pain in the lower abdomen and back as the products of conception are expelled. In most cases development of the foetus has been abnormal, and has arrested at an early stage. The only dangers are haemorrhage and infection. If the miscarriage has been incomplete, and matter has been retained, bleeding will continue; admission to hospital is needed, so that the uterus can be cleared by a simple operation. Infection is only likely if the miscarriage has been self-induced, or induced by an unqualified person, and it requires hospital treatment. A miscarriage does not mean that subsequent pregnancies will be unsuccessful.

Mites: minute parasites of the order *Acarina* that live on the skin. The mite that makes its presence most felt is the *Sarcoptes scabei*, the scabies or itch mite. The female burrows into the skin, both clean and dirty, and lays eggs;

the burrows and vesicles caused are found on the webs between the fingers, the wrists, elbows, armpits, round the line of the belt and by the umbilicus, the penis and scrotum, and the buttocks and thighs. The vesicles may become infected by scratching, for the mites set up a severe itching, a reaction to their saliva and droppings. They are spread by direct contact, and may therefore spread in the family, in schools and institutions, and in the armed forces. Personal hygiene is not a factor. Infection has occurred in pandemics in 30-year cycles, but the mite may appear at any time and has a worldwide distribution. Treatment is the application to the whole body of lotions of benzyl benzoate or lindane, which is more suitable for children. Monosulfiram is also used, but has the disadvantage that it may react with ingested alcohol to produce an effect like disulfiram (q.v.), so that it is probably better reserved for children. Crotamiton cream or lotion is also effective. Other mites are the follicle mite, *Demodex folliculorum*, which lives in association with hair follicles, and *D. brevis*, which lives in the sebaceous glands; they are found around the nose and the eyebrows, but do not appear to be responsible for any disease. There are mites which live in sugar, flour, straw and grain, which may infest people who handle these substances in quantities causing such conditions as miller's itch or grocer's itch. Scrub mites or jiggers can infest people and spread the disease scrub typhus. House mites may play a part in the precipitation of attacks of asthma or eczema.

Mithridatism: King Mithridates of Bythinia (120–63 BC) tried to acquire an immunity to poisons by habitually eating small quantities of them, starting with minute doses which he gradually increased. Such a process has been named after him.

Mitochondria: found in the cytoplasm of cells, mitochondria are separate bodies shaped like threads or granules; there are thousands of them in each cell, and they are in constant motion. They contain enzymes and are responsible for the metabolism of the cell and the release of energy. They also contain ribonucleic and deoxyribonucleic acid and can reduplicate their own proteins.

Mitosis: the process by which the cell divides in such a way as to produce two daughter cells each with the same number of chromosomes as the original cell. *Cf.* Meiosis.

Mitral Stenosis: narrowing of the mitral valve of the heart. *See* Heart.

Mixture: a combination of two or more different drugs put up usually in water. The modern tendency in prescribing is to use one specific drug in the form of a tablet or capsule, but there are many conditions in which the precise diagnosis proves elusive where mixtures of various colours have been found very useful.

MMR Vaccine: a combined vaccine against measles, mumps and rubella, to be given to children between the ages of one and two; if this opportunity is missed, it should be given before starting primary school. There may be a slight reaction about a week after vaccination, when the temperature is elevated, the child feels unwell, and there is a slight rash; occasionally after three weeks there may be slight swelling of the parotid glands, as in mumps. These reactions are not harmful, nor is the child infectious.

Molar: a solution containing in a litre the amount of a substance in grams equal to its molecular weight. Also the three back teeth.

Mole (abbrev., mol): the amount in grams of a substance equal to its molecular weight. Also a pigmented spot on the skin, usually raised and sometimes hairy. Moles should not be interfered with except by a surgeon; if they appear to change size, or bleed, the advice of a doctor should be sought.

Molluscum Contagiosum: a skin condition usually seen in children; it is caused by a poxvirus. There are small, round, nodular white swellings about the size of a split pea, which may occur on the arms and legs, the buttocks and abdomen, and sometimes on the face. They have a little dent on top, and contain a soft creamy material;

they are painless and harmless, but may be disfiguring. The infection is spread by contact, and may be picked up in such places as schools and swimming baths. The swellings may be scraped off painlessly with a curette, removed by squeezing out the contents and coagulating with silver nitrate, or abolished by the application of 12% salicylic acid in collodion.

Molluscum Fibrosum: *see* Neurofibromatosis.

Mongolism: *see* Down's Syndrome.

Monilia: the former name for a fungus now called *Candida*. *See* Candidiasis.

Monoamine Oxidase Inhibitors: *see* MAOIs.

Monocyte: the largest of the white cells in the blood, and normally the least common. Formed in the bone marrow, monocytes circulate in the blood until they migrate into the tissues, where they become macrophages with the function of ingesting particles of matter such as bacteria and broken-down red blood cells. They also play a part in the immune system.

Mononucleosis: an increase in the number of mono-nuclear cells, that is cells with one nucleus, in the blood. *See* Infectious Mononucleosis.

Morbid Anatomy: the anatomy of disease processes, a branch of pathology.

Morbidity: the sickness rate, the ratio of sick to well people in the community.

Morning Sickness: nausea and vomiting experienced by normally healthy women in the first months of pregnancy. Of uncertain origin, it may be exacerbated by psycho-logical factors and present difficulty in treatment, for it is unwise to give any drugs in pregnancy unless the risk of not giving them is greater than the risk to the foetus. Consequently the treatment of morning sickness must be reassurance and the obvious advice to avoid fried food; fruit juice and a carbohydrate diet is best. Occasionally morning sickness is so bad that the patient is best admitted to hospital, when the condition often resolves without treatment other than attention to dehydration and electrolyte balance.

Moron: an out-of-date term for a category of mentally subnormal people with a mental age between seven and nine.

Morphine: a powerful narcotic analgesic drug derived from opium. Its actions are to calm those in severe pain and diminish the pain felt, to diminish anxiety and induce sleep. It also depresses the respiratory centre and the cough centre in the brain, and may produce nausea and vomiting. It is constipating, and may cause retention of urine; it contracts the pupil of the eye. Morphine may be injected or taken by mouth. Being a drug of addiction, it must be used with caution; nevertheless it has a unique place in the relief of pain, and the possibility of addiction is immaterial when it is used in a terminal illness.

Mortality: the ratio of deaths to the number of the population in a year, often expressed as deaths per thousand of the population. The mortality rate of a disease is the ratio of deaths from the disease to the total number of cases.

Mosquito: an insect of the order *Diptera*, the family *Culicidae*. They have larvae which develop in water. The medically important genera are *Anopheles*, *Culex* and *Aëdes*. The first transmits malaria and filariasis; the second, filariasis and virus infections; the third, the virus infections yellow fever, filariasis, dengue fever and types of encephalitis caused by arboviruses.

Motion Sickness: nausea and vomiting caused mainly by the effect on the inner ear of angular and linear accelerations and decelerations set up by the motion of the ship, aircraft or car in which the victim is travelling. The eyes also play an important part, and in a car it helps to keep the eyes focused on distant objects rather than those passing nearby, or to keep the eyes closed and the head still. A number of drugs have been used to ward off the malady, one of the most effective being hyoscine in an (adult) dose of 300 μg thirty minutes before travelling. It should be noted that hyoscine may cause sleepiness and potentiate the effects of alcohol, as well as impairing driving skill. A drug which has less marked unwanted effects is cinnarizine, an antihistamine; other antihistamine drugs have been used, but they tend to produce drowsiness.

Motor Neurone Disease: amyotrophic lateral sclerosis, a progressive form of paralysis that affects patients above the age of 50, more often men than women, with cases more numerous at 70 and then decreasing. The cause is not known; there is degeneration of the anterior horn cells of the motor nerves. The hand is often first affected, and becomes weak and clumsy. There may be painful cramp in the arms, and the muscles show fasciculation, a quivering of groups of muscle fibres. The disease may affect the muscles supplied by the cranial nerves (q.v.) so that swallowing becomes difficult, and speech is disturbed. Increasing weakness of the limbs follows, and breathing may become difficult. Control of the sphincters is not affected. The disease runs its course in under five years, and there is no effective treatment.

Motor System: that part of the nervous system that is concerned with movement, as opposed to the sensory system which is concerned with sensation.

Mould: caused by the growth of various fungi, of which some common ones are *Aspergillus*, *Rhizopus*, *Penicillium*, and *Mucor*. The fungi grow as filaments on grain and various foods, and form spores. Some are very useful, for various antibiotic drugs are made from them; some are a nuisance, for they grow where they are not wanted; and some can produce disease, such as farmer's lung, by setting up reactions in the lungs when they are breathed in. A very few are poisonous when eaten.

Moulding: a term used in obstetrics to describe the adaptation of the baby's head to the confines of the birth canal.

Moxibustion: the burning of a little bundle of soft inflammable material on the skin in order to provide counter-irritation.

Mucous Membranes: membranes which secrete mucus, and form the internal lining of the body; they are composed of various sorts of epithelial cells according to the different functions they have to carry out. *See* Epithelium.

Mucus: the slimy secretion of the epithelial goblet cells.

Multipara: a woman who has had two or more pregnancies resulting in the birth of viable children.

Multiple Sclerosis (disseminated sclerosis): a disease of the central nervous system in which there is a loss of the myelin sheath which normally surrounds the nerve fibres, with loss of function and consequent scarring. The cause is still unknown, but suggestions include auto-immune disease and infection from an undiscovered virus. A disorder of fat metabolism has also been suggested, for the myelin sheath contains fatty substances. The disease attacks people in their youth, often in their twenties or early thirties, very rarely after fifty; it is found only in temperate climates. The areas in the nervous system of demyelination, loss of the myelin sheaths, are called plaques, and they range in size from a few millimetres to patches a centimetre or so across. As the name disseminated sclerosis suggests, they are found anywhere in the central nervous system, often in the optic nerves, the upper spinal cord and the brain stem. In the optic nerves the plaques produce interference with vision, and the head of the optic nerve, which can be seen with the ophthalmoscope, becomes pale. This may be the first sign of the disease; the vision commonly improves, and for a long time nothing further may be found. The disease is disseminated, or scattered, in time as well as space, and characteristically develops in a series of disabling episodes punctuated by remissions during which the disability may improve. There is commonly tingling in the feet, spreading to the waist, double vision, and weakness of one or both legs. There may be giddiness, disturbance of control of the bladder, loss of position sense in the arms, and unsteadiness. In a minority of cases the disease progresses without remissions. The course of the disease is in most cases uncertain, and may take many years, but in the end the symptoms are less relieved by remissions and the patient cannot walk properly, the arms are clumsy and there may be difficulty in the control of the bladder and bowels. Because the cause of the disease is unknown, specific treatment is not possible. This does not mean to say that nothing can be done. The patients can be helped a great deal both by the doctor and the family to continue to do what they can as long as it is humanly possible for them to carry on, and must be given every encouragement to keep going. Physiotherapy can be very useful in keeping walking possible. A number of drugs and other treatments have been tried, and apart from the use of steroids in an acute attack none have been shown to be of definite value. A diet low in animal fat and high in polyunsaturated fat may, in early cases, make relapses less severe. Judgement of the effects of treatment is made doubly difficult by the nature of the disease, with its natural remissions which can be attributed mistakenly to successful therapy. There is no specific test for the disease.

Mumps: also called epidemic parotitis, mumps is an infection with a paramyxovirus mainly affecting children. The parotid glands, which lie in front of and below the ear and cover the angle of the jaw, swell painfully and the patient runs a temperature; one of the signs that make the diagnosis certain is that the lobe of the ear is lifted up. The swelling lasts for about a week. The incubation period is between 14 and 18 days, and the patient with mumps carries the virus in the saliva for about 10 days. The infection is spread by droplets in the breath. Although the obvious sign of mumps is the swelling of the parotid glands, the virus is present in the saliva a few days before this happens, having spread throughout the body in the bloodstream before it settles in the glands. It may also settle in the testes, often only on one side; this is uncommon in boys before puberty, but if it should happen in adolescents or adults it does not damage the testes to such an extent that they become sterile, except in very uncommon cases. Mumps may cause meningitis, which is usually mild and recovers completely, or rarely encephalitis in which case the patient may become confused or even comatose. Very little is required in the way of treatment, for in most cases the illness recovers completely in about a week; if the testicles should be affected it may be necessary to give strong painkillers for a day or two. A vaccine is available, which should be given to children between the ages of one and two (*see* MMR vaccine).

Murmur: a noise heard through a stethoscope placed over the heart, in addition to the normal heart sounds. Murmurs are made by vibrations set up by the action of the heart and by the turbulence of the blood passing through the chambers and valves of the heart. They are of varying significance; their presence does not necessarily mean that the heart is diseased.

Muscle: there are three types of muscle in the human body differing both in structure and function. They are striped or striate, smooth or involuntary, and heart muscle which is in a category of its own. Striped muscle is the type found in the ordinary muscles of the body, over which there is voluntary control. Smooth muscle is found in the intestines, the bladder and the blood vessels, and is under the control of the autonomic nervous system. Striped muscle is composed of a large number of cells held together by loose connective tissue, which is condensed on the outside of the muscle to form a sheath. The muscle cells are very long, perhaps up to 10 cm, and have thousands of nuclei; each receives at its centre a fibre from a motor nerve at a neuro-muscular end plate. The outer membrane of the cell is called the sarcolemma, and the cytoplasm within the cell is the sarcoplasm, which contains long filaments of protein called myofilaments. The myofilaments have three types of protein: tropomyosins, which act as support, and those concerned in contraction, actin and myosin. Actin and myosin protein molecules aggregate to form filaments, and lying in parallel the heads of the myosin molecules are attracted to the actin molecules to produce contraction. The two types of filaments are held together in a regular pattern, which results in cross-striations appearing when the muscle fibres are examined through a light microscope. The filaments are arranged together to form a sarcomere, a unit able to contract more than 50% of its length. There are two types of muscle fibres: the first is concerned with posture, and reacts more slowly than the second type which has a fast reaction to stimulation. In smooth muscle, the filaments are not held together in a regular pattern, the cells are short, and there is no striation under the microscope. The filaments can slide past each other; smooth muscle contracts slowly, but can remain contracted for a long time. It has the property of responding to stretching by contraction. Cardiac muscle cells are much shorter than the cells of striated muscle, and they stick to each other. Striations appear under the microscope. These cells each have their own rhythm of contraction, and as they are joined together the wave of contraction spreads through them all, taking its timing from the cells with the fastest rhythm, which are in the sinu-atrial node (see Heart). If these cells should prove ineffective the remaining cells are capable of maintaining the heartbeat at a slower pace.

Contraction of voluntary and smooth muscle is stimulated by the release of acetylcholine at the nerve endings in the neuro-muscular end plates, accompanied by a change of electrical potential. The biochemical reactions that accompany contraction are very complicated, but basically creatine phosphate is changed to creatine and phosphate in the presence of calcium, and adenosine diphosphate is formed from adenosine triphosphate. The breakdown of the phosphate bonds releases energy.

Each end of a voluntary muscle is attached to a bone, and contraction draws the two ends together, thus producing flexion (bending) or extension (straightening) of a joint. The muscle has to shorten to about 40% of its extended length to produce full movement at the joint over which it acts. The attachment of a muscle to a less movable bone is called its origin, the attachment to the more mobile bone the insertion. Thus the calf muscles originate from the bones of the leg and are inserted into the heel. Sensation is relayed from the muscles to the nervous system by muscle spindles, sensory organs which are arranged in parallel with the muscle fibres. They are present in large numbers in striated muscle, and provide information about the state of contraction of the muscles, and hence the posture of the body. They are the sensory side of the reflex arc that produces a jerk in the muscle when it is suddenly stretched. Pressure and stretching in excess produce pain in muscles, as does accumulation of the waste products of metabolism in deficiency of blood circulation, but cutting does not.

Muscle Relaxants: a number of drugs act upon the neuro-muscular end plates (*see* Muscle *above*) to prevent muscles contracting, and so provide relaxation for surgical operations. The majority act by competing for acetyl-choline at the receptors in the end plates, and are known as non-depolarising relaxants. They have their origin in curare, an extract of plants employed by South American Indians on their arrow-tips to paralyse their prey. When used in conjunction with general anaesthetics the drugs relax the vocal cords, and enable tubes to be passed into the trachea; they relax the muscles of the diaphragm and abdominal wall, but as the muscles of respiration are also paralysed the patient's breathing must be assisted by a breathing machine. The amount of general anaesthetic that is required is reduced. The other muscle relaxants are called depolarising agents, and block the neuro-muscular end plates. The drug commonly used in this group is suxamethonium, which has a short action of about five minutes, as opposed to the non-depolarising agents whose action lasts up to half an hour, and it may be used to pass an endotracheal tube. The anti-cholinesterase drug neostigmine is used to counteract the effects of the non-depolarising agents, but has no effect on depolarising drugs.

Mustard Gas: sulphur mustard was used as an agent of chemical warfare in the First World War. It produces nausea and vomiting, inflammation and blistering of the skin, and inflammation of the lungs, and has been found to be a cause of cancer of the lung.

425

Mutation: chromosomes, which are responsible for the passing on of inherited characteristics, are made mostly of the substance deoxyribonucleic acid (DNA). An alteration of the DNA at a particular place in the chromosome (the gene) will result in a change of inherited characteristics so that the offspring differs from its parents in some particular. The change in the DNA is called a mutation; mutations can occur in nature, or can be brought about by such external agents as ionising radiation or the administration of nitrogen mustard; most are not an advantage to the offspring, and some indeed are lethal, but a very few strengthen the offspring in some way and so become established in time by the process of natural selection.

Mutism: dumbness, occurring naturally or wilfully.

Myalgia: pain in the muscles.

Myasthenia Gravis: a rare condition in which the muscles become quickly fatigued. It occurs in women more than men, usually in young adults, and it may be associated with thyrotoxicosis (q.v.). It has been found to be an auto-immune disease, for patients show an antibody to the receptor of acetylcholine in the muscles. The antibody is produced by T lymphocytes (*see* Lymphocyte) which originate in the thymus gland. Weakness develops in the ocular muscles, giving rise to double vision and drooping of the eyelids, worse when the patient is tired. There may then be weakness in the muscles of the throat, resulting in difficulty in swallowing and speaking, and the muscles of the neck weaken, allowing the head to hang forwards; the muscles about the shoulder may become affected, so that it is difficult to raise the arms. In severe cases the weakness spreads to include the limbs and the muscles of respiration. The diagnosis is confirmed by the use of the drug edrophonium which has an anti-cholinesterase action, and therefore helps the action of acetylcholine at the neuro-muscular end plates (*see* Acetylcholine, Muscle) and by immunological studies. Treatment has been by the drugs neostigmine or pyridostigmine, both anti-cholinesterase drugs with a longer action than edrophonium, but it is also possible to use corticosteroids with the immunosuppressive drug azothiaprine. The removal of the thymus gland has for at least 40 years been known to improve the condition, and the operation may be performed on suitable patients.

Mycobacteria: thin, slightly curved, rod-shaped bacteria, two kinds of which cause tuberculosis and leprosy.

Mycotic Disease: disease caused by a fungus, e.g. ringworm.

Mydriatics: drugs which cause dilatation of the pupil of the eye, such as atropine or hyoscine.

Myelin: a fatty substance which forms the sheath round nerve fibres, or axons, with a diameter greater than 2 μm, to insulate them from the surrounding tissues. Smaller unmyelinated nerve fibres conduct impulses more slowly. Myelinated fibres form the greater part of the white matter of the brain and spinal cord, and of the peripheral nerves.

Myelitis: inflammation of the spinal cord, or inflammation of the bone marrow.

Myelocele: the spinal cord may protrude or herniate through a congenital defect in the bones of the spinal column, called spina bifida, to form a swelling known as a myelocele. The condition may be associated with hydrocephalus.

Myelography: the X-ray examination of the spinal cord after a radio-opaque liquid heavier than the cerebrospinal fluid has been introduced into the subarachnoid space by lumbar puncture. If there is a block to the passage of the liquid, or any swelling of the spinal cord or surrounding structures, it will be seen as the position of the patient is altered to allow the liquid to run up or down.

Myeloid Leukaemia: *see* Leukaemia.

Myeloma: a tumour of the bone marrow. The tumour erodes bone, and produces pain in the back and ribs.

There are usually multiple tumours, and they are liable to form in the ribs, skull, pelvis and vertebrae – the bones containing active blood-forming marrow. The areas of erosion are seen on X-rays, and classically the Bence–Jones protein is found in the urine, which when the urine is heated precipitates at 50–60°C, dissolves as the urine comes to the boil, and precipitates again as it cools. The treatment of a solitary tumour is radiotherapy; multiple tumours are treated by cytotoxic drugs, perhaps reinforced by radiotherapy, which relieves bone pain. Whole body radiation has been used for multiple tumours instead of cytotoxic drugs.

Myiasis: infestation by maggots. The ox suffers from warble-fly maggots, and the horse from bot-fly, but man is only infested by fly larvae by accident. The commonest conditions for producing infestation by maggots are found in the tropics, although in any climate open wounds and discharges may attract flies to lay their eggs. It is true that infestation of wounds with maggots is not as bad as it might appear, for they scavenge freely and a maggoty wound is a clean wound. In Africa the mango-fly lays its eggs on the ground, and they are sometimes picked up by human beings into whose skin the larvae burrow, and produce painful swellings; in tropical America the 'human' warble-fly attaches its eggs to mosquitoes who pass them on to man. It has been known in this country for warble-flies to lay their eggs on man; the result is a boil on the skin that contains maggots.

Myocardial Infarction: the blockage of a coronary artery supplying blood to the heart muscle and consequent mortification of the area of muscle supplied. It is a common cause of death. Coronary arteries (q.v.) which are affected by atheroma are narrowed, and may suddenly become blocked. The effect is that the patient feels a sudden severe pain in the chest, which may radiate to the throat and jaw, and down the left arm. The pain may be felt in the upper abdomen, and in some cases is mistaken for an acute attack of indigestion. The patient collapses, becomes pale, and in many cases breathless. In a very serious case the pulse may disappear and the patient appear dead, but the ventricular muscle has begun to fibrillate and external cardiac massage and mouth to mouth artificial respiration may keep the patient alive until a defibrillator can be used to restore the normal rhythm. Where the pulse can be felt, but the rhythm is disturbed, intravenous lignocaine may steady the heart. The early injection of streptokinase may help in reducing the extent of the clot in the coronary artery. In less severe cases the immediate aim is to relieve the pain, and if possible intramuscular or intravenous morphine or diamorphine is used. In some places a 50% mixture of nitrous oxide and oxygen (Entonox) may be available and can be used, and in any case if possible oxygen should be given. Usually patients are admitted to hospital, where a special coronary care unit may be found, but in cases of minor severity the patient may be cared for at home. Strict rest in bed for any length of time is now not considered advisable, and patients with no disturbances of heart rhythm or signs of failure may be out of bed in three days or so. Patients admitted to hospital who do not develop signs of failure or disturbances of heart rhythm after twelve hours may be discharged in a week. In severe disease, after one month between 40% and 50% of cases of myocardial infarction have died, and of these many cases die in the first hour or two because of untreated ventricular fibrillation. The disease affects about three times as many men as women, and is more common in the north of the UK than the south; it is, perhaps contrary to popular opinion, more common among unskilled and manual workers than among sedentary workers.

Myocarditis: inflammation of the heart muscle. It may be caused by viruses, for example the influenza virus, or the Epstein–Barr virus of glandular fever; by bacteria, as in diphtheria or scarlet fever, where the haemolytic streptococcus is the infecting organism; or possibly by immunological reactions following infection.

Myoclonus: involuntary contractions of a group of muscles, one muscle or part of a muscle. The contractions may be associated with various diseases of the nervous system, including epilepsy, or may have no obvious cause, as in the facial spasms which may affect middle-aged or elderly women. Starting round the eye, the spasms spread to involve the mouth and then the whole of one side of the face.

Myoma: a tumour, nearly always benign, which grows from muscle fibres. Myomata are common in the uterus, where they contain fibrous as well as muscular tissue and are known as fibroids.

Myopathy: disease of muscle not due to a defect in the nervous system. The myopathies are rare, and are otherwise known as muscular dystrophies. They are hereditary, and a degenerative process wastes the affected muscle groups although the motor nerves are normal.

Myopia: short sight. The length of the eye is such that distant objects come into focus in front of the retina. It is corrected by concave lenses. *See* Eye.

Myositis: inflammation of the muscles. This may be due to virus infection, for example with the influenza virus or the Coxsackie virus of Bornholm disease; bacteria may infect wounds, notably *Clostridium welchii* which causes gas gangrene; or parasites may invade the muscles. The commonest parasite is *Trichinella spiralis*, a nematode worm usually acquired by eating badly cooked pork or horse meat, which makes its way from the intestine into the muscles about a week after infected food has been eaten, causing pain and weakness; complete recovery is the rule. Cysticercosis (q.v.) may follow the consumption of undercooked pork infected by the tapeworm *Taenia solium*. Polymyositis is an auto-immune disease, where lymphocytes become sensitised against muscle tissue, and the resulting inflammation causes pain and weakness; it may be associated with a cancer elsewhere in the body.

Myotonia Congenita: a rare inherited disease in which the patient's muscles do not relax after they have contracted, so that the subject may not be able to let go after shaking hands, or may be burnt because hot objects cannot be put down. It is worse in cold weather, but improved by exercise.

Myringotomy: an incision through the ear-drum, once commonly made for the relief of pus in the middle ear before the advent of antibiotics made such cases rare.

Myxoedema: a condition resulting from deficiency of thyroid hormones, otherwise known as hypothyroidism. It usually affects women in middle age, but may be found in men, and at any time of life from birth onwards. The symptoms are insidious, vague and difficult to identify, but basically the patient is inclined to be slow and easily tired. The skin may be thickened, the hair thin, and the eyelids, wrists and ankles swollen; the patient may complain of constipation, menstrual troubles or aches and pains in the joints. She may be abnormally sensitive to the cold; she may be found to be anaemic. The pulse is slow. On laboratory examination of the blood, the thyroid hormones are found to be low, and the level of the pituitary thyroid stimulating hormone, TSH, high. The cause of hypothyroidism may be the removal of part, or the whole, of the gland surgically, irradiation of the gland with ^{131}I in the treatment of thyrotoxicosis caused by overaction of the gland, or disease of the gland; but the commonest cause is an auto-immune reaction in which antibodies damage the gland and block the production of thyroid hormones. Treatment is replacement of the missing hormone with thyroxine, the dose being regulated by the biochemical changes in the blood. The hormone must be taken for life, and not discontinued as soon as the patient has returned to normal.

N

Naevus: a birthmark composed of blood vessels. *See* Birthmark.

Nails: composed of keratin, like hair, fingernails grow at the rate of one centimetre in three months; toenails take three or more times longer. They can be affected by a number of conditions. Bacterial infection is common; minor cuts and abrasions become contaminated, and collections of pus form in relation to the nail folds and under the nail. The infection is called a paronychia, may be acute or chronic, and is often very painful. If pus has formed, it must be released by incision or removal of part or the whole of the nail; before pus forms it may be possible to abort the infection by the use of antibiotics. Chronic infection is common among people whose work means that their hands are continually damp, and treatment is very difficult unless the hands can be kept dry and clean. The nails can be infected by fungus, more commonly on the toes than the fingers; local applications of antifungal ointment are not satisfactory, and the only treatment is the use of the drug griseofulvin, which has to be taken by mouth for months to be effective. As the infection is usually painless and does no harm, treatment is not in the majority of cases necessary.

Injuries to the nails are common, and often blows or crushing injuries result in the formation of a blood clot under the nail, which can be very painful unless it is released by making a hole in the nail. Often after such an injury the nail eventually comes off, but it will grow again; if the nail bed at the root has been injured, it may grow irregularly and be deformed. Ingrowing nails usually affect the great toe. Because of ill-fitting shoes, or cutting the nail too short, the corners as they grow cut into the flesh of the nail folds and cause pain or even infection. The flesh must be lifted away from the nail, and kept back from its corners until it has grown clear. In severe cases it may be necessary to remove the nail, and let it grow again. Great toe nails should be cut square across, clear of the nail folds, to prevent the condition. Nails have something to tell of a patient's health: in iron deficiency anaemia they may be spoon-shaped and soft, and the colour is pale; in heart or lung disease they may be tinged with blue, and they may be 'clubbed', when the end of the finger is thickened, the angle between the nail and the nail bed is increased, and the nail is more curved than usual; they may be pitted, as in psoriasis, which also produces ridges. Other causes of ridges are infection or serious general illness.

Naloxone: a drug used to counteract the effects of opioid analgesics such as morphine which depress the respiration and produce coma. It is given intravenously or by intra-muscular injection, but must be used cautiously in cases of addiction for it may precipitate a reaction.

Napkin Rash: dermatitis in the area covered by the napkin (nappy) is caused usually by irritation from urine broken down by micro-organisms occurring in the faeces to ammoniacal compounds. The affected area should be covered by a simple zinc cream, and the napkins sterilised by boiling. If possible, nappies should be left off until the rash has gone. A rash may be due to candida infection, which is treated by nystatin cream.

Narcissism: love of self, usually regarded as a normal stage of development which becomes abnormal if carried to excess in later life.

Narcoanalysis: the technique of using a drug such as thiopentone sodium to aid in psychoanalysis by releasing inhibitions.

Narcolepsy: in this condition the subject experiences excessive daytime sleepiness, with an irresistible urge to go to sleep at inappropriate moments. Narcolepsy may appear in adolescents or young adults, and may be accompanied by cataplexy, a short period of temporary paralysis brought on by emotional disturbance. It is one of the few conditions in which amphetamine is useful in treatment.

Narcotics: drugs which produce stupor or unconsciousness (narcosis) by their action on the central nervous system.

Naso-pharynx: that part of the throat which lies behind the nose, above the soft palate.

Naturopathy: a method of healing that uses no drugs but relies on the remedies of nature and a diet of 'natural' food.

Nausea: the unpleasant feeling that precedes vomiting.

Navel: the umbilicus, the scar in the centre of the abdominal wall where the umbilical cord joined the foetus to the placenta in the womb.

Nebuliser: apparatus for administering a drug in the form of a spray or cloud of droplets.

Necator: a genus of nematode parasites. *Necator americanus* is a hookworm found in wet tropical countries in Central America and Africa. *See* Worms.

Neck: that part of the body joining the base of the skull to the upper part of the chest. Its main contents are the throat, the thyroid and parathyroid glands, the larynx (voice-box), the trachea and oesophagus (the tubes for air and food), the blood vessels going to and from the head and brain, the seven cervical vertebrae and their muscles, and the cervical part of the spinal cord. The pharynx, the cavity of the throat, lies in front of the spinal column from the base of the skull to the level of the sixth cervical vertebra, at which point it is continuous with the oesophagus. The larynx opens forwards at the level of the fourth to sixth vertebrae, and is continuous with the trachea which is crossed by the isthmus of the thyroid gland joining the two lobes which lie one on either side. The main muscle of the front of the neck is the sternomastoid, which runs from the mastoid process behind the ear to the upper end of the sternum, the breastbone, and the inner end of the clavicle, the collar-bone. It covers the sheath containing the carotid arteries, the internal jugular vein, the vagus nerve and lymph nodes. The external and anterior jugular veins run superficially. The cervical vertebrae containing the spinal cord and the muscles that support and move the head and neck take up two-thirds of the volume of the neck. The brachial plexus of nerves leaves the lower part of the spinal cord to run out behind the clavicle into the arm, and the phrenic nerve, which comes from the upper part of the cord, runs down into the root of the neck on its way to the diaphragm; the cervical chain of autonomic nervous fibres runs in front of the fascial sheath covering the muscles.

Necropsy: autopsy, or post-mortem examination.

Negativism: in psychiatry, the refusal of a patient to attend to the examiner, or a tendency to do the opposite of what is asked or what normal feelings would indicate.

Neisseria: a genus of micro-organisms including those responsible for gonorrhoea and meningitis. Named after Albert Neisser (1855–1916), the German bacteriologist who discovered the organism of gonorrhoea.

Nematode: a roundworm or threadworm. *See* Worms.

Neomycin: an antibiotic derived from bacteria of the streptomyces group. It is active against Gram-negative organisms, but is too toxic to be given by injection. As it is not absorbed by the gut, it can be used in bowel infections and to sterilise the gut; it can be used superficially for eye and ear infections, and on the skin in powders, ointments and creams. It has, however, a tendency to sensitise the skin.

Neonatal: the term applied to matters arising in the first four weeks after birth.

Neoplasm: new growth or tumour, malignant or benign.

Neostigmine: an anti-cholinesterase drug; as it acts to block the action of the enzyme which destroys cholines-terase, it may be used in myasthenia gravis (q.v.) and to reverse the action of muscle relaxants (q.v.) of the non-depolarising group.

Nephrectomy: the surgical removal of a kidney.

Nephritis: inflammation of the kidney. Used by itself, nephritis is understood to mean glomerulonephritis, a condition which impairs the function of the glomeruli in ridding the blood of waste products (*see* Kidney). The consequences of glomerular damage are: diminution of filtration of the blood, with retention of water and salts; passage of red blood cells in the urine; passage of proteins in the urine; and possibly kidney failure. The patient may feel pain in the loin, suffer from headache and generalised pains in the bones, and develop swelling of the ankles and wrists; there may be a number of other symptoms, including diarrhoea and vomiting. The blood pressure may be raised. The basic damage to the glomeruli in glomerulonephritis is caused by an accumulation of antibody–antigen complexes arising in a number of conditions, for example scarlet fever, a streptococcal throat infection associated with a rash, although this is becoming increasingly rare. The damage to the glomeruli is variable, differing according to the disease setting up the immune reaction; in some cases the nephritis recovers completely, but in others progresses to kidney failure which requires renal dialysis, and possibly renal transplant. *See* Immune System.

Nephrolithiasis: stones in the kidney.

Nephrotic Syndrome: resulting from damage to the glomerular filtering system in the kidney arising from nephritis, there is such a great loss of albumin in the urine that the level of protein in the blood falls, and oedema develops, an accumulation of fluid in the tissues. This may be slight, and confined to the ankles, or may be so pronounced as to be disabling. There may also be a rise of blood pressure. Treatment includes restriction of salt intake and the use of diuretics such as frusemide.

Nephrostomy: the operation of making an artificial opening into the pelvis of the kidney in order to drain it.

Nephrotomy: the operation of cutting into the kidney, for example to remove a stone.

Nerve Gas: organophosphorus compounds inhibit the action of cholinesterase, the enzyme that destroys acetylcholine (q.v.), and thus produce an accumulation of acetylcholine which gives rise to a number of distressing symptoms, culminating in paralysis of the muscles of respiration. Such compounds have been developed as gases and liquids for use in war. The antidote is atropine, given by intravenous or intramuscular injection as soon as possible after exposure, to which may be added intravenous pralidoxime, a reactivator of cholinesterase.

Nerves: nerve fibres form bundles which are contained in a sheath of connective tissue, constituting white structures like cords which run from the central nervous system to the muscles, skin and other organs of the body, conveying motor or sensory impulses. Inside the nerve each fibre has its own independent function. The word 'nerves' is used loosely in general to mean neurotic symptoms, which have nothing to do with the nerves of the nervous system. A 'nervous breakdown' is an acute emotional or mental disturbance, and is the concern of the psychiatrist rather than the neurologist.

Nervous System: divided into the central nervous system, which includes the brain and spinal cord, the peripheral nervous system, and the autonomic nervous system which comprises the sympathetic and parasympathetic systems. The brain, which is contained in the skull, is divided into cerebrum, cerebellum and brain stem. The bulk of the brain is formed by the two cerebral hemispheres; below them emerges the brain stem, and to the rear of the brain stem lies the cerebellum. Together with the spinal cord, the brain is made up of neurones, nerve cells having long or short processes by which they interconnect, and cells of the neuroglia, the supporting tissue. The central nervous system weighs 1.5 kg. Its structure and functions are of the utmost complexity, and no attempt will be made here to describe them in detail. Roughly speaking the brain is the seat of consciousness and the originator of the nervous impulses upon which the life of the body depends. If the brain is destroyed the body cannot by itself survive, a self-evident fact which has with the advent of life-support systems and transplant surgery become of philosophical importance. The brain has an outer cortex or rind which is grey; this covers a mass of white matter, which forms the bulk of the brain and has deep within it the basal ganglia and the thalamus. These are large areas of grey matter made up of cell relay stations; they have many intricate connections with each other and the cortex. The cortex of the brain is made up of cell bodies; its surface is convoluted like a walnut, so that its area is greater than is apparent, and from the cells run the processes forming the white matter. Inside the brain are cavities called ventricles, which are full of cerebrospinal fluid formed by masses of small blood vessels, the choroid plexuses, which lie inside the ventricles. There are two lateral ventricles, one inside each cerebral hemisphere, one below and between them, which connects with the lateral ventricles and is called the third ventricle, and below that the fourth ventricle, connected with the third by a passage called the aqueduct. From the fourth ventricle the cerebrospinal fluid is discharged into the subarachnoid space to run up over the surface of the brain and down over the spinal cord.

The brain is covered by three membranes, the dura, arachnoid and pia (*see* Meninges), and derives its blood supply from the internal carotid and vertebral arteries, which join to make a ring at the base of the brain called the circle of Willis (Thomas Willis, 1621–75) through which the major cerebral arteries communicate with each other. The veins of the brain drain into large venous spaces in the dura mater, the venous sinuses, which conduct the blood out of the skull and into the internal jugular vein.

From the brain stem emerge twelve cranial nerves (q.v.), and from the spinal cord 31 pairs of mixed sensory and motor nerves which run to all parts of the body. Sense organs in the skin, muscles, joints, and the internal organs, as well as the organs of sight, hearing and smell, set up impulses when they are stimulated which are carried to the brain. Some of the impulses are recognised in consciousness; some, without rising to the conscious level, set in progress reflex responses. Reflex pathways, connections between sensory and motor nerves, occur in the spinal cord as well as higher in the brain. The result is that stimuli acting upon the sensory nervous system result consciously or unconsciously in observable action. Impulses travel back along the motor nerves to set muscles in motion, or to relax them. In a primitive organism the process is fairly obvious – poke it and it moves – but the complexity of man has imposed upon it the unfathomable possibilities of free will. Nevertheless, it is useful to regard the brain as functioning on more than one level: the lower, the old brain, regulating the mechanical and vegetative functions of the body, and the higher, the new brain, being the seat of the intellect. The cerebral hemispheres may be thought of as being essential for the functioning of the intellect, and the base of the brain, cerebellum and brain stem as being essential for the processes of life. The cerebral hemispheres spend a good deal of their time in keeping the old brain in check.

The autonomic nervous system carries impulses to and from the internal organs, blood vessels and glands of the body. It has two components, separated according to their anatomy and function, called the sympathetic and parasympathetic systems. The parasympathetic nerves emerge from the head and tail ends of the nervous system through the cranial nerves and the sacral nerves and find their way all over the body, while the sympathetic fibres emerge from the spinal cord between the first thoracic and upper lumbar segments. They form a chain of ganglia, relay stations, beside the spinal column on each side of the body, from which connections pass to the sweat glands of the skin, the erector muscles of the hairs, the heart, lungs, intestines, the other internal organs and the blood vessels. Both systems are regulated by the brain, in a manner which is far from clear. In general the two autonomic nervous systems are mutually antagonistic in their actions. The sympathetic system prepares the body for action; it stiffens the sinews and summons up the blood; while the action of the parasympathetic produces the old man after dinner, sleepy, slow and snoring.

No satisfactory model of the brain has been produced. Although its activity is accompanied by changes in electrical potential, this does not mean that it works by electricity, and the analogies of the telephone exchange and computer leave much unexplained. In general, attempts to explain the actions of the central nervous system on physiological grounds end up by postulating a biological computer, and those founded on psychology seem to imply that there is a ghost in the machine.

Nettle Rash: *see* Urticaria.

Neuralgia: paroxysmal pain originating in a nerve. It may be the sequel of herpes zoster (q.v.) or be confined to the fifth cranial nerve, the trigeminal nerve, which is the sensory nerve of the face. The cause of trigeminal neuralgia is not known; it is a disease of age, and is rarely seen before the fifties. The trigeminal nerve has three divisions: the first supplies the eye, the forehead, the front of the head and the nose; the second, the cheek and upper jaw; the third, the lower part of the face and the lower jaw. The pain is usually felt in one division, on one side of the face. It is agonising, and comes in paroxysms that last seconds. It may cause the sufferer to screw up the face, and has therefore the name *tic doloreux*. A variety of stimuli may provoke the pain, for example a cold draught, touching the face, or washing it. In some cases the disease can be recognised because the affected side of the face is discoloured or unshaven. Sometimes there are distinct trigger spots on the face, which when touched set off the pain. At first the pain comes at intervals, and there may be remissions lasting for months, but the progress of the condition is steady and the attacks start to strike at decreasing intervals. The pain may spread from one division of the nerve to another. The drug carbamazepine is used to treat the condition; in many cases it renders life tolerable, but in resistant cases it may be necessary to destroy the affected division of the nerve by thermocoagulation, or by open operation. Anaesthesia of the affected area follows, and if this includes the eye special measures are needed to prevent damage resulting from the loss of sensation.

Neurasthenia: an imprecise and old-fashioned diagnosis, implying fatigue, depression, loss of appetite and other ill-defined symptoms. It can be very useful in making out medical certificates.

Neurectomy: the surgical removal of part of a nerve.

Neurilemma: the thin membrane which surrounds the axon, the nerve fibre that is the extension of nerve cells through which impulses are transmitted.

Neurinoma: a benign tumour arising from the sheath of a nerve; otherwise called a neurofibroma.

Neuritis: inflammation of a nerve. The term is also used to mean a condition more properly referred to as neuropathy, in which there is a destruction of the cell body and the axon, the nerve fibre which is its extension. The loss may start in the axon, and extend back to the cell body; it may be caused by disease affecting the myelin, a fatty substance which surrounds each axon, and serves to insulate it and preserve its powers of conduction. One nerve may be affected, usually as the result of local damage caused by injury, or many nerves in generalised conditions such as disease, poisoning, abnormal immune reactions or dietary deficiency. A common disease causing neuropathy is diabetes mellitus; poisoning by arsenic, lead or mercury may be at fault; deficiency of vitamin B produces beri-beri, a reversible disease of the axons, and chronic alcoholism produces a similar state. Function is lost in the nerves affected, and abnormal sensations may arise, such as numbness and tingling in the hands and feet, or intensified sensations of pain. When pain sensation is lost, minor injuries go unnoticed and ulceration may develop. Loss of position sense results in difficulty in walking and clumsiness of the hands. Treatment depends on the treatment of the underlying condition.

Neurofibroma: a benign tumour of the sheath of a nerve.

Neurofibromatosis: molluscum fibrosum, or von Recklinghausen's disease. Inherited as a Mendelian dominant trait, there are multiple fibrous tumours which grow in association with the nerves, often just under the skin, and also patches of pigmented skin called *café au lait* spots. There is no specific treatment for the condition, but neurofibromas which are causing trouble may be removed surgically; sometimes they are disfiguring, or dangerous, according to their site. Kyphosis (q.v.) may be associated with neurofibromatosis, as may other tumours, for example meningiomas. (Freidrich von Recklinghausen, 1833–1910)

Neuroglia: the supporting tissue of the central nervous system, made up of three types of branched cells: astroglia, oligodendroglia, and microglia.

Neurology: the specialty that deals with the nervous system. It is not concerned with mental diseases that have no known pathological basis.

Neuroma: a tumour composed of nerve cells or nerve fibres; a tumour growing from a nerve.

Neurone: the nerve cell, with short processes, called dendrites, and a long process, the axon, which is enclosed in a sheath as the nerve fibre.

Neurosis: mental illness that differs from psychosis in that patients retain insight; they know that there is something wrong, whereas in psychosis there is no such awareness. The symptoms of neurosis are less severe than those of psychosis. Neuroses fall into three groups: anxiety, hysterical and obsessional. Anxiety is common, and it may be accompanied by such symptoms of overactivity of the autonomic nervous system as excessive sweating, palpitations, headaches, dry mouth, loose bowels, and frequency of micturition; these are all within normal experience when circumstances justify them, but in an anxiety neurosis they are incessant, and brought on by apprehension out of all proportion to the true situation. In hysteria, symptoms appear to be those of a physical illness, but there are no corresponding signs of illness; for example, in a limb that is declared useless all the muscles can be demonstrated to be functioning normally, and areas of the skin said to be without feeling will change during an examination. Epileptic attacks may be imitated, but there is no incontinence nor is the tongue bitten. Sudden loss of memory is sometimes a complaint, often linked to an emotional shock or other incident. In general, some advantage is gained from an hysterical illness. In obsessional neurosis intruding unpleasant thoughts and compulsions come into the mind, for example the conviction that the subject is contaminated with infectious matter or dirt, which leads to continual hand-washing. The seeds of the neuroses can be found in all normal people, and indeed these traits are often approved of by society, as in the case of the housewife who is meticulous in her house cleaning, or the man who thinks of nothing but his work and succeeds in business. It is useful in treatment to point out that the neuroses are on the whole an exaggeration of normal feelings; patients must be persuaded to look at themselves honestly and understand their difficulties in order to deal with them. Anxiety neuroses are often only short lived, and may be relieved by the use of the benzodiazepine anxiolytic drugs; but these must only be used for a few weeks, for they are addictive. They are, however, useful for helping people to get over the worst of their troubles and facing up to their circumstances. Drugs are not very useful in hysterical cases, which usually recover quickly, nor in obsessions, when psychiatric advice may be needed.

Neurosurgery: the surgery of the central nervous system.

Neutropenia: a fall in the number of neutrophilic white cells circulating in the blood to an abnormally low level. *See* Leucocyte.

Nicotine: an alkaloid present in the leaves of the plant *Nicotiana tabacum*. It has been used as a pesticide, and is poisonous if taken in small quantities by mouth, first stimulating then paralysing the autonomic nervous system, thus producing headache, nausea and vomiting, giddiness and eventually a running pulse, sweating, pain in the abdomen and collapse. It is, when smoked, addictive, but probably not responsible for the worst effects of smoking, which are due to the tar and carbon monoxide in tobacco smoke. It has therefore been used in chewing gum and in patients dependent on tobacco smoking may help in giving up the dangerous habit.

Nicotinic Acid: part of the vitamin B complex, it is essential for health; deficiency causes the disease pellagra, the symptoms of which are diarrhoea, dermatitis and dementia, but a normal Western diet supplies more than adequate quantities. Pellagra is associated with the cultivation and exclusive consumption of maize, which is a poor source of nicotinic acid.

Niehan's Cell Therapy: a form of rejuvenating treatment based on the belief that if any organ in the body is not functioning correctly it can be revitalised by the injection of fresh cells from the corresponding organ of a young or preferably unborn animal. The young healthy cells, it is claimed, find their way to the affected part of the body. There is unfortunately no evidence to show that this is so.

Night Blindness: caused by deficiency of vitamin A, which is responsible for the formation of rhodopsin, or visual purple, contained in the rods of the retina, by which dim light is perceived. Vision in bright light remains normal, although vision in poor illumination is uncertain. *See* Eye.

Nightmares: fearful dreams, common at any age, usually occurring in the later part of the night during the stage of paradoxical sleep (q.v.). Night terrors are experienced by children, and happen in the early part of the night; they may be accompanied by shouting or screaming, but often the child does not wake up, and falls into normal sleep again. No memory remains of the event. Nightmares may be caused by drugs, and are not uncommon after sleep-inducing drugs have been discontinued.

Night Sweats: characteristic of tuberculosis, and found in various low fevers such as that of Hodgkin's disease and polymyalgia rheumatica.

Nipples: *see* Breast.

Nitrates: used for their effect in dilating the coronary arteries in the treatment of angina. The most commonly used preparation is glyceryl trinitrate in tablets placed underneath the tongue. It has a quick action, lasting for about 30 minutes. It should be remembered that the tablets remain active for only eight weeks, after which they should be renewed. Longer-acting preparations are available, as are sprays and self-adhesive plasters containing the drug, which is then absorbed through the skin. Isosorbide dinitrate is more stable than glyceryl trinitrate, and is available in short and long acting preparations. Both drugs can be given by injection if necessary.

Nitrazepam: a short-acting benzodiazepine used for insomnia. It is only useful in short courses, for tolerance develops as well as dependence; if it has been taken for any length of time, sudden withdrawal may cause insomnia or in some cases confusion.

Nitrofurantoin: an antibacterial drug used in infections of the urinary tract.

Nitrogen: an almost inert colourless gas, not able to support life although its compounds make life possible; it makes up about four-fifths of the air we breathe. It is soluble in the blood, and when divers have been breathing air under increased pressure injudicious speed in rising to the surface may decrease the pressure too quickly so that bubbles of the gas form in the blood and produce various symptoms. *See* Caisson Disease.

Nitrous Oxide: laughing gas, used in 1844 as the first general anaesthetic, a property which makes it very useful for short operations such as opening an abscess or extracting a tooth, for the patient does not have to be made deeply unconscious. It is difficult to produce general anaesthesia with nitrous oxide gas and air without depriving the patient of oxygen, so that if it is given for any length of time it must be given with oxygen. It is often used in combination with volatile anaesthetic drugs and oxygen, the proportions being chosen to give the required effect. *See* Anaesthesia.

Nits: the egg containers of lice (*see* Louse).

Nocturnal Enuresis: *see* Bed-wetting.

Non-specific Urethritis: one of the most commonly encountered sexually transmitted diseases which produces frequency of micturition, some pain and a discharge. It is in many cases caused by the organism *Chlamydia trachomatis*, the organism of trachoma, in others possibly by *Ureaplasma urealyticum*; the treatment is by tetracyclines or erythromycin.

Non-viable: not capable of independent life. Used of the foetus, which without help does not normally survive before the 28th week, but with modern techniques may survive when 27 or even 26 weeks old.

Noradrenaline: substance believed to be responsible for the transmission of impulses in the sympathetic nervous system. *See* Nervous System.

Normoblast: immature red blood cell which still has a nucleus. As the cell matures and enters the bloodstream, the nucleus breaks up; the cell is then called a reticulocyte, for it contains the remains of the nucleus. Finally, when it is mature, the red blood cell has no nucleus. Normoblasts are only seen in the circulation when new red cells are being formed abnormally quickly.

Nose: inspired air passing through the nose is warmed, filtered to a certain extent and humidified by the mucous membrane with which the nose is lined; special cells in the upper part of the nose are sensitive to molecules in the air and give rise to the sensation of smell. Fibres from them run through the ethmoid bone in the roof of the nose to form the first cranial nerve, the olfactory nerve. Air has to the turbinate bones; there are three on each side project into the nasal cavity and are curved dow The cavity of the nose is separated into two sides nasal septum, a partition made in its lower part of car and in its upper part of bone. Turbinate bones and sep are covered by mucous membrane. On each side of the nose lie the maxillary sinuses, cavities in the bone of the upper jaw which communicate with the nose by passages below the middle turbinate bone, and above the nose on each side are the frontal air sinuses, cavities in the frontal bone of the forehead which communicate with the nose through air cells contained in the ethmoid bone in the roof of the nose. There is also an air sinus in the sphenoid bone which communicates with the ethmoid. The duct draining the frontal and ethmoid air cavities opens below the middle turbinate bone. Blockage of these ducts means that the air in the sinuses cannot communicate with air at atmospheric pressure, and as the air is absorbed pressure in the sinuses falls, giving rise to considerable pain. As such a block is commonly caused by infection which makes the mucous membranes swell it is not surprising that flying when suffering from a severe cold may produce a headache during the descent from altitude. Other ducts opening into the nose are the naso-lacrimal duct draining tears from the eyes and the Eustachian tube which communicates with the middle ear. Infection of the nose is usually caused by viruses, as in the common cold. Swelling of the mucous membranes may be caused by allergic reactions, as in hay fever, or by vasomotor rhinitis, a chronic irritation of the blood vessels in the nose caused by such factors as air pollution, smoking, and central heating. Although it is tempting to use inhaled anticongestant drugs such as xylometazoline or ephedrine, over-use may result in the rebound phenomenon, a worsening of the symptoms when the drug is discontinued, or in chronic irritation of the mucous membrane producing yet further rhinitis and a vicious circle. Chronic inflammation of the mucous membranes may result in polyps being formed, obstructive swellings which can be removed surgically. Infections of the nasal sinuses are not uncommon, and are treated by the appropriate antibiotics; chronic infections, usually of

NOSE
pass over
which
wards.
the
age
m

y need washing out, and even an
e drainage. Obstruction of the
may arise from nasal polyps,
membranes of the turbinate
eviation of the septum from
of a fracture of the nose.
cated. Foreign bodies in
ecially in children, and
blowing the nose will
em out usually drive
he nose *see* Epistaxis.

communicable diseases such
measles are by law notifiable to the
local   alth officer.

NSAID: an acronym for non-steroidal anti-inflammatory
drug. NSAIDs are a group of drugs that have the actions
of diminishing pain and inhibiting the formation of prostaglandins, substances ubiquitous in the body with many
only partly understood functions, which include a part
in the processes of pain and inflammation. The drugs are
therefore used in the treatment of painful inflammatory
conditions, principally rheumatic and arthritic. How great
the demand for relief is from such disease can be seen from
the fact that there are at least 20 different compounds on the
market, including aspirin, the forerunner of the group. The
NSAIDs differ from each other to a certain extent and have
to be chosen to suit each patient, but all have unwanted
effects, principally on the gastro-intestinal tract where they
may produce peptic ulceration, nausea and diarrhoea.
They are also liable to produce hypersensitivity reactions
such as asthma, rashes and urticaria, and fluid retention.
There may be an increased tendency to bleeding, and there
have been blood disorders. These unwanted effects vary,
and some, such as the tendency to peptic ulceration or
upper abdominal discomfort, may be diminished by taking
the drug with a meal.

Nuclear Magnetic Resonance Imaging: a technique
recently established for producing images of the internal
structures of the body. It depends on the fact that the

nuclei of some atoms show electromagnetic activity on being exposed to strong magnetic fields. Nuclei align with each other in such a magnetic field, and their axis of spin is tilted and rotated. A radio-frequency pulse applied at 90° to the field changes the axis of rotation. Immediately after the radio-frequency pulse the nuclei return to their original state, emitting electromagnetic waves which can be measured and used to make up an image. Hydrogen nuclei behave as single protons, and as the water and fat in the body contain hydrogen atoms they can be used to make the images detected by magnetic resonance. The technique does not interfere with the patient at all, and uses no ionising radiation. The patient lies inside a coil surrounded by a magnet, and is not conscious of the rapidly changing magnetic fields and radio-frequency pulses to which the body is subjected. Magnetic resonance imaging has been used on the central nervous system, where it has the advantage that compact bone produces no signal. It has also been used in investigating the heart and other organs, and will doubtless be widely developed; at present however the apparatus is very costly.

Nuclear Medicine: the use of radioactive substances in medicine. It is possible to trace the circulation and concentration of sources of radioactivity introduced into the body, for example radioactive iodine which is concentrated in the thyroid gland. It is also possible to add a radioactive substance to drugs or biochemical compounds to trace their use in the body, and for this purpose technetium-99m is commonly used. The same radioactive indicator can be attached to a patient's red blood cells to aid in investigation of the circulation. A common use of a radioactive substance in the treatment of disease is the use of radioactive iodine in thyrotoxicosis (q.v.).

Nucleus: the body inside the cells which contains within a membrane the chromosomes, the nucleolus and the nucleoplasm. The nucleolus is concerned with the production of ribonucleic acid (RNA), which is involved with the organisation of protein molecules by deoxyribonucleic acid, the carrier of genetic information. It is only when the cell is ready to divide that the chromosomes become visible inside the nucleus (*see* Cell). Another meaning of nucleus is a collection of nerve cells with a special function in the central nervous system.

Nucleus Pulposus: the soft centre of an intervertebral disc, formed by white and yellow connective tissue fibres and surrounded by the annulus fibrosus. It is because of the elasticity of these structures that the spinal vertebrae can to a limited extent move in relation to each other.

Nullipara: a woman who has not borne children.

Nursing: the profession of nursing as it is now understood dates from the middle of the nineteenth century, a time when the discovery of general anaesthetics and the growth of knowledge of pathology, which included the understanding of bacterial infection, laid the foundations of modern medicine and surgery. In early times there were hospitals for the sick poor in Egypt, India, Greece and Rome, with attendants rather than nurses. The early Christian Church to a certain extent cared for the sick, and male and female attendants were recruited from the religious orders. In London St Thomas's and St Bartholomew's hospitals were founded in the twelfth century; it was not until the Reformation in this country that nursing came to be separated in some measure from religion. Properly trained nurses, however, as contrasted with those who simply learned their work from experience in the wards, are a creation of the nineteenth century. The system developed in Germany under Pastor Fleidner, whose Institute of Protestant Deaconesses was founded at Kaiserworth in 1836. Florence Nightingale spent some time there. Two years later an institute was founded in Philadelphia, and in another two years Elizabeth Fry had founded one in London, the nurses being trained at Guy's and St Thomas's hospitals. The first nurses' training school was founded at St Thomas's in 1860. It was not until 1919 that the system of state registration was introduced, in great part due to the efforts of Mrs Bedford Fenwick. Her name was the first on the register of the General Nursing Council, which was set up in 1919 to be replaced in 1983 by the United Kingdom Central Council for

Nurses, Midwives and Health Visitors. Although nursing has traditionally been a female profession, since the Second World War an increasing number of men have chosen to become registered nurses, and now about one in six nurses are male.

Nux Vomica: obtained from the dried seed of *Strychnos nux-vomica*, it contains a small amount of strychnine; it has been used as a tincture or extract to improve the appetite.

Nyctalopia: night blindness.

Nystagmus: a rapid involuntary movement of the eyeballs from side to side, or less commonly up and down; there may be a rotary movement which is a combination of the two.

Nystatin: named after the New York State Department of Health, where it was originated, nystatin is a drug obtained from the fungus *Streptomyces noursei* which is active against a number of fungi and yeasts, and is commonly used in infections of the mucous membranes and skin with *Candida albicans*, or thrush. It is applied directly to the affected area in creams, suppositories or as a suspension. It may be used by mouth in the treatment of candidiasis of the intestine.

O

Oath: for Hippocratic Oath, *see* Hippocrates.

Obesity: excess of fat in the body; overweight is the term used for those who weigh 110% above the standard weight for height tables, obese for those who weigh 120% more. Various diseases may be associated with obesity: diabetes, gall-bladder disease, varicose veins, high blood pressure, atheromatous disease of the arteries, hiatus hernia, arthritis, and in women menstrual disorders and an increased tendency to develop malignant disease of the uterus and breast. Smoking increases the likelihood of coronary artery disease; while it is true that giving up smoking may result in an increase of weight, the increased weight is less dangerous than the consequences of smoking. There is an inherited factor in obesity: thin parents tend to have thin children, and obese parents fat children. Obese people do not necessarily eat more than thinner people, but must pay more attention to their diet. Apart from the obvious avoidance of falling for the temptation of sweet drinks, snacks between meals and so on, it is worth while asking for skilled advice on a diet, but it must be remembered that on an adequate well-balanced diet weight loss may be slow, and to be successful the diet must be continued; weight lost will be regained if a satisfactory diet is abandoned. If the family's eating habits are not modified as a whole, it is unlikely that an individual within the family will be able to stick to a special diet. Drugs designed to suppress the appetite may be recommended in selected patients, but they are only used in conjunction with a diet, and do little to help in most cases. There is no doubt that reduction of the weight alone will bring many cases of high blood pressure under control, and reduce the risks associated with it.

Obsession: *see* Neurosis.

Obstetrics: that branch of medicine concerned with midwifery.

Obstruction: usually used to mean a blockage of the intestines. This may be caused by a tumour, an inflammatory process, twisting of the intestine around itself (volvulus) or round an adhesion, or because the intestine is caught in a hernial sac. Acute obstruction shows itself by colicky pain in the abdomen, vomiting, constipation, distension of the abdomen and collapse. The treatment is surgical.

Occipital Lobe: the portion of the cerebrum that lies at the back of the brain; it is concerned with vision.

Occiput: the back of the head.

Occupational Disease: few trades or professions are free from the risk of specific diseases connected with each particular pursuit. This has been known and written about since classical times; the Swiss physician Paracelsus (1493–1541) wrote a monograph on *Miners' Sickness and other Miners' Diseases*, but possibly the first specialist in industrial medicine was the Italian Bernardino Ramazzini (1633–1714) who in 1700 published *Diseases of Tradesmen*. The Industrial Revolution brought with it overcrowding, insanitary working conditions and more industrial disease; Charles Thackrah (1795–1833), a physician in Leeds, described the effects of inhaling dust from cutlery-grinding in shortening the lives of the workmen, and he wrote of the short lives of miners. The Factory Act of 1833, which was an Act 'to Regulate the Labour of Children in the Mills and Factories', was the first to appoint Factory Inspectors. After this other measures were introduced over the years to control conditions leading to industrial disease, until in 1974 the Health and Safety at Work Act was passed to bring about a unified system of law to secure the health, safety and welfare of persons at work, to cover the storage and use of dangerous substances, emissions into the atmosphere, control of processes which may threaten the safety and health of the general public, and the disposal of waste. The Health and Safety Executive is responsible to the Health and Safety Commission for carrying out its recommendations and enforcing the law. The medical work is carried out by the Employment Medical Advisory Service. People who have contracted certain diseases known as Prescribed Diseases as a result of their work are entitled to benefits under the Social Security Act of 1975 and amended regulations of 1983 as long as they have worked in an occupation scheduled as carrying a risk of the disease. The list of prescribed diseases is long, and includes those caused by physical agents, infections, poisons, agents causing cancers, and those causing asthma. Under the Reporting of Injuries, Diseases and Dangerous Occurrences Regulations of 1985 the responsibility for reporting cases of disease is placed on employers after they have received a written diagnosis from the doctor.

Occupational Therapy: originating with the teaching of handicrafts, occupational therapy now takes many forms, from work designed to exercise particular groups of muscles to the encouragement of free expression painting in psychiatric cases. The object is to master disabilities and enable the patient to work again or take his or her place in normal society.

Oculentum: an ointment for the eye.

Oedema: a swelling due to the accumulation of excess tissue fluid. It may be due to local causes, such as interference with lymphatic or venous drainage, or to generalised conditions such as heart or kidney failure. In these cases the collection of fluid is largely determined by gravity, and it tends to affect the feet, ankles and legs. It is within normal bounds for the feet and ankles to swell by the end of the day, particularly in hot weather or after standing or sitting in one position for a length of time, as in an aircraft; but the swelling should have disappeared after a night in bed.

Oedipus Complex: Oedipus was a fabled Greek king, brought up by a foster parent. As a man he killed his real father and married his mother. On finding what he had done, he put out his eyes. In Freudian theory, the Oedipus complex is the subconscious desire of a child for the parent of the opposite sex.

Oesophagus: the gullet, a tube connecting the throat with the stomach. It runs through the chest and the diaphragm. Diseases affecting it are cancer, hiatus hernia (q.v.) and spasm at the lower end, and rarely varicosities caused by high pressure in the portal system of veins, which may occur in cirrhosis of the liver. Strictures can be caused by swallowing corrosive fluids, or by injury, as in one case where a sword-swallower made a mistake.

Oestrogen: oestradiol is the hormone naturally secreted by the ovaries, and any substance which has a similar action to this hormone is called an oestrogen. The effects of the oestrogens are the development of the female secondary sexual characteristics at puberty, stimulation of the beginning of the cyclical changes in the uterus and breasts, and the suppression of ovulation (*see* Menstruation). Oestrogens may be natural or synthetic, and they are used in the contraceptive pill, for the treatment of various cases of menstrual troubles such as dysmenorrhoea and menorrhagia, for menopausal symptoms and osteoporosis, and in the control of certain malignant growths of the prostate and the breast. They can be used for local application in cases of vaginal or vulval trouble at the menopause. Oestrogens are associated with an increased risk of clotting in the blood vessels, and with a risk of the development of carcinoma of the uterus, so that they are used in combination with progestogens except in cases where the uterus has been removed.

Ointment: a preparation for application to the skin, greasy and usually made of soft paraffin, which may be combined with liquid and hard paraffin. Such ointments are not soluble in water, but some modern ointments containing macrogols are, and can be washed off. Various medicinal compounds may be included in ointments, and they are used in treating chronic dry conditions. Creams are less greasy than ointments.

Olecranon: the bony tip of the elbow.

Olfactory Nerve: the nerve which conveys the sensations of smell from the nose to the brain. It is the first cranial nerve, and it runs from the upper part of the nose (q.v.) through the cribriform plate of the ethmoid bone which is perforated by many small holes to relay in the olfactory bulbs which pass back into the brain. It may be damaged by head injuries involving the ethmoid bone, or by the pressure of tumours arising from the brain or the meninges. The sense of smell is then lost.

Oliguria: diminished flow of urine, the result of severe dehydration or failure of the kidneys in severe renal disease. It may follow high voltage electrical shock, or in some cases snakebite.

Omentum: the apron of peritoneum containing fat which hangs from the stomach and colon to lie in front of the intestines. It has been called the abdominal policeman, for it may adhere to inflamed areas to wall them off from the rest of the abdominal cavity.

Omphalos: the umbilicus.

Onchocerciasis: infestation with the nematode *Onchocerca volvulus*, found in tropical Africa and Central America, where it may have been introduced by the slave trade. The larvae are carried by the blackfly *Simulium damnosum*, which lives in flowing water, and the adult worms come to lie under the skin or deep between the muscles. Of themselves they appear to do no harm, but their microfilariae, which appear about a year or 18 months after the larvae have been acquired, cause an itching rash in the skin centred on the buttock or shoulder where the adult worm may lie. The lymph glands may be enlarged in the groin or armpit. More seriously, the worms may lie under the skin of the head and the microfilariae invade the eyes, where they may cause blindness (African river blindness). Treatment is by the drug ivermectin.

Oncology: the study of malignant tumours. An oncologist is a specialist in the diagnosis and treatment of cancer.

Onychia: inflammation of a nail bed.

Onychogryphosis: gross thickening, overgrowth and deformity of a nail, usually a toenail, due to chronic inflammation or injury to the nail bed. The treatment is surgical removal; if it recurs when the nail grows again the nail bed must be removed.

Onychomycosis: a fungus infection of the nails.

Oophorectomy: the removal of one or both ovaries.

Oophoritis: inflammation of the ovary. It may be due to salpingitis, other infection in the pelvis such as appendicitis, or mumps.

Operable: the term applied by the surgeon to cases in which operation is technically possible and has a good chance of curing the condition.

Ophthalmia: inflammation of the eye or of the conjunctiva, usually applied only to severe conditions such as ophthalmia neonatorum, a purulent conjunctivitis of the newborn due to direct infection with gonorrhoea from a diseased mother, or sympathetic ophthalmia, in which damage to the uveal tract in one eye leads to inflammation of the uveal tract in the good eye. *See* Eye.

Ophthalmic: to do with the eye.

Ophthalmology: the study of the eye and its diseases. An ophthalmologist is a specialist in eye diseases.

Ophthalmoplegia: paralysis affecting the eye. It is external when one or more of the muscles moving the eye are affected, for they lie outside the eyeball, and internal when it affects the ciliary muscle of the lens, or the muscle of the iris.

Ophthalmoscope: an instrument for examining the interior of the eye, consisting of a system of lenses through which the examiner looks along a beam of light projected from the instrument. The lenses can be changed to bring the retina at the back of the eye into focus; a wider view of the retina is obtained if eye-drops of tropicamide are used to dilate the patient's pupil before the examination.

Opisthotonus: a position characteristic of severe tetanus and strychnine poisoning, when all the muscles go into spasm. The extensor muscles are more powerful than the flexor, except in the arms, so that the elbows are flexed; but the spine and hips are fully extended, and in extreme cases the back is arched so that the patient rests on the heels and the back of the head.

Opium: the dried juice of the unripe seed capsule of the poppy *Papaver somniferum*. Many alkaloids are contained in it, the principal ones being morphine, codeine, noscapine and papaverine. Together they may be used under the name papaveretum as a premedication. Codeine and morphine are dealt with under separate headings; noscapine may be used in cough mixtures. Papaverine has no analgesic action, but relaxes smooth muscle. Opium is one of the most valuable drugs we have, and one of the oldest; but it is addictive and has been for centuries liable to misuse.

Opsonisation: antibodies alter the state of antigenic particles so that they are more easily engulfed by the leucocytes and macrophages of the tissue spaces. The process is called opsonisation.

Optic Nerve: the nerve of sight, the second cranial nerve. It starts in the centre of the retina of the eye, where it can be seen through the ophthalmoscope as a pale round area called the optic disc, from which the blood vessels of the retina fan out. Passing back from the eyeball the nerves enter the skull through the optic foramina, and the two nerves join in the optic chiasm, where the fibres from the inner halves of the retina cross over; after the chiasm the fibres form the optic tracts, so that the left and right visual fields are represented in the left and right tracts. The nerves may be affected by atrophy, caused by diseases such as multiple sclerosis or tertiary syphilis, or by injury or compression by a tumour, when the head of the nerve becomes very much paler than normal. Increased pressure inside the skull caused by a tumour or other space-occupying condition may make the optic nerves swell, so that the head of the nerve can be seen to be swollen and reddened, possibly with small haemorrhages round it. This appearance is known as papilloedema. Interference with the nerves or tracts by a tumour, possibly arising from the pituitary gland which lies just below the chiasm, may interfere with vision in a manner that enables the neurologist to know where the tumour lies.

Oral Contraceptive: *see* Contraception.

Orbit: the socket in the skull that contains the eye. It is made up of parts of eight bones.

Orchidectomy: the removal of one or both testicles.

Orchitis: inflammation of the testicles.

Orf: a poxvirus infection of sheep, goats and cattle, who develop a pustular dermatitis of the lips and sometimes the tongue. It is common in lambs and kids, and can be passed on to shepherds and those who handle wool. A maculo-papular rash is followed by a blister which breaks down, forming a crusted scab which may persist for about six weeks, and then heals. The lesion is usually on the hands or arms. It can be treated by the application of idoxuridine in dimethyl sulphoxide, but will in most cases resolve harmlessly without treatment. Orf in humans is not infectious.

Organic Disease: essentially this means a disease which can be demonstrated to be present, as opposed to functional disease in which there is no demonstrable disease to be found.

Organic Substances: those which are found in living matter, or are related to it.

Organophosphorus Compounds: these compounds are used as insecticides, and some are so dangerous that they can be used as nerve gases in war. They block the action of acetylcholinesterase, an enzyme which breaks down acetylcholine (q.v.) and is essential for the proper working of the nervous system. The symptoms of poisoning are headache, weakness, sweating, abdominal pain and vomiting, excessive secretion of saliva, and a slow pulse, followed by muscular twitching, diarrhoea, difficulty in breathing, constriction of the pupils which may interfere with vision, and confusion. In severe cases the patient may become comatose and even die. Treatment is the injection of atropine, repeated as necessary, and subsequent injection of pralidoxime mesylate (P2S). The skin should be washed, for the chemical is absorbed by the skin, and contaminated clothes removed. Organophosphorus compounds produced commercially and used for pest control are tested for toxicity, and if used carefully in accordance with the instructions are not dangerous. If there is a question of poisoning, the blood cholinesterase can be determined.

Orgasm: the climax of sexual pleasure accompanied in men by the emission of semen and in women by reaching a height of excitement with contractions of the vagina, followed in both by a sudden decline in tension.

Oriental Sore: cutaneous leishmaniasis. *See* Kala-azar.

Ornithosis: a disease carried by birds and transmitted to man, caused by the organism *Chlamydia psittaci*. The organisms can be carried by pigeons, sea-birds and poultry; parrots, budgerigars and other exotic birds also carry it, and when caught from parrots the disease is called psittacosis. The organism causes headache, fever and coughing, and the infection may proceed to pneumonia, or enlargement of the liver and spleen. The incubation period is one or two weeks, and the illness may last for a number of weeks, and is liable to relapse. The organism is sensitive to tetracycline and erythromycin. Regulations affecting the importation of parrots and budgerigars have helped control psittacosis in this country.

Orthodontics: that part of dentistry concerned with treating irregularity and inaccurate opposition of the upper and lower teeth.

Orthopaedics: that branch of surgery concerned with the treatment of diseases, injuries and deformities of the bones, joints and muscles.

Orthopnoea: the term applied to the state of a patient who is unable to breathe without distress unless sitting up. It is a symptom of severe heart failure.

Orthoptics: a method of remedial exercises for the eye muscles in cases of squint. The object is to align the axes of the eyes correctly.

Ossicles: small bones; usually used to refer to the small bones of the middle ear.

Ossification: the formation of bone. It is laid down by cells called osteoblasts, which are closely related to the cells which form fibrous tissue and cartilage, and shaped by osteoclasts, which absorb bone. As the bone is formed osteoblasts are incorporated in its substance, and are then referred to as osteocytes; they are responsible for the nutrition of the bone.

Osteitis: inflammation of bone.

Osteoarthritis: a condition of the synovial joints in which there is loss of the articular cartilage and change in the underlying bone. It begins in middle age and affects women more than men, and worsens with age. It may run in families, and is very common. The underlying causes of the disease are not fully understood, but it may follow abnormal stress put on the joints for years, as in the hips and backs of miners, or injuries. The joints, particularly the large weight-bearing joints, become painful and stiff; after resting it may take some time to get them moving again. Movement is limited, and the joints creak or grate. The fingers may be affected, and small bony swellings develop on each side of the last finger joints called Heberden's

461

nodes (William Heberden 1767–1845). If the thumb is affected the grip becomes painful and weak. Pain and limitation of movement in the knees or hips may make walking increasingly difficult. X-ray examination of the affected joints is not in all cases necessary to make a diagnosis, and in any case the correlation between radiological appearances and pain is surprisingly poor. The disease cannot be cured, but treatment is possible, and is aimed at keeping the patient active. Physiotherapy helps a great deal, and the NSAID group of drugs (q.v.) can be used. In very severe cases surgical replacement of the hip with an artificial joint has revolutionised the treatment of the disease, and similar operations are possible on the knee.

Osteoarthropathy: disease affecting the bones and joints.

Osteochondritis: literally inflammation of the bone and cartilage; usually applied to a disease of the epiphyseal cartilage in children, from which the developing bones grow. The disease involves a degeneration of the cartilage, followed by regeneration. The group of diseases has various names according to its site, for example disease of the head of the femur is Perthes disease, of the thoracic vertebrae Scheuermann's disease, of the tuberosity of the tibia just below the knee Osgood–Schlatter disease. It may occur in the scaphoid bone in the wrist, in the heel, in the second metatarsal bone of the foot or in the navicular bone in the ankle, or in the ilium in the pelvis. The main importance of the disease is that it may be painful. In most cases the condition resolves in time, but in the case of the head of the femur it may lead to deformity of the hip joint and when the thoracic spine is affected very severely a kyphus may form. In osteochondritis dissecans small pieces of cartilage may split away, and become loose bodies in the shoulder or knee joint. It may also affect the elbow or ankle joints.

Osteoclast: a cell which is able to absorb bony tissue, which plays a large part in shaping bones according to the mechanical stress. The cells are active in reshaping bone after a fracture. They make calcium available in the body, and increase in response to the parathyroid hormone. The word also means a surgical instrument for breaking bones.

Osteoclastoma: a tumour of bone which behaves midway between a malignant and a benign tumour. It tends to invade tissues round about it, but rarely forms metastatic deposits in other parts of the body. The treatment is removal of the tumour with the surrounding tissues.

Osteogenesis Imperfecta: also known as fragilitas ossium, this is a rare inherited disorder of the bones, which are brittle. In one type of the disease, the baby is born with multiple fractures and consequent deformities, and may not survive. In another type, the fractures are fewer and occur later in life; in such cases the whites of the eyes may be blue, the teeth are badly formed, and there may be deafness. In a third type the limbs grow shorter than normal, and bowed; the spine and skull are deformed, and the patient cannot walk.

Osteology: the study of bones.

Osteoma: a benign tumour of bone, which may grow on the skull or the long bones. It is as hard as ivory, and need only be removed if it is disfiguring, or blocking an air sinus or the orifice of the ear, for it is not dangerous.

Osteomalacia: softening of the bones due to lack of vitamin D. In children it is called rickets. The deficiency may be in the diet, and it may be compounded by inadequate exposure to sunlight, for vitamin D is formed by the action of ultraviolet light on a sterol in the skin. Vitamin D may be poorly absorbed in coeliac disease or disease of the biliary tract, and absorption may be impaired after surgery on the stomach or intestine; it is also deficient in some cases of kidney disease. Osteomalacia causes pain in the bones and deformities of the pelvis, spine and chest; there may be weakness of the muscles of the arms and legs. Rickets leads to stunted growth and bowing of the long bones, with enlargement of the joints between the ribs and their cartilages known as a rickety rosary, together with prominent bosses on the frontal and parietal bones of the skull. There is a form of rickets which is hereditary, and is passed on by the X chromosome, so that half the children of an affected mother will have the disease, but none of the sons of an affected father, although his daughters will. Treatment of osteomalacia and rickets is the administration of calciferol, vitamin D_2; in those cases due to renal disorder, and in the inherited form of the disease, phosphate may be needed as well as calcitriol, which is used rather than calciferol.

Osteomyelitis: inflammation of the bone marrow due to staphylococci or streptococci. Once a serious and even dangerous condition – there are men who lost limbs in the Second World War, especially in Germany and Russia, because it was safer to amputate for an open fracture than to wait, when it might become infected – it has lost its menace as the result of antibiotic therapy, and is now uncommon.

Osteopathy: a system of medicine founded in 1874 by an American, Andrew Taylor Still (1828–1917), based on the theory that as long as it is in correct mechanical adjustment, the body will make the remedies necessary to protect itself against disease. The theory of maladjustment is not accepted by orthodox medical opinion, which does not believe that all pathological processes are caused by structural derangement of the skeleton, or indeed that diseases have one basic cause or can be cured by a single basic method. Nevertheless, the skill in manipulative surgery and the knowledge of bones and joints required in osteopathy is greater than that possessed by many orthodox practitioners. In theory, anyone can set up as an osteopath, but there are four schools of osteopathy approved by the General Council and Register of Osteopaths, and the degree of skill attained is shown by membership of the Osteopathic Association of Great Britain and inclusion in the Register of Osteopaths.

Osteophyte: an excrescence growing from a bone.

Osteoporosis: there is a loss of bone mass after the age of 50, which is more marked in women, although the chemical composition of the bone does not alter. There is a lack of balance between the processes of absorption and formation of bone, processes which continue throughout life. The consequence is that the cortex of the bone becomes thinner, and the internal buttressing, the trabeculation, less marked; the bones are more liable to fracture, and in the case of the vertebrae to collapse. There are a number of conditions other than age which can cause osteoporosis, but none as important. The cause of the loss of bone mass in elderly women, with the accompanying liability to fracture of the hip and forearm and painful and deforming collapse of the thoracic vertebrae, would appear to be related to the lack of oestrogen after the menopause, but the use of replacement oestrogen carries its own dangers, which are lessened if it is combined with progestogen (*see* Oestrogen). Replacement hormone therapy is undoubtedly important in those women who have had the ovaries removed, and, as this operation is usually accompanied by removal of the uterus, oestrogen alone can be used. The prevention of osteoporosis and its treatment are the subject of much research, for the high occurrence of broken bones in the elderly after a relatively minor fall presents many economic and social problems.

Osteosarcoma: a malignant tumour of bone.

Osteotomy: the surgical operation of cutting a bone.

Otitis: inflammation of the ear. Otitis externa involves the external opening and passage as far as the eardrum, otitis media involves the middle ear and otitis interna the inner ear. Otitis externa is usually due to an eczema of the skin lining the canal, and a simple eczematous discharge may respond to careful cleaning alone or corticosteroid ear-drops or ointment may be used. It may become infected and painful, but a local antibiotic such as chloramphenicol or gentamycin can be added to the drops. Occasionally a small boil forms, which is very painful, and systemic antibiotics may have to be used. In some cases the condition is complicated by a fungus infection, when it can become chronic and need specialist attention. Otitis media is a common infection in children between the ages of two and seven. The child is restless, complains of earache, often pulling at the lobe of the ear, and may have a temperature; there may be an accompanying cold. On examination with the otoscope, the drum is seen to be inflamed. Treatment is by antibiotics; the condition may recur, and may be connected with enlarged adenoids and tonsillar infections, in which case these may need attention, although removal of the tonsils and adenoids is avoided if possible, and any operation may be confined to removal of the adenoids. Middle ear infections may be followed by the development of chronic secretory otitis media, or glue ear, (q.v.). The complication of inflammation of the mastoid air cells, once common, has become rare. Infection of the inner ear is rare, and is caused by a virus; it is accompanied by severe giddiness, nausea and vomiting. It can be a complication of mumps.

Otolaryngology: sometimes called otorhinolaryngology, this specialty is concerned with the diseases and treatment of the throat, nose and ear.

Otology: the study of the ear considered as a single specialty.

Otorrhoea: a discharge from the ear, often caused by chronic otitis externa or media.

Otosclerosis: a common cause of deafness; the stapes, one of the ossicles of the middle ear, becomes bound to the oval window (*see* Ear) by new bone formation so that it can no longer move and transmit sound vibrations to the inner ear. The condition may be familial; it can be helped by operations designed to remove the adherent part of the stapes and replace it by an artificial footplate.

Otoscope: an instrument for examining the outer canal of the ear and the ear-drum.

Ovaries: the female sex glands. They are shaped like almonds, and measure about 4 cm long by 2 cm by 1 cm. In women who have not had children they lie applied to the side wall of the pelvis in front of the division of the iliac arteries, attached to the broad ligament, the double fold of peritoneum which covers the uterus and the two Fallopian tubes which run from the upper corners of the uterus to a position near the ovaries. The ovaries are attached to the uterus by the ovarian ligaments. In women who have had children the position of the ovaries varies, but the openings of the Fallopian tubes are always nearby. The ovaries have a cortex and medulla, and are covered by a thin layer of epithelium continuous with the peritoneum, and a thin layer of connective tissue. The cortex forms the bulk of the organ, and contains many germ cells arranged in follicles. Surrounding each germ cell there is a layer of cells called the granulosa layer, while cells next to them form the theca interna. A small cavity containing follicular fluid develops between the granulosa cells. One, or sometimes two, of the forming follicles continues to develop, and the others regress, so that usually only one follicle becomes mature each month. The fluid as it increases pushes the germ cell to one side, where it lies in a small clump of granulosa cells. The enlarging follicle attains a diameter of about 10 to 30 millimetres, having grown a thousand times bigger than the follicle from which it developed. It eventually ruptures, and discharges the germ cell onto the surface of the ovary near the opening of the Fallopian tube, into which it passes to become fertilised. The empty follicle collapses, and the granulosa cells multiply to form the corpus luteum, a yellow body which secretes the hormone progesterone. If fertilisation does not occur, the corpus luteum becomes inactive and degenerates into a mass called the corpus albicans. The ovarian hormones are discussed under the heading Menstruation (q.v.). The ovaries may be the seat of disease. Inflammation may spread from neighbouring structures, such as the Fallopian tubes or the appendix; mumps may affect the ovaries. Deposits of endometrial tissue may form (*see* Endometriosis), and cysts of the ovary are common. The majority are benign, and form between the ages of 30 and 60, often causing no symptoms until they grow large enough to cause a swelling in the abdomen, or press on the bladder to cause frequent passage of water or on the pelvic veins so that the legs swell. They may twist on their pedicle, or stalk, and cause considerable pain and vomiting; bleeding into the cyst, or rupture of the cyst, may cause pain and abdominal tenderness. Occasionally the cyst may be malignant. Treatment is surgical, with radiotherapy or chemotherapy in the case of malignant tumours.

Over-use Syndrome: *see* Tenosynovitis.

Ovulation: the shedding of an ovum, the germ cell, from the ovary each month, on or about the 15th day of each menstrual cycle.

Oxalates: oxalates are sometimes found in the urine after eating strawberries or rhubarb, and rarely there is an inherited error of metabolism in which oxalates are formed. Such patients suffer from kidney stones of calcium oxalate, and crystals may form in other tissues. Apart from this condition, kidney stones of calcium oxalate are common, and usually no biochemical reason is found for their formation. Oxalic acid itself is an irritant poison.

Oxidation: the combination of a substance with oxygen, or the removal of hydrogen; the increase of positive charges on an atom or the loss of negative charges. Univalent oxidation is the loss of one electron, divalent the loss of two.

Oxycephaly: a condition in which the head is more pointed than normal; also called steeple head.

Oxygen: a colourless, odourless gas which forms one-fifth of the air we breathe. It is the commonest element on earth; its atomic number is 8. It is essential for life, producing energy by the metabolism of glucose, and being transported to the tissues from the lungs in combination with the blood pigment haemoglobin. It is used in medicine for diseases of the lung, blood and circulation, when the take-up of oxygen from the air or its distribution in the body is impaired, and in anaesthesia.

Oxymel: a homemade medicine compounded of honey and vinegar, used for coughs, colds and sore throats; at one time recommended as a cure-all without any justification, it is harmless.

Oxytetracycline: an antibiotic; *see* Tetracycline.

Oxytocin: one of the two hormones synthesised in the hypothalamus and transferred to the posterior lobe of the pituitary gland, whence it is released. Its action is on the uterus and breasts; during suckling, it produces contraction of the muscular fibres in the milk ducts, causing the ejection of milk. It stimulates contraction of the uterus; it can be used to induce labour, and to reinforce the contractions; it can also be used in cases of bleeding after labour or incomplete abortion, when it is commonly combined with ergometrine. It is given intravenously or intramuscularly by injection.

Oxyuriasis: infestation with threadworm or pinworm. *See* Worms.

Ozaena: chronic disease of the nose in which there is atrophy of the lining, with the formation of foul-smelling discharge and crusts.

Ozone: a more active form of molecular oxygen, having three atoms instead of two; its chemical formula is O_3, while oxygen is O_2. It has a typical salty odour, but is poisonous in large quantities, for it irritates the lungs; air contains very small amounts. It is a powerful deodorant and germicide.

P

Pacemakers: are used in cases where the normal impulse-conducting system in the heart is blocked, and the heart rate falls to such an extent (the pulse rate may fall below 30 a minute) that the patient suffers from attacks of dizziness or loss of consciousness, known as a Stokes–Adams attack, or heart failure. The reason for the abnormal heart rate may not be known, but it may be associated with congenital defects or disease of the conduction system in the heart, coronary artery disease, or disease of the heart muscle. Digitalis or similar drugs may slow the pulse. The condition affects patients about the age of 70. The pacemaker consists of an electrode which is placed in the right ventricle of the heart and a small unit containing a battery and an electronic circuit producing the stimulating signal which is inserted under the skin of the left chest. The electrode is introduced into the subclavian vein or the central cephalic vein in the root of the neck, and under radiological control passed through the right atrium to lie at the apex of the right ventricle. The tip of the electrode lead is anchored to the muscular ridges inside the ventricle to keep the electrode in place; the operation can be carried out under local anaesthetic. The special batteries used last up to 10 years. The electronic circuit is so arranged that it will pick up impulses from the heart; if the heart rate returns to normal the pacemaker's impulse will cut out, and if the rate falls the pacing is resumed. Often the pacemaker is made so that it can be programmed by magnetic or radio signals to function according to the patient's needs. Advanced pacemakers may use two electrodes, one in the atrium and one in the ventricle, to stimulate more closely the normal conducting mechanism of the heart (q.v.).

Pachymeningitis: inflammation of the dura mater of the brain. *See* Meningitis.

Pacinian Corpuscle: a small structure about 4 mm long found below the skin and in other parts of the body, which in section is like an oval onion. It is attached to a sensory nerve fibre, and is sensitive to pressure. Named after Filippo Pacini, Italian anatomist (1812–83).

Paediatrics: that branch of medicine dealing with the diseases of children.

Paget's Disease (osteitis deformans): James Paget (1814–99), a London surgeon, described a number of diseases, the best known being a disease of bone. This is a disorganised absorption and generation of bone, commoner in men than women, occurring after the age of 40. The affected bones are enlarged and painful, and any bone can be involved, although the disease is commonest in the shin, the skull, the pelvis and the spine. The shins, and perhaps the thigh-bones, become bowed, and the joints arthritic; the thickening of the bone of the skull may lead to deafness, or other cranial nerve palsies. Fractures of the bones are liable to occur, and in some cases a sarcoma of the humerus may develop. The medical treatment of the disease requires the use of painkilling drugs, and in advanced cases may include the use of plicamycin, which is a cytotoxic drug, calcitonin or salcatonin which play a part in the regulation of bone destruction and formation, and disodium editronate, which slows down the rate of bone change. Paget's disease of the nipple is an inflammatory condition of the skin round the nipple which is due to an underlying malignant tumour.

Pain: the precise nature of pain is not fully understood. It is easy to say that it is an unpleasant sensation that arises when the body is damaged, but this is not the whole story; it is, for example, a matter of common observation that those who are injured by sudden violence may feel little pain for a considerable time, and that sensitivity to pain depends a great deal on the state of mind. In general it appears that the sensation of pain is originated by particular nerve endings called nociceptors, and carried by small myelinated sensory nerve fibres, called A delta fibres, and small unmyelinated fibres called C fibres. These fibres run in the sensory peripheral nerves to the spinal cord, where they have connections with many other nerve fibres, including some running down from the brain.

The connections take place in the region of the spinal cord called the dorsal horn; they are very complex, and the incoming impulses are locally organised, with the liberation of substance P, which transmits pain impulses, and a substance called encephalin which prevents its release. Some of the nerve impulses pass to motor nerve fibres which supply muscles, and some to the fibres of the sympathetic nervous system which supply blood vessels, abdominal organs and sweat glands, while others are transmitted to the brain. The impulses transmitted to the brain travel in fibres that transmit quickly, running in the spinothalamic tracts which lie in the antero-lateral part of the spinal cord, crossing from side to side, so that impulses set up in the right side of the body travel in the left side of the spinal cord and *vice versa*. From the thalamus in the brain the impulses travel to the cortex; they convey information about the occurrence of an injury, its location and extent, so that the appropriate action can be taken. Sensory impulses from the head are relayed through the fifth cranial nerve to the thalamus and cortex.

Although most tissues of the body are susceptible to pain, not all are sensitive; the brain itself, the liver and lungs cannot give rise to pain. The other tissues react to a variety of stimuli; hollow organs, such as the intestines and the ureters, are painful when distended; the mesentery of the intestine when stretched; heart muscle when the blood supply is disturbed; and the skin, being the outer covering of the body, reacts to many factors by feeling pain. The character of pain differs: that arising in the skin is sharp, and makes the subject move quickly away from the source of the injury, while that arising in the deeper structures is recognised as such and tends to keep the subject still. Pain may be sharply localised, but may be referred to a part removed from the true source of the pain, as when the pain from heart disease is referred to the left arm, the shoulder or the neck, or pain arising in the diaphragm is felt in the point of the shoulder. Pain arising in joints may be referred to surrounding parts of the limb. Pain is referred from deep to superficial structures.

The treatment of pain may be simple or extremely difficult, depending on whether it is acute or chronic. Chronic pain may be defined as that lasting for more than a month, continuing in spite of treatment. Acute pain draws attention to injury or disease, and is relieved by the treatment and healing of the underlying condition; in most cases it can be controlled by pain-killing drugs. For mild and moderate pain, aspirin or paracetamol are recommended; paracetamol may be compounded with codeine, dihydrocodeine or dextropropoxyphene, for which the names co-codamol, co-dydramol and co-proxamol have been adopted. NSAIDs (q.v.) are also used. For moderate to severe pain opioid analgesics are necessary, such as morphine, pethidine, and dextromoramide; there are a number of others which can be used as indicated. All may cause dependence, and in chronic pain, except that due to terminal illness, this means that they have to be used with caution.

Special pain clinics have been set up in recent years; in many cases there is no single way in which the problem of severe chronic pain can be treated, and not infrequently it requires the collaboration of more than one specialist. The subject is one in which considerable advances continue to be made.

Painter's Colic: when most paint contained lead, painters were liable to develop colic from lead-poisoning.

Palaeopathology: the study of disease processes shown in ancient remains.

Palate: the roof of the mouth, which is also the floor of the cavity of the nose. It consists of the hard palate in front, made of bone and covered by mucous membrane, and the soft palate behind, composed of muscle. When food is swallowed, the soft palate is drawn up to shut off the back of the nose.

Palliative Treatment: that undertaken to relieve distressing and painful symptoms occurring in a disease which is incurable.

Palpation: examination by touching.

Palpebrae: the eyelids.

Palpitations: an awareness of the heartbeat, felt in the neck or in the chest. The action of the heart is not normally felt, but may rise into consciousness if the force of the beat is increased, for example by strong emotion, or if it is irregular. The commonest type of irregularity is the extrasystole, a beat occurring outside the normal rhythm, which may happen in perfectly healthy people. The doubled rate in paroxysmal tachycardia (q.v.) may be felt as palpitations, as may other disturbances of rhythm due to cardiac abnormality, but in many cases palpitations are a symptom of anxiety; and once the heartbeat becomes conscious, as it may on lying in bed, it can be difficult to disregard it.

Palsy: an old word for paralysis.

Paludrine: the proprietary name for proguanil, a drug used for the prophylaxis of malaria (q.v.).

Panacea: a universal remedy.

Pancreas: a large mixed gland lying across the back wall of the upper abdominal cavity behind the stomach; its exocrine secretion is passed through the pancreatic duct into the duodenum, and its endocrine secretion passes directly into the bloodstream. It is elongated, about 15 cm long; it has a large head and a long body and tail. The head fits into the curve of the duodenum, and is on the right; the body passes to the left across the aorta, the left suprarenal gland and the left kidney, renal artery and vein. The tail continues upwards towards the spleen. The pancreas takes its blood supply from the splenic, hepatic and superior mesenteric arteries, with each of which it comes into close relationship. The pancreatic duct runs the length of the gland, collects the exocrine secretions from the lobules of the gland, and opens into the duodenum with the bile duct, which it joins just before the common orifice on the duodenal papilla in the second part of the duodenum. There may be an accessory duct draining directly into the duodenum. The gland contains many lobules which have a number of passages coming to blind ends called acini, lined with secreting cells which secrete the pancreatic juice. This is alkaline, and contains the forerunners of the enzymes trypsin and chymotripsin, which are activated by the intestinal juice, the enzymes amylase and lipase, and the chlorides of sodium, calcium and potassium. The enzymes play a large part in the digestion of food in the small intestine. The endocrine secretion of the pancreas is elaborated in small collections of cells called the islets of Langerhans (Paul Langerhans, 1847–88) which centre on capillary blood vessels and secrete insulin and glucagon, hormones concerned with carbohydrate metabolism. *See* Diabetes Mellitus.

Pancreatitis: inflammation of the pancreas. Acute attacks are associated with gall-bladder disease and gallstones, with alcoholism, with virus infections such as mumps, with various drugs and with high levels of fatty substances in the blood (hyperlipidaemia). The severity of the disease varies a great deal from relatively mild, with upper abdominal pain, nausea and vomiting, to rapidly fatal. Complications include the formation of cysts or abscesses, liver failure and jaundice, peritonitis, difficulty in breathing, kidney failure and paralysis of the small intestine. Occasionally blood seeps through into the left flank to produce discoloration of the skin. Treatment is of the symptoms as they arise; where there is an association with gallstones, surgery may be needed. In chronic pancreatitis there is inflammation resulting in progressive destruction of the gland, leading to disturbances of digestion and absorption of food and possibly diabetes. It is associated with alcoholism and malnutrition. Pain is a prominent feature of the condition; treatment is directed towards the relief of pain, and additionally requires the use of pancreatic enzymes to replace those lost. Control of the diabetes depends largely on the success of the replacement therapy for the impaired digestive processes. The patient must obviously abstain from alcohol.

Pandemic: an epidemic affecting a large area, for example a continent.

Panhysterectomy: the complete surgical removal of the uterus and its appendages.

Panophthalmitis: inflammation of all the structures of the eyeball.

Papilla: a small elevation shaped like a nipple.

Papilloedema: swelling and congestion of the head of the optic nerve as it enters the back of the eye, due to increased pressure inside the skull, clotting of the central vein of the retina, or high blood pressure.

Papilloma: a small tumour growing from the free surface of epithelium (q.v.). Papillomas are benign, and may be found on the skin, in the bladder, in the colon or rectum and in the pelvis of the kidney. Occasionally they may undergo malignant change to become a papillary adenocarcinoma. Treatment is according to their position: a simple papilloma on the skin is of little consequence, but those in the bladder or renal pelvis may bleed and have to be destroyed, and those in the large intestine are best removed.

Papovirus: there are two genera of papoviruses, both of which infect man. The commonest is the *papillomavirus* which produces warts on the feet (*verrucae plantares*), on the hands and knees (*verrucae vulgares*), on the genitals (*condylomata accuminata*), plane or juvenile warts (*verrucae planae*) and, rarely, warts in the mouth or in the larynx. *Polyomaviruses* have been found in the urinary tract of patients, particularly those with immune system deficiencies, and rarely in the brain where they cause a demyelinating disease. *See* Warts.

Papule: a small solid elevation of the skin; a pimple.

Paracentesis: the puncturing with a hollow needle of a body cavity in order to withdraw abnormal fluid for the relief of symptoms or for pathological examination.

Paracetamol: a widely used painkiller, which has an action similar to aspirin, but has no anti-inflammatory activity. It is less likely to irritate the stomach but in overdose may cause serious damage to the liver, which takes a few days to become apparent. It should be used in preference to aspirin for children under 12.

Paracusis: any alteration in the sense of hearing.

Paraesthesia: an abnormal sensation in the skin, which may be described as pins and needles, tingling, a feeling that ants are crawling over the skin (formication), or burning.

Paraffin: a mixture of hydrocarbons derived from petroleum which may be solid or liquid. It is used in medicine as a basis for ointments. Liquid paraffin was used as a laxative, but it has unwanted effects; it dissolves fat-soluble vitamins, if breathed in can give rise to pneumonia, and may produce granulomatous tumours known as paraffinomas in the mesenteric lymph nodes, the liver or the spleen, and in the mucosa of the intestine. It therefore should not be used.

Paragonimus: the lung fluke, a trematode worm, common in the East; it needs two intermediate hosts, the first being a freshwater snail and the second a freshwater crab or crayfish. If the crab is eaten raw or badly cooked, the paragonimus escapes into the intestines, makes its way through the wall of the gut, and journeys up through the abdominal cavity to reach the diaphragm, which it pierces to creep into the lungs. The treatment is praziquantel.

Paraldehyde: a colourless liquid of ethereal odour and nauseating taste which was used as a safe and powerful hypnotic, but is now reserved for cases of status epilepticus (repeated epileptic convulsions with no intervening period of consciousness) when it may be given rectally or by injection.

Paralysis: a loss of muscular power or the capacity to move, due to impairment of the nervous system or the muscular mechanism.

Paralysis Agitans: Parkinson's disease (q.v.).

Paralytic Ileus: a condition of the small intestine in which there is paralysis of the muscle of the gut due to peritonitis, injury or bleeding into the abdominal cavity. It may follow an abdominal operation.

Paramnesia: distortion or falsification of memory.

Paranasal Sinuses: the cavities in the frontal, sphenoid, ethmoid and maxillary bones, lined with mucous membrane and filled with air, that are in communication with the nose (q.v.).

Paranoia: the term paranoid indicates that the subject has ideas about relationships with other people that have no foundation in reality; the ideas are often about persecution, but not exclusively, although they involve some grievance; situations and words take on a meaning far from their true significance. This may be quite compatible with leading a normal life, although it is trying for colleagues and friends, but when exaggerated it is characteristic of a form of schizophrenia which is rare but may be dangerous if the delusions are directed against an individual.

Paraphimosis: if the foreskin is tight, and is drawn back beyond the corona of the penis, it may happen that the end of the penis becomes engorged and swollen so that the foreskin cannot be replaced. As the swelling increases because of the constriction a vicious circle is set up. It may be possible to replace the foreskin by steady pressure, but if it is not the foreskin can be surgically divided under general anaesthetic, and possibly later removed to prevent a recurrence.

Paraphrenia: some elderly patients, possibly women living alone, of a previously paranoid or depressed character, may develop symptoms of a frankly schizophrenic nature, although the original personality is retained. The state may be called late paraphrenia.

Paraplegia: paralysis of both sides of the body from the waist down.

Paraquat: a bipiridillium herbicide which is harmless if used with care, although irritating to the skin, but extremely poisonous if swallowed, producing irreversible damage to the lungs. There is no specific antidote.

Parasite: an organism which lives upon or within another organism, obtaining some advantage without conferring any in return. Man is the host for many parasitic organisms, including bacteria, viruses, protozoa (one-celled organisms), fungi, insects and worms.

Parasympathetic Nervous System: part of the autonomic nervous system. *See* Nervous System.

Parathyroid Glands: there are four parathyroid glands; they are attached to the back surface of the thyroid gland, two on each side, at the level of the middle of the gland and at its lower margin. They are small yellow bodies, measuring about 5 x 4 mm, and their function is to secrete the hormone parathormone, which regulates the use of calcium in the body, preventing the level in the blood becoming too low. Calcium is essential for many processes in the body, notably neuro-muscular function, and low levels lead to the development of tetany and convulsions. It is also essential for the secretion and action of hormones, and many other intracellular activities. Parathormone is secreted if the blood level of calcium falls, and has an action on the kidney to increase the reabsorption of calcium by the tubules and stimulate the production of calcitriol, vitamin D_3, which increases the absorption of calcium by the intestines. It also has an action on the bones, which contain the bulk of calcium in the body, stimulating the osteoclasts to absorb calcium and release it to the bloodstream. Over-secretion of the parathyroid hormone may result from tumours of the gland, and increases the amount of calcium in the blood. This commonly encourages the formation of stones in the urinary tract; other symptoms are vague, and include pains in the bones, fatigue and nausea. The tumour may be removed surgically. Deficiency of the hormone is commonly the result of removal of parathyroid tissue during operations on the thyroid gland, and results in a low level of calcium in the blood, with the development of tetany, which is spasm of the muscles usually of the forearm and leg, resulting in spasmodic flexion of the wrist and ankles, mental changes, and possibly convulsions. The treatment is by calcitriol or alfacalcidol, which are derivatives of vitamin D, with calcium.

Paratyphoid Fever: an enteric fever milder than typhoid (q.v.) caused by *Salmonella* organisms other than *Salmonella typhi*.

Paregoric: camphorated tincture of opium, which was used in cough mixtures and for diarrhoea.

Parenchyma: the functional tissue in an organ or gland, as distinct from the tissue forming the framework (stroma).

Parenteral: a method of administering drugs other than by the alimentary canal, for example by injection.

Paresis: weakness, as opposed to paralysis which is total loss of function.

Parietal: pertaining to the walls of a cavity; the parietal bones form the walls of the skull; the parietal pleura is the membrane that lies against the inside of the wall of the chest.

Parkinson's Disease: paralysis agitans, a disease of the nervous system occurring in late middle age, first described by the London physician James Parkinson (1775–1824). Recent work has shown it to be due to a degenerative process in the substantia nigra, a pigmented nucleus in the brain stem, which employs the substance dopamine as the transmitter of nerve impulses to the corpus striatum, one of the basal ganglia of the brain, in which there is consequently a deficiency of dopamine. The corpus striatum is part of the extrapyramidal motor nervous system; nerve fibres from the motor cortex of the brain run in the pyramidal tracts of the spinal cord (q.v.), but there are other motor nerve fibres running in the spinal cord outside the pyramidal tracts, and disease of this extrapyramidal system gives rise to stiffness of the muscles with loss of movement, as well as involuntary abnormal movements. The reason for the degeneration of the substantia nigra is not known. Parkinson's description of paralysis agitans runs (in part): 'involuntary tremulous motion, with lessened muscular power, in parts not in action and even when supported; with a propensity to bend the trunk forwards, and to pass from a walking to a running pace, the senses and intellect being uninjured'. The face loses expression, and the voice becomes weak; the patient slows down, and finds it hard to start walking, and then can only shuffle, although the pace may become uncontrollably fast. The tremor disappears in action, and in sleep, but is increased by emotion and excitement. The handwriting becomes increasingly small. The treatment of the disease has been revolutionised by the introduction of levadopa, which is converted to dopamine in the brain; its action is increased by combination with carbidopa or benserazide, which prevent it being broken down before it reaches the brain. Selegiline may also be used in conjunction with levadopa, particularly if the action of levadopa begins to fail. Bromocriptine can also be of use, but the dosage of levadopa has to be reduced if it is introduced. The drugs are more effective in reducing muscular stiffness and slowness than influencing the tremor. Physiotherapy can be most helpful in making the most of what movement is possible, and advice should be sought on the provision of aids to ease life at home.

Paronychia: an infection of the fold of flesh beside the nail.

Parotid Gland: the largest of the salivary glands, situated just in front of the ear and the angle of the lower jaw. It has a duct which opens into the mouth opposite the second last tooth of the upper jaw. The gland may be enlarged by mumps, when it forms a characteristic swelling raising the lobe of the ear, by other inflammation or because the duct is blocked by a stone; this produces a swelling which may vary in size, being worst just before a meal. The stone can often be shifted by sucking a lemon, or acid-drops, to increase the secretion of the gland.

Paroxysmal Nocturnal Dyspnoea (cardiac asthma): sudden breathlessness during the night, which may overtake patients suffering from heart failure. It is usually found in those who find it easier to breathe when sitting up (orthopnoea); when they slip down from their pillows at night, they wake up breathless, and can only get breath back by sitting up on the edge of the bed.

Paroxysmal Tachycardia: a disturbance in the normal rhythm of the heart, due to an extra conducting pathway between the atria and the ventricles (see Heart). This means that an impulse arising in the atrioventricular node can be passed back to the atrium from the ventricle, and if one pathway is capable of conduction while the other is in a resting phase and an extrasystole arises, that is a beat outside the normal rhythm (which can arise in a normal heart), a circle of impulses is set up which causes the heart to beat at twice its normal rate. The effect is that the patient suddenly feels the heart rate double, may feel breathless and uncomfortable, and may have to rest. The attack may last for an hour or more, and then go as suddenly as it started. It is likely to be brought on by over-exertion or fatigue. The condition usually affects hearts that are otherwise quite normal, and has no serious consequences. An attack can sometimes be stopped by pressure on the neck over the carotid sinus below the angle of the jaw, but usually stops on its own. It can often be prevented to a large extent by regular use of small doses of a beta-blocking drug such as propranolol or sotalol.

Parturition: the act of giving birth.

Pasteurisation: a process named after the French bacteriologist Louis Pasteur (1822–95), who founded the science of bacteriology and upon whose work is based a great deal of medical theory and practice, although he himself was not a physician. Pasteurisation is partial sterilisation, especially of milk, by heating, usually to a temperature of 60°C for 30 minutes; this is enough to kill most organisms of disease and delay the growth of other bacteria, thus prolonging the keeping time of milk and rendering it harmless. The same effect is realised by heating to 72°C for 15 seconds.

Patella: the kneecap.

Patent Ductus Arteriosus: a congenital condition in which the communication between the aorta and the pulmonary artery, which bypasses the lungs in the foetus, remains open at birth. The treatment is surgical; the open duct is tied off.

Pathogen: an organism, or other agent, capable of causing disease.

Pathognomonic: characteristic of a particular disease.

Pathology: the study of the nature of disease and the changes in structure and function brought about by disease.

Paul–Bunnell Test: a blood test for infectious mononucleosis (q.v.) (glandular fever). John Paul (1893–1971) and W.W. Bunnell (1902–1966), American physicians.

Pectoral: relating to the chest.

Pediculosis: infestation with lice. *See* Louse.

Pellagra: a deficiency disease resulting from lack of vitamin B$_3$. It was shown by Dr Joseph Goldberger (1874–1929), working in the southern part of the United States, that pellagra was due to a dietary deficiency of a substance soluble in water and unchanged by heat. He died before the substance was identified as nicotinic acid, a member of the vitamin B group, in 1937. Pellagra is found in places where the staple diet is maize, which is not only deficient in nicotinic acid but contains no tryptophan, an amino-acid from which the body can produce nicotinic acid. Otherwise it is found in those with digestive conditions that prevent the absorption of nicotinic acid and those whose diet is abnormally poor, for example alcoholics. The symptoms of pellagra are the three

Ds: diarrhoea, dermatitis and dementia. The treatment is the administration of nicotinic acid or nicotinamide.

Pelotherapy: the therapeutic use of mud.

Pelvimetry: measurement of the pelvis, particularly of its outlet, made by the obstetrician in order to estimate the chances of a normal delivery in cases where there may be disproportion between the head of the baby and the bony part of the birth canal.

Pelvis: the pelvis is the large complex of bones shaped rather like a basin which connects the spine with the legs and contains the lowest part of the abdominal cavity. It is formed of the two hip-bones, the sacrum and the coccyx; in front the two hip-bones meet each other at the symphysis pubis, and behind they join the sacrum, a curved wedge-shaped bone lying in the midline, made up from five fused vertebral bodies. The hip-bones are made up of three bones, separate in the child but fused in the adult, the ilium, pubis and ischium. On the outer surface of the bone is the acetabulum, the socket of the ball-and-socket hip joint. The ilium forms the crest of the pelvis, which can be felt below the waist, and the ischium the rounded tuberosity upon which one sits. In front of the tuberosity the ischium splits into two branches, the rami, which join the two rami of the pubic bone; these join in front, and the right and left pubic bones meet in the midline and are bound together at the pubic symphysis. Between the rami of the ischium and pubis is an aperture, the obturator foramen. At the back, the two hip-bones make right and left sacro-iliac joints, which involve the upper three segments of the sacrum. They are large joints which follow the curve of the sacrum, and the bones are bound together by strong ligaments, for the joints carry the weight of the upper body; the upper surface of the sacrum makes a joint with the fifth lumbar vertebra of the spinal column. The coccyx is a small bone made up of three of four incomplete vertebrae fused together, the last being only a nodule. It joins the lower part of the sacrum, and is a vestigial tail. The pelvis lies at an angle, for the lumbar spine and the sacrum meet at about 140–150° and the pelvis is tilted forwards; the plane of its inlet is about 50° to the horizontal. There are differences between the male and female pelvis: the female pelvis is wider, and tends to a more cylindrical than funnel shape.

Pemphigus: a term used for skin diseases in which blisters develop.

Penicillin: the first antibiotic drug, discovered in London by Alexander Fleming in 1928 in the mould *Penicillium notatum*. In 1938 Ernst Chain drew the attention of Howard Florey to Fleming's work, and together they established that penicillin cured streptococcal infection in mice. In 1941 it was used successfully in human infections. Since then a large number of derivatives have been made, and they have completely revolutionised the treatment of infections with staphylococci, streptococci, some spirochaetes, including those responsible for syphilis, and various fungi. Fleming, Florey and Chain received the Nobel Prize in 1945; Fleming (1881–1955) and Chain (1906–79) were knighted, and Florey (1898–1968) died a life peer.

Penis: the male sex organ through which semen and urine are discharged by way of the urethra. The shaft of the penis contains spongy tissue which fills with blood during sexual excitement: the ensuing erection makes sexual intercourse possible.

Pepsin: an enzyme secreted by the stomach which breaks down protein in the food to polypeptides.

Peptic Ulcer: ulcers in the stomach and duodenum are referred to as peptic ulcers. Duodenal ulcers are more common than those in the stomach, and more common in men than women, who are more liable to develop duodenal ulcers after the menopause. The exact cause of the ulcer is not known, although it appears to have become more common at the beginning of this century; the severity of the condition now appears to be becoming less. The 'stress of modern life' is often blamed for the development of an ulcer, but in truth life has always been full of anxiety, and ulcers appear in some people but not in others exposed to the same strains. There is an increased tendency to have a higher acid content in the stomach, and the food is passed out of the stomach into the duodenum faster in duodenal ulcer patients than is normal, so that there is less food to neutralise the acid in the duodenum. An organism, *Campylobacter pylori*, has been found in the duodenum and linked to the development of ulcers. Smoking and alcohol have also been linked with ulcers, and the NSAIDs (q.v.) are liable to cause ulceration.

The symptom of ulceration is pain related to food, felt in the upper abdomen and worse at night. Complications include bleeding from the ulcer and perforation of the duodenum with peritonitis, but they are comparatively rare, bleeding being more common than perforation. Diagnosis is made by endoscopy or X-ray examination, using barium as a contrast medium, for the intestines and stomach are radio-translucent.

Gastric ulcers may be caused by a combination of acidity and a tendency for the contents of the duodenum to flow backwards into the stomach, for the duodenal juice contains bile and a number of enzymes which can damage the lining of the stomach. They may also be caused by NSAIDs. They give rise to pain in the upper abdomen, and it is particularly important that they should be examined through the gastroscope, for the diagnosis must be made between a simple ulcer and an early malignant ulceration.

Duodenal and gastric ulcers are treated in the same way, first by the advice to eat little and often, and to give up smoking and use alcohol in moderation. Simple antacids, of which there are many, including aluminium hydroxide, magnesium carbonate and trisilicate and sodium bicarbonate, are best taken an hour or so after food, and the dose repeated if the pain recurs, for if they are taken directly after food they are lost when the stomach empties. Antacids do not unfortunately cure ulcers, although they relieve the pain; but there are ways of decreasing the secretion of acid in the stomach, controlled by the vagus nerve, which rely on blocking the stimulating agents, acetylcholine and histamine. Pirenzepine is an anti-cholinergic drug which inhibits the secretion of acid and pepsin, and the action of histamine is inhibited by cimetidine, nizatidine, ranitidine and famotidine. Histamine has an action throughout the body, but there are two types of receptors through which it works: H_1 and H_2. The receptors in the stomach are of the H_2 type, and the drugs named above only antagonise H_2 receptors, thus having little effect on the rest of the body. Cimetidine, the oldest of the drugs, is the most liable to produce unwanted effects.

Treatment by these drugs is effective in the majority of cases, but peptic ulcers tend to recur, and in some cases medical treatment is ineffective. In such instances surgical treatment may be required, as it is in cases where the ulcer perforates or bleeds uncontrollably. The operation commonly carried out for resistant duodenal ulcers is division of the vagus nerve, which may be combined with a procedure to ensure adequate emptying of the stomach such as a plastic operation on the pylorus of the stomach (pyloroplasty) or an artificial connection between the stomach and the small intestine (gastro-enterostomy). Alternatively a selective division of the vagus may be undertaken, leaving the nervous supply of the emptying mechanism untouched but interrupting the fibres controlling the secretory cells of the stomach. Resistant gastric ulcers are usually treated by partial removal of the stomach (partial gastrectomy).

Percussion: the procedure of tapping the body with the fingers to detect the resonance of structures lying below the surface. Usually one hand with the fingers spread is placed on the body, and the middle finger tapped with the middle finger of the other hand. A flat sound indicates that the tissue below is solid, a resonant note that it is hollow. Percussion over a healthy lung gives a resonant sound, while over a lung consolidated by pneumonia, or over an effusion of fluid in the chest, the note is flat.

Perforation: piercing a hole, or the resulting hole itself. Perforations may be made by sharp instruments, or may occur through disease, as with the perforations in the stomach or duodenum resulting from ulceration.

Periarteritis Nodosa: inflammation of the outer part of the wall of an artery and the tissues immediately round about. Also *see* Polyarteritis.

Periarthritis: inflammation of the tissues surrounding a joint.

Pericarditis: inflammation of the pericardium, the membrane surrounding the heart. It may occur in association with coronary thrombosis, virus infection, tuberculosis, rheumatic heart disease or bacterial infection, or as the result of injury. There is pain in the chest, and if there is an effusion of fluid between the two layers of the pericardium the action of the heart may be affected. It may then be necessary to aspirate the fluid.

Pericardium: the membranous sac which contains the heart. It has two layers, between which is a capillary space containing a film of fluid. This provides lubrication to assist the free movement of the heart in relation to neighbouring structures. The outermost part of the pericardium is fibrous.

Perichondrium: the thin membrane which covers cartilage, except on free joint surfaces.

Pericranium: the periosteal membrane covering the skull.

Perilymph: the fluid found in the inner ear separating the membrane of the labyrinth from the surrounding bone. It does not communicate with the endolymph, the fluid inside the membranous labyrinth. *See* Ear.

Perimetry: measurement of the outer limits of the field of vision of each eye.

Perinephric: surrounding the kidney.

Perineum: the fork, strictly the region between the genital organs in front and the anus behind. Extended to mean the area bounded by the pubic symphysis, the ischial tuberosities and the coccyx.

Periods: *see* Menstruation.

Periodic Disease: recurrent polyserositis: a disease of unknown cause, inherited as a recessive trait, commonest among Arabs, Armenians, Jews and Turks, which usually starts before the age of 20; the patient suffers a variety of symptoms. It may resemble acute peritonitis, with abdominal pain, vomiting, and a raised temperature and pulse; the condition lasts for a day or two. There may be pain in the chest, resembling pleurisy, pains in the joints, a red skin rash over the legs and ankles, and severe headache. As the name indicates, the symptoms recur from time to time. Acute attacks are treated with colchicine. The disease is not dangerous, but a certain number of patients develop amyloid disease (q.v.).

Periosteum: the thin membrane of connective tissue that surrounds the bones.

Periostitis: inflammation of the periosteum. It may follow injury, when the periosteum is stripped from the bone and there is an extravasation of blood, an open fracture, or bacterial infection in neighbouring tissues; it can be caused by tuberculosis and syphilis.

Peripheral: a term applied to structures towards the outer parts or extremities, for example the peripheral as opposed to the central nervous system.

Peristalsis: the process by which the contents are propelled along tubular organs, as in the intestines; contractions of the muscle in the walls of the gut pass in a wave-like motion along its length, being controlled by the nervous plexus present there.

Peritoneoscopy (laparoscopy): the examination of the peritoneal cavity and abdominal organs through an endoscope passed through the abdominal wall.

Peritoneum: the membrane covering the inner walls of the abdominal cavity and the organs it contains. There are two layers: the membrane covering the wall of the cavity is the parietal layer, and that covering the abdominal organs the visceral layer. Between the two layers is a thin film of fluid which acts as a lubricant and allows the organs to move in relation to each other and the abdominal walls. The peritoneum forms various folds by which the organs are suspended, and one large fold in front called the omentum, an apron containing fat which hangs down from the stomach. To the back of it is applied the transverse colon, which lies just below the stomach. The small intestine is attached to the back wall of the abdomen by a fold of peritoneum called the mesentery, in which run the blood vessels and lymphatics of the gut. The kidneys, ureters and bladder lie outside the peritoneum, with only part of their surfaces covered by the membrane. The visceral peritoneum covering the duodenum, ascending and descending colon fuses with the parietal peritoneum where these structures lie against the posterior abdominal wall, except for that part of the descending colon called the sigmoid, which has a free mesentery. The peritoneal cavity extends from the diaphragm to the floor of the pelvis; in the male it is closed, but in the female the cavity communicates with the exterior through the openings of the uterine (Fallopian) tubes. The folds of the peritoneum formed to contain the various organs make up interconnecting compartments, the most important of which are the lesser sac lying behind the stomach and the greater sac which comprises the rest of the cavity. In disease pus or blood may collect in a compartment and give a clue to its origin, for example a gastric ulcer may perforate in the posterior wall of the stomach into the lesser sac. When inflamed locally the peritoneum may produce a sticky exudate to which the omentum adheres, thus sealing off the area, or the peritoneum may itself seal off the infection.

Peritonitis: inflammation of the peritoneum. In the acute form, most cases occur as a result of disease of an abdominal organ, for example appendicitis or diverticulitis, perforation of a peptic ulcer, or perforation of the bowel due to an obstruction or a malignant tumour. There is an exudate from the peritoneum, paralysis of the bowel, abdominal pain with vomiting and spasm of the muscles of the abdominal wall. The patient becomes shocked, with a rising pulse rate and falling blood pressure. The condition is a surgical emergency. Chronic peritonitis may be the result of tuberculosis, when the symptoms are insidious; the patient loses weight, runs a temperature, and may develop a protruding abdomen due to the collection of fluid within the peritoneal cavity. There may be pain and diarrhoea. Treatment is by anti-tuberculous drugs.

Peritonsillar Abscess (quinsy): an abscess round the tonsil, usually occurring as the result of acute infection of the tonsils. The abscess forms behind the upper part of the tonsil, and as it develops the tissues become swollen, there is increasing pain, with difficulty in swallowing, and a feeling of choking. There is a high temperature. The abscess may burst of itself, or have to be opened by a slight operation which can be carried out under a local anaesthetic, and antibiotics are given according to the infecting organism. Quinsies may recur, and consideration must then be given to the advisability of removing the tonsils when the infection has resolved.

Pernicious Anaemia: a megaloblastic anaemia, that is, with red cells larger than normal, first described by Thomas Addison (1793–1860), a London physician, and sometimes known as Addisonian anaemia. It is due to deficiency of vitamin B_{12}, a water-soluble vitamin, without which red cells cannot properly be formed in the bone marrow. Vitamin B_{12} in the food combines with a substance called intrinsic factor, secreted by the stomach, and the combination is absorbed in the ileum, whence the B_{12} is transported to the liver while the intrinsic factor is digested in the absorbing cell. In the blood plasma the vitamin is combined with another substance called transcobalamin. In pernicious anaemia, there is an atrophy of the stomach cells which can no longer secrete acid or the intrinsic factor, and to this extent it is a disease of the stomach rather than the blood. An immune reaction has been suggested as the basis of the condition, for antibodies are found to the intrinsic factor in the serum. It is a disease of late middle age, and is said to be more common in northern Europeans and those with blue eyes. The symptoms are those of anaemia, with fatigue, breathlessness and weakness to which may be added a sore tongue and involvement of the nervous system, resulting in numbness and pins and needles in the legs and feet, with unsteadiness and difficulty in walking. Treatment is by the injection of vitamin B_{12} (hydroxycobalamin); after the first course, when it is given five or six times over a few weeks at intervals of a few days, it should be given by intramuscular injection every three months for life. Other types of macrocytic anaemia may be due to deficiency of vitamin B_{12} or folate, another water-soluble vitamin without which red blood cells cannot be formed normally. It is present in most foods, but especially in liver, fresh vegetables and fruit, and those on poor diets may develop a folate deficiency, as may those suffering from diseases causing malabsorption such as sprue or coeliac disease. In pregnancy there is an increased need for folate, which may not be met, and folic acid should be given routinely during pregnancy. Some drugs may cause deficiency of B_{12} such as barbiturates and alcohol, although beer drinkers find enough in the beer which has a high content; but it may occur in alcoholic cirrhosis of the liver. The diagnosis is made on biochemical examination of the blood, and the deficiency is made good by folic acid.

Pernio: a chilblain.

Peroneal: the name given to the structures of the outer side of the leg: perone, which means a pin, is the Greek name for the fibula.

Peroxide of Hydrogen: H_2O_2, a colourless and odourless liquid, which gives up bubbles of oxygen, and is an antiseptic and cleaning agent. It can be used as a mouth-wash in a 6% solution mixed with water, or for cleaning and disinfecting ulcers and wounds. A solution in warm water can be very useful in removing dressings that have stuck, without disturbing the wound. It may also be used to remove wax from the ears.

Perspiration: sweat is secreted by glands in the skin, which are distributed all over the body; they number three or four million, and secrete a watery fluid which evaporates from the skin and by doing so cools the body when it is exposed to heat, or is subject to a higher temperature than normal, as when the metabolic rate is increased in exercise or fever. The glands are more frequent in the palms of the hands and the soles of the feet. They are supplied by the sympathetic nervous system under the control of the hypothalamic area of the brain; the nerve fibres release acetylcholine to activate them. Under normal circumstances about half a litre of water is lost unnoticed every day by insensible perspiration, but the sweat glands can produce up to two or three litres an hour. The cooling effect of the evaporation of sweat is most important in regulating the body temperature in hot climates, but sodium chloride may be lost in the sweat. It is therefore sensible to take more salt if sweating is excessive. Sweating caused by a warm atmosphere occurs over the whole of the body, but is more obvious on the forehead, the upper lip, the neck and the chest. Sweating can also be caused by emotion or anxiety, especially in young people, and then it is more obvious on the palms, the soles of the feet and in the armpits. It may be worrying because of the breakdown of the fluid by bacteria on the skin or clothes, which produces a smell; this is worse in hot weather or hot surroundings. In such cases the obvious treatment is the avoidance of anxiety and hot surroundings, but this is easier said than done. Loose clothes, preferably cotton, frequent changes of socks, the avoidance of shoes which prevent the circulation of air, and frequent washing all help, and in severe cases the drug propantheline, which counteracts the action of acetylcholine, may be used. Local application to a dry skin of aluminium chloride hexahydrate in alcohol or aluminium hydroxychloride in a cream or gel stops excessive sweating, and may be used in the armpits; a solution of 3% formalin may be used for soaking the feet for 10 minutes. In cases of uncontrollable excessive sweating in the armpits the nervous supply to the glands may be interrupted surgically, or the part of skin containing the overacting glands removed.

Pertussis (whooping cough): a disease of children caused by bacterial infection of the respiratory tract by *Bordatella pertussis*, an organism which attacks the ciliated epithelial cells of the air passages. These are cells with constantly moving hairlike processes which clear the air passages of foreign matter, and pass secretions upwards so that they can be coughed out. If this process is impaired, an unproductive dry hacking cough develops which lasts for weeks. Whooping cough starts about a week after infection with a catarrhal phase which is similar to any mild upper respiratory infection, and then the cough develops. There is a mild fever and loss of appetite, and the child feels ill. After a week or so, the cough becomes paroxysmal, and a bout of coughing is followed by the characteristic whoop which is caused by trying to breathe in through partially closed vocal cords. Vomiting may occur, and nose bleeding or haemorrhages across the whites of the eyes. In infants there may be no whoop, but the paroxysm of coughing can be followed by a period of apnoea, that is, they stop breathing and may go blue. The most common complications are pneumonia and infection of the middle ear, areas of collapse in the lungs and convulsions. In very rare cases there may be serious damage to the central nervous system. Paroxysmal coughing lasts between two weeks and a month, but coughing lasts for much longer, and the whoop may return if the child develops a simple upper respiratory infection. The infection is spread by droplets; it is possible for adults to spread the infection, although in older people the disease does not go beyond the catarrhal stage. The organisms of whooping cough are sensitive to the antibiotics erythromycin and tetracycline, but the latter is best avoided in children as it stains the teeth. Unfortunately antibiotics are not effective in shortening the course of the disease once it has reached the stage of paroxysmal coughing, but they will prevent the spread of infection, and can be given to contacts who have not been immunised. Figures from the USA and Canada show that vaccination has been extremely effective in controlling the disease, but the use of the vaccine in the UK has been the subject of controversy; the period during which the vaccine was unpopular showed an increase in the number of cases. The vaccine does sometimes cause local reactions and fever, and has been held to be responsible for extremely rare cases of damage to the central nervous system; nevertheless serious reactions to the vaccine are far outnumbered by the serious consequences of this distressing disease.

Pes Cavus: a foot with an exaggerated arch in the longitudinal axis, often associated with claw toes. It is usually congenital, but may be associated with disease of the nervous system, for example poliomyelitis. There may be real difficulty in finding shoes to fit, but if this can be done there are usually no symptoms. Very severe cases may need surgical treatment.

Pessary: an instrument in various forms, usually a ring, designed to support a prolapsed womb from inside the vagina. Alternatively, it means a vaginal suppository.

Pestis: plague (q.v.).

Petechia: a pinpoint red or purple spot in the skin or mucous membrane due to a tiny haemorrhage from a capillary blood vessel.

Pethidine: a synthetic drug with a narcotic painkilling action, similar to morphine but less powerful and lasting for a shorter time, used often in obstetrics and as a premedication for general anaesthesia. It is a drug of addiction.

Petit Mal: a form of minor epilepsy (q.v.).

Peyotl: a substance produced from the Mexican cactus *Anhalonium lewenii*. It has an action similar to that of mescaline (q.v.).

pH: a measure of acidity; pH 7 is neutral: less than pH 7 is acid, and more than pH 7 alkaline. The pH expresses the concentration of hydrogen ions in a solution as the negative logarithm to the base 10.

Phaeochromocytoma: a rare tumour of the medulla of the suprarenal gland, which secretes adrenaline and noradrenaline in excess, causing paroxysmal attacks of high blood pressure, headache and palpitations. A similar tumour may develop in a ganglion of the sympathetic nervous system, when it is known as a paraganglioma.

Phage: or bacteriophage is a virus which can only reproduce itself in a bacterium.

Phagocyte: any cell able to engulf foreign matter such as bacteria; in particular, polymorphonuclear white blood cells, monocytes, and macrophages.

Phalanx: the phalanges are the small straight bones of the fingers and toes.

Phalloidin: the toxin of the poisonous fungus *Amanita phalloides*, which produces necrosis of the liver and kidneys if eaten in mistake for an edible mushroom. The only treatment is renal dialysis undertaken within 24 hours.

Phantom Limb: after a limb has been amputated, the patient often has the sensation that it is still there. Usually the phantom disappears after a time, but in rare cases it persists and becomes painful, presenting a difficult problem. There is, however, a natural tendency for the pain to improve and eventually go.

Pharmacology: the study of the action of chemical substances on living organisms. The clinical pharmacologist studies their action in man. It was not until the nineteenth century that developments in chemistry and in the understanding of disease enabled pharmacology to begin to emerge from the mass of untidy and often useless formulae that had accumulated over the centuries, and at the turn of this century an ever-increasing stream of drugs began to emerge from the laboratories; it has never stopped, and does not look like stopping. As the understanding of physiology, the way organisms work, extends, and the way the processes are disturbed by disease become clearer, so the scientific basis of clinical pharmacology becomes firmer. An idea of the rate of change in the last 50 years may be gained from the fact that of 110 widely used efficient drugs listed recently to treat common diseases, only 15 were available in 1945.

Pharmacopoea: the official list of drugs. The British Pharmacopoea is the responsibility of the British Pharmacopoea Commission, set up under the Medicines Act of 1968. A handbook for medical practitioners is published by the British Medical Association and the Royal Pharmaceutical Society as the British National Formulary, and is revised every six months.

Pharmacy: the technique or art of preparing and dispensing medicines, and the place where they are prepared or sold.

Pharyngitis: inflammation of the pharynx, a common accompaniment of upper respiratory infections.

Pharynx: in front, the pharynx is continuous with the nasal cavity and the mouth. Above, the pharynx reaches to the base of the skull behind the upper part of the nose, and below it is continuous with the larynx and the oesophagus. In its upper part the Eustachian tubes, which run from the middle ear, open on each side, and from the back wall grow the adenoids, masses of lymphatic tissue. The pharynx has three constrictor muscles: when food is swallowed, the soft palate rises to shut the nasal cavity, the epiglottis rises to shut off the larynx, and the constrictor muscles direct the food into the oesophagus.

Phenacetin: a mild analgesic drug similar in action to aspirin, used for many years but found to be liable if used over a period of time to produce damage to the kidneys. It is no longer used.

Phenergan: the proprietary name for the antihistamine drug promethazine hydrochloride. *See* Antihistamines.

Phenindione: a drug which can be taken by mouth to reduce the clotting power of blood; it antagonises the effect of vitamin K. It is liable to excite various sensitivity reactions such as skin rashes and diarrhoea, and it colours the urine pink.

Phenobarbitone: a sedative and antiepileptic drug now controlled under the Misuse of Drugs Regulations because of the addictive properties of the barbiturates. The use of phenobarbitone is confined to the control of epilepsy.

Phenol (carbolic acid): a crystalline derivative of coal tar. When water is added it becomes a powerful disinfectant and antiseptic. It was the substance used by Lord Lister in his original antiseptic surgical technique, which revolutionised surgery, but is now used less in medicine. It is extremely poisonous if swallowed.

Phenolphthalein: a laxative substance, liable to cause skin rashes, and for that reason better not used. It turns alkaline urine pink, and because it is recycled in the liver its action may last for several days.

Phenylbutazone: one of the NSAID group of drugs, formerly used for rheumatic diseases and gout but found to have serious unwanted effects: it may cause peptic ulcers, interfere with the formation of the blood cells, and lead to fluid retention severe enough to precipitate heart failure in patients with heart disease. It has therefore fallen into disuse except in certain special cases.

Phenylketonuria: an inherited inborn error of metabolism, in which the enzyme which should break down the amino-acid phenylalanine is absent; accumulation of this substance in the body impairs the development of the nervous system and although babies with the condition appear normal at birth they show a considerable mental handicap as they grow up. They tend to be fair, with blond hair and blue eyes. Babies should be tested for phenylketonuria at the age of six days, using the Guthrie test carried out on a dried spot of blood on a filter paper. The treatment is by a special diet which contains a reduced amount of phenylalanine; it has to be well controlled, as a deficiency of phenylalanine leads to further mental impairment and other symptoms, so that it is necessary to estimate the amount of phenylalanine in the blood at regular intervals. The special diet has to continue at least to the age of 10, and if possible to the age of about 16. After that the patient has to stay on a diet restricted in protein.

Phenytoin: an anticonvulsant drug used widely in the treatment of epilepsy, sometimes in combination with phenobarbitone. It may coarsen the skin of the face, or produce acne, as well as excessive growth of hair; the gums may become enlarged and prone to bleed. Some cases of trigeminal neuralgia that do not respond well to carbamazepine may be suited by phenytoin, or the two drugs may be used in combination.

Phimosis: the opening of the foreskin may be too small for it to be drawn over the end of the penis. This is quite common in little boys, but it must be remembered that the foreskin may not be entirely free from the underlying glans penis until the age of three or four. Phimosis is often thought to be an indication for circumcision, but this is not necessarily so, unless it leads to infection (balanitis) or irreducible paraphimosis (q.v.).

Phlebitis: inflammation of a vein. It may happen as the result of injury or infection, but the term is commonly applied to the condition of superficial venous thrombosis, clotting of a vein just under the skin, which commonly happens in varicose veins of the leg. It is not dangerous, and is best treated by NSAI drugs (q.v.). Suitable varicose veins can be treated by inducing them to thrombose by an injection of a sclerosing solution such as ethanolamine oleate, for the clot is followed by scarring of the vein which eventually becomes a fibrous cord.

Phlebolith: a stone in a vein. Concretions are not uncommon, especially in the veins of the pelvis, where they have been mistaken for stones in the ureter on radiographs.

Phlebotomus: the sandfly, a small biting fly found in subtropical and tropical countries. The female sandfly carries the organisms of leishmaniasis (q.v.) and sandfly fever, an acute fever lasting for a few days caused by a virus.

Phlebotomy: the incision of a vein in blood letting, or to insert a cannula.

Phlyctenula: a very small blister or ulcer on the conjunctiva or cornea.

Phobia: abnormal fear. A compound word is often made with phobia as the suffix to the name of the object feared, for example agoraphobia, fear of being in the open, or claustrophobia, fear of being shut up.

Phocomelia: a congenital malformation in which the limbs do not develop, and the hands or feet are attached to the body. This was a common malformation caused by thalidomide.

Phonocardiogram: a record of the sound vibrations made by the action of the heart.

Phosgene (carbonyl chloride): a colourless gas known since 1812, used by the German army in the First World War as a war gas which attacked the lungs. It is heavier than air and therefore collects in trenches and dug-outs.

Phosphorus: at one time the cause of 'phossy jaw', a necrosis of the lower jaw found in workers in chemical and match factories, phosphorus in its yellow waxy form is now used in making fireworks and similar products and rarely in rat poison. It is very poisonous if swallowed, and can produce burns if it comes in contact with the skin. The red form is not dangerous.

Photophobia: fear of the light. It is a symptom of some eye diseases and of irritation of the meninges, the membranes surrounding the brain, for example in meningitis.

Photosensitivity: excessive sensitivity of the skin to light, particularly the light of the sun. It is a feature of the inborn error of metabolism called porphyria, a fairly rare disease, and may be caused by a number of drugs including sulphonamides, tetracyclines, the antimalarial chloroquine, some phenothiazines used in psychotic disorders, the diuretic bendrofluazide and other thiazides, and rarely the oral antidiabetic sulphonylureas.

Photosynthesis: the process by which green plants, using the pigment chlorophyll, synthesise carbohydrates from carbon dioxide and water, using energy derived from the sun.

Phrenic Nerve: the nerve which supplies the muscle of the diaphragm. Because the diaphragm develops from the tissues of the neck and during the course of development passes down from the region of the neck to lie between the chest cavity and the abdomen, the phrenic nerve takes its origin from the nerve plexus in the neck, called the cervical plexus, and passes down through the chest to reach the diaphragm. Pain arising in the diaphragm is often referred to the tip of the shoulder.

Phrenology: a pseudoscience founded in about 1800 by Franz Gall (1758–1828) in Vienna, who maintained that anatomical studies showed that there are 37 areas of the brain responsible for traits of character, and that these areas are reflected by lumps on the surface of the skull; he therefore concluded that character could be deduced from examination of the head. The doctrine, once fashionable, has no basis in fact.

Phthirius Pubis: the crab louse.

Phthisis: wasting; because it was so often associated with pulmonary tuberculosis, the word was frequently used as a synonym for the disease.

Physics: scientists working in physics have a large part to play in many different fields of medicine, including computer science, radiation physics, ultrasonics, electronics, biological engineering, the measurement of physiological functions, nuclear magnetic resonance and the application of lasers. There is obviously enormous potential in the application of physics to medicine.

Physiology: the study of the functional processes of living organisms.

Physiotherapy: treatment by physical methods, including

active and passive movements, exercises, massage, the use of electrical stimulation, and heat. The profession of physiotherapy is under the control of the Chartered Society of Physiotherapists. It is essential for the practice of medicine both in and out of hospital, not only in the treatment of diseases of the joints, muscles and ligaments, but also in the treatment of diseases of the nervous system and the respiratory system, the difficulties of old age and of terminal illness.

Physostigmine: eserine (q.v.).

Pia Mater: the innermost of the three membranes that cover the spinal cord and brain. It dips down between the convolutions of the cortex, and forms a sheath round the blood vessels of the brain as they enter its substance. It is very delicate, and is separated from the arachnoid mater by a space containing the cerebrospinal fluid. There are many fibrous connections between the two membranes.

Pica: a perversion of appetite, which may be found in children and adults, usually pregnant women. It may occur in iron deficiency anaemia. Things are eaten which would not normally be considered fit to eat, such as soap, clay or coal.

Piles: *see* Haemorrhoids.

Pilocarpine: an alkaloid derived from the leaves of the plant *Pilocarpus microphyllus* or *jaborandi*. Its action mimics stimulation of the parasympathetic nervous system, and it is used in eye-drops in the treatment of glaucoma, when it constricts the pupil of the eye.

Pilonidal Sinus: a small abnormal opening in the skin in the midline about 3 cm behind the anus which contains hairs. It is often infected, when it becomes painful and swollen. Never seen in children, it is in some way connected with the development of body hair, but the precise way it forms is obscure. It may be similar to the sinuses which form on the hands of barbers because hairs are driven into the skin;

it may be congenital. The treatment is surgical excision.

Pineal Body: a small structure in the brain, formed by a projection from the back wall of the third ventricle (*see* Nervous System). It was thought by Descartes to be the seat of the soul, by others to be a third eye; in animals it has been found to influence the sexual cycle and the pigmentation of the skin; but in man its significance is unknown. Children who develop a tumour of the gland, which is rare, may be retarded in their sexual development according to one report, or undergo precocious puberty according to another.

Pinguecula: a yellowish spot which forms in the conjunctiva of the eye on the nasal side of the cornea in elderly people. It is harmless.

Pink Disease: a disease in which young children between six months and three years become irritable, develop a rash and dislike of the light (photophobia) and painful, swollen and cold hands and feet. The nose, ears and cheeks are red. It was found that this condition was caused by mercury used in teething powders, and as soon as this was realised and the use of mercury in children's medicine abandoned, the disease disappeared.

Pinkeye: a contagious epidemic type of conjunctivitis, in which the membrane covering the white of the eye becomes red, painful and swollen. It is due to a virus infection, and is spread by direct contact with hands that have been rubbing itching and sore eyes as well as through towels and face-flannels. It resolves spontaneously, but chloramphenicol or gentamycin eye-drops or ointment may be used to stop secondary bacterial infection. Ointments should be applied to the eyelids; they will stop crusting at night and prevent the eyelids from sticking together. Eye-drops should be used every two hours or so, for they are quickly lost in the tears; they should be dropped into the outer angle of the eye.

Pinta: a skin disease found in Central and South America, caused by a spirochaete *Treponema carateum* which is very like the organism of syphilis, *T. pallidum*, and that which causes yaws, *T. pertenue*. All are spread by direct contact and are sensitive to penicillin.

Pinworm: threadworm. *See* Worms.

Piperazine: a drug active against threadworms and roundworms; the worms are paralysed and passed in the motions.

Pituitary Gland: also called the hypophysis, this gland lies at the base of the brain, to which it is attached by a stalk. It is about the size of a large pea, and is contained in its own well-protected bony cavity, the pituitary fossa, just above and behind the cavity of the nose. Its name is derived from the Latin *pituita*, mucus, for it was once thought that it secreted mucus into the nose. In fact it elaborates several hormones which act on many distant parts of the body, and are of great importance. The gland is divided into an anterior lobe, an intermediate part and a posterior lobe. The anterior lobe secretes eight hormones, which are: growth hormone (GH), thyrotrophin (TSH), prolactin (PRL), follicle stimulating hormone (FSH), luteinising hormone (LH), adrenocorticotrophin (ACTH), beta-lipotrophin (beta-LPH), and gamma-lipotrophin (gamma-LPH). The posterior lobe secretes vasopressin or antidiuretic hormone (ADH) and oxytocin. The growth hormone is essential for the normal growth of the body: it stimulates the reproduction of cells and the growth of cartilage, and conserves the body's stores of protein by mobilising fat to be used as fuel, and decreasing the breakdown of amino-acids. Overproduction of GH associated with tumours of the pituitary causes acromegaly, and a lack of the hormone causes dwarfism. TSH regulates the activity of the thyroid gland, and deficiency is rare. The level in the blood is low in cases of thyrotoxicosis, overaction of the thyroid gland, and high in cases of thyroid deficiency. Prolactin is needed for normal development of the breast and the secretion of milk in nursing mothers. FSH is in great part responsible for the formation of sperm in the male, and in the female stimulates the formation of follicles in the ovulatory cycle. LH, with FSH, stimulates the secretion of testosterone in the male and takes part in the formation of sperm, and in the female is responsible for the rupture of the ovarian follicle in mid-cycle (*see* Ovaries). ACTH stimulates the production of steroids in the adrenal cortex, and also has an action in stimulating the production of the pigment melanin. The actions of beta-LPH and gamma-LPH are uncertain. The secretion of all these hormones is controlled by the hypothalamus in the brain, to which the pituitary gland is connected by its stalk; there is no direct connection with the anterior pituitary, but a portal system of blood vessels carries various releasing factors to the gland. The known factors are: growth hormone releasing factor (GHRF), to which there is an inhibiting hormone (GHRIH), thyrotrophin-releasing hormone (TRH), gonadotrophin-releasing hormone (GnRH) which controls LH and FSH, and corticotrophin-releasing factor (CRF). The posterior lobe of the pituitary is connected directly to the hypothalamus, and the two hormones, ADH and oxytocin, are formed in the hypothalamus and transported to the gland. ADH acts on the tubules of the kidney to increase the reabsorption of water and produce a concentrated urine. It also causes contraction of smooth muscle, thus raising the blood pressure by constricting the arteries, but has this action only in amounts greater than occur in nature. Its secretion is inhibited by cold and alcohol, among other factors, thus leading to increased production of dilute urine. Deficiency of the hormone leads to diabetes insipidus. Oxytocin causes contraction of the milk ducts in the lactating breast in response to stimuli from the nipples during suckling. It also causes contraction of the muscle of the uterus; it must play an important part in labour, but the mechanism by which it does so is unknown.

Pityriasis: a skin condition in which scaling takes place. *Pityriasis alba* is found in children; it is a mild dry eczema which leaves a white patch. It is of no consequence. *Pityriasis rosea* causes a rash of red oval patches, and starts with one herald patch followed after about a week by generalised spread. The rash may irritate, and lasts for about a month. *Pityriasis versicolor* is caused by a skin infection with the yeast *Malassezia furfur*, and is common in the tropics, but is also found in temperate climates. It affects the arms, neck and trunk. The rash may be paler or darker than the surrounding skin, and may or may not irritate. Local application of clotrimazole, econazole, or miconazole may be used in treatment. *Pityriasis capitis* is commonly known as dandruff; shampoos containing coal tar extract are useful in treatment.

Placebo: a harmless inactive medicine given not for any pharmacological effect but to please the patient, as the name suggests. A placebo may be used in clinical trials of a new drug as a control treatment to nullify the 'placebo effect' which makes patients believe that a pill is doing them good merely because they are taking some kind of treatment.

Placenta: the organ by which the mammalian foetus in the womb is connected to the mother. Through it the foetus is supplied with oxygen and nourishment, and the waste products are taken away. It is a fleshy disc about 3 cm thick and 18 cm in diameter, and when fully developed weighs about 500 gm. It is developed from foetal tissue. The umbilical cord runs from the foetus to the placenta carrying blood, which is separated from the mother's blood by the placental membrane: oxygen and nutrients can pass in one direction, carbon dioxide and urea in the other. Cells cannot normally pass from one circulation to the other (but *see* Haemolytic Disease of the Newborn). The placenta produces hormones, human placental lactogen (HPL), progesterone and oestrogens necessary for a normal pregnancy. Abnormalities may affect the placenta: it may separate before its time, or fail to separate when it should. It may cover the outlet of the uterus (placenta praevia) or be split into two lobes. Some disease organisms can pass the placenta, notably those of syphilis and rubella (German measles), and affect the foetus, and some drugs can reach the foetal circulation, a fact which means that drugs must be used with great care during pregnancy, particularly during the first three months. The placenta is normally extruded from the uterus as the afterbirth during the third stage of labour.

Plague: due to infection with the bacterium *Yersinia pestis*, plague still exists in the world, and there have been cases in the United States, Central and Southern America, many parts of Africa, and South-East Asia. It is primarily a disease of rodents, spread by fleas; when the flea bites an infected rodent the organisms multiply in its oesophagus and block it. When the flea bites another creature it regurgitates the organisms and so infects it. There are about 200 different kinds of rodents that can be infected with plague, and 30 different kinds of fleas capable of carrying the infection. In the wild, many foci of infection exist, and unless man ventures into such an area plague does not present any danger. The precise causes of outbreaks of plague in the past are obscure, but once the disease, usually carried by rats which live in contact with man, is introduced into a community it spreads quickly. Infected fleas are the danger, except in the case of pneumonic plague when the organism can be coughed out by the victim and the disease spreads by droplet infection. Plague takes two main forms, bubonic and pneumonic. In bubonic plague the lymph nodes, usually in the groin, become enlarged and suppurate; the nodes in the armpit or the neck may be affected. The temperature rises, and a severe headache develops, with pains all over the body; the patient becomes confused and shocked, and if left untreated in many cases dies on about the fourth or fifth day. If patients survive for a week they may recover. Some patients die without developing a bubo, but may pass on the infection in their breath to another who develops pneumonic plague, where the infection centres in the lungs and the sputum is full of organisms and highly infectious. Treatment is the early use of tetracycline, streptomycin or chloramphenicol. Sulphonamides may be used, but are not effective in pneumonic cases. The disease does not respond to penicillin. Patients with buboes are not infective, providing they are not carrying fleas, but patients with pneumonic plague are highly infective. Control of the disease rests mainly on the control of fleas: if rats are killed, the fleas leave them and can still spread infection. An outbreak of plague may be heralded by the appearance of dead rats in the streets. A vaccine for immunisation is available, made from killed plague organisms.

Plaque: plate, flat area or patch. It is the name given to the area of pathological change in the central nervous system in multiple sclerosis. Dental plaque is a deposit which forms on the teeth; it contains a mass of micro-organisms and is a starting point of dental disease.

Plasma: in medicine, the fluid part of the blood in which the blood cells are suspended; the fluid left after the blood has clotted is called serum.

Plasmodium: the organism of malaria (q.v.). It is a protozoal parasite.

Plaster: a piece of fabric coated with a medicinal substance for application to the skin; an adhesive plaster is coated with a substance having adherent properties and is used for the application of dressings. Plaster of Paris is a powder made by heating gypsum, calcium sulphate dihydrate, so that about three-quarters of the water of crystallisation is driven off. If it is mixed with water it sets hard, and is used in impregnated bandages to make immobilising and supportive casts.

Plastic Surgery: that branch of surgery concerned with the correction of congenital or acquired deformities in order to improve appearance and function. Although operations to improve the appearance of the face after disfiguring wounds or disease have been recorded since ancient times, in common with the rest of surgery full development had to wait until the discovery of anaesthetics and aseptic techniques in the nineteenth century. A major impetus to the establishment of plastic surgery as a specialty was the First World War, but it was not until the Second World War that the number of specialists began to grow; in 1955 the first Congress of the newly formed International Association of Plastic Surgeons was held in Stockholm. Recent advances in the subject include the development of microsurgery, by which technique avulsed fingers and even arms have been replaced. Cosmetic surgery is only a part of the field covered by the plastic surgeon, although it is perhaps the work by which he or she is best known.

Platelets (thrombocytes): blood cells, the smallest cells in the body, their average diameter being 2–4 μm. They are made by bone marrow cells called megakaryocytes, and have no nucleus; they play an important part in the coagulation of blood, and adhere to the walls of injured capillary vessels and arterioles to seal them off. They number $150–350 × 10^9/l$. Recent research suggests that anti-tumour or anti-microbial agents may be introduced into a patient's platelets removed in a blood sample; the platelets are replaced in the circulation to deliver directly to the macrophages, cells which engulf damaged and degenerating cells, substances to aid in their function of destroying bacteria and tumour cells. *See* Thrombocytopenic Purpura.

Plating: a technique used in orthopaedic surgery to treat an unstable fracture by fastening a metal plate to the bone to hold the broken ends in place. It is also the technique of inoculating a plate of nutrient medium with bacteria.

Platysma: a thin sheet of muscle lying just under the skin, running from the lower jaw to the upper part of the chest. It is thought to correspond to the *panniculus carnosus*, a muscular sheet found in animals just under the skin.

Pleura: the membrane covering the lungs and the interior of the chest wall. The layers are continuous with each other; the membrane covering the chest wall is called parietal, that covering the lungs, visceral or pulmonary. Between the two membranes is a capillary space filled with fluid, which enables the lungs to move freely in the chest. The parietal membrane is reflected from the lower part of the chest wall to cover the upper surface of the diaphragm, and in the midline it covers the mediastinum, the partition which separates the two sides of the chest cavity and contains the heart, great blood vessels and the other structures which run through the thorax.

Pleurisy: inflammation of the pleura, caused by infection spreading from the lung, for example in pneumonia, abscess of the lung or tuberculosis, or irritation without infection as with a tumour or an embolism of the lung (*see* Pulmonary Embolism). There is a sharp pain in the chest, worse on movement and aggravated by breathing and coughing, arising from the parietal pleura which lines the inside of the chest wall. The roughened pleural surfaces can be heard rubbing together through the stethoscope. The patient takes shallow breaths because of the pain and tries to move the chest wall as little as possible. If the diaphragmatic pleura is involved, the pain is felt in the side of the neck and the tip of the shoulder; if this is the case, pain can often be relieved by injecting local anaesthetic into the area over the shoulder to which the pain is referred. Pain can arise in the chest wall and resemble pleurisy in Bornholm disease (q.v.) or in developing herpes zoster before the rash appears. If dry pleurisy progresses to the exudate of fluid and a pleural effusion, the sharpness of the pain fades and is replaced by an aching pain. The treatment of pleurisy is the treatment of the underlying condition. Pleural effusions are demonstrated by radiography, and may be aspirated through a needle passed through the chest wall under local anaesthesia.

Pleurodynia: pain on taking a deep breath, often used as a synonym for Bornholm disease (q.v.).

Plexus: a network of structures, applied to nerves, blood vessels or lymphatic vessels.

Plumbism: lead-poisoning.

Pneumoconiosis: a disease of the lung caused by exposure to mineral dust. Coal miner's pneumoconiosis is caused by inhaling various kinds of dust arising from coal, silica, mica and other minerals. The dust sets up numerous inflammatory foci in the acini and lobules of the lungs, which progress to fibrosis; the worst offenders are carbon and quartz dusts. Simple uncomplicated pneumoconiosis may produce no signs of illness, but if the small foci coalesce, or larger areas are affected by inflammation, the area of lung tissue available for gas exchange is restricted, emphysema may develop, and the airways become restricted. The disease in this severe stage is called progressive massive fibrosis. Other types of pneumoconiosis can be caused by the inhalation of silica, as in slate quarrying, working with granite or sandblasting, kaolin, talc, mica, and asbestos, the last being responsible in some cases for the development of malignant tumours. However, asbestos is only dangerous to those who have worked with it for years, and occasional accidental exposure is not of consequence. The prevention of pneumoconiosis is the prevention of dust in the air. A British Pneumoconiosis Panel exists for the purpose of assessing disablement and compensatory benefit payments.

Pneumocystis: *Pneumocystis carinii* is an organism which causes disease of the lung in patients suffering from immune system deficiencies, particularly AIDS (q.v.). About 75% of normally healthy people develop an antibody to the organism by the age of four, and it is found in the lungs in healthy people with no evidence of disease. The organism is confined to the lungs, and is sensitive to co-trimoxazole.

Pneumonectomy: the removal of a lung.

Pneumonia: inflammation of the lungs caused by microorganisms. The commonest organism is *Streptococcus pneumoniae*, but there are a number of others, among them *Legionella*, *Haemophilus influenzae*, *Staphyloccus aureus* and the respiratory syncytial virus. In a number of cases no definite organism is found, but almost any organism can cause pneumonia if the conditions are suitable. The disease is commonest in winter, and patients develop a headache, a high temperature, general aches and pains, a cough, often with pain in the chest (*see* Pleurisy) and vomiting. There may be blood in the sputum, and the patient may become confused. Not infrequently at the beginning of the infection there is no cough, and the patient just feels very ill with a severe headache. Before the advent of antibiotics the illness was full of drama, with a week's fever and even delirium preceding the crisis, in which the patient would break out in a sweat, the fever would fall, and peaceful sleep and recovery follow. Now, while pneumonia remains a severe and in some cases a dangerous disease, most cases respond quickly to amoxycillin and rest in bed and

511

are treated at home. Some cases, however, need hospital treatment particularly if pneumonia complicates an attack of influenza or an attack of chicken-pox in an adult.

Pneumonitis: inflammation of the lung caused by micro-organisms or any other agent, including the inhalation of noxious vapours.

Pneumoperitoneum: air in the peritoneal cavity, which may be introduced for diagnostic purposes in radiography or laparoscopy, or may be the result of injury or the rupture of a diseased part of the gastro-intestinal tract. It was once used in the treatment of tuberculosis to raise the diaphragm and so rest the base of a diseased lung

Pneumothorax: air in the pleural space surrounding the lungs. It was formerly introduced artificially to collapse and so rest tuberculous lungs and prevent the spread of infection, but now the common causes of a pneumothorax, apart from those induced to permit endoscopic examinations of the pleural cavity, are spontaneous rupture of an enlarged air sac or injury to the lung or chest wall. Normally expansion of the chest produces a negative pressure in the airtight potential space between the pleural membrane lining the chest wall and that covering the lungs, and air at atmospheric pressure enters the lungs. If however the space is not airtight because of a communication with the air passages of the lungs or with the air outside the chest wall, the elastic lung collapses as air at atmospheric pressure enters the pleural space. If the communication remains open, the air in the space remains at atmospheric pressure; but if the communicating passage, usually a tear in the chest wall or the lung, develops a valvular action, opening on inspiration and closing on expiration, the pressure in the pneumothorax builds up and a tension pneumothorax ensues, which begins to shift the heart to one side, and if left produces a fatal collapse of the circulation. The breathing becomes increasingly difficult, and the patient increasingly distressed. The pneumothorax caused by the rupture of enlarged air sacs, known as spontaneous pneumothorax, may occur in healthy young men with no obvious cause; the rupture commonly seals itself when the lung collapses, and if left the air is slowly absorbed, but often it is found expedient to remove the air by introducing a needle into the affected pleural space through the chest wall connected to a tube opening under water, so that the air bubbles out on expiration but cannot be drawn in on inspiration. Enlarged air sacs may develop in asthmatics or those with emphysema, and if they rupture are treated the same way. Injuries of the chest wall may result in pneumothorax if the wound penetrates the lung, or if the end of a broken rib tears the lung; they may be associated with bleeding into the pleural cavity. Air may be sucked in through a damaged chest wall. In all cases the possibility of a tension pneumothorax must be kept in mind and, if one develops, it must be relieved by the introduction of a needle through the chest wall. Drainage can be left until the emergency has been overcome.

Podagra: pain caused by gout in the great toe.

Podophyllin: if the root of the plant *Podophyllum peltatum* is dried and powdered the resin can be used to shrivel certain papillomas and warts that grow on the skin.

Poisoning: there is no satisfactory definition of a poison, but it is usually taken to mean a substance which in relatively small amounts is dangerous to life, or injures health, its effect being produced chemically and by absorption into the bloodstream. There is hardly any substance which could not, taken in sufficient amounts, produce poisonous effects, and it is well known that in allergic states generally innocuous substances can prove deadly to those who are sensitive to them. While the majority of cases are acute, it must not be forgotten that exposure to noxious substances over a period of time can cause chronic poisoning. Acute poisoning is in the case of adults very often self-induced, and in the case of children accidental. The majority of cases of self-induced poisoning in adults are female, and of these many are in their teens or twenties. By no means all of these cases are truly suicidal; very many have been characterised as a cry for help. Drugs of various sorts are commonly used in suicide attempts, often those which have been prescribed for anxiety, depression or insomnia, either for the patient or someone in the household, and in many cases, particularly in men, liberal amounts of alcohol have also been taken to wash the pills down. In the case of children, accidental swallowings of household products or drugs are common causes of poisoning; in the country various berries are often eaten, some of which can be poisonous. The poison which causes most deaths by far in children is however carbon monoxide (q.v.). Popular belief has it that poisons are best treated by specific antidotes, but unfortunately this is not so. Antidotes do exist in some cases: naloxone counteracts morphine or other opioid analgesics, poisoning by carbon monoxide requires oxygen, by cyanides dicobalt edetate, by heavy metals sodium calciumedetate or dimercaprol, by organophosphorus compounds atropine, paracetamol poisoning is treated with methionine, and desferrioxamine is given for poisoning by iron salts. General care is most important in the unconscious patient; the breathing may be obstructed or impaired, so that the airway must be cleared and if necessary artificial respiration (q.v.) started. The blood pressure may be low so that the head should be lower than the feet, or the legs raised up; if the patient has been unconscious for any length of time the body temperature may have fallen, and the patient should be covered by blankets. Hot water bottles should not be used. In conscious patients, especially children, ipecacuanha can be given to induce vomiting, except in cases where a corrosive poison or a derivative of petroleum such as a metal polish is in question, for they are dangerous to the lungs and there is a risk of inhalation. In adults the stomach may be washed out, and activated charcoal given to decrease absorption from the stomach. In all cases a search should be made for the source of the poison, and any containers or remaining material found taken to hospital with the patient; in the case of carbon monoxide poisoning, a full description of the circumstances in which the patient was found may be very important.

Poisonous Plants and Fungi: the most poisonous fungus is the mushroom death cap, *Amanita phalloides*; one may be fatal. It not only looks like an edible mushroom, but is said to have an attractive taste. The symptoms of poisoning may be delayed for over six hours, and include abdominal pain and vomiting and diarrhoea, followed by jaundice and liver failure; if there is any doubt that a poisonous mushroom has been eaten, the sooner the doctor is called the better, for successful treatment depends on speed. Other mushrooms of the genus *Amanita* are poisonous, for example fly agaric, *Amanita muscaria*, which produces symptoms in about 15 minutes of drowsiness, vomiting and hallucinations. In general it is wise to avoid any mushrooms with white gills. There are many plants which can be poisonous, and it is impossible to give a complete list; they may produce dermatitis (like stinging nettles or poison ivy), disturbance of the stomach or intestines if eaten (like narcissus, wisteria, yew, privet, holly, buttercups and others), disturbance of the heartbeat (like foxglove or lily-of-the-valley), effects like nicotine (for example, the tobacco plant or laburnum), effects like atropine (for example, deadly nightshade), and there are those which produce hallucinations (like Indian hemp and morning glory). Children of an enquiring nature not infrequently eat berries, and may light on deadly nightshade, yew or laburnum seeds, but several have to be eaten to produce much effect. The adult searching for herbal remedies without an adequate knowledge of botany may concoct a poisonous mixture. Those who take herbal remedies should be aware that some interact with orthodox medicines; it is not wise to take both at the same time.

Poliomyelitis (infantile paralysis): a disease of the central nervous system, caused by an enterovirus, the poliovirus, which has three types. The infection is spread by pollution of food and water with sewage or human ordure, by the spread of infected matter by flies, or occasionally by droplet infection from the nose; it is commonest in warm climates where hygiene is poor. In such circumstances children are infected. If hygiene improves, the infection may die out for a time, but if it returns the average age of those infected is higher. The infection starts with a sore throat, fever and malaise. This passes, and then the patient may develop headache, fever, and general pains in the muscles, with neck stiffness indicating a meningitis; this may last about a week. In some cases paralysis develops with the fever; groups of spinal cord motor cells are affected which supply the muscles of the limbs, and in severe cases the muscles of respiration. The legs are affected more often than the arms, and the paralysis is worse if exercise has been taken during the incubation period. In the worst form of the disease the brain stem is affected, and the muscles supplied by the cranial nerves are paralysed, together with the brain centres concerned with breathing and the circulation.

In many countries, including the United Kingdom, the disease has virtually disappeared following widespread immunisation programmes. Vaccines are prepared against all three types of the virus, and there are two types of vaccine, inactivated and live attenuated; the latter is given by mouth, and used routinely in infant immunisation in three doses; further doses should be given on beginning and leaving school. The inactivated virus is given to those with immunodeficiency disease, or may be used during pregnancy. Mothers with babies given the live vaccine should be careful to wash their hands well when dealing with nappies. Travellers to countries where the disease has not been controlled can be given the oral vaccine if they have not been immunised in the last 10 years.

Polyarteritis: a disease in which the walls of the arteries undergo an inflammatory process; it affects the smaller and medium-sized vessels, and leads to blockage of the artery, clotting, or destruction of the vessel wall. It does not affect the whole length of the vessel. The cause is obscure, but it may be the result of abnormal immune reactions. It may affect any part of the body, and damage any organ; often the kidneys are affected, with a consequent rise to deafness, the lungs with coughing, difficulty in breathing and blood in the sputum, or the muscles and joints, with accompanying pain. If the eyes are affected the vision deteriorates. The disease may take weeks to develop, during which time the patient feels ill, runs a temperature, and loses appetite; there may be pains in the muscles and joints. The treatment is by steroids, at first in high doses, then reducing according to the patient's progress. In severe cases the immunosuppressive drugs azathiaprine or cyclophosphamide are added to the steroids.

516

Polycystic Disease: an inherited disease affecting the kidneys and liver. There are two forms, one of which affects babies and children, the other adults. The form affecting children shows multiple cysts in the kidneys and often the liver. The changes lead to kidney failure which has to be treated by renal dialysis or kidney transplant, but liver failure may supervene later. In adults, the disease is again inherited, but shows itself in the thirties or forties by kidney infections, the passage of blood in the urine, stones, or kidney failure. The liver is enlarged. Both the kidneys and liver show multiple cysts. The treatment is again renal dialysis or transplant. The disease that occurs in children is inherited as a recessive characteristic, but the adult disease is inherited as a dominant trait; because it shows itself later in life, children may have been born before the disease has been recognised, and they have to be warned that they may pass the condition on to their children as well as possibly developing the condition themselves.

Polycythaemia: an increase in the number of circulating red blood cells. This may be caused by a chronic shortage of oxygen, as in those who live at high altitudes, impaired circulation of the blood in certain congenital abnormalities of the heart, or inefficient exchange of oxygen in the lungs because of chronic lung disease. Polycythaemia may also be found without any obvious cause, when it is called polycythaemia vera; there is an overproduction of red cells in the bone marrow, rather as in leukaemia there is an overproduction of white cells. The disease is not common; it shows itself in middle age, possibly by headaches and dizziness, or a tendency to bruising or nose bleeding. Because the blood becomes thick and viscous the patient is liable to suffer from thromboses, haemorrhage or heart failure; one of these complications may be the first sign of the disease. The treatment is removal of the surplus red blood cells by drawing off a quantity of blood, a procedure which needs to be repeated from time to time according to the blood count. In addition, the overactivity of the bone marrow may be reduced by the injection of radioactive phosphorus or by the use of the drug busulphan.

Polydactyly: the congenital abnormality of having more than five fingers or toes.

Polymorph: an abbreviation for polymorphonuclear leucocyte. *See* Leucocyte.

Polymyalgia Rheumatica: a disease found most commonly in people over 60, with twice as many women being affected as men. The cause is not known; it produces pain and stiffness in the muscles, usually those of the shoulders and pelvis, worst on waking. It may be bad enough to prevent the patient moving without the greatest difficulty. It is accompanied by a greatly raised erythrocyte sedimentation rate (*see* Sedimentation Rate) and treated with the corticosteroid prednisolone

Polyneuritis: inflammation of several nerves together. *See* Neuritis.

Polyp: a growth arising from mucous membrane. Usually applied to greyish overgrowths of the mucous membrane lining the nose and paranasal sinuses which may follow chronic infection. Polyps may also occur in the bladder or the bowel, or elsewhere where there is mucous membrane. If they are troublesome they are removed; they may bleed, or cause obstruction to the air passages in the nose.

Polypharmacy: a term applied to the prescription of a number of drugs at the same time, which is in most cases unreasonable.

Polyuria: the passage of abnormally large amounts of urine.

Polyunsaturated Fats: fats which have fatty acids in which there is more than one double bond between the carbon atoms. In saturated fats there are no double bonds. It is thought that a high ratio of unsaturated to saturated fat in the diet reduces the level of blood cholesterol and decreases the clotting time. A recommended ratio is 0.8; the best source of unsaturated fat is vegetable oil. Saturated fats are found in meat and dairy products. *See* Cholesterol.

Pomphylix: an eczematous skin condition with very small blister formation on the hands and feet; that occurring on the hands may be linked with an infection with *Taenia pedis*, athlete's foot, although there is no infection in the pomphylix.

Pons: that part of the brain stem that lies in front of the cerebellum and below the cerebral hemispheres. Below, it is continuous with the medulla and above the cerebral peduncles emerge from it and run into the cerebrum.

Porencephaly: a cyst arising in the brain as the result of an infarct or other damage.

Porocephalosis (pentastomiasis): infestation with the blood-sucking parasites *Linguatula* or *Armillifer*. The first infest dogs, wolves and foxes, which are the definitive hosts, and pass on the herbivores which are the intermediate hosts. If an ovum is eaten by a human being, cysts form, usually in the liver, without producing symptoms. If, however, a cyst is eaten, larvae escape from it in the stomach and find their way through the oesophagus into the naso-pharynx, where they set up an intense reaction resulting in coughing and sneezing, with discharge and bleeding from the nose, difficulty in breathing and swallowing, and vomiting. This illness is known as halzoun, and occurs in the Middle East. *Armillifer* infests snakes, and herbivores are the intermediate hosts. If humans acquire the ova by drinking water in which an infested snake has been, or eat uncooked snake meat, the eggs develop into larvae which in turn become nymphs. They may be found in the tissues, and usually produce no symptoms, but encyst and calcify so that they are seen on X-ray plates. In a few cases serious symptoms have been produced by inflammation set up in various organs. The parasite is found in Africa, India and the Far East, in the Philippines and Australia.

Porphyria: a defect of metabolism in which porphyrins are overproduced in the body, mainly in the liver and bone marrow, and excreted in the urine and faeces. Porphyrin with iron makes up haem which, combined with the protein globin, forms haemoglobin, the red pigment responsible for carrying oxygen to the tissues. Combined with magnesium, porphyrin makes the pigment chlorophyll, which is responsible for the synthesis of carbohydrates under the influence of the sun's rays in plants. There are two types of porphyria, acute and non-acute. The acute disease is inherited as a dominant trait, and produces acute abdominal pain with vomiting, which may be mistaken for an acute abdominal condition requiring surgery. It also affects the nervous system, producing cramps and paralyses of the muscles, mostly in the arms, but the weakness can affect the muscles of respiration. There may be sensory and mental changes, and even epileptiform fits. The pulse rate rises, as does the blood pressure. The urine becomes brown or red if left standing in the light. The attacks recur, and are seen mainly in young adults; they may be precipitated by a number of drugs, among them oral contraceptives, tetracyclines, sulphonamides, barbiturates and alcohol. There is a long list. In some attacks, called mixed attacks, the skin becomes sensitive to sunlight, and blisters form. The treatment of an attack calls for a high carbohydrate diet, removal of any precipitating drug, and treatment of the symptoms of pain and mental disturbance. Non-acute porphyria is usually acquired, and the fault lies in the liver. Most cases are the result of alcoholism, and the skin symptoms are marked; exposure to sunlight causes reddening and the formation of large blisters. Porphyrins have been used in the treatment of malignant growths by laser, for they are more readily absorbed by cancerous than by normal tissues; the malignant cells are then sensitive to the presence of light.

Portal Vein: the vein that carries blood from the spleen, pancreas, stomach and intestines to the liver.

Port-wine Stain: a birthmark whose name is descriptive; it is a haemangioma of the capillary vessels. The majority persist for life.

Positron Emission Tomography: radioactive isotopes can be used to label substances introduced into the body in order to follow their progress, concentration in various organs, and their use, and so observe normal function and function in disease. In order to investigate normally occurring substances it is necessary to label naturally occurring elements, but all have a short half-life; the gamma ray emitting form of oxygen has a half-life of 2.1 minutes, of nitrogen 10 minutes and of carbon 20.1 minutes. Instead of hydrogen, which has no form which emits gamma rays, fluorine has been substituted with a half-life of 110 minutes. In order to measure and demonstrate the distribution of the elements in the tissues, detectors of radiation are placed round the body. When the isotopes decay, they emit positively charged electrons called positrons. These collide with negative electrons, and when they do so gamma rays are emitted at 180° to each other. The radiation detectors pick up the radiation, and the readings are submitted to computer analysis, similar to that employed in computerised axial tomography by X-rays (see CAT). In this way the processes of metabolism can be studied in health and disease. The name of the technique is often abbreviated to PET.

Positive Pressure Ventilator: a breathing machine used to inflate and oxygenate the lungs of an unconscious or paralysed patient. If it has to be used for any length of time, the machine is connected through a tracheostomy, an artificial opening into the windpipe.

Posterior Fossa: the compartment in the rear of the skull, below the cerebral hemispheres, which contains the cerebellum and the brain stem.

Posterior Root Ganglia: each nerve running out from the spinal cord has two roots, anterior (ventral) and posterior (dorsal); the anterior carries motor fibres, the posterior sensory fibres. Before the two roots join to form a nerve, the posterior root has upon it a ganglion, a collection of sensory nerve cell bodies; from these posterior root ganglia cells one fibre runs out along the nerve to end in a sensory organ, the other runs into the spinal cord. The posterior, or dorsal, root ganglia lie in the spaces between the vertebral bodies, the intervertebral foramina, through which the nerves leave the spinal column.

Post-mature: over-developed; used of an infant born after its time.

Post-mortem: after death.

Postnatal Depression: it is not uncommon for mothers to experience emotional disturbances directly after childbirth, and it is quite normal. Depression can be compounded by worry or tiredness, particularly if the child was unwanted or unexpected, and the patient may feel that she is quite unable to cope. Mothers in this condition need considerable support. The use of drugs to help the condition is not recommended. Occasionally a true psychotic state develops after childbirth, especially in those who have had a mental illness previously, and psychiatric treatment is needed.

Postpartum: after childbirth.

Post-traumatic: following injury.

Postural Drainage: used in conditions where there is a collection of mucus or sputum in the main air passages in the lungs, postural drainage means putting the patient in such a position that the secretions drain by gravity. The patient may be positioned head-down over the side of the bed, while the physiotherapist taps the chest to help dislodge the sputum.

Post-viral Syndrome: a condition of chronic malaise following an infection by a virus. It has long been known that influenza, for example, may be followed by depression and a feeling of ill health for many weeks. This kind of condition is familiar to most doctors who have spent much time in general practice. In spite of research, no laboratory tests have been found which could identify such an illness and the diagnosis of post-viral syndrome remains one which can only be made on clinical grounds;

it cannot be proved or refuted. The best that can be said is that the post-viral syndrome is a complex inter-relationship between social, psychological and physical factors.

Potassium: a metallic element that plays a most important part in the transmission of nerve impulses to the muscles. A shortage of potassium (hypokalaemia) results in weakness of the muscles, including the heart, and paralysis of the intestines. It may occur because of excessive loss of electrolytes in diarrhoea and vomiting, or in various other conditions. The use of diuretics may increase the excretion of potassium by the kidneys; the advisability of giving routine potassium supplements with diuretics has been the subject of controversy, but they are probably only needed in cases where there is liver disease or an irregularity of heart rhythm.

Pott's Disease: tuberculosis of the spine, which may collapse vertebrae and result in curvature of the spine or hunchback deformity. It was described in 1779 by Percival Pott, a London surgeon (1714–88).

Pott's Fracture: a fracture dislocation of the ankle, the result of turning the foot outwards. The fibula is broken above the ankle, and the tip of the tibia torn off or the medial ligament of the ankle ruptured. It was described by Percival Pott in 1750 (*see above*), who is said to have suffered from such a fracture while walking across London Bridge.

Poultice: a soft, moist preparation applied to the skin while hot in order to increase the flow of blood to boils or carbuncles, or to provide counter-irritation in painful conditions. The most satisfactory poultice is made of kaolin, which can be impregnated with various antiseptics or counter-irritant substances, is not messy and can be heated under the grill.

Pox: a disease with pustular eruptions on the skin; once used to signify the great pox, syphilis.

Pralidoxime: a substance which reactivates cholinesterase after it has been attacked by organophosphorus compounds (q.v.); it is used with atropine in cases of poisoning by these chemicals.

Precordium: the region in front of the heart, the left lower part of the front of the chest.

Prednisolone: synthetic corticosteroid, given by mouth for its anti-inflammatory action. *See* Corticosteroids.

Pre-eclampsia: *see* Eclampsia.

Pre-frontal Leucotomy: *see* Leucotomy.

Pregnancy: the average duration of pregnancy in the human being is from 274 to 280 days, the commonest early signs of its existence being the cessation of the periods, enlargement of the breasts, sometimes nausea in the mornings and frequency in passing urine. A firm diagnosis of pregnancy can be made after the second week by testing for the presence of hormones in the urine, but it may be possible that hospital laboratories are not able to offer such a test unless there are medical reasons; there are, however, pregnancy testing kits available over the counter in the pharmacist's shop. The nipples and surrounding areola start to become darker about the third month and quickening, or movements of the foetus, may be felt from about the eighteenth week. From the third month onwards the pregnant womb begins to rise out of the pelvis and can be felt through the abdominal wall. When a pregnancy has been confirmed, the first visit to the antenatal clinic should take place in the 12th week, when the blood pressure, weight and height will be measured, and blood taken for grouping, testing for rhesus and rubella antibodies and VDRL tests. At subsequent visits the blood pressure is checked, the urine tested for sugar and albumin, and the weight measured; normally the gain in weight should not be more than 2 kg in a month. A gain of 3 kg is expected during the first 20 weeks, 3 kg between the 20th and 30th weeks, and between 3 and 3.5 kg from the 30th to the 40th week, making a total of 9.5 kg. The height of the pregnant uterus in the abdomen is examined, the way the foetus is lying, and the sound of its heart. Older mothers will be offered an amniocentesis (q.v.) to screen for Down's syndrome at 16 weeks, although it is becoming increasingly possible for hospitals to undertake chorionic villus sampling between eight and ten weeks to exclude the possibility of genetic defects. Ultrasound examination of the foetus is widely used to make sure all is well and to discover the presence of twins. Anaemia is a constant risk during pregnancy, and supplements of iron and folic acid should be taken as a routine. There is a formidable list of drugs that must be avoided during pregnancy, and all drugs should be avoided if possible during the first three months; the rule is that the possible risk to the foetus must be less than the possible benefit to the mother. Alcohol should only be taken in occasional single drinks, and is best avoided, as is smoking.

Premature Birth: a baby that weighs less than 5½ lb or 2.5 kg at birth is regarded as premature, however many days the pregnancy is thought to have lasted. If the baby weighs less than 2½ lb, or 1.1 kg, the expected weight at 28 weeks, survival is possible but not certain. At 26 weeks survival is at present not possible. The vast majority of babies born live weighing over 4½ lb, or 2 kg, will survive with proper care. The causes of premature birth are in many cases not understood, but in about two-thirds of cases the birth is hastened by conditions such as multiple pregnancy, bleeding and pre-eclampsia. Prematurity is also associated with poverty.

Premedication: various drugs are used to prepare a patient for general anaesthesia; they usually include atropine or hyoscine (scopolamine) to dry up the secretions of the lungs and salivary glands, and an opium derivative such as papaveretum or a benzodiazepine such as diazepam or temazepam, which has a shorter action, to reduce anxiety and make the patient sleepy. The choice will depend on various factors; in emergencies and minor operations the premedication may be dispensed with, and atropine or hyoscine given at the induction of anaesthesia. Benzodiazepines are useful because they have an amnesic effect, that is they cloud the memory, and they can be used in doses too small to produce complete unconsciousness for operations under local anaesthesia or for endoscopies.

Premenstrual Tension: *see* Menstruation.

Prepatellar Bursitis: *see* Housemaid's Knee.

Presbyacusis: progressive hearing loss associated with old age. It can be helped by a hearing aid.

Presbyopia: the elasticity of the lens of the eye is gradually lost with age, so that the power of focusing is impaired and near vision lost. Spectacles are needed for reading and close work.

Prescription: the directions written by the doctor to the pharmacist for the preparation, administration and supply of medicines. They are written in a particular form, giving the patient's name and address, the date, and the doctor's name and address. The name of the drug or formula for the medicine is given; the amount of the dose and when it is to be taken follows, and the amount to be supplied is clearly stated. Many medicines can only be supplied on a doctor's prescription, and in particular prescriptions for drugs controlled under the Misuse of Drugs Regulations 1985 schedules 2 and 3 must be signed and dated by the prescriber, and written in ink in the prescriber's own handwriting. The total amount of the drug to be supplied must be given in figures and words.

Presentation: in general, this means the combination of symptoms and signs which mark the beginning of a disease. In obstetrics, it means the part of the foetus which is positioned at the opening of the birth canal at the beginning of labour. The commonest presentation is the left occipito-anterior, that is the foetus is ready to emerge head first with the neck slightly bent so that the left side of the back of the head is in front. If the chin is to the front, the birth is more difficult; in about 3% of cases the baby sits down to be born, rather than standing on its head, and this is called a breech presentation. The obstetrician may be able to turn the baby before birth, for although a breech birth is normally successful it may be more difficult, and in some cases require a Caesarean section.

Priapism: condition in which there is a persistent, often painful erection of the male organ without any sexual desire. It may occur in a number of disorders, among them sickle-cell anaemia, chronic leukaemia and polycythaemia vera. Priapus was the classical god of procreation.

Prickly Heat: exposure to a hot climate in those unaccustomed to it may cause the sweat gland ducts to become blocked; they rupture, sweat escapes into the skin, and a papular itchy rash develops. This may happen quickly, or only appear after a couple of months. It is worse if the clothes are unsuitable; they should be light and loose. If possible, the subject should avoid the heat, staying in the shade or in air-conditioned places, and avoid scratching the rash, for boils may develop if the skin becomes infected. Calamine lotion helps by increasing evaporation from the skin; some recommend taking vitamin C 1 gm a day. Baths of tepid water are useful, but soap should be of a good quality and not likely to irritate the skin. The condition usually goes quite quickly, but may recur. Special attention should be taken to keep the skin folds, such as those in the groin, dry; this is particularly important in infants, who are often more liable to develop a heat rash than adults.

Primaquine: drug used in the treatment of malaria caused by *P. vivax* or *P. ovale*. *See* Malaria.

Primidone: drug used in the treatment of epilepsy.

Primigravida: a woman pregnant for the first time.

Primipara: a woman who has borne one child.

Probang: a flexible rod with a ball, sponge or tuft of bristles at the end, invented in the seventeenth century as a surgical instrument for use in the throat and oesophagus.

Probenecid: a drug which increases the excretion of uric acid in the urine, and is therefore used in the treatment of gout to cut down the number of attacks. When first given it may precipitate an attack, and must be combined with another drug to treat this, such as colchicine or an NSAID. It must be taken indefinitely. It also has the action of decreasing the excretion of penicillins and cephalosporins, and so promotes a higher concentration of these drugs in the blood.

Procaine: introduced as a local anaesthetic in 1905, after many years procaine has been superseded by newer drugs such as lignocaine and is now seldom used.

Procidentia: the complete prolapse of the uterus or rectum.

Proctalgia: pain in the anus and rectum. No cause is known for the severe pain in *proctalgia fugax*, which may last for up to 10 minutes, and no treatment is possible.

Proctitis: inflammation of the rectum.

Proctology: the study of diseases of the rectum and anus.

Proctoscope: an instrument for examining the interior of the anal canal and the lower part of the rectum.

Prodromal: a symptom or sign that precedes the full development of a disease.

Progeria: premature changes of old age, seen in the rare inherited Werner's syndrome which may affect young adults.

Progesterone: a naturally occurring hormone which prepares the lining of the uterus for implantation of the fertilised ovum. It is used in the contraceptive pill. *See* Ovary.

Prognosis: a forecast of the probable course and outcome of an illness.

Progressive Muscular Atrophy: *see* Motor Neurone Disease.

Proguanil: a drug used in the preventive treatment of malaria (q.v.).

Prolactin: a hormone secreted by the anterior part of the pituitary gland (q.v.). It stimulates the production of milk in nursing mothers.

Prolapse: the falling downwards or forwards of an organ; usually used of the uterus, which may become displaced downwards as the result of weakening of the muscles of the floor of the pelvis in women who have borne children. It may be accompanied by incontinence of urine when the pressure in the abdomen is raised by coughing or straining (stress incontinence). Treatment is if possible by surgical operation.

Prolapsed Intervertebral Disc: between each of the vertebral bodies in the spine is a disc of elastic tissue which has a centre of softer tissue, the nucleus pulposus, surrounded by the annulus fibrosus, a ring of denser stronger fibrous tissue which binds the bodies of the vertebrae together. Under strain the softer centre of the disc can bulge through the outer fibrous ring, and come to press on a nerve root issuing out between the vertebral bodies from the spinal cord. If this happens pain results, both locally and in the area supplied by the nerve, possibly with weakness of the muscles. Prolapse of a disc is most likely to occur in the lower back, between the fourth and fifth or third and fourth vertebrae, when it gives rise to lumbago and sciatica. The strain most likely to result in a prolapse is sustained in bending forwards and picking up a heavy object; the annulus fibrosus is likely to give way towards the back of the vertebral body. Prolapse of a disc is often said to be the cause of low back pain, but the diagnosis should really be reserved for those cases in which interference with the nerves can be demonstrated by neurological examination, for there are many structures in the back which when strained can cause pain. Treatment is rest; in persistent cases physiotherapy is needed, and if the diagnosis is clear, in suitable cases an operation can be performed to remove the bulging part of the disc. As in all cases of low back pain, the bed should be hard or at the least firm; in acute cases boards under the mattress, or a mattress on the floor, are best. Prolapse of the discs in the neck can occur, but prolapse of the discs in the thorax is uncommon. The condition is sometimes referred to as a slipped disc. Once it has occurred it is likely to recur, and bending forward to pick up anything heavy must be avoided by those who have had low back pain. It is best to squat, and let the legs do the work.

Pronation: the movement of turning the hand palm down or facing backwards. The prone position is lying with the face downwards.

Prontosil: the proprietary name for the first sulphonamide, which was introduced in 1932.

Prophylaxis: treatment undertaken to prevent a disease; the prevention of disease.

Propranolol: a beta-blocking drug (q.v.).

Proprietary Drugs and Medicines: those which are protected as to their composition, method of manufacture and name by patent, trademark or copyright. They bear a brand name by which they are prescribed, as against the generic name by which the drug is known in the Pharmacopoeia. A patent protects a new drug for 20 years in the UK, a period which runs from the date when the patent is granted and includes the time taken for development and testing.

Proprioception: the perception of impulses from the sensory organs (proprioceptors) that give information about the position and movements of the body; they are found mostly in the muscles and tendons. Information is also derived from the labyrinth of the ear (q.v.) and the eyes.

Proptosis: displacement forwards, usually used of the eyeball (exophthalmos).

Prostaglandins: substances first found in the seminal
fluid of men and sheep, but present throughout the
body. They are divided into groups named from A to
F. They act as local hormones, regulating the action of
other hormones and playing a part in the processes of
metabolism, and have many effects, involving for example
the secretion of acid in the stomach, the blood pressure,
and the body temperature. They increase the contraction
of smooth muscle, particularly in the uterus, and are used
in obstetrics to induce abortion; the drugs dinoprost or
dinoprostone are injected into or outside the amniotic sac.
Dinoprostone can also be used to induce labour at term; it
is available in vaginal tablets or gel, or it can be given
by mouth. Mysoprostol, a synthetic prostaglandin E, is
used to decrease the secretion of acid in the stomach and
so promote the healing of peptic ulcers.

Prostate: the gland surrounding the neck of the bladder
and beginning of the urethra in men. It has three lobes,
a middle and two lateral, and it measures about $3 \times 2.5
\times 4$ cm. It contains smooth muscle fibres, as well as cells
which secrete a fluid which goes to make up the seminal
plasma which is ejaculated in the sexual act. It is in later
life liable to benign enlargement, which slowly obstructs
the free flow of urine from the bladder, causing difficulty
in starting to pass urine, a poor stream, dribbling and
frequency, and predisposing to infection of the urine. If the
symptoms warrant it, the enlarged gland may be removed,
either by open operation through the lower abdominal
wall or by resection through the operating cystoscope. If
left, the enlarged prostate may cause a complete urinary
obstruction with acute retention of urine, which must be
relieved by the passage of a catheter and subsequent
operation. After the operation men are usually sterile,
but not impotent. The prostate may suffer a malignant
change, which is liable to produce secondary deposits
in the bones, so that the first indication of its presence
may be an abnormal fracture. Commonly, however, it
produces the same symptom as a benign enlargement,
obstruction which may need operative relief. Measures
can be undertaken to deprive the tumour of testosterone
and so affect its growth; removal of the testicles has this

effect. More commonly stilboestrol tablets are used, or cyproterone, which has an anti-androgen action. Buserelin and goserelin at first increase the secretion of testosterone, and then cut it off. They are given by injection followed in the case of buserelin by a nasal spray. The prostate is sometimes the site of infection which produces pain and in some cases a discharge. The only antibiotics which reach the infected prostatic secretions are tetracyclines, erythromycin and trimethoprim. Stones may form in the gland after an infection, but may not be harmful.

Prosthesis: an artificial substitute for a missing part, for example false teeth or an artificial limb.

Proteins: complicated large molecules made up of a combination of thousands of amino-acids joined together; they contain nitrogen, carbon, hydrogen and oxygen and in many cases sulphur. There are about 20 basic amino-acids, which are made from inorganic substances by chlorophyll-containing plants and some bacteria; the amino-acids essential in a human diet are isoleucine, leucine, lysine, phenylalanine, tyrosine, methionine, cystine, threonine, tryptophan and valine; histidine is essential for infants. These are all present in a normally varied diet, and other amino-acids required are synthesised in the body. Proteins are either simple or conjugated, that is, combined with another substance as in haemoglobin; they can be burnt for energy, but are essential for maintaining the structure of the body and growth. The metabolism of proteins requires many enzymes, which in rare inherited diseases may be absent, in which case the condition is known as an inborn error of metabolism; acquired errors of metabolism may be caused by such conditions as vitamin deficiencies, where co-enzymes may be lacking.

Prothrombin: known as Factor II, it is the precursor of thrombin, the enzyme concerned with the conversion of fibrinogen into fibrin during the process of blood clotting. *See* Coagulation of the Blood.

Protoplasm: the material of which all living cells consist.

Protozoa: micro-organisms with one cell which form the lowest division of the animal kingdom. They differ from bacteria, for the characteristics of the protozoan cell resemble closely the characteristics of the cells from which multicellular creatures are made. About 30 protozoa are known to exist as parasites on man, but half of these are harmless. The others are responsible for such diseases as malaria, amoebic dysentery, sleeping sickness, kala-azar, toxoplasmosis, trichomoniasis and giardiasis. Infection is passed on in several ways: by insects, by the contamination of food and water, and by direct contact. Protozoa are found as parasites throughout the animal and plant kingdoms, and in any place where there is water.

Proximal: describes anything which is nearer to a given point of reference; things farther away are called distal. The knee, for example, is proximal to the foot, and the foot is distal to the knee, for in anatomy the centre point of the body is taken as the reference point.

Prurigo: an itching condition characterised by nodules deep in the skin, commonly seen in the upper part of the back.

Pruritus: itching, a sensation which makes the subject want to scratch. It is found in many conditions ranging from insect bites to obstructive jaundice. Treatment varies according to the cause, but if no cause can be found, overheating of the skin must be avoided, and the clothes should be loose. Calamine lotion can be used to cool the skin. Pruritus is often worse at night when the body is warm; the lighter the bedclothes the better. Patches of irritating dry skin can be covered with a simple emollient such as aqueous cream, which can also be used instead of soap, which may be irritating. Antihistamines by mouth reduce the sensation of itching, but must not be used as a local application.

Pseudocyesis: false pregnancy, in which the signs of pregnancy are present but the uterus is empty.

Pseudogout: a condition occurring in the elderly in which the symptoms are similar to gout, but the crystals deposited in the joints are calcium salts and not urate crystals. It is commonly confined to one joint, usually the knee.

Pseudomonas: a genus of gram-negative bacilli, of which one, *Pseudomonas aeruginosa*, is liable to cause infection of wounds and burns, particularly in hospitals, for it is resistant to most of the common antibiotics and antiseptics, and once established it is difficult to eradicate. It may cause other serious types of infection in debilitated patients or those with immunodeficiency syndromes. Some penicillins, ticarcillin, azlocillin and piperacillin, are active against *Pseudomonas aeruginosa*, but must be given by injection. Carfecillin may be given by mouth for infections of the urinary tract. The aminoglycosides gentamicin and tobramycin are also active against the organism.

Psittacosis: *see* Ornithosis.

Psoriasis: a skin disease, more common in white-skinned people and temperate climates, where it affects up to 2% of the white population and tends to run in families. There is very rapid growth of the cells of the epidermal layer of the skin, which pass upwards quickly without developing a horny layer, and are lost; the cause is not known. The disease can affect all ages but is commonest in young adults, producing red areas with sharp margins covered with silvery scales, often on the elbows, knees, back and scalp, although they can occur anywhere; usually they do not itch. There are spontaneous remissions. The areas of psoriasis may occur in patterns, which are named: in guttate psoriasis they are very small and scattered like drops all over the body, a pattern which is common in children; in nummular discoid, round symmetrically distributed larger areas appear. The nails may become pitted, and lifted away from the nail bed. On the palms of the hands and the soles of the feet the areas may be cracked and infected. A proportion of patients develop arthritis which resembles rheumatoid arthritis. A number of treatments are used: the oldest is coal tar, made up as an ointment, cream or lotion. Dithranol is effective, but may stain the skin and clothes; it is made up as a paste, cream, ointment or wax application. It may be applied after taking a bath in weak coal-tar solution. PUVA therapy, which is the exposure to long-wave ultraviolet light (UVA) with a psoralen taken beforehand to sensitise the skin, is based on the fact that exposure to sunlight helps many patients. In many cases it is effective in a month or six weeks, but it is only available in special clinics, and there is a risk of long-term effects which include cataracts and skin cancers. The filtered sunlight which shines on the Dead Sea is especially effective, and many patients are treated there. In severe cases of psoriasis the cytotoxic drug methotrexate may be given to older patients, and in younger adults etretinate may be used by mouth; but etretinate produces deformities in the foetus, and must not be taken if there is any likelihood of pregnancy or during pregnancy. The possibility of pregnancy must be avoided for two years after treatment, and blood may not be donated for transfusion during the same period.

Psychedelic: from the Greek *psyche*, the soul, and *delos*, clear, the word is applied to drugs which are thought to make the soul manifest by confusing perception and thereby releasing the spirit from the bounds of reality. Others would say that the drugs produce hallucinations, delusions, and psychotic states.

Psychiatry: that branch of medicine which deals with mental illness.

Psychoanalysis: method of treatment of mental disturbances based on the theories of Sigmund Freud (1856–1939), which held that mental illness is to be explained in terms of a conflict between primitive emotions in the unconscious mind and the more civilised and learned tendencies in the conscious mind. The personality is divided into the 'id', which is the unconscious, containing primitive and repressed impulses, the conscious 'ego', and the half-conscious, half-unconscious 'super-ego' which may roughly be equated with the conscience. Thus all behaviour is the result of a three-cornered struggle between the ego, representing reality, the super-ego representing the social impulses, and the id representing primitive

535

desires. Initially the child is entirely primitive, but growing up is a process of slowly putting away childish ways and learning to repress unsuitable behaviour or sublimate it into something more useful; if this process fails, neurosis may develop in later life and the individual's relationships with others suffer. The first persons to whom the child has to relate are of course the parents, and psychoanalysis attaches great importance to this as the prototype of all later relationships; for example, a child who hates the father may grow up with an unreasoning hatred of all authority, or a child who is unloved will be unable to form any genuine love relationships later. The main instincts are sexual and aggressive; from these all the others arise, the word sexual being used in the widest possible sense to include, for instance, the infant's pleasure in sucking or in its bowel movements. In psychoanalysis the patient's problems are analysed by the method of free association: the patient lies on a couch and says whatever comes into his or her head, and this enables the psychoanalyst to unravel the sources of trouble. The method takes a great deal of time, up to an hour, five days a week, perhaps for a year or more, and can only be employed successfully by those especially trained in the technique.

Psychology: that branch of science as opposed to medicine which deals with the workings of the normal mind and is concerned with the study of normal behaviour. It clearly overlaps medical work, and clinical psychologists work with doctors to an increasing extent in what has become known as 'behavioural' medicine.

Psychoneurosis: synonymous with neurosis (q.v.).

Psychopathic: adjective applied to many forms of abnormal behaviour; a psychopath is one who is in some respect at odds with society, and the disturbance takes the form of antisocial actions, irresponsible and self-seeking, which are a trouble to others rather than to the psychopath.

Psychopathology: the study of the processes and nature of mental disorders.

Psychopharmacology: the branch of pharmacology that deals with the effects of drugs on the mind and behaviour.

Psychosis: the more serious and profound mental disorders such as schizophrenia and manic-depressive illness are known as psychoses; in general, a patient suffering from a psychosis does not recognise that there is anything wrong, that is to say there is no insight into the condition, while one suffering from a neurosis knows that there is something wrong, and has insight.

Psychosomatic Disease: disease affecting both the mind and body. Most diseases in fact involve both, because they affect sentient human beings, but some are influenced if not determined by the state of mind, such as peptic ulcer, asthma, colitis, migraine and certain skin conditions. It is likely that emotions such as anxiety acting through the brain on the autonomic nervous system exacerbate such diseases; every patient must be considered as a whole rather than just a vehicle for a particular disease.

Psychosurgery: surgery performed on the brain in order to modify the behaviour in severe mental disturbances. *See* Leucotomy.

Psychotherapy: the treatment of mental disorders by methods which do not involve the use of drugs, surgery or electroconvulsive treatment. It is not necessarily the same as psychoanalysis, and one psychotherapist can treat patients in small groups using the therapeutic possibilities of interactions between members of the group. There are a number of different techniques in psychotherapy based on different theories, but most derive from Freud. *See* Psychoanalysis.

Psychrotrophic Bacteria: bacteria that are able to spoil food and cause poisoning after being exposed to low temperatures. Examples are: *Clostridium botulinum*, which will withstand temperatures down to 3.3°C and causes botulism (q.v.); *Yersinia enterocolitica*, withstanding 1°C and causing diarrhoea and abdominal pain, especially in children; *Escherichia coli* of the type that causes traveller's diarrhoea (q.v.) which withstands 4°C; *Aeronomas hydrophila*, which can cause acute diarrhoea and withstand a temperature of −0.4°C; and *Listeria monocytogenes* (q.v.) which withstands −0.1°C. These bacteria are killed by cooking, but the temperature must be at least 70°C for two minutes. *L. monocytogenes* may need temperatures of 90°C. Psychrotrophic bacteria have come into prominence with the advent of 'cook-chill' catering.

Pterygium: a fold of membrane that is the shape of a wing in the conjunctiva of the eye, extending from the cornea across the sclera, the white of the eye, to the corner of the eyelid.

Ptomaine: a nitrogenous substance, otherwise called a putrefactive alkaloid, formed by the action of bacteria on dead animal matter. It was once held to be responsible for food poisoning.

Ptosis: the downward displacement of an organ; usually used to mean drooping of the upper eyelid.

Ptyalin: enzyme contained in saliva which breaks starch down into glucose and maltose.

Puberty: the beginning of the period of life when reproduction is possible, marked by the development of the secondary sexual characteristics and in girls by the beginning of menstruation. In boys it usually happens between 10 and 15, in girls at about 12 with a wide variation between 10 and 17.

Pubis: the bone felt at the bottom of the abdomen in the midline. It is the bone through which the hip-bone or os coxae joins its fellow on the opposite side, and the joint is called the pubic symphysis. *See* Pelvis.

Puerperal Fever: childbed fever, a septicaemia which was up to the middle of the last century widely fatal. Ignaz Semmelweiss (1818–65), while working in Vienna in 1846, noticed that the incidence of the fever was greater in labour wards where students rather than nurses examined patients. Suspecting that the students were carrying a contagion from the dissecting rooms, he made them wash their hands, and thereby greatly reduced the spread of the disease; but his efforts were not popular, nor accepted. Oliver Wendell Holmes (1809–94) in Boston observed and described the fact that the disease was contagious. It is in fact caused by infection of the uterus after childbirth by micro-organisms, mostly group A *streptococci*, and it was controlled to a great extent by antiseptics and scrupulous cleanliness on the part of the attendants at a labour when the principles of antiseptic and aseptic surgery were understood, but it was only reduced to its present low incidence by the advent of antibiotics.

Puerperium: the period of recovery after childbirth.

Pulmonary: to do with the lungs.

Pulmonary Embolism: the blocking of a branch of the pulmonary artery by a blood clot (*see* Embolism). The clot commonly forms in a deep vein in the leg as the result of damage to the vein wall, a sluggish circulation or an abnormality of coagulation. Circumstances favouring these conditions are confinement to bed, operations on the abdomen or pelvis, taking oestrogens in the contraceptive pill, or pregnancy. Injury to the leg may set up a deep vein thrombosis. Pulmonary embolism may be a complication of surgical operations after which a patient is confined to bed; the shorter the time, the less risk of a clot forming. The embolism may be minor or massive. In the case of a minor embolism there may be pain in the chest on breathing, caused by inflammation of the pleural membrane in the area of the embolism, and blood in the sputum; treatment is the administration of anticoagulant drugs usually starting with heparin and continuing with warfarin. In massive pulmonary embolism, which may have been preceded by a minor embolism, the patient may collapse and die. If the first shock is survived, right heart failure supervenes, with breathlessness and central pain in the chest which at first may look very like a coronary thrombosis; but patients with a thrombosis find it easier to breathe sitting up, whereas those with a pulmonary embolism find it easier lying down, for the venous return to the right heart is diminished by sitting up. The diagnosis is confirmed by electrocardiography and chest X-ray, and the extent of the thrombosis may be confirmed by cardiac catheterisation and pulmonary arteriography. Anticoagulant drugs are used, with streptokinase, which promotes the formation of plasmin and so breaks up clots (*see* Coagulation of the Blood), except in cases where there has been a major operation within five days or a hip replacement operation within ten days and in certain other cases, including the delivery of a child, within ten days. In such cases surgical operation to remove the clot must be considered, as it will be in cases where treatment with streptokinase is ineffective. If patients who have had a pulmonary embolism or a deep vein thrombosis in the leg have to undergo a subsequent operation or be confined to bed they can be given anticoagulants to prevent the formation of clots. Patients in whom a thrombosis and embolism has been associated with the contraceptive pill must clearly find another method of birth control.

Pulmonectomy: the surgical removal of a lung.

Pulp Infection: the pulp meant in this term is the pulp of the fingertip; such an infection can have serious consequences if it is not dealt with quickly and adequately, but antibiotics have made it far less difficult to treat than once it was.

Pulse: the expansion and contraction of a blood vessel in response to fluctuations in blood pressure as the heart beats. The arterial pulse can be felt at the wrist where the radial artery lies over the bone below the base of the thumb, and can also be felt in the temple or in the neck; the venous pulse can usually be seen just above the inner part of the collar-bone. The arterial pulse should be regular, and in men the rate is about 70–72 a minute, while in women it may be a little faster at about 78. A large number of types of pulse are described beside slow, fast or irregular, such as water-hammer, abrupt, running, vermicular, pistol-shot and others; a great deal can be learnt from the feel of the pulse.

Punch Drunk: it has been known for a very long time that some old boxers, particularly those who have not been very successful, become forgetful, unsteady on their feet and uncertain in their speech; this is the result of repeated injury to the brain, shown by characteristic changes found at post-mortem examination. The same condition can overtake others who in the course of their sport may receive repeated minor head injuries.

Pupil: the normally circular opening in the iris of the eye (q.v.).

Purgatives: *see* Constipation.

Purpura: haemorrhages from the capillaries which cause purple spots to appear in the skin. The condition may be divided into two classes, one of which is due to a deficiency in the number of platelets circulating in the blood (*see* Thrombocytopenic Purpura) and the other an abnormality of the capillary blood vessels resulting from infections, drugs, immunological reactions or scurvy. Elderly people are liable to bruise very easily, because of fragility of the capillaries, and in children the paroxysmal coughing of whooping cough can produce purpura because the pressure in the veins is raised.

Pus: tissue fluid containing the products of inflammation: dead white blood cells, bacteria and broken-down tissues.

Pyaemia: septicaemia, in which pus-forming organisms multiply in the blood and set up abscesses in parts of the body far removed from the original infection.

Pyelitis: inflammation of the pelvis of the kidney. It is rarely found on its own, but is usually associated with inflammation of the substance of the kidney. *See* Pyelonephritis.

Pyelography: the radiological examination of the pelvis of the kidney after it has been outlined by a radio-opaque substance. The outlining may be achieved in two ways: in the first, intravenous or excretory pyelography, a compound containing iodine is injected into a vein after a plain X-ray has been taken of the abdomen, and further pictures are taken after 5, 10, 15 and 30 minutes. The kidney concentrates and secretes the compound into the urine, and so outlines first the kidney, then the renal pelvis, the ureter and the bladder. Some idea of the function of the kidney can be obtained from the time taken to excrete the contrast medium and the degree of concentration achieved. The second method is retrograde pyelography, in which a cystoscope is passed into the bladder, and fine catheters introduced into the ureters through which dye can be injected to fill the urinary tract. The picture obtained is sharper, with a better outline of any abnormality, but the function of the kidneys is not revealed.

Pyelonephritis: inflammation of the kidney and the renal pelvis. Commonly the infecting organism is *Escherichia coli*, which is normally found in the lower part of the bowel. It is thought that infection ascends the urinary tract from contamination from the anus *via* the skin of the perineum separating the anus from the opening of the urethra, for urinary tract infection is commoner in infants with napkins and in women. Often the infection shows as cystitis, where it appears to be confined to the bladder, but infection of the urine means infection of the whole urinary tract, and particularly when there is any difficulty in passing urine, as in pregnancy or obstruction from an enlarged prostate, infection of the kidney becomes manifest, with pain in the loins, fever and shivering, and often the passage of blood-stained urine. Once the infecting organism has been identified by bacteriological examination of the urine, the appropriate antibiotic can be used.

Pyknolepsy: the name given to petit mal when the attacks are very frequent. *See* Epilepsy.

Pyloric Stenosis: a narrowing of the pylorus, the outlet from the stomach. In babies this may be congenital; it usually occurs in baby boys, often the firstborn, showing itself between the second and sixth weeks by vomiting often described as projectile. It may be noticed that the wind the baby brings up has a foul smell. There is no diarrhoea with the vomiting; the baby is constipated, loses weight and becomes dry. At operation the muscle surrounding the pylorus is found to be over-developed; after it has been divided the baby makes a good recovery and takes food in a matter of hours. In adults, pyloric stenosis is usually caused by scarring from a duodenal ulcer, but occasionally the obstruction is due to a malignant growth of the stomach; it leads to vomiting, often of large quantities of undigested food. The treatment is surgical; the lower part of the stomach may be removed and a new opening made into the small intestine (partial gastrectomy), or a bypass may be made into the small intestine (gastro-enterostomy).

Pylorospasm: a spasm of the muscle at the pylorous, usually caused by a duodenal ulcer.

Pylorus: the aperture in the stomach through which food passes into the duodenum. It is surrounded by a ring of muscle.

Pyogenic: anything which produces pus, usually applied to micro-organisms.

Pyorrhoea: the discharge of pus; pyorrhoea alveolaris is a disease of the gums and teeth in which pus is continually discharged and the teeth become loose.

Pyrethrum: an insecticidal powder.

Pyrexia: fever.

Pyridoxine: vitamin B_6.

Pyrimethamine: a drug used in cases of chloroquine-resistant malaria (q.v.).

Pyrogen: any substance which provokes a fever.

Pyuria: the passage of pus in the urine.

Q

Q Fever: an acute febrile illness caused by infection with the micro-organism *Coxiella burnetii*, a species of *Rickettsia*. There is weakness and headache, with a fever, pains in the muscles and general malaise, and patients often develop pneumonia; there may be inflammation of the liver, with jaundice. The incubation period is about three weeks, and the fever lasts for a week or two. The organism normally infects sheep, cattle and goats, passing to them from wild animals via ticks and lice, but humans acquire the infection by inhaling dust from dried excreta or drinking infected milk. *Coxiella burnetii* is sensitive to chloramphenicol and tetracycline.

Quadriceps: the large muscle covering the front of the thigh. It is a combination of four muscles, the vastus medialis, vastus intermedius, vastus lateralis and rectus femoris. The rectus femoris takes origin from the pelvis, the other three muscles from the femur, and the combination forms a common tendon, the quadriceps tendon, which contains a sesamoid bone, the kneecap or patella, and is inserted into the upper part of the tibia. The action of the muscle is to extend the knee.

Quadriplegia: paralysis of all four limbs.

Quarantine: the isolation of people who are suspected of having a communicable disease or who have been in contact with one. Ships were originally held for 40 days if they were suspected of carrying disease, and the term arose from the French *quarante*. It is now mostly used for the compulsory six months' detention of animals brought from abroad into the United Kingdom; this is to prevent the spread of rabies. *See* Incubation Period.

Quartan Fever: fever recurring at 72-hour intervals; malaria caused by *Plasmodium malariae*.

Quassia: the bitter-tasting wood of a tropical tree from which an infusion can be made which was in the eighteenth century used as a remedy for fevers; it was also used as an enema to treat worms.

Quickening: the first movements of the foetus, usually felt by the mother at about the 20th week.

Quinidine: a drug obtained from the cinchona tree and used to treat irregular heart action.

Quinine: an alkaloid made from the bark of the South American cinchona tree, which has for many years been used as a remedy for malaria; it is still used against chloroquine-resistant strains of *Plasmodium falciparum*, the organism of malignant malaria, and can be given by mouth or by intravenous infusion. It can also be used for the relief of night cramps.

Quinolines: the derivatives of quinoline include quinine, chloroquine, amodiaquine, primaquine and mefloquine, all used in the treatment of malaria.

Quinolones: 4-quinolones are a group of antibiotics which comprise nalidixic acid and cinoxacin, used in urinary infections, ciprofloxacin, used in Gram-negative and some Gram-positive infections that are resistant to other antibiotics, and enoxacin, which is used in skin infections, shigella infections, gonorrhoea and urinary infections.

Quinsy: *see* Peritonsillar Abscess.

Quotidian Fever: fever recurring every day, as in malaria when the infection is mixed.

R

Rabies: a virus disease endemic in many parts of the world among wild animals, including foxes, wolves, jackals, mongooses, raccoons, skunks and bats. It may be passed on to domestic animals, particularly dogs, although cats can be infected. In Central and South America vampire bats are responsible for up to a million deaths a year in cattle they infect with rabies. It is difficult to estimate the number of human deaths from rabies each year in the world, but it is thought that there are well over 10,000 in India, about 70 in Mexico, and less than 6 in the United States. Only one or two a year are known in continental Europe, despite the fact that since the last world war there has been a spread of infection among foxes from Poland towards the English Channel.

The rabies virus is one of the rhabdovirus group, and it advances from the site of infection through the peripheral nerves to the central nervous system as well as to the rest of the body, and produces two groups of cases, the furious and the paralytic. In dogs only one out of four develop furious rabies, but in cats the proportion is three out of four. The incubation period is between three and twelve weeks, although it may be as short as a week or as long as a year. The infection is spread to man by the bite of a rabid animal; the incubation period is usually the same, but is shorter after a bite on the face than after a bite on the limbs. The illness begins with pain or itching in the healed bite, with fever, headache, general malaise and anxiety; if the infection has spread mainly to the spinal cord, paralytic rabies follows, but more commonly the infection is worst in the brain and the furious form of rabies develops. Hydrophobia, the fear of water, is characteristic, and there are generalised muscle spasms, hallucinations, aggressive irrational behaviour and manifestations of terror. The condition is fatal in most cases, but there is a chance of recovery in a modern intensive care unit.

Early treatment of a possibly infected bite is essential; the wound is cleaned surgically, and a course of immunising injections given, both passive and active. If the animal that inflicted the bite proves to be healthy for five days the course of injections may be stopped, but if the animal was wild, or observation is impossible, the full course must be given. Active immunisation against rabies is possible: three injections are given, the second a month after the first and the third six months later, with reinforcing injections every year or three years according to the risk of infection. Several countries including the United Kingdom have controlled rabies by strict regulations concerning the importation of animals, and in countries where rabies is prevalent domestic dogs can be immunised; vaccines have been laid down in bait to spread immunity in wild animals.

Rachitic: rickety. *See* Osteomalacia.

Radiation: the emission of waves, rays or particles. Radiations may be ionising or non-ionising. Non-ionising radiations liable to affect human beings are those of ultraviolet light which can in excess cause skin cancer, powerful ultrasonic waves which can damage the tissues by heating, and radio frequency electromagnetic waves such as those used in microwave ovens which can cause burning by induction heating. There is no evidence to suggest that the use of ultrasound of the power used in medical diagnostic procedures is harmful, nor is there much evidence that exposure to the radiation from strong magnetic fields is dangerous, although the use of nuclear magnetic resonance imaging (q.v.) has led to limits being recommended until there is more experience in the matter.

Ionising radiations are, however, different. They impart enough energy to an irradiated substance to cause ionisation, that is, an electron is displaced from the atoms making up a molecule, which may damage the molecules which make up a cell and so damage the cells themselves. Ionising radiations may be X-rays which are electromagnetic waves of a very short wavelength, gamma rays which are the same as X-rays but given off by radioactive atoms, or particulate, the particles being given off by atomic disintegration or produced by electrical particle accelerators. X-rays were discovered by Wilhelm Röntgen (1845-1923), the German physicist, in 1895; used by doctors ever since, they are the greatest source of artificial irradiation. Others are nuclear reactors and the nuclear bomb. There are many natural sources of ionising radiations, ranging from cosmic rays emanating from the sun and other parts of the universe, to which we are all exposed, to radon in the soil and granite. The units used to measure the dose of ionising radiation absorbed are the *rad* and the *gray*. The rad equals 0.01 joules of energy absorbed in 1 kg of tissue, and the gray 1 joule absorbed in 1 kg tissue. Biological activity is measured differently: 1 *rem* is the amount of any radiation taken to produce the effect of 1 rad of gamma rays; one *sievert* (Sv) the amount required to produce the effect of 1 gray of gamma rays.

The effect of ionising radiation on tissues depends on the linear energy transfer (LET). X-rays and gamma rays have a low LET; they produce few interactions along their path, they travel far into or through the body, and their effect depends on the rate at which the dose is received. The damage they do to the larger molecules varies according to the chemical state of the molecule, which can increase or decrease the effect. Charged particles have a high LET; they produce many interactions and do not penetrate far into the body, but their biological effect is pronounced, and is less dependent on rate of dosage. The effect of irradiation of the whole human body ranges from a drop in the number of lymphocytes in the blood after a dose of 0.1 Sv to death after a dose of 10 Sv or more as a single exposure. The effect of irradiation of the testis may be sterility after a dose of 2 Sv or more, and a temporary drop in the sperm count after 0.15 Sv. The effect on the ovary is sterility after a dose of 2.0–3.0 Sv, and temporary sterility after 1.5–2.0 Sv. It is estimated that damage to the genes, and therefore the risk of mutation in offspring, is incurred after a dose of 0.2–2.5 Sv, which is enough to cause temporary or permanent sterility in potential parents. The long-term effects of irradiation include the development of all kinds of cancer, but the growths that result have no distinguishing feature and it is therefore impossible to estimate their number. It is, however, known that leukaemia, usually of the acute myeloid type, is a disease that can follow irradiation, as are skin cancers and cancer of the breast.

As was said above, the greatest source of radiation in everyday life is medical diagnostic radiography. Limits have therefore been set on the amount of radiation people should receive in any one year. They are for whole body irradiation 0.5 rem, subject to an average for any one year of 0.1 rem, so that the total dose received in a lifetime does not exceed 7 rem. Higher doses can be given if only a part of the body is irradiated, but care is always taken that the dose should be as small as possible. Other dose limits are observed for radiation workers.

Radiculitis: inflammation of a root, applied to inflammation of a nerve root.

Radiography: the demonstration on photographic plates or fluorescent screens of the images formed by the passage of short-wave radiation from X-rays through an object. In medical radiography, the radiographer is responsible for the production of the X-ray plates; the radiologist is a medically qualified specialist who examines and reports on the films.

Radiology: the medical specialty concerned with the use of electromagnetic radiation to produce images of parts of the body. The electromagnetic waves used may be X-rays, the gamma rays given off by radioactive materials, or ultrasonic waves. In nuclear magnetic resonance imaging (q.v.) magnetic waves are used. Radiology has been, and continues to be, basic to many advances in surgery and medicine.

Radiotherapy: the use of ionising radiation in the treatment of disease. It depends on the fact that rapidly dividing tumour cells are more susceptible to the effects of radiation than normal cells. The radiations used are electromagnetic, (X-ray or gamma radiation), or accelerated particles. *See* Radiation.

Radium: a rare element which is radioactive. Radioactivity was discovered by Pierre (1859–1906) and Marie (1867–1934) Curie who described the alpha, beta and gamma radiation given off by the element, which they isolated for the first time. Radium has been used a great deal in the past in radiotherapy, but has been superseded by various artificially produced isotopes.

Radius: bone of the forearm which lies on the outer side when the arm is by the side with the palm facing forwards. It is able to rotate round the ulna, the other forearm bone, so that the movements of pronation and supination are possible. It plays a small part in the formation of the elbow joint, but a large part in the wrist joint. It is often fractured in falls on the outstretched hand (Colles' fracture).

Radon: a radioactive gas, the product of the breakdown of radium. It may be found in the soil.

Râle: a sound heard through the stethoscope in diseases of the lung and air passages. Râles are described as moist or dry, being produced by the passage of air over or through dry or wet secretions or by the expansion of sticky alveoli. Rhonchi are more coarse snoring or wheezing noises caused by obstructions in the air passages, and crepitations are finer, more crackling sounds than râles.

Ramus: a branch. Used in anatomy to describe a smaller branch given off by a larger structure, or the smaller branches into which a structure divides.

Ranitidine: a drug used in the treatment of peptic ulcers (q.v.).

Ranula: a cyst lying under the tongue, developing as the result of a blocked salivary or mucous gland. It is not dangerous and can easily be treated surgically.

Rash: a temporary eruption or discoloration of the skin, often associated with an infectious fever. Salient characteristics of such rashes are:
   Measles: first small greyish spots appear inside the mouth on the inside of the cheeks (Koplik's spots). About three days later the skin rash starts as small red raised spots on the forehead and behind the ears which spread onto the face and so down over the trunk and the whole body.

It is fully developed in two days, and darkens; as it does so, the spots tend to run together and form blotches. It lasts about a week.

Rubella, or German measles, has a rash of small red spots starting on the face and spreading to the trunk, but it only lasts a couple of days. There are no spots inside the mouth, but the lymph nodes behind the ear and in the neck are enlarged. Neither of these rashes itches.

Varicella or chicken-pox: the rash starts on the trunk and is most marked on those parts of the body that are normally covered. It begins as small flat spots, which become pimples and then small blisters which become yellow, burst and scab over. The rash itches a good deal, and lasts about a week. The pocks form in crops and take about a day to turn from small flat spots to pustules.

Scarlet fever is now a very mild condition associated with a streptococcal infection, usually of the throat, although within living memory it was a dangerous disease. The skin reddens, and upon it are small red spots starting on the chest, arms and neck, and spreading outwards and downwards. It does not itch, and nowadays is usually so mild that it almost escapes attention. The tongue becomes covered with a white fur, which peels off to leave the surface red.

RAST: radio-allergosorbent test carried out on blood to detect allergy to bee or wasp venoms or other substances.

Rat Bite Fever: there are two types of rat bite fever, one caused by infection with *Streptobacillus moniliformis*, the other with *Spirillum minor*. The first, caused by rat bites or contact with rats, may also be acquired by drinking milk or eating food contaminated by rats. The fever takes a few days to develop, and produces a headache with pains in the muscles and vomiting. There may be a rash on the back of the limbs and on the palms and soles, and pain and swelling of the large joints. In the second type of infection, particularly found in Japan, the incubation period is more than a week, and the fever is severe. The original bite becomes inflamed. There may be pains in the joints, but no swelling. The rash is dark. Both types of fever are treated by penicillin or erythromycin.

Rauwolfia: a genus of tropical shrubs and trees from which arrow poisons were made. From the roots of *Rauwolfia serpentina* a substance was made which was for many years used in India to quieten excited patients, and which came into use in Europe in the eighteenth century. After the Second World War the alkaloids isolated from rauwolfia, in particular reserpine, came into use both in psychiatry and in the treatment of high blood pressure; it was in its time a revolutionary drug, but has now been superseded by a number of new compounds, although it remains available for use in cases where other treatments fail or cannot be used.

Raynaud's Disease: described by Maurice Raynaud (1834–81), a French physician; it occurs usually in young women, in whom the fingers and toes become cold and white, or blue, when exposed to cold. They go numb, and may tingle and even be painful. They go red when warmed, and may again be painful as the circulation recovers. The cause is spasm of the arterioles supplying the fingers and toes, but why this should happen is not clear. A similar condition called Raynaud's phenomenon may occur as a consequence of various diseases, or in those who have used pneumatic hammers or chain saws. It may be caused by certain drugs including ergot. In severe cases the skin over the fingertips may become pitted or, rarely, gangrenous. There is no specific treatment, but various drugs have been used, including nifedipine. Obviously the hands and feet must be kept warm. In serious cases affecting the legs, surgical interruption of the sympathetic nervous supply has been successful, but in cases affecting the arms similar operations have been disappointing.

RBC: an abbreviation for red blood cell.

Rectum: the last part of the intestine which joins the anal canal. It begins at the level of the third part of the sacrum, being continuous with the pelvic colon, and is about 12 cm long. It is most of the time empty, for the passage of faeces into the rectum sets up the desire to defecate.

Reflex: an automatic, involuntary reaction to a stimulus. A reflex arc in the nervous system consists of the receptor of the stimulus, the nerve which conducts the sensory impulse, the connection between the nerve and the nerve cell supplying the organ or muscle which responds, and the nerve running from the cell to the responding structure.

Reflux: a flow of fluid in a direction opposite to the normal flow.

Refraction: the deviation of light rays from a straight path when passing obliquely through the junction between two media of different optical density. In medicine, the determination of refractive errors in the eye and their correction by lenses.

Regional Ileitis: *see* Ileitis.

Rehabilitation: the restoration of a patient after injury or illness to a state in which he or she can be self-sufficient, even if the occupation has to be changed. It includes retraining for employment as well as physiotherapy and the provision of aids to daily living.

Reiter's Disease: first described by Hans Reiter (1881–1969), a German physician, this condition mostly affects young males, and produces non-specific urethritis, conjunctivitis and arthritis, often of the knee but also affecting other joints. There may be pain in the feet caused by inflammation of the plantar fascia, the connective tissue in the soles of the feet, or in the ankle because of inflammation of the Achilles tendon. The skin of the soles of the feet may be thickened, and the nails may be affected. The urethritis, which produces a discharge and some discomfort on passing water, and the conjunctivitis are of less importance than the arthritis, which may be disabling. The disease may be acquired sexually, but it may follow an attack of bacillary dysentery; no specific organism has been found responsible, although *Mycoplasma hominis* and *Chlamydia trachomatis* have been implicated. Tetracyclines are given for the non-specific urethritis, and the arthritis is treated with NSAIDS.

Rejection: the destruction of grafted tissues which are not immunologically compatible with the host.

Relapsing Fever: there are two forms of relapsing fever, one spread by lice, the other by ticks. The louse-borne form is caused by the spirochaete *Borrelia recurrentis*, and the body louse *Pediculus humanus* becomes infected by biting an infected patient. Lice flourish where there is overcrowding and dirt, and relapsing fever is a disease of war and poverty. It is endemic in Ethiopia, but may occur anywhere. Tick-borne relapsing fever is found more often in tropical and subtropical countries, and various species of *Borrelia* are involved. The incubation period is about a week; the fever arises suddenly, with severe headache, generalised pains, and vomiting. The liver is involved, and there may be jaundice, as well as a rash on the trunk. In the louse-borne disease the fever lasts for about a week, there is an intermission of about a week, and then up to five relapses of fever with remissions; the tick-borne disease is less severe and the fever only lasts for about three days, but there may be up to a dozen relapses. Tetracycline or erythromycin are used in treatment; the tick-borne disease is more difficult to cure and the course of tetracycline must continue for 10 days.

Relaxant: a drug that reduces tension; muscle relaxants are used during general anaesthesia to produce muscular relaxation without increasing the dose of the anaesthetic agent. They may also be used in the treatment of tetanus.

Remission: an abatement of symptoms during the course of a disease.

Renal Calculus: stone in the kidney. Most stones are made of calcium oxalate, some are mixed calcium oxalate and phosphate, some consist of magnesium ammonium phosphate, a few of uric acid, and some are mixed calcium and phosphate. A very few contain cystine. Normal urine contains substances which prevent the formation of crystals, and the balance between these and the amount of salts in the urine which can form stones determines the likelihood of stones beginning to form. Calcium oxalate stones are usually small, and are passed without much trouble. Calcium and phosphate stones are larger, and may remain in the pelvis of the kidney. Stones are harmful if they obstruct the passage of urine through the urinary tract, creating back-pressure, or if they lead to chronic urinary infection. Just under half of all stones that are formed pass spontaneously into the ureter and so into the bladder. In their passage down the ureter they may cause intense colicky pain in the flank and abdomen, which can be ameliorated by the use of hyoscine or atropine to relax the smooth muscle of the ureter. The amount of urine passed should be increased by drinking large amounts of water. If stones become stuck, they can be dislodged by cystoscopy and ureteric catheterisation. The passage of a stone into the bladder may be accompanied by blood in the urine and frequency of passing urine, but it is usually passed safely out of the bladder through the urethra. About a fifth of the stones lodge in the bladder, where they may cause frequency of micturition, blood in the urine, difficulty in passing urine and infection, but can be seen and dealt with by cystoscopy. The larger stones that remain in the pelvis of the kidney may give rise to urinary tract infection and pain in the loin, and if they are undetected may lead to damage to the kidney itself. Infections are treated with the appropriate antibiotics. The stones can be removed in a number of ways: open operation on the kidney is possible, but it is also possible to approach the stone through a small incision in the flank through which a track is made to the kidney; through this an ultrasound probe can be passed to break up the stone, and the fragments can be removed through an endoscope. Another method which does not require any surgical intervention is extracorporeal shock wave lithotripsy (*see* Lithotripsy). Those who suffer from recurrent renal stones should be investigated for factors that increase the likelihood of stone formation such as the excretion of excess calcium. If it is found, it may be treated by dietary restrictions, for example on dairy products; tea and fruit, which contain oxalates, should be taken in moderation. The intake of water must be kept fairly high at over three litres a day.

Renal Dialysis: if the function of the kidneys is impaired to the extent that they are no longer able to rid the body of water and waste products, death is inevitable unless these functions are taken over by an artificial kidney or a kidney transplant. The principle of renal dialysis which makes the artificial kidney possible, that is the use of a tube made of a semipermeable membrane through which the waste products of the blood can pass into a solution surrounding the tube while the proteins and cells are retained, was described in America in 1913, but it was not until the Second World War that W.J. Kolff (born 1911) in Holland produced a successful machine. Since that time great advances have been made in the design and application of artificial kidneys, and now a patient treated by renal dialysis can continue to lead a working life for years.

An artificial connection is made surgically between the radial artery in the forearm and a superficial vein. Arterial blood then can be drawn off from the superficial vein through a needle, and pumped into the artificial kidney machine where it passes through the tube of semipermeable membrane, washed down by dialysis fluid. This fluid contains sodium, dextrose and other substances in the same concentrations as are found in the blood, which prevents some essential constituents of the blood passing the membrane; the concentrations can be varied according to the needs of the patient. The blood is then returned to the patient. Dialysis of the blood as a rule takes place three times a week for between four and six hours. Dialysis is also possible through the natural membrane of the peritoneum, when the dialysis fluid is introduced into the peritoneal cavity through a catheter implanted into the abdominal wall and left there for a period of time. It is then drained off and replaced. This has to be done every four hours. Two litres of fluid are used at a time, supplied in a plastic bag. When the bag has been emptied into the peritoneal cavity it is worn in a belt, and then used to drain off the fluid; it is discarded, and a new bag fitted, the process taking well under an hour. This technique is very effective, and patients can be independent, but it needs scrupulous attention to detail for there is a risk of peritonitis. A variant is the use of peritoneal dialysis only at night, the fluid being drained and replaced by a machine; the catheter connection is then disturbed only once a day, and the risk of peritonitis is diminished. It remains true, however, that the best and the most economical treatment for kidney failure is a kidney transplant.

Repellants: usually applied to substances that repel insects, such as dimethylphthalate (DMP) and dimethyl-toluamide (DET).

Repetitive Strain Injury: *see* Cramp, Tenosynovitis.

Reserpine: *see* Rauwolfia.

Resolution: in medicine, the process of healing; for example, 'The pneumonia resolved quickly, and the patient is now well.'

Respiration: the process of breathing. It includes the muscular movements of the chest wall and diaphragm whereby the lungs are filled with air, and the exchange of gases in the lungs between the air and the blood. In health the normal respiratory rate at rest is about 18–20 a minute.

Respirators: machines that help paralysed patients to breathe. They may be divided into two classes, those which pump air or gases into the lungs under positive pressure, and those which enclose the patient's chest and produce a drop in the atmospheric pressure, thus drawing air under atmospheric pressure into the lungs through the mouth and nose, which are outside the apparatus in which the partial vacuum is induced. These were used in cases of chronic paralysis of the muscles of respiration, which are uncommon now that poliomyelitis has been controlled by general immunisation. The iron lung was of this type. Positive pressure respirators, now commonly referred to as ventilators, are used in a number of conditions besides weakness of the muscles of respiration, for example head injuries and drug poisoning, and are essential equipment in intensive care units. They are also used by anaesthetists in the operating theatre in conjunction with the muscle-relaxing drugs, and in various operations where the breathing has to be supported artificially. For temporary use, the positive pressure ventilator is connected to an endotracheal tube, a tube passed through the larynx into the windpipe, but for extended use a tracheostomy is made, an opening into the trachea below the larynx.

Respiratory Distress Syndrome: in adults, this term refers to acutely difficult or inadequate respiration occurring in patients with previously normal lungs. It may be caused by a number of unrelated conditions, such as injury, severe infection of the lungs, poisoning by gases, or by drugs. In newborn children, particularly those born prematurely, by Caesarean section, or to a diabetic mother, the disease is due to inadequate exchange of gases in the alveoli of the lung, which are filled with a hyaline material. Normally the alveoli of the newborn contain a lipoprotein called surfactant, which has the property of decreasing the surface tension at the interface between air and fluid, thus facilitating the expansion of the alveoli. If surfactant is not synthesised, the lungs do not expand properly, and the consequence is the respiratory distress syndrome. The disease is also called hyaline membrane disease, from the appearance of the material filling the lungs. The condition develops shortly after birth, and is characterised by rapid, laboured breathing; the baby is blue and exhausted. Highly specialised and constant care may allow the baby to survive, and after the first few days a gradual recovery takes place as the alveoli expand and adequate gas exchange becomes possible. Recently surfactant substitutes have been developed to be given to premature babies; they have been approved for use in the USA and are currently undergoing trials in Britain.

Resuscitation: properly applied to the process of reviving the apparently dead, that is those in whom the heartbeat and breathing have stopped, the term has been extended to cover the treatment of surgical shock.

Retention: the process of keeping back or maintaining in position; usually applied to the involuntary retention of urine because of an obstruction, such as an enlarged prostate gland.

Reticulocyte: a newly formed red blood cell, so called because it shows on microscopical examination after staining a fine network which is thought to be the remains of a nucleus; the mature red cell has no nucleus. Increased numbers of reticulocytes are seen in the circulation in cases where a large number of red cells have been lost in a haemorrhage, or where they are being destroyed, as in a haemolytic anaemia.

Reticulo-endothelial System: name given to a system of cells scattered throughout the body which have the special function of phagocytosis, that is they eat up foreign material, such as bacteria, and the remains of dead cells. These phagocytic cells are called macrophages, and originate in the bone marrow; they circulate in the bloodstream as monocytes before becoming fixed in the tissues, principally in the spleen, liver, lymph nodes and bone marrow. The endothelial cells lining the blood vessels are also phagocytic and regarded as part of the reticulo-endothelial system. The monocytes play a part in the immune system, and produce humoral agents called monokines, which among other actions promote the formation of antibodies and in inflammation produce fever by influencing the hypothalamus in the brain.

Retinal Detachment: the retina (*see* Eye) is a membrane lining the eye which is sensitive to light. It has two layers, one composed of nerve cells and the other pigmented. The nerve cells are transparent and lie on the inner part of the eye, with the pigmented layer as a backing. If a hole or tear develops in the nerve cell layer as the result of injury, degeneration or severe short-sight, the fluid in the eye may separate the nerve cells from the pigmented layer and the sight is impaired. The condition is treated by sealing the holes, usually now by the use of a laser beam. It may be done by local freezing (cryotherapy).

Retinitis Pigmentosa: a condition inherited as a dominant or recessive characteristic, or one linked to the X chromosome. It produces night blindness and constriction of the visual field.

Retinopathy: disease of the retina.

Retrobulbar Neuritis: inflammation of the optic nerve behind the eye; it is a common presenting sign in multiple sclerosis, and is detected by the pale appearance of the optic disc on examination of the eye by ophthalmoscopy.

Retroflexion: the backward bending of an organ or structure, applied especially to the bending backwards of the body of the uterus in relation to the cervix.

Retrograde Amnesia: loss of memory for a period of time preceding a particular incident. The term is generally applied to the type of memory loss that follows a severe blow to the head resulting in loss of consciousness. *See* Amnesia.

Retrolental Fibroplasia: this condition develops in newborn infants in whom the blood vessels of the retina undergo spasm and the tissues of the retina consequently degenerate and scar. It is due to excessive oxygen in the blood, and this means that oxygen has to be administered to infants with great care.

Retropharyngeal Abscess: a rare form of abscess which collects behind the back of the pharynx, and is due to tuberculosis of the vertebrae of the neck.

Retroversion: the displacement backwards of an organ, usually used to refer to the uterus which normally lies with the body slightly inclined forwards from the vertical. It may take up a position with the body pointing more to the rear at puberty, when it grows to adult size, but the condition gives rise to no trouble except rarely during pregnancy when it may fail to rise easily out of the pelvis as it enlarges and have to be assisted to do so by manipulation. Retroversion may follow pregnancy, and unless the uterus was retroverted before the pregnancy it may cause discomfort. If it is replaced and perhaps supported by a pessary the uterus usually regains its normal position. Operations can be performed in cases where there is chronic discomfort attributed to retroversion.

Retrovirus: a group of viruses of which HIV, the virus responsible for AIDS, is a member.

Reye's Syndrome: a rare disorder of the liver in children in which there is severe vomiting and drowsiness, which may proceed to coma and death, occurring after a virus infection such as measles or chicken-pox; the precise cause is not known, but it has been associated with various drugs, the most commonly used being aspirin. The use of aspirin for children under 12 years old has therefore been abandoned in the United Kingdom and the USA.

Rhabdovirus: a group of viruses which includes the organism responsible for rabies.

Rhesus Factor: *see* Haemolytic Disease of the Newborn.

Rheumatic Fever: a disease which has become far less common in the Western world in the last 60 or 70 years, but remains widespread in the less developed countries. It is associated with infection by a haemolytic group A *Streptococcus*, which commonly produces a sore throat, and appears to be due to an abnormal immune response to the infection. It affects children between four and fifteen years old; the joints become painful, but most importantly the heart is involved, with the mitral valves being damaged and the heart muscle weakened. The aortic and tricuspid valves are less commonly damaged. In a few cases the central nervous system is involved and the patients develop chorea, that is clumsiness with abnormal involuntary jerky movements. The streptococcus is sensitive to penicillin, and aspirin is used for the joint pain, an exception to the rule that it should not be given to children under 12 (*see* Reye's Syndrome). Strict rest is necessary until the symptoms have disappeared and laboratory blood tests are satisfactory; this may take two or more months. The disease is liable to recur, and long-term use of penicillin is advised either by mouth or by injection at set intervals for up to 10 years. The damage to the mitral valve results in incompetence of the valve which may require cardiac surgery.

Rheumatism: a term loosely applied to pain and inflammation of the joints and muscles which causes stiffness and difficulty in moving. It includes many diseases, principally osteoarthritis and rheumatoid arthritis (*see below*).

Rheumatoid Arthritis: a disease affecting the joints, over twice as common in women as it is in men. The cause is not certain, but it is thought to be due to an abnormality of the immune system involving an auto-immune reaction, that is a reaction to one of the body's own constituents. It occurs at any age, but is most common between 35 and 55 in women and 40 to 60 in men, and may come on suddenly or insidiously. The joints most commonly affected are the hands, wrists, ankles and knees, and those in the neck. There is pain and swelling, with difficulty in movement, worse in the morning and after a period of inactivity. The tendon sheaths may become inflamed, producing pain on movement, and the feet are painful when walking. The hands and feet may become deformed. In advanced cases the knees become unstable and walking becomes still more difficult, while the elbows become stiff and fixed in flexion. Patients may develop pleurisy or pericarditis, and may be anaemic. Treatment is aimed at enabling the patient to make the best possible use of the function that remains, and may include surgery as well as physiotherapy and the use of splints and aids at home. The NSAIDs (q.v.) are used, but the results may be disappointing and it may be difficult to select the drug which suits each patient best. There are a number of slow-acting anti-rheumatic drugs which may be used, among them gold salts, penicillamine, chloroquine and azothiaprine. All have to be used over a considerable time, and all have unwanted effects which mean that they can only be used under constant medical supervision. The corticosteroids are not used in the treatment of rheumatoid arthritis.

Rhinitis: inflammation of the mucous membrane of the nose, as in the common cold. When chronic it may lead to the formation of nasal polyps, and may be associated with inflammation of the sinuses. It may be of allergic origin, as in hay fever or sensitivity to the house dust mite or animal hair or fur.

Rhinophyma: a form of rosacea in which the nose becomes red, nodular and enlarged. It is disfiguring. *See* Acne Rosacea.

Rhinorrhoea: a discharge from the nose. This may be due to allergic rhinitis, the allergy commonly being to pollen, house dust mite, moulds and animal dander. The treatment includes, if possible, the avoidance of the allergen, and the suppression of the symptoms by antihistamines such as terfanadine or astemizole; the use of sodium cromoglycate has to be continuous, for it prevents rather than cures the condition, and has to be used four or six times a day as a nasal spray or drops. In adults and older children corticosteroid nasal sprays are very effective (*see* Hay Fever). Vasomotor rhinitis (q.v.) is a condition that causes a clear discharge from the nose all the year round; in children, enlarged adenoids may cause a degree of rhinorrhoea, as may the development of nasal polyps in adults.

Rhinoscopy: the examination of the interior of the nose.

Rhinovirus: a group of viruses which produce the common cold.

Rhodopsin: visual purple, present in the rods of the retina. It is derived from vitamin A, and is responsible for vision in dim light.

Rhonchus: a noise heard through the stethoscope when there is a partial block of the air passages; it is a whistling, wheezing or snoring sound, coarser than a râle (q.v.).

Rhubarb: the root of *Rheum officinale* or *palmatum* was once popular as a purgative, especially for children.

Riboflavin: vitamin B_2. Normal diets have an adequate content of this vitamin, but deficiency leads to cracked lips, a sore tongue, and itching dermatitis of the genitalia.

Ribonucleic Acid (RNA); a substance included in all living cells by which information contained in the inherited DNA (deoxyribonucleic acid) is used in the formation of protein molecules. DNA is found in the cell nucleus; RNA in the ribosomes. It is through this mechanism that hereditary characteristics are handed down from generation to generation.

Ribosomes: granules in the substance of living cells which contain RNA and proteins. The synthesis of proteins takes place in the ribosomes.

Ribs: curved, long, thin bones that run from the thoracic vertebrae behind towards the sternum or breastbone in front. There are twelve; they increase in length from the first to the seventh, and then decrease. Only the first seven reach the breastbone, to which they are joined by the costal cartilages, short lengths of cartilage extending from the ends of the ribs. The lower five ribs are progressively shorter, the upper three cartilages articulating with the one above, the lower two extremities being free. The space between the ribs contains the intercostal arteries, veins and nerves and the intercostal muscles. The ribs contain active red marrow. They are fairly easily broken by a blow to the chest, and the broken ends if displaced inwards may injure the lung (*see* Pneumothorax). The treatment of a simple fracture of a rib is to leave it; an injection of local anaesthetic will ease the pain and make breathing easier. Multiple fractures may need surgery. If the lower chest is injured, it must not be forgotten that there may be an underlying internal injury to the liver, spleen or gut.

Rickets: *see* Osteomalacia.

Rickettsiae: small micro-organisms which were at one time considered to be halfway between bacteria and viruses; they cannot live outside living cells. They are now classified as bacteria. They are carried by ticks, mites, fleas and lice, and are responsible for typhus, Q fever, and Rocky Mountain spotted fever. Rickettsiae are sensitive to chloramphenicol and tetracyclines.

Rifampicin: an antibiotic drug used in the treatment of tuberculosis and leprosy. It reduces the effectiveness of the contraceptive pill.

Rigor: an attack of shivering and a sensation of cold, suffered during a sharp rise in temperature in a fever. Rigor mortis is the stiffening of the muscles that takes place after death.

Ringworm: a superficial fungus infection of the skin, so called because the centre of the infection heals while the spread is centrifugal, so forming a circle. *See* Tinea.

Rinne's Test: named after the German surgeon Heinrich Rinne (1819–63) who described it, the test involves alternately holding a vibrating tuning fork half an inch from the ear and placing its foot on the mastoid bone behind the ear until it can no longer be heard in one of the two positions. The other ear is closed while the test is made. Normally the note is heard longer when conducted through the air than through the bone, but when there is some impediment to the conduction of sound in the outer or middle ear, and the inner ear and auditory nerve are normal, the reverse is true. *See* Ear, Weber's Test.

RNA: *see* Ribonucleic Acid.

Rocky Mountain Spotted Fever: tick typhus, caused by *Rickettsia rickettsii*, found mostly in America, particularly in the southern Atlantic States and in southern central States of the USA. Ticks once infected remain infected for life; they may live on dogs and small animals, and so reach human beings. The disease has an incubation period of about a week. It causes fever with headache, and a rash which appears on the fourth day of the illness, which lasts for about three weeks. The treatment is with tetracycline or chloramphenicol.

Rodent Ulcer: a malignant tumour of the skin arising from the basal cells (*see* Skin). It is usually found on the face, particularly in those who have been exposed to the sun, for it is caused by ultraviolet light; it looks like a small raised ulcer that will not heal. It is only locally malignant, and does not give rise to secondary growths in other parts of the body, but if it is left it is capable of spreading into the bone beneath the skin. It can be treated with complete success by surgical removal or radiotherapy.

Romberg's Sign: named after Moritz Romberg (1795–1873), the German physician who first described it, Romberg's sign is present when a patient cannot stand with the eyes closed and the feet together without swaying or falling. It is due to a loss of position sense in the legs, classically in tabes dorsalis, a manifestation of the third stage of syphilis.

Röntgen: a unit of gamma or X radiation; it is the amount which will produce in 1 cubic centimetre of air 1 electrostatic unit of electrical charge of either sign. It has been superseded by new units (*see* Radiation). It was named after the German physicist Wilhelm Röntgen (1845–1923) who discovered X-rays in 1895.

Rorschach Test: devised by the Swiss psychiatrist Hermann Rorschach (1884–1922) for investigating intelligence and personality; otherwise known as the 'ink-blot' test, for patients are asked to say what impressions they gain from examining a series of patterns made from ink-blots.

Rosacea: *see* Acne Rosacea.

Roundworm: *see* Worms.

Rubefacients: substances that produce reddening of the skin by increasing the blood flow. They are used to rub into the skin over painful muscles and joints, and act by counter-irritation; they are contained in various liniments and creams.

Rubella: German measles. A mild infection, its importance lies in the fact that infection of pregnant women can result in congenital deformities of the foetus. It is a virus disease, causing a mild fever, sore throat, enlargement of the lymph nodes in the neck and behind the ear, and a pink rash. The incubation period is between two and three weeks, and it is spread by droplet infection on the breath. Damage to the foetus by maternal rubella may be extensive, showing itself in the newborn by eye and heart defects, jaundice, and encephalitis; in infancy by stunted growth, microcephaly, which is an undersized head, and paralyses; and as the child grows older by deafness, with impaired speech and perhaps autism. There are a number of other possible abnormalities. The virus reaches the foetus by crossing the placenta, and infection is most dangerous in the first two months of pregnancy; after infection in the third month the commonest defect is deafness, and after the fourth month defects are rarer. In many cases a pregnant woman developing rubella in the first three months of her pregnancy is advised to have the pregnancy terminated, for there is a 50% chance of the foetus being affected. Now that a vaccine is available, all female children should be vaccinated. The vaccine is combined with those for mumps and measles as MMR vaccine and is offered for all children as a routine between one and two years old, and on entering primary school. One attack of rubella confers immunity; it is possible to test the blood for immunity to rubella, and if in doubt those who plan to have children can be tested and vaccinated. As the vaccine is made from the live virus, pregnancy after vaccination must be avoided for at least one month. Women who are tested during pregnancy and found to have no immunity should be vaccinated after the child is born.

Rupture: a hernia (q.v.)

S

Sabin Vaccine: poliomyelitis vaccine made from live but attenuated viruses. In the UK such vaccine is made from a mixture of strains 1, 2 and 3 of the poliovirus and offered routinely for all infants and children; it is given by mouth in three doses, at three months old, eight weeks later, and six months later. Further doses are given on entering and leaving school. Reinforcing doses may be given to adults at intervals of 10 years. *See* Salk Vaccine. (Albert Sabin, American virologist, born 1906)

Sacro-iliac Joints: the joints between the sacrum and the iliac bones of the pelvis. The joints are bound together by strong ligaments, for through them the weight of the body is transferred to the legs. The joints may give rise to pain, particularly in ankylosing spondylitis and during the latter part of pregnancy when the ligaments become lax in order to allow the pelvis to expand during childbirth.

Sacrum: a triangular bone formed by the fusion of five vertebrae, lying at the base of the spinal column. Above, it forms a joint with the fifth lumbar vertebra, and below with the coccyx; on each side it forms joints with the iliac bones, in which there is no movement; the ligaments are strong and bind the two sides of the pelvis together.

Sadism: a sexual perversion in which pleasure is derived from inflicting pain on others. Named after the Marquis de Sade (1740–1814), a notorious degenerate.

Safe Period: the period during which it is assumed that conception after sexual intercourse will not occur. This method of contraception is based on the assumption that there are only certain days in the menstrual cycle during which a woman can become pregnant. Ovulation (q.v.) normally takes place 15 days before the next menstrual period is due; if 5 days are added on each side of this date to allow for errors, the fertile period is likely to be from the

8th to the 18th day of the normal 28-day cycle. Any time outside this is said to be in the safe period, but because menstruation tends to be irregular and because ovulation is influenced by emotional and other factors, the idea of a safe period is a misconception.

St Vitus's Dance: Sydenham's chorea. *See* Chorea.

Salbutamol: a drug widely used to dilate the air passages in asthma. It is very effective, and is given by mouth, by injection or in an inhaler; the inhaler is preferred. Patients may be tempted to overdose themselves, but the drug has unwanted effects which include an increasing pulse rate, trembling of the hands, headache and irritability; in some cases the patient may become confused.

Salicylates: the bark of the willow *Salix alba* is an old remedy for fevers, and during the nineteenth century the active principle salicylin was isolated, from which salicylic acid was obtained, and sodium salicylate was used to reduce fever and relieve pain. At the turn of the century acetyl salicylic acid was found to be more effective, and the Bayer company of Germany who discovered the drug called it Aspirin (q.v.) from the German for salicylic acid, *spirsäure*. Salicylic acid itself is used as an application to scaling conditions of the skin and to hardened skin, and for the removal of warts. It may also be used in fungus infections of the skin, and in combination with sulphur for acne. Sodium salicylate is still used in the treatment of rheumatic disease, as is choline magnesium trisalicylate.

Saliva: the secretion of the parotid, submandibular and sublingual glands, as well as many smaller glands in the mouth. Saliva contains ptyalin, which breaks down starch to sugar, as well as mucus which moistens the food and the inside of the mouth and gullet and makes swallowing possible. It is secreted in response to the presence of food, or in anticipation of food, by a nervous reflex.

Salk Vaccine: a vaccine containing poliovirus types 1, 2 and 3 inactivated by formaldehyde. It is given by injection, and has certain drawbacks; it is therefore reserved for those with deficiencies of the immune system. *See* Sabin Vaccine. (Jonas Salk, American physician, born 1914)

Salmonella: bacteria of many species responsible for paratyphoid and typhoid infections. Named after Daniel Salmon (1850–1914), an American bacteriologist. *See* Food Poisoning.

Salpingitis: inflammation of the Fallopian, or uterine, tubes. It is commonly the result of infection travelling from the vagina through the uterine cervix and uterus, and may be due to gonorrhoea or infection with *Chlamydia trachomatis* or *Mycoplasma hominis*. The infection may be mixed. It is possible that infections may arise as complications of termination of pregnancy, or the fitting of an intrauterine contraceptive device. The symptoms are pain in the lower abdomen, with tenderness on both sides. The pain is worse in gonorrhoeal infections, and there may be a raised temperature; the menstrual flow may be heavy. The patient is therefore likely to seek treatment more quickly than in other tubal infections, and treatment can be started sooner with more chance of success than in the other cases which may become chronic before the patient is seen. In some cases the diagnosis may only become clear on laparoscopy, examination of the lower abdomen through an endoscope. Treatment for gonorrhoea is with ampicillin or amoxycillin; in other cases these penicillins are used, with doxycycline and metronidazole added. The complications of salpingitis include the formation of an abscess in the tube, and the consequences may be an increased likelihood of ectopic pregnancy (q.v.) or sterility if the ends of the tubes adjacent to the ovary become obstructed. In some cases the infection becomes chronic, with intermittent pain and backache and frequent excessive periods. Treatment may be difficult.

Salt: common salt is sodium chloride, a substance essential for life. When it is deficient, the blood volume and pressure fall, there are muscular cramps, dizziness and fainting, and sometimes confusion. Normally there is a comfortable excess of salt in everyday food, but in a hot climate, especially after a good deal of sweating or a bout of diarrhoea, during which salt is lost, it is sensible to take considerably more salt with the food than usual.

Salvarsan (arsphenamine): a drug devised by the German Nobel Prize winner Paul Ehrlich (1854–1915), originally designed to destroy trypanosomes, the organisms of sleeping sickness, but found to be specific for syphilis. It has been replaced by penicillin.

Sanatorium: a special hospital for the treatment of tuberculosis. Since the introduction of chemotherapy for the disease, such hospitals have become unnecessary.

Sandfly Fever: also called phlebotomus fever, a virus disease transmitted to man by *Phlebotomus pappatasi* midges found on the shores of the Mediterranean and other subtropical places including Turkey and India. The virus is found in gerbils, sheep and cattle; in man it causes a fever which lasts from three to five days with headache, general aches and pains and diarrhoea. Apart from the discomfort the disease is harmless, and there is no specific treatment. Once it has bitten a patient with the disease, the midge remains infective for the rest of its life.

Saphenous Vein: the long saphenous vein can be seen under the skin running up the inside of the leg from the ankle to the groin, and the short saphenous vein from the outside of the ankle to the back of the knee. The long saphenous vein is the longest vein in the body, and is often used in vascular surgery to provide the source for a graft. The saphenous veins are in about one out of five people the site of varicosities. They connect with the deep veins of the leg through communicating veins which have one-way valves, normally allowing blood to flow only from the superficial to the deep vessels. If the valves are defective the superficial veins dilate to form varicosities. *See* Varicose Veins.

Saprophyte: any micro-organism that lives upon dead or decaying matter.

Sarcoidosis: a chronic disease in which granulomas are formed in various parts of the body. A granuloma is a nodule of tissue composed of cells which collect in response to chronic infection or irritation, derived from the white cells of the blood and comprising monocytes, macrophages, lymphocytes and epithelioid cells (*see* Epithelium). Similar collections of cells are found in tuberculosis and leprosy, but no organisms have been identified in sarcoidosis. In tuberculosis, the centre of the granuloma breaks down, a process known as caseation, but this does not happen in sarcoidosis: the granulomas either resolve or become fibrosed. Most of the cases affect the lungs, and come to light because chest X-rays show a characteristic appearance. The patient may have no symptoms, or may have a cough, sometimes with a mild fever and malaise. In other cases the disease affects the skin, producing tender red swellings on the shins called erythema nodosum, and there may also be pains in the joints, especially the knees and ankles. The eyes may be affected, damage being produced in the uveal tract, that is the iris, ciliary body and choroid (*see* Eye), possibly leading to a disturbance of vision, and the lymph nodes may be enlarged. The liver, spleen, and the bones of the hands and feet can be involved, as can many other parts of the body. In many cases of disease affecting the lungs the X-ray appearances slowly resolve, and judging from the number that are unexpectedly recognised on routine chest X-rays and X-rays taken for unrelated reasons it is likely that a number of cases go undetected. Treatment in cases where symptoms require it is difficult because the cause of the disease remains obscure, but corticosteroids are used with good effect, and hydroxychloroquine has been used.

Sarcoma: a malignant tumour arising in structures derived from mesoderm, which include bones, muscles and connective tissue. Sarcomas may be named after the tissue in which they arise, for example osteosarcomas affect bone, fibrosarcomas the fibrous tissue, lymphosarcomas the lymphatic tissue; or they may be named after the type of cells they contain: for example, round cell sarcoma or spindle cell sarcoma. The tumours may spread by metastasis through the bloodstream, often to the lungs, through the lymphatics or by direct invasion of neighbouring tissues.

Sarcoptes: a genus of acarids, which includes *Sarcoptes scabiei*, the itch mite which causes scabies. *See* Mites.

Scabies: a skin disease caused by *Sarcoptes scabiei*. *See* Mites.

Scan: the picture produced by a scanner, a recording apparatus used to depict the results of examining the body by X-rays, ultrasound, or other radiations. The scanner measures different areas in turn and integrates the results.

Scaphoid: one of the eight small bones of the wrist. It articulates with the radius, and is the largest member of the proximal row of bones. Its particular importance is that it is sometimes fractured by a fall on the outstretched hand or by a severe blow on the palm; the fracture line is difficult to see in an X-ray, and it may not be until a week after the injury that it becomes clear, as the bone rarefies where it has been fractured. Such fractures require immobilisation of the wrist, and may take up to three months to heal.

Scapula: the shoulder-blade.

Scar: fibrous tissue formed during the healing of an injury.

Scarlatina (scarlet fever): an infection with group A *Streptococcus pyogenes*, usually of the throat in children, associated with a skin rash which consists of red spots all over the body developing after 24 hours and sore throat, fever, shivering, nausea and vomiting. The tongue is covered with a white fur through which the red papillae project, the 'strawberry' tongue. Soon the white coating disappears, leaving the tongue red, the 'raspberry' tongue. The rash fades after a few days, and the skin begins to scale. The treatment is with penicillin. During the last hundred years the severity of the disease has declined from being a common cause of death in children to a mild condition that may pass unnoticed.

Schistosomiasis: *see* Bilharzia.

Schizont: a stage in the development of the malaria parasite. *See* Malaria.

Schizophrenia: *see* Mental Illness.

Sciatica: pain in the distribution of the sciatic nerve, which supplies sensation to the back of the thigh and the outer side of the leg and foot. The sciatic nerve is the largest nerve in the body, and it originates from the lumbo-sacral plexus of nerves, with contributions from the fourth and fifth lumbar and the first, second and third sacral nerve roots. As well as carrying sensory fibres it carries motor nerve fibres to the hamstring muscles and the muscles of the leg and foot. Pain felt in the area supplied by the nerve may be provoked by a number of factors, but the commonest cause is interference with the sensory nerve roots as they emerge from the spinal cord and run between the vertebrae to the lumbo-sacral plexus. Interference may be the result of prolapse of the intervertebral discs between the fourth and fifth lumbar vertebrae or the fifth lumbar and first sacral vertebrae (*see* Prolapsed Intervertebral Disc) or of osteoarthritic changes in the vertebrae. Pain may be referred from the hip or from the sacro-iliac joints, or may be caused by uncommon diseases such as tumours which have to be taken into consideration. Treatment of sciatica is the treatment of the underlying condition, if this is possible, but in many cases it comes down to rest and analgesic drugs.

Scintillation: the radiations given off by a radioactive substance can be measured by the effect they have on a phosphor, which gives off light in response to radiation; the light flashes are counted by converting them into electrical impulses.

Sclera: the white fibrous outer covering of the eyeball, continuous behind with the sheath of the optic nerve and in front with the translucent cornea. It forms the white of the eye.

Scleroderma: an uncommon disease in which there is thickening of the skin due to overproduction of collagen by fibrous tissue cells, with diminution in the capillary circulation. It is part of a generalised condition called systemic sclerosis, other symptoms of which are difficulty in swallowing and diarrhoea; it may affect the joints, muscles, kidneys, heart and lungs. The disease is thought to be due to a malfunction of the immune system.

Sclerosis: hardening of a tissue, used particularly of the nervous system in multiple or disseminated sclerosis and of the walls of the arteries in atherosclerosis.

Scolex: the head and neck of a tapeworm; the part by which it attaches itself to the wall of the gut.

Scoliosis: deformity of the spine due to curvature to one side. It may be consequent upon disease of the spine, weakness of the spinal muscles, hip disease, a habit of bad posture, rickets, sciatica or a difference in the length of the legs. If possible it is treated by physiotherapy to improve the posture.

Scopolamine: alternative name for hyoscine. *See* Hyoscyamus.

Scorpion: a venomous arachnid carrying a sting which may occasionally prove fatal; it is found in tropical and subtropical parts of the world, including North Africa and the Middle East, India, in the Americas and in Trinidad. An anti-venom is available.

Scotoma: a patch of diminished or lost vision, which may be seen as a shadow within the visual field.

Scrapie: a disease of sheep and goats which has been used in research into slow virus encephalopathies. The viruses, also called prions, are quite distinct from usual viruses, but they can produce a characteristic disease after being subjected to filtration and inoculation into susceptible animals. The disease is thought to be linked in some way to certain human diseases, for example Alzheimer's disease, motor neurone disease, Creutzfeldt–Jacob disease and Parkinson's disease, because of similar degeneration of the nervous system discovered on microscopical examination and similarities between proteins found in the involved nervous tissue. The nature of the link between these diseases is obscure, and subject to intense research; recently the matter has been brought to public attention by the incidence of the related spongiform encephalopathy in cattle.

Scrofula: tuberculosis of the lymph nodes in the neck, in which the disease may slowly progress to the formation of fistulous openings. *See* King's Evil.

Scrotum: a pouch of skin below the root of the penis which contains the testes and accessory structures. It is divided into two halves by a partition of fibrous tissue, and the thin skin has in it a layer of smooth muscle, called the dartos muscle, which contracts in response to cold. Normally the testes are placed so that they are maintained at a slightly lower temperature than the rest of the body.

Scruple: a unit of weight in the apothecaries' system, equal to 20 grains or 1.296 g.

Scurvy: a vitamin C deficiency disease. At one time common in ships' crews undertaking long voyages without fresh fruit or vegetables, it was prevented in the later eighteenth-century Royal Navy by the regular issue of lime juice. Those affected become weak, wounds fail to heal, the gums bleed, and the skin bruises easily. In children, bleeding may take place under the periosteum, the membrane covering the bones, which become tender. Vitamin C was synthesised in 1928 and named ascorbic acid; there is an adequate amount in a normal diet, the vitamin being contained in fresh fruit and vegetables, but it is soluble in water and destroyed by heat, so that some is lost in cooking.

Seasickness: *see* Motion Sickness.

Sebaceous Cyst: a common cyst formed under the skin by blockage of the duct of a sebaceous gland (*see below*). The secreted sebum collects behind the block, and the cysts so formed may be as big as a golf ball. These cysts are common on the scalp, but may form anywhere; they may be multiple. They are easily removed, usually under local anaesthetic.

Sebaceous Gland: set in the skin, usually in association with a hair in the angle between the hair follicle and the erector pilae muscle, the muscle which makes the hair stand on end, sebaceous glands secrete a fatty material called sebum which prevents the skin becoming dry. The glands become more active at puberty, and their development is complete by the 25th year. Abnormalities affecting the glands include the formation of sebaceous cysts, acne vulgaris, and seborrhoea, a condition in which there is excessive secretion of sebum, sometimes associated with seborrhoeic dermatitis, an itching rash of the skin, commonest in the skin flexures, on the forehead over the eyebrows, beside the nose, on the chest and in the scalp, where it causes cradle cap in babies and dandruff in adults.

Seborrhoeic Dermatitis: *see above*.

Secretion: the process by which a gland elaborates the particular substance for which it is responsible. These substances are called secretions; they may be from exocrine glands, which discharge onto a surface such as the skin or the lining of the intestinal tract, or from endocrine glands, which discharge into the bloodstream. Eccrine secretions are those which are pumped through the cell membranes, apocrine secretions those which accumulate in part of the cell and then break off; in holocrine secretions the secreted matter is contained within the whole of the cell and the cell together with the secreted substance forms the secretion, as in the sebaceous glands. Some glands secrete continuously, others are controlled by hormones, nerves, and by body chemistry.

Sedative: any drug used to quieten and relax a patient.

Sedimentation Rate: if a specimen of whole blood is prevented from clotting by an agent such as sodium citrate and allowed to stand, the red blood cells will in time sink to the bottom of the container leaving a clear column of plasma above them. The rate at which the cells fall is the erythrocyte sedimentation rate (ESR). A specimen of blood is drawn up into a thin clear tube, which is left to stand vertically for an hour; the distance between the red cells and the meniscus at the top of the column of plasma is measured in millimetres. A number of factors are involved in influencing the rate of fall, among them gravity and the extent to which the cells clump together, which in turn is related to the amount of fibrinogen and globulins in the blood. The ESR is used as a guide to the presence of disease in the body; it is normally below 10 mm an hour, and is increased in infections, malignant disease, rheumatoid arthritis and other collagen diseases, and other conditions; it is not specific, but can give an indication of the progress of a disease and the effect of treatment.

Sella Turcica: the pituitary fossa in the sphenoid bone at the base of the skull, so called because of its fancied resemblance to a Turkish saddle.

Semen: the male genital fluid, containing spermatozoa with the secretions of the prostate gland and the seminal vesicles.

Semicircular Canals: *see* Ear.

Seminal Vesicle: there are two seminal vesicles, lying one on each side above the prostate gland at the base of the bladder. Their ducts join the vas deferens, the tube through which spermatozoa are brought from the testes, and they secrete a sticky fluid which becomes part of the semen.

Seminoma: a malignant tumour of the testis.

Senna: the dried leaf of *Cassia acutifolia*, made up as a syrup, fluid extract, tablets or granules and used as a laxative.

Sensitivity: awareness and response to tactile or other stimuli; also a state in which there is an abnormal reaction to certain stimuli. Patients are said to be sensitive to penicillin, for example, when they suffer skin rashes or other disturbances as a result of taking it, or sensitive to nickel when contact causes a rash. It is also used to indicate the reaction of a micro-organism to a drug which kills it or prevents its multiplication, for example many staphylococci are sensitive to penicillin.

Sepsis: infection of the tissues or the blood by micro-organisms.

Sepsis Violacea: the dung-fly.

Septicaemia: the presence in the blood of bacterial toxins.

Septum: in anatomy, a partition between two sides of a structure, for example the interventricular septum dividing the two ventricles of the heart, or the nasal septum dividing the right from the left nostril.

Sequestrum: a piece of dead bone which has become separated from the blood supply of the living bone as the result of injury or infection.

Serum: the clear fluid that separates from whole blood when it clots. It is plasma with the fibrinogen removed. Serum contains antibodies and antitoxins, which can be used in the treatment of certain diseases such as tetanus. Serology is the study of antibody–antigen reactions.

Serum Sickness: immune reaction to the injection of foreign serum. Serum taken from horses that had been actively immunised against tetanus was once used in the treatment and prevention of the disease in humans, and it was not uncommonly the cause of serum sickness, which produced fever, pains in the joints and a skin rash about a week after the injection. Horse serum is no longer used, as active immunisation against tetanus is a routine, and human immunoglobulins are available for passive immunisation.

Sesamoid Bone: short bone found embedded in joint capsules or tendons, for example the kneecap or patella.

Sex and Sexual Problems: it was for long the custom to think of sex as an impulse arising at puberty and dying out in women at the change of life and in men some time later. This totally false belief caused many to feel that any manifestation of sex before or after these ages must be abnormal, but it is now realised that the impulse is present in various forms from the earliest months until the end of life. Quite apart from the Freudian theory that sucking and defecation are both forms of sexuality in the widest sense, infants evince interest in their sexual organs, and their interest is carried on throughout childhood with the special characteristic that at this age the main interest is auto-erotic, that is, centred on the child's own body. Masturbation is thus a feature, an almost universal practice which causes no mental or physical harm in spite of warnings dating from Victorian times. It is, however, necessary to note that masturbation carried out to excess may well be a sign of something wrong, usually indicating extreme anxiety rather than excessive sexuality. Just before puberty there is a brief homosexual stage which may or may not be marked by physical manifestations of interest in the same sex. Ordinarily this is the time when schoolgirls develop 'crushes' for older girls or schoolteachers, and schoolboys have their heroes. There are few people who have not at some time or another manifested homosexual tendencies and there is not necessarily anything abnormal about this, since the natural development of sex is from the self through the similar to the quite different: that is, the other sex.

At puberty the interest normally becomes heterosexual, and at the same time the body matures so that parenthood becomes possible, the menstrual periods beginning in girls and nocturnal emissions in boys. Such emissions are normal, and in no way weaken the body or sap the strength, any more than intercourse does in adults. The periods need equally be no cause for distress in girls, but it is still true that certain cases of dysmenorrhoea, pain with the periods, are related to faulty teaching which associates them with guilt or shame. The proper way to educate children in sex matters is to answer from the earliest days every question the child asks about sex, and to answer truthfully; to answer only what has been asked, without elaborating or giving lectures; and to ensure that lectures are given at the proper time and place, in biology classes at school. Otherwise children learn the 'facts of life' in a garbled version from their comrades, and the choice is not between some information and none but between accurate fact and inaccurate nonsense. Faulty upbringing has a great deal to do with difficulties in sexual relationships in later life.

In regard to adult sexual behaviour, there are no real standards by which to judge whether it is adequate or normal, unless individuals are considered in relation to their own needs, which means that the matter is inextricably linked with their subjective states. Difficulties in sexual relations are almost always difficulties in personal relationships showing up in a sexual guise: impotence on the part of the man is rarely due to a physical disease, such as diabetes, but more likely to be the result of fear of failure or lack of genuine interest in his partner. Although few men fail to reach orgasm on some occasion, failure to do so worries many women, although it is true that perhaps as many as a half rarely reach that point. The failure to reach orgasm while still obtaining some pleasure from sexual congress is perfectly compatible with a happy married relationship. Sexual technique is not everything in marriage, although sex and affection cannot be separated from each other; affection and mutual understanding are far more important than sex.

Homosexuality is not uncommon; it is said that 4% of the total population, male and female, is exclusively homosexual. There is no discernable reason for this in the physical make-up of individuals, and the reasons must be psychological. It has already been said that a homosexual period is normal in development, but in most cases passes into heterosexuality. In some cases it does not.

Sexually Transmitted Disease (venereal disease, STD): the diseases include syphilis, gonorrhoea, non-specific urethritis, herpes simplex genital infection, venereal warts, trichomoniasis, candidiasis, scabies, louse infection with *Pthirus pubis*, chancroid, and lymphogranuloma venereum, which are described under separate headings. A variety of other infections, which are not necessarily venereal, can be transmitted during sexual intercourse, such as AIDS, hepatitis A and B, and certain virus, bacterial and protozoan infections found in the intestines and liable to be passed on particularly by male homosexuals.

Shaking Palsy: paralysis agitans, Parkinson's disease (q.v.).

Shellfish: in certain susceptible people shellfish are liable to set up allergic reactions, varying from severe vomiting and diarrhoea to irritating skin rashes. Food-poisoning organisms may also be contained in shellfish, for the places where they exist can be contaminated with sewage; they have also been implicated in cases of poisoning caused by certain algae and by the flagellate protozoon *Gonyaulax catanella* which forms a destructive red tide in the sea and upon which the shellfish may feed.

Shell Shock: the name given in the First World War to the state of battle exhaustion, for it was thought to be due to the physical effect of shell explosions rather than psychological distress.

Shigella: genus of micro-organisms that cause dysentery.

Shingles: *see* Herpes Zoster.

Shock: acute failure of the circulation, with low blood pressure, cold sweaty pale skin, blue fingers and toes, a rapid but weak pulse, fast shallow breathing, prostration and confusion. The state may be caused by grave injury, haemorrhage, burns, myocardial infarction, pulmonary embolism, severe intestinal infection with loss of fluid, spreading sepsis, and other acute dangerous conditions. The patient's state is worsened by pain and cold, and morphine should be given if necessary and the patient kept warm; failure of the circulation from haemorrhage or loss of fluid must be counteracted by transfusion of blood, plasma or electrolytes. In anaphylactic shock hypersensitivity to a foreign substance or drug produces acute and profound depression of the blood pressure and the escape of fluid into the tissues; the treatment is the immediate injection of adrenaline. Those injured in an accident should be kept warm and as comfortable as possible; unless they have abdominal injuries, those conscious should be encouraged to drink any fluid except alcohol. Shock is a word commonly used to describe the mental distress caused by any disagreeable event, but this is quite different from the medical meaning of shock.

Shoulder: whereas the hip joint and pelvis are designed to carry weight, and are large and relatively fixed, the joints of the shoulder girdle are mobile and designed to place the hand where it is wanted. The shoulder girdle consists of the scapula, the shoulder-blade, and the clavicle, the collar-bone. The scapula forms a ball-and-socket joint with the humerus, the bone of the upper arm. Unlike the pelvic bones, the scapulae are not joined together but are free to move over the back of the upper part of the chest wall, to which they are joined by muscles; the clavicle makes a joint at its outer end with the scapula, and at its inner end with the breastbone, the sternum; it keeps the arm propped out from the chest wall and attached to the skeleton. The muscles which keep the shoulder girdle attached to the skeleton in front are the pectoralis minor, the subclavius and the serratus anterior, and those behind the trapezius, the rhomboids, and the levator scapulae. The shoulder joint itself is crossed by a number of muscles which add to its stability; they are the deltoid, teres major and minor, supra- and infraspinatus, and subscapularis running between the scapula and the upper arm. These muscles between them give the shoulder its strength and mobility. Common injuries to the shoulder girdle are fractures of the clavicle and dislocations of the shoulder joint. The humerus may be broken just below the joint. *See* Frozen Shoulder.

Shunt: in medicine, the term used for a short-circuit, usually between blood vessels, which may occur naturally but may be made surgically, for example in preparing the forearm vessels for renal dialysis.

Sialitis: inflammation of a salivary gland or duct.

Sialolithiasis: the formation of concretions in the duct of a salivary gland. The obstruction causes the gland to swell, but the stones can often be washed out if the patient can be persuaded to suck acid-drops or lemons.

Sibling: a brother or sister.

Sickle-cell Disease: an inherited disorder of haemoglobin formation in which the molecule is abnormal. It is found in areas where *Plasmodium falciparum* or malignant malaria is prevalent, for the abnormality offers partial protection against the disease; about 50 million Africans carry the trait, with another 10 million people in India, Arabia, Turkey and Greece. Sickle-cell disease occurs when both parents pass on the condition, for the trait itself is harmless, but when it is inherited from both parents haemoglobin S is formed. This results in the red blood cells becoming deformed or sickled, in which state they survive for only a short time, and tend to clump together to the extent that they can clog small blood vessels and hold up the circulation; in severe cases the blood supply to sections of tissue can be cut off so that they die (infarction). The short survival of sickle cells means that patients are anaemic; the severity varies from individual to individual. The course of sickle-cell disease in severe cases is marked by sickle-cell crises, during which patients suffer great pain in the bones, and sometimes in the abdomen, while the lungs can be affected, causing breathlessness and pain, and damage to the brain can cause fits. The crises are due to multiple infarctions. In babies and children in particular, great numbers of sickle cells may become collected in the spleen and liver, causing a potentially fatal anaemia. Patients with sickle-cell disease may be very prone to develop an acute infection, which in some cases proves fatal if it is associated with a crisis. The treatment of the crises therefore involves identification and treatment of any underlying infection, together with the administration of painkilling drugs and oxygen to make the best of the oxygen-carrying capability of the diminished red blood cells; in severely anaemic cases transfusions of normal blood are necessary. Methods are available for prenatal diagnosis of the condition.

Side-effects: drugs may have effects on the body which include some which are not wanted, although part of their total action: antihistamines produce drowsiness, the analgesic codeine produces constipation. All drugs are liable to produce unwanted effects and in prescribing, the judgement has to be made whether these outweigh the advantages that the drug offers.

Sigmoid: a structure shaped like an S, for example the sigmoid colon.

Sigmoidoscopy: the endoscopic examination of the interior of the sigmoid colon; the instrument used is called a sigmoidoscope.

Silicosis: *see* Pneumoconiosis.

Silver: silver sulphadiazine is an effective antibacterial applied to the skin, and can be used for burns, wounds and ulcers. Silver nitrate can be used as a caustic application to over-exuberant granulation tissue formed during the healing of ulcers, or as a 0.5% solution for suppurating wounds.

Sinus: the air cavities within the skull in association with the nose; the venous spaces within the skull; a blind abnormal opening on the skin through which pus is discharged.

Sinusitis: inflammation of the mucous membrane of the sinuses, the air spaces in the bones of the skull associated with the nose (q.v.). Those commonly infected are the maxillary sinuses or antra in the cheek, less commonly the frontal sinuses in the forehead. There is pain and tenderness over the infected sinus; antibiotics are commonly used in the treatment, with inhalations designed to shrink and humidify the swollen mucous membrane, but if they are unsuccessful the antrum may have to be washed out. In chronic cases an operation to establish free drainage may be necessary. Infections of the frontal sinus may prove dangerous if the long drainage duct is blocked, for it is possible for the infection to reach the interior of the skull or the orbit; in such cases an operation may be needed. The frontal sinuses may become infected after swimming or diving with a cold. Infections of the ethmoid sinus, while rare, are also dangerous; the root of the nose becomes swollen, with the eyelids, but the prompt use of antibiotics, if necessary intravenously, is usually successful.

SI Units: *see* Weights and Measures.

Skeleton: the bony framework which supports the soft parts of the body.

Skin: the skin covers the outer surface of the body, and is continuous with the mucous membranes which cover the interior surfaces of the body at all the natural orifices. It is tied loosely down to the underlying connective tissue except over the joints, where the attachment is firmer over the flexor surfaces. The skin has two layers, the outer epidermis and the inner dermis. In the dermis, the inner layer which supports the epidermis, there is a papillary layer which looks like a great number of minute hills and valleys upon which the epidermis lies, and a reticular layer. The dermis contains fibrous tissue and fibroblasts and other cells which can multiply rapidly after an injury, and elastic fibres which give the skin its elasticity. It also contains the blood vessels, nerves and lymphatic vessels of the skin, the sweat glands, hairs and sebaceous glands. The dermis is the main part of the skin. The epidermis lying on it has a basal layer of cells which migrate outwards, losing their nuclei and changing shape from the basal cells, which are nucleated and cylindrical, and have between them melanocytes whose function is to synthesise dark melanin pigment, to the flat dead cells on the surface. The cells form the fibrous protein keratin as they approach the surface, and this binds them together to form a tough membrane, thickest over the pressure points on the soles of the feet and the hands. This layer is called the stratum corneum. From the time that new cells are formed in the basal layer of the epidermis to the time that the keratinised skin is formed is about two weeks; the cells die and are shed after about another two weeks, so that the skin is continually renewed. Keratin also forms the nails and the hair; in animals it forms the hooves, claws, horns and feathers. Apart from forming keratin, the epidermis also forms vitamin D under the influence of sunlight.

The skin has a rich blood supply, the vessels looping up into the papillary processes of the dermis. The function of the blood vessels in the skin is not only to nourish the tissues, but also to act as a surface radiator or heat exchange system; the arterioles have muscle in their walls so that they can be shut down when heat is to be conserved. There are also a number of short-circuits between the arterioles and venules in the face and ears, fingers and toes, and palms and soles, called glomus bodies, which bypass the capillary circulation and are concerned with heat regulation.

As well as protection and heat regulation another prime function of the skin is the provision of sensory information about the surroundings of the body, and it therefore has a rich nerve supply, with pain receptors, pressure receptors, and touch and temperature receptors. It is not clear how the sensation of itching arises, but it is thought to be caused by stimuli which are sufficient to damage the skin and release histamine or enzymes but not to produce pain.

Certain substances can pass through the epidermis; it is impermeable to water, but substances soluble in fats such as alcohol can dissolve the cell walls and pass through, absorption being increased at higher skin temperatures and high rates of blood flow, as well as by wetting the keratin layer. Absorption takes place readily through areas of damaged or inflamed skin.

Skull: the skull or cranium is formed by a number of bones which are locked together to form a casing for the brain. The vault of the skull is made up of the frontal, parietal and occipital bones, and the base of the frontal, ethmoid, sphenoid, temporal and occipital bones. In the base of the skull are a number of holes or foramina through which structures run out of the skull, the largest being the foramen magnum through which the spinal cord passes into the vertebral column. The skull contains the brain, its membranes and blood vessels, and is rigid; it is liable to injury, but fractures of the vault of the skull, unless they are depressed and so injure the brain, are not of themselves important except that they give an indication of the force transmitted to the brain (*see* Concussion). Fractures of the base of the skull may open passages between the nose and the interior of the skull, through which cerebrospinal fluid may escape or infection ascend, or into the ear, and fracture of the temporal bone may involve the middle meningeal artery which may bleed outside the dura mater and compress the brain (*see* Extradural Haemorrhage, Head Injuries).

Sleep: For about eight hours out of the twenty-four we withdraw from the world of consciousness and movement into sleep, a state which is far from understood. It is not unconsciousness, for we can be woken up; the mind is not inactive, for we can selectively pick up signals that will wake us – a mother will in her sleep recognise the cry of her child, picking it out from any number of other noises. Lack of sleep is not fatal, but the longer one stays awake the more irritable and slow one is liable to become, and after about two days awake one tends to have delusions of a minor sort. During sleep the blood pressure falls, the pulse rate slows, the muscles relax and the electro-encephalogram, the record of the electrical activity of the brain, changes. Slow waves at 1–3 a second become prominent, and there are groups of waves at 12–14 a second. The pattern changes at intervals; the eyes begin to move rapidly and the electro-encephalogram resembles its waking activity, while the muscles relax further, with occasional jerky movements, and the breathing and pulse may be irregular. This stage of sleep is called paradoxical, or REM sleep, and it occurs about every hour and a half; it is thought by some to be the phase of sleep in which we dream. If subjects are prevented from sleeping during the phase of slow-wave sleep or during REM sleep, they afterwards spend more time in the phase of sleep that they missed. The function of sleep is obscure, but it is true that the pattern of hormonal activity during waking hours is more inclined to favour the breaking down of tissues, and that during sleep the higher levels of growth hormone, testosterone and prolactin encourage the formation of protein. *See* Insomnia.

Sleeping Sickness: *see* Trypanosomiasis.

Slimming: *see* Obesity.

Sling: the one important thing about a sling is that the hand should always be higher than the elbow.

Slipped Disc: *see* Prolapsed Intervertebral Disc.

Slough: dead tissue which separates from healthy tissue as the result of ulceration or inflammation.

Smallpox (variola): an acute and dangerous virus infection known for its fatal effects for centuries. It has finally been eradicated from the world, and the World Health Organization was able to issue a declaration of its extinction in 1980. Vaccination, to which this deliverance is due, was discovered by the Englishmen Benjamin Jesty (1737–1816) and Edward Jenner (1749–1823).

Smelling Salts: ammonium carbonate or sal volatile, an old remedy for fainting.

Smoking: a burning cigarette produces tar and carbon monoxide, which are absorbed into the body through the lungs and produce lung cancer, bronchitis and emphysema, atherosclerosis leading to heart disease and arterial disease, high blood pressure, cancer of the bladder and stunting of foetal growth. One-third of all cancer deaths and a great number of deaths through heart disease could be avoided by not smoking. The death rate of middle-aged smokers of over 20 cigarettes a day is twice that of non-smokers, taking all diseases into account. It is obviously better not to smoke tobacco; best not to start, but having started it may be difficult to stop. Various ways are suggested, but the best way is to stop suddenly on the spur of the moment and stick to it. A safe way to take tobacco is as snuff, for it is not burnt and produces neither tar nor carbon monoxide.

Snakes: *see* Bites and Stings.

Soap: a compound of fatty acids and an alkali. All soap is antiseptic, so the addition of another antiseptic is of doubtful value. In cases where soap irritates the skin, aqueous cream may be used.

Sodium: a soft white metallic element normally found in combination with other elements. It is essential for life, and forms the principal cation in the extracellular fluids. It is commonly taken in the form of sodium chloride, or salt (q.v.).

Sodium Cromoglycate: a drug which prevents the development of allergic reactions. Its action is not fully understood, but it acts locally. It is very useful in asthma, when it is given by inhalation to act on the air passages. In cases of hay fever it is given by nasal spray or drops, and in allergic conjunctivitis, such as occurs in hay fever, in eye drops. It can also be used in food allergies, when it is given in capsules. It has no effect on an existing allergic attack, but when used regularly prevents such attacks from developing.

Soft Sore: chancroid (q.v.).

Solar Plexus: the name given to the great upper abdominal plexus of sympathetic nerves which lies behind the stomach at the level of the first lumbar vertebra. Its fibres, which include the coeliac and mesenteric plexuses, were thought to radiate like the rays of the sun.

Solvent Abuse: *see* Glue Sniffing.

Somatotypes: a classification of types of bodily build according to certain physical characteristics was made in 1940; *see* Ectomorph, Endomorph and Mesomorph.

Sonne Dysentery: dysentery caused by the micro-organism *Shigella sonnei*. *See* Dysentery.

Sore Throat: *see* Throat.

Spanish Fly: *see* Cantharides.

Spastic: the term applied to that type of paralysis in which the muscles are stiff rather than limp, a condition caused by damage to the upper motor neurones of the brain usually in the cortex or in the internal capsule, where the motor nerve fibres are gathered together as they pass downwards from the cortex to the brain stem and spinal cord. A spastic condition of the legs called Little's disease (William Little, London physician, 1810–94) or spastic diplegia, may affect children, especially those born prematurely. In this disease the legs are weak but straight, and tend to become crossed when the child walks. The arms are relatively normal but the speech may be affected, although the intelligence is not. These children are sometimes referred to as 'spastics', as are those suffering from other birth injuries to the cerebral hemispheres causing spastic paralyses.

Spatula: a blunt flat tool used for mixing ointments and other substances; often used to refer to the flat piece of wood or metal the doctor uses to keep the tongue down when inspecting a patient's throat.

Spectacles: there are four types of errors in vision which are improved by the use of lenses in spectacles: myopia, which is short-sight, hypermetropia or long-sight, astigmatism and presbyopia. Short-sight is caused by the refractive power of the eye bringing the image to a focus in front of the retina, long-sight by the opposite error, so that the image is focused behind the retina. In myopia a concave lens is used to correct the fault, for objects at a distance cannot be seen clearly; in hypermetropia, distance vision is not affected, but convex lenses may be needed for near work. In astigmatism the curvature of the cornea or lens is not symmetrical, so that rays of light in one plane cannot be brought to a focus at the same time as rays at right angles to that plane; near and far sight are affected, and circles appear elliptical and blurred at two points opposite each other. A lens to correct this type of defect must be cylindrical, that is, flat in one plane and curved in the plane at right angles to it. Astigmatism may exist with short or long sight, and mixed astigmatism may result in the eye being long-sighted in one meridian and short-sighted in the other. In presbyopia, changes due to age cause the lens to lose its elasticity, and therefore its ability to accommodate for near vision, so that lenses are necessary for close work and reading. This is the case with many people over the age of 50.

Speculum: an instrument used to inspect the interior of natural body passages, often fitted with a light or mirror. Its range is limited, in contrast to an endoscope, which is fitted with lenses and often made with fibreoptics so that it can be passed deep into the body. The speculum is used for examining the interior of the vagina, rectum, nasal cavity or outer ear.

Speech Disorders: when due to brain damage, in right-handed people, it follows damage to the left side of the brain, and *vice versa*. There are two main areas of the brain concerned with speech, Broca's area and Wernicke's area. Broca's area was described by the French surgeon Paul Broca (1824–80), and is the inferior frontal cerebral convolution, which lies in the area of the temple. Wernicke's area was described by Karl Wernicke, a German neurologist (1848–1905), and is behind Broca's area in the posterior superior temporal convolution. Damage to Broca's area produces a predominantly motor disturbance, with difficulty in articulating words but the ability to recognise them, and damage to Wernicke's area predominantly a lack of comprehension, with the ability to speak but the production of often unintelligible words. This is a simplified description, for the two types of disorder may be mixed, and many other areas of the brain are concerned with comprehension and expression of speech, but it was on these observations that modern comprehension of the complicated processes of understanding and use of language were based.

Spermatocoele: a cyst of the epididymis. Spermatocoeles are quite common, being usually found in middle-aged men, although they may form at any time. They are not dangerous, but may grow quite large and become tense and uncomfortable. They are easily removed.

Sphenoid: although the word sphenoid means wedge-shaped, the sphenoid bone in the base of the skull looks more like a bat with its wings spread. The bone forms part of the floor of the middle fossa of the skull, and has in the centre of the body a depression called the sella turcica which houses the pituitary gland. The body also contains two air sinuses which communicate with the nose.

Sphincter: a ring of muscle which can constrict a natural passage or close an orifice.

Sphygmomanometer: an instrument for measuring the arterial blood pressure.

Spica: a bandage applied in a figure-of-eight so that the turns overlap each other.

Spina Bifida: the defective development of the posterior part of the spinal column, so that the arches of the vertebrae fail to meet and fuse in the midline. It may be a minor defect confined to one vertebra, and of no consequence, or of greater extent but still covered by muscle and skin, in which case there is often a tuft of hair or a naevus in the overlying skin (spina bifida occulta). In these cases symptoms of interference with the nervous system may develop, such as weakness of the legs or incontinence. In severe cases of spina bifida there is protrusion of the membranes covering the spinal cord (meningocoele) or of the membranes and a portion of the spinal cord (meningomyelocoele). In some cases the cord is laid open (rachischisis). The worst cases are associated with lack of development of the brain and the overlying bone (anencephaly). The cause of the condition is not known, but there appears to be some genetic factor, and possibly a nutritional factor. The treatment of meningocoeles is surgical excision, but a proportion of such cases progress to hydrocephalus (q.v.). The treatment of meningomyelocoeles depends on a number of factors, but even those who can be treated may be left with paralysis of the legs with loss of sensation, incontinence, spinal deformity, and hydrocephalus with some diminution of mental powers. They need specialised care. In most cases prenatal diagnosis of the condition is possible by amniocentesis and ultrasound examination.

Spinal Anaesthesia: if a local anaesthetic is injected into the subarachnoid space round the spinal cord, the body below that level will be anaesthetised, but consciousness will be maintained.

Spinal Column: the backbone. In the child there are 33 bones, but in the adult the lowest three or four fuse to form the coccyx, and the five above them unite to form the sacrum, so that there are only 26 separate bones in the adult spinal column. The separate bones are called the vertebrae, and they are arranged as follows: 7 cervical vertebrae in the neck, 12 thoracic or dorsal vertebrae with ribs attached in the chest or thoracic region, and 5 lumbar vertebrae in the small of the back. Below them are the sacrum, uniting the two hip-bones to form the pelvis, and the coccyx. The average length of the male vertebral column is 70 cm; the cervical spine is 12 cm long, the thoracic spine 28 cm, the lumbar 18 cm and the sacrum and coccyx 12 cm. The female spine is some 10 cm shorter. The spinal column seen from the side shows four curves. The cervical, or neck, curve is convex forwards, the thoracic curve concave forwards, the lumbar curve convex forwards and the pelvic curve concave forwards. The vertebral canal, in which the spinal cord runs, lies behind the bodies of the vertebrae, and is enclosed by the pedicles and laminae of the vertebrae which make an arch on each side and unite in the midline to form the spines of the vertebrae, which can be felt through the skin. The vertebral bodies are separated by discs of fibrous tissue with an elastic centre, which enable them to tilt and rotate a little on each other, although they are bound together by strong ligaments running longitudinally in front and behind. At the junction of the pedicles and laminae of the arches of the vertebrae are articular facets, above and below; the joint surfaces of the upper facets face backwards, while the lower joint surfaces face forwards. Transverse processes extend laterally on each side from the pedicles as they join the laminae. The joints made by the articular facets are enclosed in capsules and ligaments, and between the laminae run elastic ligaments, the ligamenta flava, which are continuous behind with the ligaments running between the vertebral spines and in front with the ligaments of the intervertebral joints. Muscles run the length of the vertebral column, being attached to the transverse processes and spines. Intervertebral foramina are spaces between the vertebrae through which the nerves leave the spinal cord. In front lie the intervertebral discs and the upper part of a vertebral body, above and below the margins of pedicles, and behind an intervertebral disc, so that the space the nerves pass through is limited.

Fractures of the spinal column can be caused by forced flexion or extension, direct violence, dropping on the heels from a height or diving onto the head. The most dangerous complication is damage to the spinal cord, which comes to an end opposite the second lumbar vertebra. Below that level, fractures can damage the nerves that run down from the cord to leave the spinal column at the lower spinal foramina. The commonest sites of fracture are the lumbar spine and the neck, and the commonest fracture the crush fracture of the body of a vertebra that results from violent flexion. If there is any question that victims of an accident have a broken spine, they should not be moved except by skilled hands; if it is absolutely necessary to move them, they must be carried in exactly the position in which they were found. If this is not possible, they may in grave emergency be carried face downwards so that the back is extended and cannot bend forwards; the neck must be supported so that it cannot move. It is important to remember that people who have head injuries may also have injuries to the spine, and if they are unconscious they cannot complain of pain or show signs of paralysis.

Spinal Cord: the part of the central nervous system that extends from the brain to run within the spinal column as far as the second lumbar vertebra, where it is continued by the filum terminale, a fibrous cord extending to the second piece of the sacrum, where it is anchored. In the embryo the spinal cord occupies the whole length of the spinal column, but the mesoderm which forms the bones grows faster than the nervous tissue, and the discrepancy develops. The spinal cord is surrounded by membranes as is the brain, the pia mater being the innermost, arachnoid in the middle, and the dura mater the outermost. The space between the arachnoid and pia mater is filled with cerebrospinal fluid (CSF), continuous with that which surrounds the brain. A specimen of the fluid may be withdrawn through a needle introduced between the lower lumbar vertebrae below the level of the cord, a procedure called lumbar puncture. If the cord itself is cut across in the dissecting room it is seen to be made up of white matter surrounding a mass of grey matter shaped like an H, with the ventral horns pointing forwards and the dorsal horns towards the back. The ventral horns are concerned with the motor system of nerves which supplies the muscles, and the dorsal horns with the sensory system which relays sensory information to the brain. The intermediate part of the grey matter between the first thoracic segment of the cord and the third lumbar is part of the sympathetic nervous system. The white matter is made up of bundles of nerve fibres running up and down the cord; they are all arranged in a definite order according to their function. From the spinal cord run 31 pairs of spinal nerves which between them supply the structures of the body except those of the head and part of the neck, which are supplied by the cranial nerves. The spinal nerves are segmental; their distribution is according to the segments of the embryo from which the various structures developed. Each spinal nerve has an anterior root, which carries motor fibres, and a posterior root which carries the sensory fibres. The posterior root has upon it a ganglion where sensory fibres relay. The two roots join, and emerge as a single nerve from the intervertebral foramen, the space between the vertebrae. The nerve then separates into two branches, the dorsal to supply the back and the ventral to supply the structures in the front of the body. The nerve also gives off sympathetic fibres to the chain of ganglia that runs down each side of the vertebral column. The spinal nerves that are to supply the arms and legs form large plexuses, the brachial and lumbo-sacral plexuses from which the limb nerves originate, but the nerves of the abdomen and thorax run separately round the body. Although the nerves emerge in order from between the vertebrae and are named accordingly, the first thoracic nerve for example being related to the first thoracic verte-bra, due to the discrepancy in length between the spinal column and the spinal cord, the spinal nerves run ever more obliquely inside the vertebral column to reach their points of exit at the intervertebral foramina; the leash of nerves running down from the end of the cord at the level of the second lumbar vertebra to reach the lower lumbar and sacral foramina is called the cauda equina, the horse's tail. The results of injury to the spinal column depend on the site; in the neck the cervical cord may be injured, and the resulting paralysis, loss of sensation, or both, may include everything below the neck, while it is possible to crush vertebrae in the lower lumbar spine without injuring the spinal cord at all. Tumours, both simple and malignant, may affect the spinal cord, some of which are amenable to surgery; the commonest disease to affect the cord is multiple sclerosis (q.v.).

Spirochaetes: micro-organisms shaped like spirals. Most of them are not important in medicine, but those that are include the organisms of relapsing fever (*Borrelia recurrentis*), Lyme disease (*Borrelia bergdorferi*), Weil's disease (*Leptospira interrogans*), yaws (*Treponema pertenue*), rat bite fever (*Spirillum minor*) and syphilis (*Treponema pallidum*).

Spirometer: an instrument for measuring the volume of air inhaled and expired; used in the investigation of lung disease and in assessing the effects of treatment.

Spironolactone: a diuretic drug which has the advantage of retaining potassium in the body; it may be used to increase the action of other diuretics, or by itself in the treatment of oedema.

Splanchnic: to do with the viscera, the large internal organs of the body, applied particularly to the abdominal organs. Splanchnology is the study of the viscera.

Spleen: a solid, somewhat oblong, flattened organ lying in the upper left part of the abdominal cavity behind the stomach. It is covered by the ninth, tenth and eleventh ribs and in contact with the under-surface of the diaphragm. It measures about 12 cm × 6 cm × 4 cm. It has several functions to do with the blood. In the foetus it is the origin of red blood cells, although it later gives up this activity except in emergency; it stores blood, and its cells remove and destroy imperfect and worn-out red blood cells; it is part of the reticulo-endothelial system (q.v.), and it plays a part in the immune system by producing antibodies, lymphocytes and plasma cells. It may be injured by blows to the upper abdomen even when it is healthy, but when enlarged by disease, for example malaria, it protrudes from its protected position under the lower ribs, and a man can be killed by a shrewd blow to the left upper abdomen. When injured the spleen bleeds freely, for its artery is a branch of the short thick coeliac artery which branches directly from the abdominal aorta and the venous drainage is into the portal system which has no valves. If it has to be removed surgically because of an injury, there are no ill effects except in young children, who may become unduly susceptible to infections. The treatment of certain blood diseases may entail removal of the spleen.

Splenectomy: surgical removal of the spleen.

Splenomegaly: enlargement of the spleen, which may be caused by a number of conditions. In tropical countries malaria and other parasitic infections account for many cases, while in this country the leukaemias may be responsible, as may virus infections; cirrhosis of the liver or other liver disease may lead to high pressure in the portal venous system which enlarges the spleen; heart failure may be responsible, as may some types of haemolytic anaemia, where there is excessive destruction of red blood cells.

Splints: simple supports to keep fractures still are needed in the first-aid treatment of broken bones so that the patient can be moved without causing unnecessary pain or further damage. Splints can be made from anything stiff which can be bound to a limb, but are most necessary in the case of a broken forearm or wrist, for the upper arm can be bound to the side, and the legs bound together if one is broken. If the forearm is splinted it should be supported in a sling.

Spondylitis: *see* Ankylosing Spondylitis.

Spondylolisthesis: in this condition the fifth lumbar vertebra slips forward on the sacrum, and the patient complains of low back pain and in some cases pain down the legs, for the intervertebral disc may protrude. The treatment is in the first place rest and physiotherapy; a spinal support may help. In advanced cases operation to fix the lumbar vertebra in position upon the sacrum may be advised.

Spondylosis: osteoarthritic change in the intervertebral joints is called spondylosis; the intervertebral disc loses its bulk and elasticity, the bone becomes rarefied and bony spicules, called osteophytes, grow out from the margins of the vertebral bodies. Arthritis also affects the joints between the articular facets on the pedicles of the vertebral arches (*see* Spinal Column), which adds to the pain that can be caused by spondylosis. The joints commonly affected are in the neck and the lumbar region; there is pain, worse on movement, and in the case of the neck radiating to the back of the head and the shoulders, and in the lumbar region into the buttocks and legs. The parts become stiff after rest, and the back is painful on standing or sitting for any length of time. Radiological appearances are not a good guide to the severity of the symptoms, which may vary from time to time, passing off and then returning. Treatment is directed to the relief of pain, often with the use of NSAIDs (q.v.), and may include physiotherapy. In the neck, the pain may be helped by a collar to restrict movement; in rare cases where the outgrowth of bone has interfered with the spinal cord, operations have been designed to relieve the pressure. The use of a spinal corset for the back should be avoided if possible, for it usually results in loss of muscle tone and weakness. Surgery has little to offer in the case of spondylosis of the lumbar spine, although it is possible to fuse the vertebrae to prevent painful movement.

Spongiform Encephalopathy: an appearance of the brain in certain cases which is thought to be caused by infection with an agent resembling a virus, but too small to be seen with the electron microscope. It has been suggested that the agent is composed only of protein, for which the name prion has been used. Examples of such diseases in man are Kuru, Creutzfeldt–Jacob disease and the rare Gerstmann–Straussler syndrome, which may be a variant of Creutzfeldt–Jacob disease (q.v.). Similar appearances are seen in the brains of sheep with scrapie and those of cattle with bovine spongiform encephalopathy. Many questions about the nature of spongiform encephalopathies in man and animals remain unanswered.

Spore: in bacteriology, spores are dormant forms assumed by certain bacteria which enable them to survive under environmental conditions sufficiently adverse to kill the ordinary form. The organisms of medical importance that form spores include those causing tetanus, gas gangrene and anthrax. They survive in dust and mud, and will withstand temperatures little short of boiling point, which means that eradication of spores is much more difficult than the destruction of non-sporing organisms. Spores will survive in the absence of animal or human hosts for long periods of time, and retain their infectivity.

Spotted Fever: see Rocky Mountain Spotted Fever. The term may also refer to epidemic meningococcal meningitis and typhus.

Sprain: an injury to a joint in which a ligament is torn but not completely ruptured.

Sprue: coeliac disease (q.v.) occurring in adults. Tropical sprue, or post-infective malabsorption syndrome, is a similar condition not due to gluten sensitivity affecting expatriates and the indigenous population in tropical countries excepting Africa, although for many years it was thought to affect only expatriates. The disease starts with an attack of diarrhoea, which becomes chronic. The diarrhoea may be caused by a number of organisms; no one organism is specific. The stools become bulky and offensive, with excessive passage of wind. In time the patient loses weight, and folate deficiency begins; in six months there is an accompanying deficiency of vitamin B_{12} and megaloblastic anaemia develops, with a sore tongue, weakness and oedema. The treatment is the administration of tetracyclines, folic acid and if necessary vitamin B_{12}.

Sputum: the substance coughed up from the lungs and air passages, consisting mainly of mucus, with added pus cells if there is an infection.

Squill: obtained from the bulbs of *Urginea maritima*, squill has been used as an expectorant in cough mixtures.

Squint: a condition in which the two eyes point in different directions. A squint may be divergent, with the eyes deviated outwards, convergent, where they point inwards, or vertical, when the faulty eye points up or down. Most cases are congenital, and due to imbalance of the eye muscles so that there is poor correlation between focusing and convergence of the axes of the eyes. Other cases are due to paralysis of one or more of the muscles that move the eyeball, or vision so poor that the images seen in both eyes cannot be superimposed. If a squint is present at birth and uncorrected, the vision in one eye may be mentally suppressed to avoid double vision, although the eye is normal. This condition is called amblyopia. Congenital squints are treated by orthoptic methods, which exercise the muscles of the eye, and amblyopia is corrected by shading the good eye so that the neglected eye must be used. In the course of treatment it may be necessary to operate on the muscles that move the eye in order to attain a perfect balance. Squints due to weakness of the eye muscles developing in later life are accompanied by double vision, and the treatment is that of the cause of the weakness.

Stammering: stammering and stuttering are common forms of speech disorder, occurring in male more than female children, and sometimes continuing in later life. They may appear in adolescence, or even in adults; in stammering there is difficulty in starting to pronounce words or syllables, in stuttering a repetition of the initial letter, and the two may occur together. Once the word is achieved the urgency may produce hurried speech. The cause of the difficulty is not fully understood; it is thought that there is a combination of a disturbance of the neuro-muscular mechanism concerned with speech production and a psychological factor, the latter predominating in stammering which appears later in life. There can be no doubt that stammering itself presents a psychological difficulty which can exacerbate the condition. Treatment is undertaken by speech therapists, who can help a great deal in coping with any physical difficulties and helping the accompanying anxieties. Those cases which are predominantly due to psychological causes not infrequently prove to be of short duration and amenable to treatment.

Stapes: one of the small bones of the middle ear, shaped like a stirrup. *See Ear.*

Staphylococcus: a round micro-organism (coccus) which grows in clumps that look like bunches of grapes. It is Gram-positive, and the species chiefly responsible for producing disease in man is *Staphylococcus aureus*, otherwise called *Staphylococcus pyogenes*. It is present in quantities in the general environment, and is often present in health on the skin or in the nose. Characteristically it infects superficial cuts and scratches, and produces boils, carbuncles, impetigo and other skin lesions exuding pus. If it gains access to the interior of the body it can cause abscesses, pneumonia, septicaemia and other severe septic conditions. It can contaminate food, and some strains grow in colonies which produce a poisonous toxin so that anyone eating the food on which they are growing may develop an acute attack of vomiting and diarrhoea. Staphylococci have in many instances become resistant to penicillin and other antibiotics, and can present a difficult problem. Particularly resistant are those which flourish in hospitals.

Starvation: if individuals go completely without food but have sufficient water they can survive for a variable time, on average about a month, by which time the weight has halved. If even 500 calories is taken a day, it makes a very great difference to the survival time. Emergency food should be in the form of carbohydrate rather than protein because in conditions where there is not enough food and water the kidneys are able to conserve more water if they do not have to excrete the end products of protein metabolism. In infancy, undernutrition causes irreversible damage to the developing brain and results in intellectual dullness.

Status: in medicine, a continuing state or condition, for example, status asthmaticus, in which the asthma continues with increasing breathlessness and exhaustion, as opposed to an asthmatic attack which recovers; or status epilepticus, in which the patient suffers repeated epileptic convulsions without regaining consciousness.

Steatopygia: the condition of having protruding fat buttocks.

Steatorrhoea: the passage of excessive fat in the motions. The stools become pale, frothy, bulky and offensive; the condition is characteristic of disturbances of absorption of food from the intestines. *See* Coeliac Disease, Sprue.

Stellate Ganglion: there are three sympathetic nervous ganglia in the neck, lying on the fascia covering the muscles of the vertebral column. The fibres of the sympathetic system enter the ganglia from the thoracic spinal cord, running upwards in the neck. The upper ganglion is at the level of the second and third cervical vertebrae, the middle opposite the sixth cervical vertebra, and the lowest lies above the neck of the first rib. The lowest ganglion is often joined with the first thoracic ganglion, which lies below the neck of the third rib, and this large irregular formation is called the stellate ganglion or cervico-thoracic ganglion. It supplies sympathetic nervous fibres to the arm through the brachial plexus of nerves, fibres which go to the heart, fibres which go to various structures within the skull travelling with the vertebral artery, and fibres supplying the neighbouring large branches of the subclavian artery. The sympathetic ganglia supplying the arms are sometimes removed surgically to produce dilation of the blood vessels of the arm in Raynaud's phenomenon (q.v.), but the results are disappointing; the operation may be used in cases of excessive sweating of the arms and hands. Interference with the stellate ganglion produces Horner's syndrome (q.v.).

Stenosis: the abnormal narrowing of a natural orifice or passage, for example mitral stenosis, narrowing of the mitral valve in the heart, or pyloric stenosis, narrowing of the passage from the stomach to the duodenum.

Stereoencephalotomy: the use of an instrument to guide probes and electrodes accurately to the deeper structures of the brain with the consequent production of surgical lesions.

Stereoscopic Vision: the nervous pathways running from the light-sensitive retina of the eye are so arranged that the right-hand field of vision is represented in the left cerebral hemisphere, and *vice versa*. Both eyes are normally directed to see the same thing at the same time, but they do not see it from the same point of view. The relative distance of objects from each other and from the eyes is judged from minute differences in the visual signals derived from the right and left eyes, the stimuli from one half of each retina going to the same cerebral hemisphere for analysis. Full stereoscopic vision is therefore impossible with one eye alone, a fact which can be demonstrated by trying to thread a needle with one eye closed. A single eye can, however, judge distances by recognising the angle subtended at the eye by familiar objects, and judge distance from the known size of the object; it can accurately compare the angular velocities of moving objects; but it is difficult to play cricket, although there are some very good one-eyed golfers.

Sterility: some people wish to be sterile, and undergo operations or take drugs to attain this end, while others complain that they cannot have children and seek medical advice. There are many reasons for a couple being sterile: on the male side, it is essential that the man should be capable of intercourse, that the semen should be normal, and that the spermatozoa should be present in sufficient numbers and should move freely. Normally about a 100 million spermatozoa are ejaculated into the woman's vagina, of which one million reach the uterus, a few thousand reach the uterine tubes, perhaps a hundred reach the ovum in the tubal ampulla, and one fertilises the ovum. In over 20% of cases the man is sterile, and male infertility may be a contributory factor in the sterility of many more marriages. On the female side, it is essential that ovulation should take place, that the ovum should be able to find its way into the uterine tube, and thence into the uterus, where the lining must be in the proper condition to allow the fertilised ovum to become embedded.

The reasons for male sterility range from the presence of a varicocoele (q.v.) to the results of infection or injury; in many cases no obvious cause can be found, but in any case treatment of male infertility is disappointing. The investigation of male infertility includes a full medical examination and a sperm count, which is repeated at least three times at intervals of at least a week. The count shows the amount ejaculated, the number of sperm, their motility and form, and the time of survival. There should be at least 2 ml of ejaculate, and 40 million sperm of which 60% are normally formed and motile. In the absence of fertile sperm, the only alternatives are adoption or artificial insemination by donor.

In the case of a young woman it is reasonable to wait two years after marriage before concluding that she is sterile, but in the case of older women there may be more urgency. Full medical examination may be followed by investigation to establish the patency of the uterine tubes, for in up to a fifth of cases previous inflammation has damaged them. In a further fifth of cases there is no apparent reason for sterility, but in about a sixth of cases there is an abnormality of ovulation (*see* Ovary). If there is a failure at the beginning of the cycle, drugs counteracting the effects of oestrogen such as clomiphene or tamoxifen may be used, and in mid-cycle human chorionic gonadotrophin (HCG) and follicle stimulating hormone (FSH) may bring about ovulation. Human growth hormone (HGH) has recently been used in cases where HCG therapy has failed. In some cases the failure of clomiphene may be due to the secretion in excess of the hormone prolactin; in such cases the antagonist bromocriptine is used. In cases where the uterine tubes are blocked, and in some cases where there is failure in the ovulatory cycle, the techniques of assisted conception (q.v.) may be used in specialist centres.

Sterilisation: (1) The destruction of bacteria contaminating instruments, dressings, etc., by heat, antiseptics or irradiation. (2) The operation of rendering individuals incapable of reproduction. In the male, this is accomplished by tying and dividing the vas deferens as it ascends from the testis, a simple operation that can be carried out under local anaesthetic through small incisions on both sides of the neck of the scrotum. Sterilisation is not immediate; two negative sperm counts must be obtained three months and four months after the operation. The results are meant to be permanent, and there is only an outside chance that an effective operation can be reversed by specialised surgery. Female sterilisation is a more complicated operation, and requires admission to hospital for a night or two. It is carried out under anaesthesia by laparoscopy; an endoscope is introduced through a small incision into the abdominal cavity and plastic or metal clips are placed on the uterine tubes to block them. In some cases the operation can be reversed by removing the clips and restoring the continuity of the tubes. No operation can be guaranteed to be completely effective in every case, and no operation is free of possible complications; operations for sterilisation are no exception. Neither operation has any effect on subsequent sexual activity.

Sternum: the breastbone; it has three parts, called from above downwards the manubrium, the body and the xiphoid process. The three parts have joints between them, and the manubrium is set at a slight angle with the body; the joint can be felt as a ridge. The sternum articulates with the cartilages of the upper seven ribs.

Steroids: a group of chemicals classed as lipids, which are derived in the body from cholesterol. They include the adrenal and sex hormones, the bile acids and vitamin D.

Stethoscope: an instrument through which the physician listens to sounds arising in the interior of the body, notably from the lungs and heart. It was invented in principle by the French physician Théophile Laennec (1781–1826). Before his time the physician applied his ear directly to the patient's body; Laennec interposed a wooden tube, similar to that used today in obstetrics for listening to the foetal heart. Since then the stethoscope has been modified, and has a bell or diaphragm chest-piece and flexible tubes leading from the chest-piece to the ear-pieces.

Stilboestrol: a synthetic compound which has greater activity than naturally occurring oestrogens, to which it is not chemically related. It may be used in the treatment of carcinoma of the prostate gland.

Stillbirth: if a child is born after the 28th week of pregnancy and does not breathe or show any other sign of life it is said to be stillborn.

Stokes–Adams Attack: a condition in which a patient with an abnormally slow pulse rate suddenly becomes unconscious and pulseless. In most cases the heart resumes beating; the cause is heart-block, and the use of a pacemaker (q.v.) avoids this dangerous complication. (William Stokes, Dublin physician, 1804–78, and Robert Adams, also of Dublin, 1791–1875)

Stomach: the stomach is a large pouch into which the oesophagus, the gullet, conveys food from the mouth. In health, it has a capacity of between half and one litre, and it secretes gastric juices which digest the food. It lies below the diaphragm in the left upper part of the abdomen, crossing over to the right below the liver; the oesophageal end is called the cardia, and the other end, which is continuous with the duodenum, the beginning of the small intestine, is called the pylorus; between the cardia and the pylorus is the body of the stomach, which bulges up to the left of the cardia as the fundus, which normally contains a bubble of air. The left border of the stomach, which is the longer, and bulges out to the left, is called the greater curvature, and the right border the lesser curvature. The part of the stomach before the pylorus is sometimes known as the antrum. From the greater curvature of the stomach hangs the great omentum, a fold of peritoneum containing fat which extends downwards in front of the intestines and the transverse colon, which is attached to it; above, the stomach is connected to the under-surface of the liver by a fold of peritoneum called the lesser omentum. The stomach hangs comparatively free in the abdominal cavity, and moves with the breathing; it is tethered at the cardiac end by the oesophagus and at the pylorus by the duodenum, which is attached to the posterior abdominal wall. It is lined by mucous membrane thrown up in ridges, the rugae, and the wall is well furnished with smooth muscle.

When the stomach is empty small waves of contraction pass along the wall from the cardia to the pylorus; when it is full, under the influence of the vagus nerve the contractions become more vigorous, and sweep the food down into the duodenum. The stomach collects food at irregular intervals, and passes it on more regularly to the intestine. The cells of the stomach wall secrete hydrochloric acid and pepsin, an enzyme that digests protein, but the main digestive processes occur in the intestines. Beside pepsin and hydrochloric acid, the stomach elaborates a substance called intrinsic factor which enables the digestive system to absorb vitamin B_{12}, without which megaloblastic anaemia develops. The movements and secretions of the stomach are controlled both by hormones and the autonomic nervous system, through the vagus nerve. The autonomic system is to a great extent influenced by emotions; anger increases gastric secretion, anxiety diminishes the activity of the stomach. Acute emotion can produce paralysis of the muscle and dilatation of the stomach, which gives rise to the sensation of the heart dropping into the boots; substitute stomach for heart and pelvis for boots, and the phrase is probably accurate. *See* Peptic Ulcer, Pernicious Anaemia.

Stomatitis: inflammation of the mucous membrane of the mouth. It may be caused by infection, for example by the fungus *Candida albicans*, which produces thrush, white patches on the mucous membrane, affecting infants and debilitated adults; it may follow a course of antibiotics or corticosteroid treatment, and is an early sign of AIDS. Thrush is treated by the local application of nystatin, either sucked as tablets or applied in drops. There may be bacterial infection, which produces inflammation of the gums, and is thought to be due to poor dental hygiene which attracts infection by a mixed bag of bacteria, among them *Borrelia vincenti* and *Fusobacterium fusiformis*. The gums become painful and bleed, and the breath is foul. The treatment is penicillin. The mouth is sometimes affected in severe leukaemia, especially after chemotherapy, and poisoning with gold or mercury. Herpes simplex infection produces blistering, usually confined to the lips, and is treated by the local application of idoxuridine or acyclovir. In hand, foot and mouth disease the small blisters occurring in the mouth and on the hands and feet of children are caused by the Coxsackie virus; the condition is self-limiting and needs no specific treatment. Syphilis may affect the mouth in any of its three stages; the initial infection may be on the lip or tongue; in the secondary stage, ulcers described as snail tracks develop on the tongue, lips or tonsils; and in the third stage a white patch called leucoplakia may be seen on the tongue, and a gumma may form on the tonsils, tongue or palate. Other types of leucoplakia may be caused by smoking or by friction against the teeth or dentures. Apart from various ulcerations which may occur in association with some skin diseases, or as the result of irritation by irregular teeth or ill-fitting dentures, a type of recurrent ulceration of the mouth called aphthous ulceration is very common. No definite cause has been established; it is found more frequently in females before the age of 40, and affects the edges of the tongue as well as the inside of the lips and cheeks. The condition is painful, and lasts up to two weeks; it is liable to recur at irregular intervals. The treatment is local corticosteroids, applied in a special ointment or in tablets that are kept in the mouth in contact with the ulcers. Various benign tumours may occur in the mouth, but ulceration that will not heal, especially on the tongue, must be regarded as malignant until it is proved otherwise.

Stones: these are found in the kidneys, bladder, gallbladder, prostate gland, salivary glands and elsewhere. They are formed by a number of factors, among them infection and desiccation, and usually contain calcium salts. The symptoms and treatment of the more important stones are described under the headings of the organs in which they are found.

Stools: the faeces, the waste matter discharged from the bowels.

Strabismus: a squint (q.v.).

Strangulation: *(1)* Compression of the throat, blocking the windpipe and the arteries of the neck in order to kill a victim. *(2)* Compression of the blood vessels supplying a part or organ sufficient to cut off the blood supply, for example in the case of a strangulated hernia, where the hernia becomes lodged in its sac outside the abdominal cavity, swells, and the blood vessels are obliterated.

Strangury: a state in which the urine can only be passed in slow painful drops although there is a strong desire to urinate.

Strawberry Mark: a naevus, a collection of blood vessels forming a birthmark, which slowly disappears without treatment.

Streptococcus: a round Gram-positive micro-organism which has a tendency to grow in chains. Some produce disease in man, and can be classified according to their power of haemolysis, that is, the breaking down of blood when grown on an appropriate culture medium. Alpha-haemolytic streptococci cause a partial breakdown of blood, beta-haemolytic a complete breakdown. Beta-haemolytic organisms are further divided according to their antigenic reactions: group A produces most disease in humans, and is further divided serologically into numbered types. The beta-haemolytic group A streptococci cause tonsillitis, impetigo and wound infections, septicaemia, erysipelas, scarlet fever, and some of these infections may be followed by rheumatic fever or kidney disease (glomerulonephritis). Group B causes septicaemia and endocarditis, inflammation of the lining of the heart. *Streptococcus pneumoniae* is an alpha-haemolytic streptococcus responsible for pneumonia, middle ear disease, meningitis and other infections, and other alpha-haemolytic organisms, previously called *Streptococcus viridans*, can cause endocarditis, abscesses and dental infections. Streptococci are killed by heat over 65°C and by disinfectants, and are sensitive to penicillin and other antibiotics.

Streptokinase: a drug which activates plasminogen to form plasmin (*see* Coagulation of the Blood), which attacks fibrin and dissolves clots. It is used in the treatment of deep vein thrombosis, pulmonary embolism and myocardial infarction or coronary thrombosis, and given by intravenous infusion.

Streptomycin: an antibiotic derived from the soil mould *Streptomyces griseus* discovered in 1944 by Selman Waksman (1888–1973) in the United States. It is active against many bacteria, but is now used principally for its action against the organism of tuberculosis, the treatment of which was revolutionised by its discovery. It is used in combination with other drugs, for example isoniazid, and is given by intramuscular injection. It may affect the eighth cranial nerve, the auditory nerve, and produce giddiness and deafness.

Stria: a groove or line in the skin, caused by weakening of the elastic fibres of the skin consequent upon stretching. Striae are seen in the abdominal skin of women after pregnancy, or after the abdomen has been distended for any cause.

Stricture: abnormal narrowing of a natural passage such as the urethra, bowel or oesophagus, caused by scarring after injury or infection, or by a tumour.

Stridor: the noise made by the breath in passing an obstruction in the larynx, caused for example by diphtheria, inflammation of the larynx and trachea in virus infection, or an inhaled foreign body.

Stroke: apoplexy (q.v.).

Stroma: the tissue that forms the supporting framework of an organ, as distinct from the parenchyma, the functioning tissue.

Strongyloides: *Strongyloides stercoralis* is a roundworm that may infest man, found in subtropical and tropical countries. *See* Worms.

Struma: goitre.

Strychnine: an alkaloid derived from the seeds of the tropical tree *Strychnos nux vomica*. It aids transmission of impulses at the synapses of the central nervous system, and was prescribed in small doses as a tonic for many years; it was also used as a bitter stimulant to the appetite. In larger doses it is poisonous, and causes convulsions similar to those of tetanus which may prove fatal.

Stupor: a state of incomplete unconsciousness in which painful stimuli will cause the subject to react.

Stuttering: *see* Stammering.

Stye: An infection of a sebaceous gland in the edge of the eyelid. The infecting organism is usually a staphylococcus, and a small abscess forms, which may be helped to discharge by removal of the eyelash which is commonly found protruding from its centre, and by the application of heat. Chloramphenicol eye ointment may be used.

Subacute Bacterial Endocarditis: *see* Endocarditis.

Subacute Myelo-optic Neuropathy (SMON): a disease occurring mainly in Japan, in which unpleasant numbness and weakness in the legs is associated with impairment of vision; the disease starts with abdominal pain and diarrhoea, and may spread to involve the sensation and power of the arms and produce changes in consciousness and sometimes convulsions; it may lead to green discoloration of the tongue. After many efforts to find an infective agent it was suspected that the drug clioquinol (Enterovioform) used as an anti-diarrhoeal agent was responsible for the disease, and since the drug was banned in Japan in September 1970 the incidence has markedly decreased.

Subarachnoid Haemorrhage: bleeding into the subarachnoid space (*see* Meninges), which is normally filled with cerebrospinal fluid. The blood comes from a ruptured aneurysm (q.v.) on the arterial anastomosis at the base of the brain, called the circle of Willis (Thomas Willis, 1621–75), from an aneurysm on another cerebral artery, or from a leaking arterio-venous malformation in the cerebral circulation. Subarachnoid bleeding may follow a head injury, but in this case the bleeding is not of the first significance. Spontaneous bleeding causes a sudden severe headache, often felt at the back of the head, which may be followed by loss of consciousness; if the patient comes round, there will be neck stiffness and dislike of the light because of the irritation of the meninges. Other neurological signs may be found depending on the site of the aneurysm and the damage done by the bleeding. One quarter of the attacks are fatal within 24 hours, and another quarter will prove fatal within a month. A brain scan will confirm the diagnosis; lumbar puncture will demonstrate blood in the cerebrospinal fluid. Angiography is used to demonstrate the site of bleeding and if possible early operation undertaken to clip off the aneurysm or deal with a bleeding arterio-venous malformation. If the bleeding has come from a source near the division of the internal carotid artery into its branches, the carotid artery may be tied in the neck to reduce the risk of further haemorrhage.

Subclavian: under the collar-bone or clavicle, e.g. sub-clavian artery.

Subclinical: it is possible for people to develop infections and overcome them without falling ill. Such unnoticed infections are termed subclinical, and are the way most of us acquire resistance to common diseases.

Subcutaneous: under the skin, usually applied to in-jections.

Subdural Haematoma: bleeding under the dura mater, the outermost of the three membranes enclosing the brain. Unlike the bleeding in an extradural haemorrhage (q.v.), the blood in this case comes from the veins. The precipitating head injury may appear to be comparatively minor, especially in older people, and the bleeding is slow because the normal pressure inside the head is high enough to depress the rate of venous bleeding. The true state of affairs may not show itself for many days or even weeks, but as the blood clot breaks down it forms an area of high osmotic pressure and attracts fluid into itself, swelling gradually until it takes up enough space to give rise to symptoms. The patient, who may have forgotten all about the bump on the head, suffers from increasing headaches, becomes forgetful and dull, and then confused or stuprose. Unconsciousness may supervene. The difficulty is often in diagnosis, but when this has been accomplished the condition is relieved by a simple operation to release the collection of altered blood.

Subluxation: a dislocation which is partial or incomplete.

Submandibular Gland: this gland secretes saliva into the mouth. Lying under cover of the lower jawbone in front of its angle, it is about the size of a walnut. Its duct runs forward to discharge from a small papilla under the tongue, and is known as Wharton's duct, under which name it figures in an unquotable anatomical mnemonic rhyme.

Subperiosteal Haematoma: a collection of blood under the membrane covering a bone. It is usually the result of an injury, such as a kick in the shin, and it can be very painful.

Suicide: since the Suicide Act of 1961 suicide or attempted suicide has ceased to be a crime, but it is still a criminal act to 'aid, abet, counsel or procure' the suicide of another person. A distinction has to be made between those who attempt suicide with the intention of killing themselves and those whose attempt is 'a cry for help'. Between these groups are a number of people who are undecided and confused. Of those who succeed in killing themselves, about one-third have made previous attempts. It is not true that those who are seriously suicidal do not talk about suicide; they do not commit the act without warning. Nearly all have some severe mental disturbance, usually depressive, and a number are alcoholics or abuse drugs. Some are schizophrenic. More men than women commit suicide, but more women than men attempt it unsuccessfully. The average age of those who commit suicide is about 50, the average age of those who attempt it about 35. About one-fifth of emergency medical admissions to hospital are attempted suicides, and about a quarter of the patients make another attempt within a year, often within three months. Patients do however recover from serious suicidal tendencies, and their case is not hopeless.

Sulphonamides: introduced in the early 1930s by Gerhard Domagk (1895–1964), who was awarded the Nobel Prize, for some years these were the only drugs active against many pathogenic bacteria that had previously been uncontrollable, and they saved countless lives. They are not without unwanted dangerous effects, notably on the kidneys and the blood, and they have to a large extent been superseded by the antibiotics, except for sulphamethoxazole in combination with trimethoprim (co-trimoxazole) which is used for various infections, in particular those of the urinary tract, typhoid fever and salmonellosis.

Sulphonylureas: drugs which increase the secretion of insulin and its effect, and are used in the treatment of diabetes (q.v.), particularly those of late onset where insulin-secreting cells are still active. The drugs are given by mouth, and are used in conjunction with control of the diet.

Sunburn: redness of the skin followed by blistering may be caused by exposure to the ultraviolet radiation of the sun for a few hours, especially in those with fair complexions; the effect of the sun is strongest at midday, and may not be fully appreciated if there is a cooling breeze. The rays are blocked by ozone and water vapour, and are most likely to be harmful at high altitudes. Titanium dioxide paste can be used to provide protection, but is thick and greasy; sunscreening lotions filter out part of the ultraviolet radiation, and usually carry an indication of the sun protection factor. This indicates the degree of protection afforded compared with the unprotected skin –

an SPF of 6 indicates for example that exposure six times longer than when unprotected should be tolerated.

Sunstroke: *see* Heatstroke.

Superfluous Hair: may be removed by depilatory creams, which destroy the hair but not the hair root, and may be irritant to the skin, and also by waxes, plucking, or electrolysis. Shaving does not make the hair grow faster or become coarser. In severe cases endocrine treatment may be used; the contraceptive pill can be used to suppress the activity of the ovaries, and the drug cyproterone acetate is an anti-androgen. Cimetidine and spironolactone have some anti-androgenic activity in addition to their primary effects, and have also been used. *See* Hirsutism.

Supination: a term applied to mean turning the hand so that the palm is upwards or forwards. Pronation is the opposite movement.

Suppository: a bullet-shaped medicated solid mass made of easily melted substance for introduction into the rectum or vagina, so that the contained medication will be absorbed through the mucous membrane or act locally.

Suppuration: the formation of pus. A suppurating wound is one discharging pus.

Suprapubic: above the pubic bone at the bottom of the abdomen; it is usually applied to operations carried out through the lowest part of the abdominal wall, for example suprapubic cystotomy, the opening of the bladder through the abdominal wall.

Suprarenal Gland: the adrenal gland.

Suprasellar: above the sella turcica, the bony depression in the base of the sphenoid bone that holds the pituitary gland. Tumours of this region, which may be congenital (suprasellar cyst) or acquired (suprasellar meningioma) very often interfere with the function of the optic nerves, which join to form the optic chiasm just above the pituitary gland. They also interfere with various functions of the hypothalamic area of the brain.

Supraspinatus Tendinitis: the supraspinatus muscle takes origin from the upper part of the back of the shoulder-blade, and its tendon is closely applied to the capsule of the shoulder joint as it runs to be inserted into the upper part of the humerus, the bone of the upper arm. It may become inflamed, or the seat of a deposit of calcium, so that the arm cannot be raised from the side for more than about 40° without pain, for the tendon comes into contact with the underside of the acromion, the bony extension of the shoulder-blade above the joint. If the arm is moved passively above the head it can be held there, but the arc between about 40° and 90° is painful. The treatment is injection of local anaesthetic and cortisone into the area, with physiotherapy. Deposits of calcium in the tendon may be removed surgically. *See* Frozen Shoulder.

Surfectant: a surface-active agent which affects the surface tension of liquids, such as a detergent. Pulmonary surfectant is a substance secreted in the alveoli which decreases the surface tension of fluid in the lungs. *See* Respiratory Distress Syndrome.

Suture: *(1)* Surgical stitch, or the insertion of a stitch, or the material used for the stitch. *(2)* The immovable fibrous joints between the bones of the skull are called sutures.

Swab: a twist of cotton wool on a stick used for taking specimens from the surface of mucous membranes or from infected areas for examination by the bacteriologist. It is also used to mean pieces of gauze or other material used to apply antiseptic to the skin, or to mop up fluids or blood, for example during the course of a surgical operation.

Sycosis Barbae: an infection of the hair follicles of the face by staphylococci, called barber's itch because it was spread by infected brushes used for shaving in the barber's shop.

Symbiosis: a condition in which two dissimilar organisms live in close association. The association may be beneficial to both, when it is called mutualism; beneficial to one but not the other, which is parasitism; beneficial to one, but without effect on the other, commensalism; or deleterious to both, synnecrosis.

Sympathetic: in medicine this refers to part of the autonomic nervous system, which regulates the unconscious automatic processes of the body. *See* Nervous System.

Symphysis: a type of joint where the opposing surfaces are united by a strong plate of fibro-cartilage, as in the symphysis pubis.

Symptom: evidence of functional change which indicates the presence of disease. It is usually applied to evidence that the patient has noticed, as opposed to evidence noted by an observer, which is called a sign.

Synapse: the place where processes of different nerve cells meet, or where processes meet the bodies of other nerve cells; it is at the synapses that nerve impulses are transmitted in the nervous system by the release of chemical substances.

Syncope: a faint, or sudden loss of consciousness due to a fall of blood pressure disturbing the circulation to the brain.

Syndrome: a set of signs and symptoms which occur together in a definite pattern.

Synousiology: the study of the science of sexual intercourse.

Synovitis: inflammation of the synovial membrane, the slippery membrane that lines joints, tendon sheaths and bursae.

Syphilis (the great pox, morbus gallicus, lues): once the worst of the sexually transmitted diseases, syphilis has with the advent of penicillin become perhaps the easiest to treat successfully, providing that treatment is started early.

The infecting bacterium is *Treponema pallidum*, a spiral organism, which produces a papule on the infected area about three weeks after infection. The papule breaks down and ulcerates; the ulcer is called a chancre, which can be a centimetre or more across and has a hard base. Chancres may be found on the penis, the vulva, the lips or in the case of homosexual men the anus. Any sore on the genitals should be examined to exclude syphilis. If left, the chancre heals in anything between three and six weeks. Six weeks to several months after this the secondary stage of the disease develops. A pale red rash breaks out over the whole body, which may extend onto the face, forehead, the palms of the hands and the soles of the feet. In the moist parts of the body the rash may form grey discs, called condylomata lata, which run together and are very infectious. Ulcers develop in the mouth and throat which are said to look like snail tracks. The rash fades, and the disease enters a latent stage during which the only sign of its presence is a positive serological test. Women may infect their unborn babies for three or four years after entering the latent stage, but expectant mothers are submitted to serological tests early in pregnancy. After a period of years the third stage of the disease may develop, with damage to the skin, the central nervous system, the bones, the heart and the aorta. Syphilis has been called 'the Great Imitator' because of the variety of its manifestations, but the late stages, such as general paralysis of the insane or locomotor ataxia (q.v.), are now rarely seen. Treatment is with penicillin, or in those sensitive to penicillin, tetracycline or erythromycin.

Syringe: an instrument for injecting or withdrawing fluid or gas into or out of the body, usually connected to a needle or tube.

Syringomyelia: an uncommon disease of the spinal cord beginning between the ages of 15 and 30, in which cavities slowly form in the substance of the cord in the neck and interfere with the sensations of heat and pain in the hands and arms so that patients tend to burn themselves without realising it. Examination shows that there is also weakness and wasting of the muscles, with absent tendon jerks, and there may be pain in the arms. The cavity in the cord may extend upwards and involve the lower cranial nerves, causing difficulty in swallowing and weakness of the voice. The face may lose sensation except for the mouth and nose. The condition usually comes on slowly, but may suddenly get worse after coughing or sneezing. It appears to be due to an interference with the normal circulation of the cerebrospinal fluid, often due to a malformation described by the Austrian pathologist Hans Chiari (1851–1916) in which the lower part of the cerebellum projects through the foramen magnum, pressing on the spinal cord as it leaves the skull and obstructing the free flow of fluid. If this is demonstrated by investigations, the pressure in the foramen magnum may be relieved by surgical operation. However, if left, most patients can live a reasonable life and die from an unrelated disease.

Systole: the contraction of the heart, as opposed to diastole, the period of relaxation.

T

Tabes: in the general sense, the word means a wasting disease; it is now applied almost exclusively to tabes dorsalis, or locomotor ataxia (q.v.).

Tachycardia: rapid heartbeat which may be due to fever, emotion, exercise, chronic infection, anaemia, haemorrhage or certain drugs. It may be due to a disorder of cardiac rhythm, as for example in paroxysmal tachycardia (q.v.).

Taenia: a genus of tapeworms. *Taenia saginata* and *Taenia solium* are those important in medicine, for man is the only natural host. The intermediate hosts of *T. saginata* are cattle; the tapeworm lives in man's small intestine, and segments containing eggs break off and are passed in the faeces. The eggs are released into the soil when the segment disintegrates, and are eaten by the cattle, where the embryos change into larvae or cysticerci. When human beings eat raw or undercooked beef, the developing worm fastens itself to the wall of the small intestine by four suckers on its scolex (head). The worms are hermaphrodites, and each segment contains both male and female reproductive organs. Living for years, and growing as long as 10 metres, the worms give rise to few symptoms. The intermediate host of *T. solium* is the pig, and it is acquired by eating raw or undercooked pork or ham. Unlike *T. saginata*, it has hooks as well as suckers on the scolex by which it attaches itself to the intestine. It may grow up to 4 metres long, and is also a hermaphrodite. *T. solium* can give rise to the condition of cysticercosis (q.v.), in which eggs develop into cysticerci in many parts of the body, including the brain. The drug praziquantel is used in the treatment of both *T. solium* and *T. saginata*.

Talipes: club-foot (q.v.).

Talus: the ankle-bone, the highest of the small bones of the ankle, which makes a joint with the tibia and fibula, the bones of the leg. It can also mean the ankle.

Tapeworm: a parasitic worm which is long and flat, like a piece of tape; it is divided into segments. *See* Taenia.

Tar: a black sticky substance obtained by heating coal or certain species of pine. It contains a mixture of ingredients, among them cresol, phenol, paraffin, naphthalene and toluene; there are many others. It is used in medicine as an application to the skin in the treatment of psoriasis and eczema, coal tar being more active than wood tar. There are many preparations on the market in the form of solutions of varying strengths, creams, ointments and paste; it may be mixed with zinc or corticosteroids. Tar can irritate the skin and make it sensitive to light.

Tarsorrhaphy: an operation in which the eyelids are sewn together to protect the eye, used in cases where the cornea has lost its sensitivity, for example after operation on the fifth cranial nerve for trigeminal neuralgia.

Tarsus: the ankle; also the flat firm plate of connective tissue which supports the eyelid.

Tartar Emetic: a mixture of antimony and potassium tartrate which was used as an emetic, but is no longer recommended. It was also used in the treatment of bilharziasis and kala-azar, but in the latter disease antimony may now be used in the form of sodium stibogluconate.

Teeth: the teeth are made of a substance called dentine, which is covered by a layer of enamel. There are no blood vessels or cells in the dentine, but otherwise it is the same as bone; enamel is a mineral containing calcium and phosphate, and it is the hardest substance in the body. Each tooth has a crown and a root, in the centre of which is the pulp, which contains a nerve and blood vessels. The root is set in the jaw; it is covered by modified bone tissue called cement, and a peridontal membrane which binds the cement and jawbone together. This membrane has blood vessels and nerves. The teeth begin to erupt at about six months; the inner incisor at the front of the mouth is the first, followed by the second incisor. The first molar tooth comes at a year, the canine at eighteen months and the second molar at two years. There are 20 milk, or deciduous, teeth. They begin to give way to the 32 permanent teeth at about six years; the first molar is the first to be replaced, followed at about yearly intervals by the first incisor, the second incisor, first pre-molar, canine, the second pre-molar and the second molar. The third molar teeth, the wisdom teeth, follow between the 13th and 25th years.

Dental caries is extremely common and can be very painful; it occurs because bacteria, notably *Streptococcus mutans*, form a film on the teeth called plaque and break down sugar to form acid. The acid dissolves the enamel and the bacteria gain access to the dentine and pulp. The ensuing infection sets up considerable pain, and may extend to the tissues round the root of the tooth and cause a dental abscess. If possible the dentist preserves the tooth by removing the decayed material and restoring the substance of the tooth with a filling, but if the infection has progressed to abscess formation the tooth may have to be removed. Prevention of dental decay rests on cleaning the teeth regularly, and denying the bacteria the sucrose necessary for them to produce acid. The addition of one part per million of fluorine to drinking water decreases the incidence of dental decay in children by over a half.

Teething: this is often given as the cause for numerous minor complaints of infancy, but the diagnosis in the majority of cases is erroneous.

Telangiectasis: a red spot on the skin formed by dilated capillary or terminal arterial blood vessels.

Temazepam: short-acting benzodiazepine, often used as a hypnotic in cases of insomnia; the use should be short term, for withdrawal symptoms are liable to occur. It may also be used as a premedication before general anaesthesia.

Temperature: the average body temperature in health is

37°C (98.6°F). It is a little lower in the morning and higher in the evening.

Tempero-mandibular Joint: the joint between the temporal bone of the skull and the lower jaw or mandible. It is just in front of the ear, and the head of the mandible can be felt moving by a finger placed in the outer passage of the ear. The joint is a sliding hinge which allows movement of the mandible from side to side, and the two bones are separated by a plate of cartilage inside the joint. This may become displaced or torn so that the jaw clicks on movement. Relatively minor incidents such as a wide yawn can dislocate the joint; but if this happens the dislocation can be reduced. The operator stands in front of the patient, places the thumbs on the back teeth and the fingers under the chin, presses the thumbs down and the fingers up, and the jaw clicks into place.

Temporal Arteritis (giant cell arteritis, cranial arteritis): seen in patients over 60, the disease produces headache or pain in the temple where the temporal artery is found to be thickened and tender. The patient may feel unwell and run a temperature as well as having various aches and pains in other parts of the body. It is important because the eyesight may be affected with blurred vision or blindness, which may be temporary or permanent. The ESR (*see* Sedimentation Rate) is markedly raised, and if the diagnosis is in doubt a biopsy of the artery is taken. As soon as the diagnosis is made, corticosteroids are given, initially in high doses, which are reduced in accordance with the progress of the signs and symptoms and the improvement of the ESR. Corticosteroids in low doses may be needed for years, but the disease does not threaten life.

Tendinitis: inflammation of a tendon.

Tendon (sinew): the cord made of dense fibrous tissue which joins muscle to bone.

Tendon Jerk: if a tendon is tapped sharply so as to stretch it, a spinal reflex causes the muscle to contract.

Tenesmus: straining painfully but ineffectively to pass a motion or pass urine.

Tennis Elbow: pain in the outer part of the elbow, radiating down the forearm. The elbow is tender over the origin of the common extensor tendon from the lateral epicondyle of the humerus: that is, the outer bony point felt at the elbow. If a definite tender spot can be found, the pain is often relieved by the injection of local anaesthetic, followed if this is successful by a corticosteroid. Golfer's elbow is a similar condition occurring on the inner side of the elbow.

Tenosynovitis: inflammation of the sheath of a tendon, usually caused by repeated minor injury or repeated awkward movement. It is painful, particularly on movement, and is treated by rest and if necessary immobilisation. In stenosing tenosynovitis the tendon sheath becomes narrowed, and the tendon may be locally thickened. This commonly affects the flexors of the fingers in the palm of the hand; the result is a trigger finger, where the finger straightens with a jerk. The narrowing can be relieved by a simple operation.

Tenotomy: the surgical division or partial division of a tendon.

Tentorium: the tentorium cerebelli is the fold of dura mater that separates the cerebral hemispheres above from the cerebellum below. In its edge, which is fixed horizontally to the interior of the skull, it splits to enclose the transverse sinus, which receives the venous blood drained from the cerebral hemisphere in the sagittal sinus and straight sinus; this bends downwards to become the sigmoid sinus and then the internal jugular vein. As the fixed edge of the tentorium continues forwards it is attached to the petrous temporal bone and encloses the superior petrosal sinus; it extends as far forwards as the posterior clinoid processes of the sphenoid bone. Through the gap between the free edge of the tentorium and the body of the sphenoid bone passes the midbrain. Because of the number of important venous sinuses that join to run in the edge of the tentorium it is possible for a blow on the back of the head to result in extensive bleeding inside the skull.

Teratoma: a tumour composed of embryonic tissues including all three layers of developing cells, endoderm, mesoderm and ectoderm. A solid teratoma may contain pieces of bone, nerve or intestine, and is usually malignant; it may develop in the testis, or in other places, and must be removed. Cystic teratomas may contain various rudimentary tissues such as skin, hair and teeth, and are not malignant; they may contain ectoderm to the exclusion of other tissues, and are then called dermoid cysts.

Term: a definite period of time, in medicine usually applied to the duration of a pregnancy; full term is 282 days from the first day of the last menstrual period. The date on which a birth can be expected is calculated by adding 7 to the date of the last menstrual period and taking away three calendar months.

Termination: commonly used to mean termination of pregnancy, or abortion. This is at present carried out surgically, but recently a drug has been used in France, mifepristone, which blocks the action of progesterone, the hormone necessary to maintain pregnancy, and so brings about abortion. Application has been made for permission to use the drug in Britain in cases not more than nine weeks pregnant.

Testicle (testis): male reproductive organ. The testicles are paired, smooth and oval, and measure about 4 cm × 3 cm × 2.5 cm. Each testicle is covered by a membrane called the tunica vaginalis, which has two layers separated normally by a thin film of fluid. Both testicles lie in the scrotum, the left usually a little lower than the right. Along the back of the testicle lies the epididymis, a long thin tube coiled and turned upon itself which has about 15 ducts opening into it from the testis through which travel the spermatozoa. Each testicle contains a large number of seminiferous tubules in which the spermatozoa are formed, and interstitial cells called Leydig cells which elaborate the male hormones (Franz von Leydig, German anatomist, 1821–1908). It takes about 70 days for a mature spermatozoon to be formed; the process is controlled by the hormone testosterone and by the pituitary hormone FSH (*see* Ovary). Interstitial cell stimulating hormone regulates the secretion of testosterone. From the epididymis the spermatozoa pass into the vas deferens, which runs in the spermatic cord into the abdominal cavity through the inguinal canal and passes into the prostate gland at the base of the bladder. Here the vas deferens joins the seminal vesicle, and from it the spermatozoa pass into the urethra through the ejaculatory duct.

The testicle may become infected and inflamed, usually by *Escherichia coli* as part of an infection of the urinary system, by *Neisseria gonorrhoeae* as part of a gonorrhoeal infection or by the tubercle bacillus. Inflammation of the testicle can be caused by mumps, and this is more common in adults than in children. The symptoms of inflammation are pain and swelling of the testicle, and treatment varies according to the cause. Sudden pain and swelling may be caused by torsion of the testicle, in which the organ is twisted so that the spermatic cord is obstructed and the blood supply cut off. The treatment is immediate surgery. Tumours of the testicle can be malignant, for example seminoma or teratoma, or simple, as for example a cyst of the epididymis. Tumours may cause an excessive amount of fluid to collect between the two layers of the membrane enclosing the testicle, forming a hydrocoele, and the same can happen as the result of inflammation. Many hydrocoeles, however, collect for no obvious reason. The fluid can be drawn off under local anaesthetic. Injury to the testicle is not uncommon, but in civilian life rarely serious enough to need surgical treatment, although a collection of blood may form after a severe blow which has to be released if it is causing an increase of pressure inside the inelastic capsule of the organ. Even relatively slight blows dealt the gland are liable to cause great pain and a degree of shock.

Testosterone: the male hormone secreted by the testis. It is necessary for the development of the secondary sexual characteristics, that is, the growth of the beard and pubic hair, the growth of the genital organs and the lowering of the voice at puberty, together with the characteristically male body shape. In the absence of testosterone before puberty the body will continue to grow in a predominantly female shape. After puberty it is responsible for the production of semen.

Test Type: printed letters used to test acuity of vision. The letters are designed to subtend a known angle at the eye when the subject stands at a specified distance from the test type, or when a test card is held at a given distance from the eye.

Test-tube Babies: *see* Assisted Conception.

Tetanus (lockjaw): a disease caused by the micro-organism *Clostridium tetani*. The spores of this organism are found in the bowels of many animals, including man, and are very common in the soil, particularly when it is cultivated and manured. The bacilli are Gram-positive and anaerobic, that is, they will only grow in the absence of oxygen. Infection occurs through a wound or abrasion in the skin; it need only be a very minor wound, and in some cases no entry wound can be found. The organism produces a toxin called tetanospasmin, which spreads to the spinal cord and the brain, both through the blood and along the nerves. The incubation period is from one to two weeks; it may be shorter or longer. The muscles become stiff, and the mouth will not open fully. There is difficulty in swallowing, and the neck becomes stiff. The abdominal muscles become rigid, and the muscles of the back, which are very strong, may contract so hard that the body arches backwards in the position called opisthotonos, supported by the heels and the back of the head. Reflex spasms of the muscles may occur, including the muscles of the larynx, so that the breath is cut off. Complications include pneumonia, irregularity of heart action, a low blood pressure and, if the spasms are severe, fractures of the thoracic spine.

The treatment is the use of human tetanus immunoglobulin, and control of the spasms and rigidity by the use of drugs such as chlorpromazine, diazepam and phenobarbitone. A tracheostomy (q.v.) may be carried out so that the airways can be kept clear by suction and the possibility of laryngeal spasm obstructing the breathing is avoided. When the facilities of an intensive care unit are available, severe cases of tetanus may be treated by paralysing all the muscles with curare or a similar drug and using an artificial breathing machine to support the respiration.

Prevention of tetanus is by active immunisation with tetanus toxoid, which is offered for all infants and children as a routine in the United Kingdom. Booster doses may be given at five-yearly intervals. If a wound is sustained that might be infected, unless an injection of toxoid has been given within a year previously a booster dose should be given. If the patient has never been immunised a course of three injections should be started, the second injection six weeks after the first and the third six months later.

Tetany: not to be confused with tetanus, tetany is a condition in which there is abnormal excitability of the nerves and muscles. In mild cases, there is numbness and tingling of the hands and feet, and round the mouth. If the blood is cut off from the forearm by a sphygmomanometer cuff, the muscles contract and the wrist is flexed, the fingers are flexed at the knuckles and extended at the finger joints; the thumb is drawn towards the palm. This sign was first described by Armand Trousseau, a French physician (1801–67), and bears his name. In severe tetany the hand assumes this position, the face grimaces, the voice becomes hoarse and the feet are drawn down at the ankles. The condition is caused by lack of calcium ions in the blood (*see* Calcium), and may be due to deficiency of the parathyroid glands, lack of vitamin D or deficient absorption of calcium; it may also be due to alkalosis of the blood from taking excess of alkalis, as may happen in the over-enthusiastic treatment of a peptic ulcer or a bout of hysterical over-breathing.

Tetracyclines: a number of antibiotic drugs were discovered by research into the properties of organisms found in the soil; hence the proprietary name Terramycin for oxytetracycline. They have a broad spectrum of activity, but many organisms have developed resistance to them and they are not as widely used as they once were. They are, however, used against chlamydia and rickettsia (q.v.) and brucella, which causes undulant fever; they are active against *Haemophilus influenzae* and are therefore used in cases of chronic bronchitis, and against *Mycoplasma pneumoniae*, which causes infection of the lungs, and *Mycoplasma hominis*, which may cause non-specific urethritis. They can be very useful in treating cases of acne, when small doses are given for three months or longer. Tetracyclines are deposited in growing bones and teeth, and stain them yellow, and are therefore not given to pregnant women, those who are breast-feeding or children under 12. Milk, alkalis, calcium, magnesium and iron salts interfere with the absorption of tetracyclines, and should therefore not be taken at the same time.

Tetraethyl Lead: used as an anti-knock additive to petrol. It has been found that lead emitted in exhaust fumes can contaminate the air and dust, be breathed in and settle on crops, and is potentially dangerous. The use of tetraethyl lead in petrol is therefore being discontinued.

Tetraplegia (quadriplegia): paralysis of all four limbs.

Thalamus: a large group of nuclei in the midbrain, where ascending sensory nerve fibres from the spinal cord relay to the cerebral cortex.

Thalassaemia: an inherited defect in the formation of haemoglobin; there are a number of types, of which the most important is beta-thalassaemia. Alpha-thalassaemia is more common, but those who suffer from it are either stillborn or if they survive have a relatively mild form of the disease. There are further types of the disease, but thalassaemia may also be classified according to its severity into major, intermediate and minor disorders. The major disease, commonly beta-thalassaemia, produces profound anaemia in children, which if not treated by transfusions is often fatal. If transfusions are given, the children at first do well, but accumulate an excess of iron which gives rise to complications culminating in damage to the heart, which may prove fatal in the second or third decade. The intermediate forms of the disease vary a great deal, and require careful observation so that treatment may be given as necessary. If the spleen becomes enlarged it may be removed. The carriers of beta-thalassaemia suffer only from the minor form of the disease, which rarely gives any trouble. Thalassaemia was first recognised in 1925; by 1936 it was realised that many cases came from the Mediterranean region, and the name thalassaemia was introduced from the Greek *thalassa*, the sea. Since then it has been found in many parts of the world, and the molecular genetics, which are complicated, continue to be a subject for research. The control of the disease depends on genetic counselling, and the detection of cases in antenatal clinics; prenatal diagnosis is possible by amniocentesis or chorionic villus biopsy.

Thalidomide: a sedative and hypnotic drug which appeared when first introduced to be useful and safe, for the effects of a large overdose were not fatal, and its action in animals showed no ill effects. Introduced in Germany in 1956, it came to the United Kingdom in 1958 and was used freely as a tranquilliser; but in 1960 it was suspected that thalidomide might be responsible for the development of myxoedema (thyroid deficiency) and neuritis, and no licence was granted for its use in the United States. By 1961 it had become clear that thalidomide had in fact been responsible for the birth of a number of deformed children, born to mothers who had taken the drug between the 24th and 40th days after conception, and it was withdrawn from use in the United Kingdom in December 1961. Many of these children suffered from phocomelia, in which the arms and legs fail to develop. The drug is now reserved for use in the painful complication of neuropathy in leprosy. Since the thalidomide tragedy the medical profession has become very wary of prescribing drugs during pregnancy, particularly during the first three months.

Theca: a sheath, used particularly of the dura mater covering the spinal cord.

Theophylline: a drug which dilates the bronchi and bronchioles; derived from tea, or made synthetically, it is used in the treatment of asthma.

Therapeutics: the study of the science of treating disease. Therapy is the treatment of disease.

Theriac: a mixture once believed to heal the bites of wild animals and protect from the effects of their venom.

Thermography: variations of temperature over the surface of the body can be recorded by using photographic film sensitive to infra-red radiation. The technique is called thermography, and the record a thermogram. Because the surface temperature of the body is determined by the state of the local circulation, and variations in the blood supply to a part can be produced by underlying disease processes, thermography may help in the diagnosis of diseases such as cancer of the breast.

Thermometer: an instrument for the measurement of temperature. Single readings of a patient's temperature, while useful, may be misleading, and the subjective sensations of a patient with a raised temperature can be more valuable in diagnosis. The pattern of repeated readings is needed to elucidate the nature and course of a disease.

Thiabendazole: a drug used in the treatment of infestation with the worm *Strongyloides stercoralis*.

Thiamine: vitamin B_1. Deficiency of this vitamin produces the disease beri-beri (q.v.).

Thiazides: diuretic drugs which act on the first part of the distal convoluted tubule of the kidney (q.v.) to block the reabsorption of sodium. They are used in the treatment of high blood pressure and heart failure.

Thigh: the function of the leg is to support the body upright and to make locomotion possible. The thigh-bone is called the femur, and it is the longest bone in the body. It runs from the hip to the knee, and bears the entire weight of the trunk. At the knee it makes a hinge joint with the tibia, the principal bone of the leg, and at the hip a ball-and-socket joint with the pelvis. The ball at the head of the femur is carried on a long neck, which is set obliquely to the shaft at an angle of 125°, and when standing upright with the knees together the shaft of the femur runs obliquely from the outer sides of the pelvis to the knee. The obliquity is greater in the female than the male because of the greater width of the female pelvis. The muscles acting on the hip joint are the abductors, the gluteal muscles of the buttock; the flexors, the iliacus, psoas, rectus femoris and sartorius; the adductors; and the extensors, the hamstrings. In addition there are muscles which rotate the femur. All these muscles act in concert to make standing and walking possible. The gluteal muscles of the buttock are attached to the greater trochanter, a projection above the junction of the neck of the femur with the shaft; the gluteus maximus also runs into the iliotibial tract, a band of strong connective tissue which runs on the outer surface of the thigh from the brim of the iliac bone of the pelvis to the knee, where it is attached to the upper end of the tibia. The iliacus and psoas run from the pelvis and the spine respectively to the femur. The rectus femoris joins the three vastus muscles arising from the femur to form the quadriceps muscle, whose tendon includes the kneecap, the patella, and is inserted into the tibia to extend the knee as well as flex the hip. The sartorius, the tailor's muscle, runs obliquely across the thigh from the crest of the pelvis to reach the tibia on the inner side of the knee. The adductor muscles, the horseman's muscles, run from the pelvis to the shaft of the femur to bring the legs together, and the extensor muscles of the thigh, the hamstrings, are also the flexors of the knee joint, running from the pelvis to the tibia and fibula at the back of the knee. It will be seen that to a great extent the movements of the hip and knee joints are interdependent. The blood vessels of the thigh are the femoral artery and vein, which run round the femur from the front of the thigh to the back of the knee, and the principal nerve is the sciatic nerve, which originates at the lumbar and sacral nerve plexuses and runs down the inner side and back of the thigh.

Thiopentone: thiopentone sodium is an intravenous anaesthetic with a rapid action commonly used to induce anaesthesia.

Thomas's Splint: named after the inventor, Hugh Thomas, a Liverpool surgeon (1834–91), the splint is used to immobilise the knee and take the weight of the body from the foot of the splint, which is in contact with the ground when the patient stands up, directly to the ischial tuberosity, the bony part of the pelvis upon which we sit. The foot can be tied to the lower end of the splint and, as the upper end is applied to the pelvis, traction on the foot stretches the whole leg including the thigh and provides a means of immobilising a fractured femur.

Thoracic Duct: the large lymph vessel that begins at the cisterna chyli, a sac between 5 and 8 cm long lying beside the aorta in the aortic opening of the diaphragm. Into this sac there run the right and left lumbar lymph trunks draining the lower limbs and the intestinal trunk from the intestines. From the cisterna chyli the thoracic duct runs up through the thorax to the neck, crossing from the right of the aorta to the left and coming to lie on the left of the oesophagus. In the root of the neck it turns to the left and forwards at the level of the seventh cervical vertebra and is joined by the left jugular and subclavian lymph trunks from the head and the arm, and the lymph trunk from the structures in the left side of the thorax. The lymph carried by the thoracic duct runs into the subclavian vein at the junction of the jugular and subclavian veins. Lymph trunks from the right arm and the right side of the thorax and head join to form the right lymphatic duct, which opens into the junction of the subclavian and jugular veins on the right.

Thoracic Outlet Syndrome: a condition in which there is compression of the nerves and blood vessels of the arm as they cross the first rib on their way into the upper part of the arm. This produces tingling and numbness in the arm, or pain; if the artery is obstructed Raynaud's phenomenon (q.v.) may occur in the affected arm. The symptoms are worse at night, when the patient is tired, and they may be brought on when heavy weights such as a pail of water are carried on the affected side, and the shoulder is depressed. The hand may become pale and painful when the arm is raised above the head for any length of time. Obstruction to the vein may cause a thrombosis, with a swollen arm.

The cause of the compression may be a cervical rib, an extra rudimentary rib on the last cervical vertebra above the first rib, or an abnormality of the plexus of nerves that supplies the arm so that it arises one segment lower than normal; in some cases no abnormality of anatomy can be found. If there is a cervical rib it can be removed; in cases where the nerve plexus is lower than usual, or when there is no obvious abnormality and exercises to strengthen the muscles of the shoulder girdle have failed to help, the first rib can be removed.

Thoracoplasty: an operation in which several ribs are partially removed, allowing the chest wall and the underlying lung to collapse. Before the advent of drugs active against tuberculosis, this operation was frequently performed.

Thoracoscopy: the inspection of the interior of the thoracic cavity through an endoscope.

Thoracotomy: the operation of opening the wall of the chest.

Thorax: the chest, which contains the heart and the lungs and through which runs the oesophagus carrying food from the mouth to the stomach. The walls of the thorax are supported by ribs, twelve on each side, which are joined to the vertebral column behind and in the case of the upper seven ribs to the breast bone, the sternum, in front. Between the ribs are intercostal muscles, nerves, arteries and veins. The chest wall is covered by muscles: the pectorals in front, and the trapezius and latissimus dorsi behind. The shoulder-blade, the scapula, and its muscles cover the upper outer part of the back of the thorax, and the clavicle, the collar-bone, lies at the junction of the neck and thorax in front. The muscles, the scapula and the clavicle are all part of the shoulder girdle which supports and moves the arm.

The thoracic cavity is separated from the abdominal cavity by the diaphragm, and into right and left sides by a central membranous partition called the mediastinum, which contains the heart, the great blood vessels entering the heart, the oesophagus, lymph nodes and in its upper part the trachea, the windpipe, which branches into right and left bronchi to enter the lungs, and the thymus gland. The heart is contained in a special sac called the pericardium, made of two layers of slippery membrane separated by a thin film of fluid which enables it to move freely, and the lungs are separated from the chest wall in a similar way by two layers of thin membrane called the pleura. The outer membrane is applied to the inside of the thoracic wall, and the inner one covers the lungs. Between the two is another very thin layer of fluid. The potential space between the pleural membranes is airtight. When the chest wall is raised by the intercostal muscles and the diaphragmatic muscle contracts, drawing the diaphragm down, air under atmospheric pressure enters the lungs; when the muscles relax, the air is driven out.

Threadworm (pinworm): *Oxyuris vermicularis*; *see* Worms.

Thrill: in medicine, a sensation felt when the hand is placed on the surface of the body over an internal structure producing a vibration. Over the heart, a thrill is an indication that there is disease of one of the valves, or a defect in the septum between the ventricles. A loud murmur will be heard through the stethoscope.

Throat: commonly the seat of infection involving the tonsils alone or more usually the whole of the throat, when it is called pharyngitis. The infection is most often due to a virus; this may be complicated by secondary infection with haemolytic streptococci, *Haemophilus influenzae* or *Streptococcus pneumoniae*. In most cases a virus infection lasts for only a few days, and needs no treatment, but if it is more severe, and causes malaise, a fever, and enlargement of the lymph nodes in the neck, bacterial infection is likely and penicillin may be used. *See* Tonsils.

Thrombin: an enzyme concerned with the conversion of fibrinogen into fibrin. *See* Coagulation of the Blood.

Thrombocytopenic Purpura: deficiency in the number of platelets circulating in the blood may lead to multiple small haemorrhages from the capillaries and small arterioles, which show as small red spots on the skin called purpura, and in severe cases may cause bleeding from the stomach or intestines, from the nose, or excessive loss at the periods in women. There may be a tendency to bruise abnormally easily. Platelets are produced in the bone marrow by cells called megakaryocytes, and they normally adhere to damaged endothelial cells lining the blood vessels, forming plugs and playing a part in the coagulation processes necessary to seal off leaking capillaries and arterioles. In certain rare inherited conditions they may be abnormal and fail to function properly, but acquired defects in the system are more common. If the bone marrow is disturbed they are not formed in sufficient quantities; conditions causing this include leukaemias, cancers involving the marrow, and some anaemias. Chronic alcoholism may decrease the formation of platelets. Some drugs, particularly thiazide diuretics (q.v.), may also have this effect, as may exposure to radiation. Virus infections such as rubella, mumps, measles or infectious mononucleosis may be followed by a deficiency in platelet formation, or cause increased destruction of platelets. It is not uncommon for a deficiency in platelets to be found during pregnancy, but this is not marked and is rarely significant; it is also possible for a mother to produce antibodies to her baby's platelets in consequence of an antigen in the platelets derived from the father, resulting in a platelet deficiency in the child. In many cases no obvious cause for the thrombocytopenic purpura can be found, and these cases are called idiopathic. The treatment for severe cases is with corticosteroids; if these fail, some cases respond to removal of the spleen.

Thrombophlebitis: inflammation of a vein with consequent thrombosis, the formation of a clot. It is quite common in varicose veins, which become red and tender and sometimes painful enough to make walking difficult. The condition normally resolves by itself in a couple of weeks, but treatment with NSAIs and a supporting bandage or elastic stocking will help.

Thrombosis: the formation of a clot or thrombus in a blood vessel. It may occur in arteries, particularly when the wall has been roughened by atherosclerosis (*see* Arterial

Disease), or in the veins, especially when the blood flow is stagnant or sluggish. This may be the case after surgical operations, particularly those for fractures of the neck of the femur and open operations on the prostate gland, when small thrombi may form in the veins of the calf. Thrombosis of the deep veins can be dangerous, for there is a risk of a piece of clot breaking off and being carried in the circulation to the lungs, where it becomes lodged in the pulmonary artery or one of its branches forming a pulmonary embolus and cutting off the supply of blood to a part of the lung. Thrombosis is encouraged by oestrogen, which is contained in contraceptive pills, so that the smallest effective dose is chosen in prescribing. The use of the anticoagulant drugs heparin and warfarin has reduced the risks of deep vein thrombosis, as has the encouragement of getting out of bed as soon as possible after surgical operations.

Thrush: candidiasis (q.v.).

Thymol: a mild antiseptic derived from oil of thyme, often used in mouthwashes.

Thymus: a gland which lies at the root of the neck behind the breastbone in the upper mediastinum (*see* Thorax). It grows from birth to puberty, and thereafter diminishes in size but remains active. It is an important part of the lymphatic system, being responsible for the formation of lymphocytes (q.v.) called T cells, which are essential in the immune reaction. The gland may be enlarged in the disease myasthenia gravis (q.v.), and may be removed surgically in the treatment of that condition, and it may be the seat of a tumour called a thymoma, of which some are malignant.

Thyroid: the thyroid is a ductless gland lying in the neck in front of the windpipe, the trachea, just below the larynx, the Adam's apple. It has two lobes, one on each side of the trachea, joined across it by an isthmus. Two parathyroid glands (q.v.) are embedded in the rear surface of the thyroid gland on each side. It secretes the important hormones thyroxine (T_3) and tri-iodothyronine (T_4) under the influence of the anterior pituitary thyroid-stimulating hormone (TSH). It also secretes the hormone calcitonin, which plays a part in bone formation. Swellings of the gland are known as goitres (q.v.); overaction results in thyrotoxicosis (*see below*) and deficiency of thyroid secretion produces myxoedema (q.v.). The normal function of the thyroid depends on an adequate intake of iodine in the diet.

Thyrotoxicosis: Graves' disease (Robert Graves, Dublin physician, 1796–1853) is the commonest cause of this overaction of the thyroid gland. It is five times more common in women than men, and is thought to be an auto-immune disease; it runs in families. The patient is nervous, emotional and overactive, loses weight, sweats freely and dislikes the heat, feels weak and may have diarrhoea. There is a fast pulse, fine tremor of the outstretched hands, and the eyes may be prominent. The thyroid gland is enlarged. Investigation shows high levels in the blood of the thyroid hormones T_3 and T_4, and a low value of the pituitary hormone TSH (*see* Thyroid). The treatment of the disease may be medical, in which case the anti-thyroid drugs propylthiouracil or carbimazole are used, which block the synthesis of thyroid hormones, with propranolol, a beta-blocker (q.v.). These drugs are used if there is a thyroid crisis or storm during which the condition suddenly becomes worse, sometimes in an infection or after surgery; in some cases there is no obvious precipitating factor. If there is a relapse after medical treatment, or the treatment is ineffective, the secretion of the gland may be cut down by destroying the secreting cells with radioactive iodine; the iodine is concentrated in the thyroid gland, and may be given by mouth. The dose required is not easy to judge, and in some cases a deficiency of thyroid secretion follows, but this can be treated by giving thyroid hormone (thyroxine) by mouth. Operative removal of most of the gland is also possible, and the results are good, but there is an increasing tendency to use radioactive iodine. Apart from Graves' disease, overactive nodules of thyroid tissue may develop in cases of goitre; the treatment is the same.

Tibia: the shin-bone.

Tic: a quick repeated spasmodic movement, usually of the face, neck or shoulder. These movements may begin at about eight years old and become a habit; they can be stopped by an effort of will, and may pass off or become chronic, being increased by anxiety. They may be associated with encephalitis, or develop after an injury. Tic doloreux is trigeminal neuralgia (*see* Neuralgia), and is so called because the lancinating pain makes the sufferer screw up the face.

Tick: a blood-sucking insect larger than a mite; both are *Arachnidae*. Hard ticks are *Ixodidae*, soft ticks *Argasidae*. Some contain a toxin which can cause paralysis, but such cases are rare, occurring in the United States and Australia, mostly in children. Ticks carry several diseases, among them encephalitis, relapsing fever, Lyme disease, typhus, spotted fever, Q fever, and babesiosis which is a protozoan parasitic disease common in wild and domestic animals in tropical and subtropical countries, passed on to man by hard ticks.

Tincture: the alcoholic solution of a drug.

Tinea: a superficial fungus infection of the skin. Tinea pedis is athlete's foot, caused by the organisms *Trichophyton rubrum* and *T. interdigitale*, which produce moist itching lesions commonest between the fourth and fifth toes, and sometimes blisters on the soles of the feet. *T. rubrum* may cause scaly patches on the toes and feet, and attack the nails. Infections of the groin are caused by *T. rubrum* or *Epidermophyton floccosum*, and are more common in males. Tinea corporis is ringworm of the arms, legs or trunk, formed in a ring because the fungus spreads outwards from the central infection. Tinea capitis is ringworm of the scalp, seen mostly in children and caused by *Microsporum canis*, which infects dogs and cats. The simplest treatment for Tinea infections is benzoic acid compound ointment, also called Whitfield's ointment; more modern are the imidazole preparations such as clotrimazole or sulconazole, and the undecenoates and tolnaftate. Chronic infections may require griseofulvin by mouth for a considerable time.

Tinnitus: incessant noise in the ears; it may be buzzing, ringing, hissing or whistling, and is common in older people. It may follow disease of the auditory nerve or the cochlea (*see* Ear), and be associated with deafness. It may be produced by large doses of quinine or salicylates. If it is loud it may be very distressing, but it is difficult to treat; there are devices which produce other noise to mask it which may be found useful.

Tissue: the tissues are the substance of the body; particular tissues such as connective or fatty tissue are collections of cells of the same type specialised in the same way to carry out a particular function. A tissue culture is a collection of cells removed from an organism and set out to grow and multiply in artificial conditions; a tissue bank is a supply of tissues stored for use, for example in grafting.

Tobacco: *see* Smoking.

Tocopherol: vitamin E, a fat-soluble substance mainly found in vegetable oils. It is responsible for maintaining the integrity of membranes, and deficiency, which may affect undernourished infants or those suffering from biliary obstruction, may produce anaemia. Without vitamin E, rats cannot reproduce, but the same has not been shown to be true of human beings.

Tolbutamide: a drug which increases the secretion of insulin, and is used in selected cases of diabetes mellitus. It is given by mouth.

Tomogram: an X-ray taken to show structures lying in a selected plane in the body.

Tomomania: a madness for cutting; unkindly applied to some surgeons.

Tongue: the tongue is made up of a number of muscles contained within its substance, called intrinsic muscles, and a number arising outside it and blending with the intrinsic muscles. They are called extrinsic muscles, and arise mainly from the hyoid bone and the lower jawbone; they move the tongue in relation to neighbouring structures. The intrinsic muscles have fibres running longitudinally, vertically and transversely and are mainly concerned with altering the shape of the tongue. There is a fibrous partition running down the centre of the tongue, and very few blood vessels cross the centre line. In between the muscle fibres are many glands with both mucous and serous secretions which open onto the surface and edges of the tongue, which is covered with stratified squamous epithelium, forming on the surface various sorts of papillae. Under the mucous membrane at the back of the tongue is a collection of lymphatic tissue, the lingual tonsil. The muscles of the tongue are supplied by the twelfth cranial nerve, the hypoglossal, and the sensory nerves are the lingual nerve for the front two-thirds and the glossopharyngeal nerve for the posterior one-third. The artery is the lingual artery, a branch of the external carotid. The tongue is liable to various disorders: glossitis, or inflammation, can result from excessive smoking, habitually taking hot or irritating food or drink, or neglecting septic teeth or gums. Anaemias resulting from iron deficiency, or deficiencies of folate or vitamin B_{12}, may cause glossitis. Small ulcers, called aphthous ulcers, may form on the edge of the tongue which are commonly self-limiting and, but for the discomfort, harmless; but any lasting ulcer of the tongue should call for medical attention, for carcinoma of the tongue is not now thought to be significant; apart from obvious disease, inspection of the tongue is most useful in estimating the degree of dryness in a dehydrated patient.

Tonics: unfortunately no such things exist, in the sense of a medicine designed to brace up the whole system. Anyone feeling unwell is either suffering from a specific disease or is psychologically upset, usually by anxiety or depression. Some have great faith in vitamins, but they are only necessary in those who lack them; normal diets contain more than enough. Anything offered as a general tonic is a placebo.

Tonsils: the tonsils are paired collections of lymphoid tissue that lie on each side of the throat just behind the back of the tongue. They filter organisms from the throat and mouth, manufacture antibodies, and play an important part in the immunological system. They reach their peak of development at about the fifth year. They are frequently infected in children of five or six, and infections continue to be a trouble up to puberty and sometimes beyond. Infections are usually started by viruses, with secondary bacterial infection by a haemolytic streptococcus; the throat is sore, the temperature rises, there is a headache and general malaise and sometimes vomiting. The tonsils can be seen to be enlarged and red. In many cases there is associated infection of the adenoids, collections of lymphoid tissue in the naso-pharynx, and sometimes infection of the middle ear. The lymph nodes in the neck are commonly enlarged and may be painful. The treatment is penicillin or erythromycin. There may be repeated attacks of tonsillitis, but these usually disappear by the time of puberty. The indications for removal of the tonsils are: enlargement of the tonsils to such an extent that they interfere with breathing, more than four attacks of tonsillitis in a year sufficiently severe to interfere with schooling, abscess formation behind the tonsils (quinsy), and repeated attacks of tonsillitis with middle-ear infection. The operation of tonsillectomy may be combined with removal of the adenoids. It should be noted that infective mononucleosis in young adults produces an appearance of the tonsils that resembles severe tonsillitis, and the unwary administration of ampicillin will produce a rash in such cases.

Tophus: a deposit of monosodium urate crystals which collects in gout, and forms swellings in the joints and tendons. Gouty tophi may be seen under the skin of the ear and over the finger joints.

Torticollis (wryneck): a condition that may develop in middle age or later, in which spasm of the sternomastoid muscle causes the head to turn to one side; the muscle runs from the mastoid process of the skull behind the ear to the inner end of the collar-bone and the top of the breastbone. Spasm of other neck muscles may draw the head back, or forwards. The cause is not known; treatment is difficult, but diazepam may help, and the patient may find some trick to relax the spasm, such as touching the jaw. A rare inherited disease, dystonia musculorum deformans, may produce torticollis as part of a more generalised spasm of the muscles, which may include writer's cramp. Occasionally a birth injury damages the sternomastoid muscle, when a hard lump appears in the side of the neck and the head is turned to one side; if the injury produces a scar which contracts, it may have to be divided surgically.

Total Allergy Syndrome: a condition in which it is supposed that patients react to so many substances that they have to live in a special environment, eat special food, and in all respects be protected from any possible factors which may precipitate an allergic reaction. It is, to say the least, extremely doubtful if any such condition exists.

Tourniquet: a band which can be tightened round a limb to compress the arteries and veins. The purpose may be to stop arterial bleeding from a wound, to prevent the spread of venom from a snakebite or to provide the surgeon with a bloodless field. The blood supply to a limb must not be cut off for more than 30 minutes; the tourniquet must be loosened for 20 seconds every half-hour, and never left on for more than two hours. If a tourniquet is applied, everyone to do with the case must be warned, and if possible a T should be marked on the patient's forehead with the time the tourniquet was first put on. A tourniquet should not be applied to a bleeding limb unless it is impossible to control the bleeding by direct pressure.

Toxaemia: the presence of bacterial toxins in the blood. Toxaemia of pregnancy is a different condition, and is now called eclampsia (q.v.).

Toxicara: *Toxicara canis* is a worm that lives in the intestines of dogs and foxes. A pregnant bitch can infect her puppies before they are born, as the larvae can cross the placenta, and the puppies can carry adult worms as early as three weeks after birth. The eggs are passed in the excreta, and if humans eat contaminated food the larvae travel through the lungs and liver but normally do no harm and die in about a year. Occasionally however they reach the eye, where they can set up a granulomatous inflammation and affect the retina, causing a squint and loss of vision. The condition is found in children about six years old. In very young children who have ingested a large number of eggs the larvae may travel widely in the viscera and set up serious illness, but in such cases the eyes are not touched. It is sensible to keep puppies well wormed, and to be careful in dealing with their excreta.

Toxicology: the study of poisons and their actions.

Toxin: a poison; usually applied to those elaborated by bacteria or animals.

Toxoid: a bacterial toxin so modified that it has lost its poisonous properties, but can still act as an antigen to provoke the formation of antibodies; tetanus toxoid is, for example, used by injection to induce immunity to tetanus, but it does not produce symptoms of the disease.

Toxoplasmosis: infection with the protozoan parasite *Toxoplasma gondii*. This exists in three forms: the trophozoite, the tissue cyst and the oocyst; trophozoites are found in many animals including birds and mice, in which they multiply and form tissue cysts. If an infected creature is eaten by a cat, sexual forms of the parasite develop in the cat's intestine and produce eggs, oocysts, which are passed in the cat's excreta and may then form spores, which persist in the soil for months and are infectious. The cat is the definitive host of the parasite, and from the oocysts in the soil many animals and birds become infected. Human beings may become infected from cats or by eating meat containing tissue cysts which has been badly cooked; the disease is common in sheep. By the age of 70 about half the population of the United Kingdom have developed a positive serological test for toxoplasmosis, showing that they have been infected; in France the figure is much greater, about three-quarters of the population being infected before the age of 20. In the vast majority of cases the infection does no harm and passes unrecognised, but in some there may be enlargement of the lymph nodes and rarely a rash, with general malaise which may last weeks; the disease resembles infectious mononucleosis. It usually resolves without trouble, but it may infect those suffering from immunosuppressive disorders such as AIDS or those who are taking immunosuppressive drugs, when the disease may affect the brain and produce encephalitis. Most importantly, however, mothers who become infected during pregnancy may pass the infection on to the child. This may result in miscarriage, or the child may be born with abnormalities of the central nervous system which are apparent at birth or become apparent later, perhaps after several years. The disease may affect the eye, giving rise to inflammation of the posterior part, in particular the retina. In some cases this does no harm, but in some, discovered usually between 10 and 20, it affects the vision. The treatment of primary infection in mother and newborn baby is a combination of pyrimethamine and sulphadiazine to which is added folinic acid, alternated with spiramycin every three to five weeks. Pregnant women who have not developed a positive serological test for the disease, and about 20% have before the age of 20, should be careful to avoid raw or undercooked meat, and be very careful how they handle cats and their litter trays.

Trachea: the windpipe, which runs from the larynx, the Adam's apple, downwards and somewhat backwards from the lower neck, into the upper mediastinum in the thorax to divide into right and left main bronchi at the level of the fifth thoracic vertebra. Its wall contains between 16 and 20 rings of cartilage, open backwards; the rear wall is of smooth muscle. The rings are joined by fibro-elastic tissue, for the trachea has to conform to the movements of the neck and breathing. It is lined by mucous membrane which has cilia, hairlike processes which move the secretions upwards towards the larynx. The oesophagus lies behind the trachea.

Tracheitis: inflammation of the trachea, usually associated with inflammation of the larynx. The infection is by a virus of the influenza or para-influenza groups, and there is a burning pain behind the breastbone on breathing, and hoarseness. In children there may be croup (q.v.). There is no specific treatment, but inhalation of steam and the use of a steam kettle in the room to provide humidified air helps diminish the discomfort. Tracheo-laryngitis is often part of a general respiratory infection which includes bronchitis.

Tracheotomy: the operation of cutting an opening into the trachea. The operation is carried out by making an incision in the midline of the neck below the larynx, and opening the trachea between the third and fourth cartilaginous rings; an oval piece may be cut out, and a tube passed into the opening. The opening into the trachea is called a tracheostomy, and it can be temporary or permanent. Although the obvious reason for making a tracheostomy is obstruction to the airway in the larynx, there are other indications for the operation, among them deep unconsciousness after a head injury, for it decreases the dead space, that is the space in the mouth and upper airway through which the air merely goes in and out without reaching the lungs, it enables secretions to be sucked out and provides a wide unobstructed airway, and it makes it possible for the patient to be connected to a positive pressure breathing machine. The hole in the trachea heals up quite quickly when it is no longer required.

Trachoma: infection of the eye by the micro-organism *Chlamydia trachomatis*, which causes conjunctivitis, with the formation of follicles and ultimate scarring. The infection may involve the white of the eye and the cornea, and lead to scarring of the cornea and blindness. The disease is common in South and Central America, Asia, Africa and the Middle East, and it is associated with poverty and the resulting overcrowding and insanitary conditions. Babies and young children are the worst affected. It is thought that between five and ten million people are blind because of trachoma. The treatment of the disease is with tetracycline, erythromycin or rifampicin ointment applied to the eyelids for some weeks, or tetracycline or erythromycin given by mouth. *Chlamydia trachomatis* may also cause non-specific urethritis in men and pelvic inflammation in women, being passed on sexually, and it is possible for newborn infants to develop an eye infection from an infected mother. This type of chlamydial infection is increasing in this country and the USA, and cases have been found of conjunctivitis and trachoma caused by infection transferred from the genitals to the eyes in adults.

Tranquillisers: a group of drugs used to sedate mentally disturbed patients. They have been divided into two classes, the major and minor tranquillisers, the major drugs being used to treat frankly psychotic states and the minor used in severe anxiety and as aids to sleep. The classes are better described as anti-psychotic, anxiolytic and hypnotic drugs. The anxiolytics and hypnotics are mostly derived from diazepine and vary in the duration and speed of their effect. They have in the past been greatly over-prescribed; although they are not as dangerous as the barbiturates which they replaced, they can lead to dependence and when they are discontinued to withdrawal symptoms which include anxiety and insomnia. These effects are similar to those for which the drugs were originally prescribed, and so lead to further prescribing. In cases where the drugs have been used for a long time in large doses, withdrawal symptoms may be very disturbing, and include confusion, delirium and convulsions. The drugs therefore have to be stopped very gradually and carefully. It is now recommended that the drugs should only be used for severe anxiety, and only be given for less than a month; if used for insomnia, they should only be given in cases where the patient is very distressed or disabled. The use of the major tranquillisers, the anti-psychotic drugs, is of course in a different category.

Transfusion: *see* Blood Groups.

Transient Global Amnesia: in this condition the patient suffers a temporary loss of memory, lasting for a few hours, during which there is no loss of consciousness and activity is normal; patients continue to mow the lawn or even drive. It is possibly due to temporary disturbance of the blood supply to the brain from the vertebral arteries. Recovery is complete except for memory of what passed during the attack. *See* Amnesia.

Transient Ischaemic Attack: the patient suddenly suffers weakness in the face, arm or leg, and numbness in the affected part with a disturbance of speech if the attack affects the dominant hemisphere. There may be double vision, disturbance of vision, giddiness, nausea and vomiting, but usually no loss of consciousness. The symptoms often start to clear up within minutes, and certainly improve within 24 hours. There may be repeated attacks. The condition is due to small clots breaking away from atherosclerotic patches in the carotid or vertebral arteries that supply the brain; in some cases the clots originate in the heart. The arteries in the brain are blocked and the nervous tissue supplied loses its function until the blood supply returns, probably through collateral or alternative arteries. The condition is the same as a minor stroke, but in a stroke there is no return of function. Transient ischaemic attacks may herald the future occurrence of a stroke. *See* Apoplexy.

Transplant Surgery: the first kidney grafts were carried out in Boston in 1955, with partial success; it was not until three years later that grafts carried out between identical twins were completely successful. It was clear that the immune reaction would reject tissue that was not identical, and after much research it was found that a combination of corticosteroids and the synthetic drug azathioprine suppressed the reaction so that grafts that were not of identical tissue would survive, although the best results were obtained with grafts taken from parents or brothers and sisters. Work on kidney grafting was helped by the fact that patients with unsuccessful grafts could be treated by the artificial kidney, so that an unsuccessful graft was not fatal. It was then found that liver transplants were less liable to rejection than kidney grafts, but heart transplants more liable, and the penalty for failure was greater because there was no artificial substitute for either; but advances in immunosuppressive drugs such as cyclosporin A led to more successful operations. The chief obstacles to organ transplantation are the drawbacks to immunosuppressive drugs, and the shortage of donors. Immunosuppressive drugs not only lower resistance to infection, but may have serious unwanted effects: azathioprine can damage the liver and bone marrow and decrease the number of white cells and platelets in the blood, and cyclosporin can damage the kidneys and cause high blood pressure. Immunosuppressive drugs will no doubt be continually improved, but the supply of donors rests with the public at large and their attitude to the removal and use of suitable organs from the dying or recently dead. If suitable organs are offered, the survival time of a kidney packed in ice is 48 hours, 10 hours for the liver and 4 hours for a heart, so that the removal of organs and subsequent operations must be carefully timed. Experiments have shown that it is possible for any organ in the body to be transplanted except the central nervous system, which will not regenerate.

Transudate: fluid which has passed through a membrane, or been exuded from tissue.

Transvestism: an unnatural wish to wear the clothes of the opposite sex; usually men wishing to wear women's clothes.

Trauma: an injury or wound.

Traveller's Diarrhoea: a term applied to the short attacks of diarrhoea which afflict many people when they first arrive in a warm country. Most cases are due to a type of *Escherichia coli* which produces a toxin which affects the bowel. The disease is short; it lasts for one or two days, and the bacteria are often resistant to antibiotics, so that rational treatment is confined to drinking plenty of water. Codeine phosphate or loperamide may be useful in relieving the diarrhoea. In more severe cases where salt may have been lost half a teaspoon of salt and six teaspoons of sugar may be added to a litre of drinking water. If antibiotics are needed, trimethoprim or ciprofloxacin are useful. In cases where prophylaxis is absolutely essential these drugs may be used, but there is a risk of inducing bacterial resistance to them.

Travel Sickness: *see* Motion Sickness.

Trematodes: flukes (q.v.). Also *see* Worms.

Tremor: shaking, which may be fine, and shown in the outstretched fingers as in hyperthyroidism, or coarse, involving the whole limb, as in Parkinson's disease. It may only appear when the patient is reaching out for something, when it is called an intention tremor, or it may disappear on purposeful movement and be present only at rest. The first happens in cerebellar or brain stem disease, the second is typical of Parkinsonism. A fine tremor can be seen in anxiety states, or may be the result of taking certain drugs, for example salbutamol used in asthma; it may occur in chronic alcoholism and in old age; occasionally such a tremor may be present in health, for it is inherent in the mechanism for maintaining posture.

Trendelenburg Operation and Position: Freidrich Trendelenburg was a German surgeon (1844–1925) who gave his name to an operation for varicose veins and to a position on the operating table, with the body sloping downwards and backwards at between 30 to 40 degrees and the knees bent and hanging down at about the same angle.

Trephine: a surgical instrument for removing a disc of bone, usually from the skull. The trepan was a cylindrical saw for the same purpose.

Treponema: a genus of spirochaetes, micro-organisms formed like a very thin coiled thread that can bend and spin on its long axis. *Treponema pertenue* causes yaws, *Treponema pallidum* syphilis and *Treponema carateum* pinta. The organisms are easily killed by antiseptics, heat, or exposure to the oxygen of the atmosphere, and are sensitive to penicillin.

Trichinosis: an infection with the worm *Trichinella spiralis*, which infects pigs and is acquired by eating undercooked pork. Most infections pass unnoticed, but some may cause diarrhoea, followed by fever, pains in the muscles and swelling of the face due to a sensitivity reaction. In most cases a full recovery ensues, but rarely the lungs, heart and central nervous system become involved. The treatment is with thiabendazole or mebendazole.

Trichomonas: *Trichomonas vaginalis* is a protozoan parasite which causes inflammation of the vagina in women and urethritis in men. It is commonly passed on in sexual intercourse, but as it can survive outside the body in moisture it is about the only organism affecting the genito-urinary system which can genuinely be picked up from a lavatory seat. The organism is sensitive to metronidazole, administered by mouth or in pessaries, or nimorazole which can be given by mouth as a a single dose. Both these drugs cause a reaction to alcohol, which should therefore be avoided during treatment.

Trichuris: the whipworm, a small roundworm. *See* Worms.

Tricyclic Antidepressants: a class of antidepressant drugs used in the more serious cases of depression. They include amitryptiline, which has a considerable sedative action, and imipramine, which has less. There are a number of drugs in this class, one of which may be selected to suit the needs of the individual patient. Amitryptiline is often used in small doses to treat nocturnal enuresis in children over seven years old.

Trigeminal Nerve: the fifth cranial nerve, the sensory nerve of the face. It has three divisions, the ophthalmic, maxillary and mandibular, or first, second and third. It also has a motor branch which supplies the muscles used in chewing.

Trigeminal Neuralgia: *see* Neuralgia.

Triorthocresyl Phosphate: used in industry as a high temperature lubricant and anti-corrosion agent: if it is taken internally it can cause irreversible damage to the nervous system. It has been found as a contaminant in cooking oil and in illegally distilled alcohol.

Trismus: a spasm of the muscles which move the jaw – lockjaw.

Trisomy: an abnormality of the chromosomes in which an extra one is present, added to one of the normal 23 pairs. Trisomy 21 is Down's syndrome (q.v.).

Trocar: a sharp instrument used for piercing a body cavity, used with a cannula which is a shorter hollow tube fitting over the trocar so that the sharp end protrudes. When the trocar and cannula have been introduced, for example through the skin of the scrotum into a hydrocoele (q.v.), the trocar is withdrawn and the fluid allowed to escape through the cannula.

Trophoblast: when the fertilized ovum begins to divide it forms a collection of cells called the morula. This acquires a central cavity, and the outer layer of cells is the trophoblast, which is responsible for implanting the ovum into the uterine endometrium. From the trophoblast develops the embryonic side of the placenta. It has recently become possible to remove a fragment of trophoblastic tissue at about the tenth week of pregnancy for examination of the cells' genetic make-up and the diagnosis of hereditary disease.

Tropical Sore: a slow-healing ulcer in the skin caused by *Leishmania major* or *Leishmania tropica. See* Leishmaniasis.

Truss: a device to keep hernias of the abdominal wall under control and prevent them from protruding. If possible, an operation for the repair of the hernia is in every way preferable to wearing a truss.

Trypanosomiasis: *Trypanosoma brucei gambiense* causes sleeping sickness in West Africa, and *Trypanosoma brucei rhodesiense* causes the disease in East Africa. Trypanosomes are small parasites spread by the tsetse fly. In West Africa the disease is almost confined to human beings, and the flies responsible for carrying the organisms live by rivers; but in East Africa the disease predominantly affects game, and the flies live in the open bush. In the West African disease, about three weeks after a bite from a tsetse fly a small swelling appears, which may ulcerate. Several weeks or even months afterwards the patient begins to feel ill and develops a fever, with enlargement of the lymph nodes of the neck. The fever may show periods of recovery and then relapses. Months or years after, signs of involvement of the central nervous system appear with increased sleepiness, personality changes, and eventually abnormal movements and convulsions. The patients waste and become stuprose.

In East Africa the symptoms are much the same, but they develop more quickly and the heart is involved earlier than the central nervous system. Treatment of the disease is with suramin or melarsoprol, but the drugs are not without their own dangers.

In South America *Trypanosoma cruzi* is responsible for Chagas' disease. Carlos Chagas (1879–1934), a Brazilian physician, discovered the organism and described the disease, which is spread by reduviid bugs; once they have bitten an infected individual they stay infective for life, passing on the infection in their droppings. A swelling may develop at the site of an infected bite, followed by enlargement of the lymph nodes and possibly the liver and spleen; rarely the heart is involved at this stage, or there may be encephalitis. Many years after infection the patient becomes ill with heart disease; there may be enlargement of the oesophagus or colon, presumably because the parasympathetic nervous system is damaged. Drugs that have been used in the acute stage of the disease are benzidazole and nifurtimox; in the later stages the heart conditions are treated as required, and if necessary the megaoesophagus and megacolon may be treated surgically. It has been suggested that Charles Darwin suffered from this disease, acquired in South America; he certainly suffered from unexplained ill health in his later years.

Tsetse Fly: *see* Trypanosomiasis *above*.

Tubal Pregnancy: *see* Ectopic Gestation.

Tuberculosis: a disease caused by infection with the

micro-organisms *Mycobacterium tuberculosis* or *Mycobacterium bovis*, of which the first is responsible for most human infections. The bacillus provokes the formation of tubercles, collections of macrophages, which are white blood cells and tissue cells able to engulf bacteria and form epithelioid cells; these may fuse to form giant cells, which are characteristic of the tubercle. The macrophages are activated by T lymphocytes (q.v.), by the invading organisms and by the activity of other macrophages. When the tubercle has formed, the centre breaks down, a process called caseation. The disease process destroys the tissues which it involves, which are principally those of the lung, for the disease is acquired by breathing in the infecting organism.

Tuberculosis is a very ancient disease, primarily one of poor nutrition and overcrowding. Until recently, most people were infected with the bacillus, but overcame the infection without falling ill, and developed a positive immunological reaction. This, or a healed lesion in the lung which left a scar visible on X-rays, was the only evidence of infection in the majority of cases. This has changed in Europe and North America, and now infection is not common, although it has remained so in the developing countries. Infection is spread by bacilli coughed out by those suffering from tuberculosis of the lungs; it can also be caught by drinking raw milk from infected cows, when the disease does not necessarily affect the lungs, but the adoption of pasteurised milk and the eradication of the disease from cattle has made bovine tuberculosis rare.

Primary tuberculous infection is usually found by X-ray examination of contacts of those suffering from known pulmonary tuberculosis. The developed disease, known as postprimary tuberculosis, shows itself by a cough, perhaps with blood in the sputum, pain in the chest, or pneumonia which does not respond to antibiotics. Some cases are found on investigation of unexplained illness. The diagnosis is made on the chest X-ray and the discovery of the tubercle bacillus in the sputum. The disease may be complicated by the development of a pleural effusion, or in severe cases a tuberculous abscess in the chest, an empyema. The lymph nodes in the mediastinum may become enlarged, but involvement of the lymph nodes elsewhere, once common in the United Kingdom, is now seen principally in those from Asia and Africa. Infection of the lymph nodes of the neck was formerly usually caused by bovine tuberculosis, but now *Mycobacterium tuberculosis* is found. Severe infections may produce miliary tuberculosis, which is a blood-borne dissemination of the disease to all parts of the body; or the disease may affect the meninges, causing tuberculous meningitis, the kidneys and urinary tract, the bones and joints, the spine, the abdomen, and the membrane enclosing the heart, the pericardium. Such cases are now seen for the most part in the developing countries.

The treatment of tuberculosis was revolutionised by the discovery of streptomycin, and the subsequent development of PAS, para-aminosalicylic acid, rifampicin and isoniazid, now the chief drug used in combination with rifampicin. Ethambutol and pyrazinamide are also used in combination with these drugs; in many countries isoniazid is used with thiacetazone. In Britain, tuberculin tests, the Mantoux and Heaf tests, are done on children between 11 and 13 years old, which show strong positive reactions if active tuberculous infection is present so that investigation and if necessary treatment can be carried out; immunisation with BCG vaccine, made from an attenuated strain of *Mycobacterium bovis*, is carried out on the children with a negative tuberculin test.

Tularaemia: a rare disease in human beings caused by the bacillus *Francisella tularensis*, named after Tulare in California where the disease was first identified. It occurs principally in rodents but may affect other animals, and is spread to man by ticks, flies and mosquitoes, or by touching infected animals. The condition has been found in Scandinavia, Russia and Japan, and manifests itself by a fever with headache and pains in the muscles. Ulcerating papules may develop, often on the hands or where a bite occurred, with enlargement of the neighbouring lymph nodes. The patient may develop tonsillitis, pneumonia, or abdominal pain with diarrhoea. The organism is sensitive to streptomycin and gentamycin.

Tulle Gras: a net of pliant material impregnated with soft paraffin which may be mixed with ointment containing an antiseptic or antibiotic; it is used for dressing raw surfaces such as burns or ulcers.

Tumour: any swelling; usually used to mean a growth, benign or malignant.

Twilight Sleep: the induction of a state of partial anaesthesia and analgesia by giving scopolamine and morphine. The technique was formerly used during childbirth.

Tympanic Membrane: the ear-drum. *See* Ear.

Typhlitis: inflammation of the caecum.

Typhoid Fever: a serious disease caused by *Salmonella typhi*, found throughout the world but commonest where sanitation and water supplies are less than first class. The infection is spread by contamination of food or water by the excreta of patients suffering or recovering from the disease, or of those carrying the disease but apparently in good health. It is confined to human beings. The incubation period is from one to three weeks. Patients complain first of headache and feeling ill, and then may develop a cough and abdominal discomfort. In some cases diarrhoea follows, with blood in the motions, and a rash may develop on the upper part of the abdomen and the lower chest. The appearance of the rash is described as rose-spots. The diagnosis may not be easy, but may become clear if the patient gives a history of having been in a place where typhoid is known to occur; culture of the stool and urine, and a blood culture, will usually confirm the disease. If not treated, typhoid lasts about a month, but complications may occur which include haemorrhage from the intestines, perforation of the bowel, pneumonia, jaundice, kidney failure and mental confusion or dullness. Treatment is with amoxycillin, chloramphenicol or ciprofloxacin, but convalescent patients may continue to excrete *Salmonella typhi* and cannot be declared free of the possibility of spreading infection until three negative cultures have been made of the urine and stools.

It is possible for people to carry the organisms for years without knowing that they have had the disease. They excrete *S. typhi* intermittently, usually having a focus of chronic infection in the gall-bladder, and if this is so the gall-bladder may be removed. A vaccine is available for travellers to places where typhoid is known to be common, and it is given in two injections four to six weeks apart, with booster doses every three years if necessary. It is no substitute for care in avoiding uncooked vegetables or fruit that cannot be peeled, and making sure that the water is safe or has been boiled.

Typhus (jail fever): an infection caused by *Rickettsia prowazekii* and spread by lice. The organism persists in man after the fever has resolved, and the excreta of infected lice lie in the dust and remain infective for a long time. It is a disease of dirt, overcrowding and poor personal hygiene, and is now found only in a few countries, but was once a great scourge. The incubation period is about a week; the patient suffers from a severe headache and fever, and develops a rash at first on the trunk, then spreading outwards, which may become confluent, break down and ulcerate. There is confusion, and possibly convulsions, stupor and coma follow. The circulation fails. Left untreated, half the patients die. The treatment is with tetracyclines and chloramphenicol. *See* Rickettsiae.

Tyrosine: an important amino-acid which is part of most proteins, and is essential for life.

U

Ulcer: a chronic defect in the epithelial surface of the skin or a mucous membrane, exposing the tissues that lie below. Ulcers are formed by the interaction of a number of factors which include a poor blood supply, inefficient drainage of the tissues, infection by micro-organisms, injury by physical agents such as cold, heat, chemicals, pressure or irradiation, malignant growths, and disease of the nervous system which, by abolishing the sense of pain, makes the skin the site of repeated minor injury. Examples of such ulceration are: varicose ulcers occurring with varicose veins, which are caused by a poor blood supply, inefficient drainage leading to waterlogging of the tissues, and minor injury; rodent ulcer of the skin, caused by a basal-cell carcinoma; syphilitic ulcer caused by infection with *Treponema pallidum*; ulcers of the feet in diabetes, caused by a poor blood supply and the numbness of neuropathy; and bedsores caused by a poor blood supply and poor tissue drainage consequent on continuous pressure, often with superadded infection. The precise reasons leading to the development of peptic ulcers are not understood, but if any imperfections in the mucous membrane lining the stomach and duodenum are continually subjected to the action of acid and the digestive juices ulceration might be expected to follow. The treatment of ulcers depends on removal of the cause: malignant ulcers are excised or irradiated, infective ulcers treated with appropriate antibiotics. Those, like varicose ulcers, that are mainly caused by poor tissue drainage aggravated by the action of gravity are treated by rest and the elevation of the affected leg, or bandaging to endeavour to decrease the accumulation of tissue fluid. Any dead tissue must be removed from an ulcer and if the epithelium will not grow over it skin grafting may be necessary. In the treatment of peptic ulcers anti-acids are used, with drugs that decrease the secretion of acid.

Ulcerative Colitis: a disease of the colon and rectum in which there is inflammation of the large bowel, possibly with ulceration. The cause of the disease is not known, although there are a number of theories ranging from infection through allergy to auto-immune reaction. It is most frequent in the Western world, although known elsewhere. The disease can start at any age but is most common among young adults; there is an attack of bloody diarrhoea, which may be mild or severe. Subsequently attacks recur at varying intervals; in rare cases the diarrhoea does not cease but becomes chronic. In consequence of the blood loss the patient may become anaemic, and in severe attacks the patient loses appetite and weight and feels ill. It was once thought that the disease had a psychosomatic basis because emotional upsets can bring on an attack, but there is no real evidence for this, and the experience of having this disease is quite enough to produce depression and emotional disturbance. There may be complications: severe bleeding can take place, and rarely perforation of the gut; in a severe attack acute dilatation of the colon may occur, with abdominal pain and distension, and collapse. Skin rashes may be associated with the disease, and a form of conjunctivitis, ulcers in the mouth, and arthritis. The diagnosis is confirmed by examination of the large bowel by endoscopy. Treatment is with corticosteroids and the drug sulphasalazine by mouth, combined with local corticosteroids in a retention enema. More severe cases need hospital admission, for intravenous therapy may be needed; perforations of the colon, or the complication of acute dilatation, need surgical treatment, which usually consists of removal of the colon and the provision of an ileostomy, an artificial opening of the end of the small intestine made through the abdominal wall. Such an operation may be needed in chronic cases, or those where there have been frequent severe attacks. It may be recommended in some cases that have lasted for more than ten years in whom it is thought that there is an increased risk of developing a malignant growth of the colon. Patients with an ileostomy can lead perfectly normal lives. It has, however, recently been found possible with an improved operation to remove the colon but preserve the rectum after its lining has been removed; the continuity of the bowel can be restored, making an ileostomy unnecessary.

Ulna: the inner of the two bones of the forearm. Its upper end makes the elbow joint with the humerus, the bone of the upper arm.

Ultrasonics: sound waves which are of a frequency above the range of audible sound, which lies between 20 and 20,000 cycles per second. Sound waves generated in the range of 1–10 million waves per second are reflected to a greater or lesser degree by changes in density of the substances through which they are passed, the degree of reflection depending on the change in density. This fact was first applied in naval work on SONAR, an acronym for Sound Navigation and Ranging, in the First World War, but it was not until after the Second World War that it began to be possible for it to be used in medicine. An apparatus was designed to emit the sound vibrations through the body and pick up the echoes, which were displayed on a cathode ray screen. The technique was developed until the strength of the returning echoes was reflected in the brightness of the image on the screen, and automatic scanners as well as hand-held scanners came into use. The Doppler effect was used to detect movement.

The effect of ultrasonic sound waves on the tissues depends on the power with which it is generated; high power ultrasound destroys tissues, but lower strengths may help healing of injuries and ulcers, possibly by warming the tissues. High-powered ultrasonic waves can be applied by small instruments to fragment the structures to which they are applied, a technique used to fragment kidney stones. Only very low-powered waves are used in diagnostic ultrasound, and they do not harm the tissues through which they pass. This means that ultrasonic examination is particularly useful in obstetrics, and examination of the developing foetus is widely used to detect any abnormalities in about the fourth month of pregnancy; the examination also shows the presence of twins and the position of the placenta. Ultrasound is used in the investigation of many parts of the body, including the heart, the liver and the kidneys, but is not so useful in examining the lungs, which are full of air, or the intestines. Interpretation of the results depends a great deal on the skill of the operator.

Ultraviolet Light: electromagnetic waves shorter than those visible to the eye but longer than X-rays; the radiation is emitted by the sun, but absorbed by the ozone and water vapour of the atmosphere. The radiation reaching earth is described as falling into three ranges: UVA, of 320–400 nanometres, UVB of 290–320 nm, and UVC of 200–290 nm. UVC can affect the skin at high altitudes, UVB is the most penetrating and is liable to produce sunburn, and UVA can affect the skin if it is sensitised by certain drugs or substances. Overexposure to the sun produces sunburn after about six hours, but screening lotions and creams are available (*see* Sunburn); chronic exposure damages the skin, making it less elastic and sometimes leading to scaling; after long exposure skin cancers, basal cell carcinomas or squamous epitheliomas may develop, but these can be cured by removal or irradiation and are most unlikely to give rise to secondary spread. Melanomas are also encouraged to develop by exposure to ultraviolet light; these do give rise to secondary deposits. They commonly arise in previously existing moles, and if one starts to grow, bleed or change in any way medical advice is needed. Natural sunlight is beneficial to the skin disease psoriasis, and artificial UVB and UVA may be used in treatment. Acting on the skin, ultraviolet light promotes the formation of vitamin D.

Umbilicus: the navel.

Unconsciousness: in all cases of unconsciousness it is of the first importance that the airway should be kept clear. In victims of accidents it is possible for the airway to be blocked by a swallowed tongue, but this can be felt by a finger in the mouth and the tongue hooked forward; if the subject can be moved, the best position is on the side or on the front with the head turned to the side so that secretions or vomit fall out of the mouth and are not inhaled; the tongue can be kept forward and the airway clear, if the patient cannot be moved, by putting the fingers behind the angle of the jaw below the ear and pulling the jaw forwards. If an unconscious person appears to be choking, a finger should be passed down the throat to see if there is an obstruction that can be removed; if this is not possible, the victim should be put face downwards, and with the arms round the chest a quick powerful squeeze may dislodge the obstruction. If an unconscious person has to be moved after an accident they should be moved in the position in which they were lying, for it is possible to make injuries worse by altering the position; it is always best to leave an injured person where they lie until skilled help arrives, once the airway has been assured. It is dangerous to try to make a semiconscious or unconscious person drink anything, especially spirits. If the unconsciousness is not the result of accident, it is worth looking through the pockets or handbag in case the person is diabetic, when there will often be a card or some sugar. Epilepsy is usually obvious, and a major fit is more frightening and dramatic than dangerous; all that is required is to make sure that the epileptic cannot be injured by the surroundings, and is not choking. In all cases efforts must principally be directed at making sure the airway is clear, and keeping the patient still and reasonably warm.

Undecenoic Acid: used, with undecenoates, in the treatment of fungus infection of the skin. *See* Tinea.

Undine: small specially shaped glass flask used for irrigating the eye.

Undulant Fever: *see* Brucellosis.

Upper Respiratory Tract: includes the nose, mouth and throat as far down as the trachea.

Uraemia (azotaemia): excess of urea and other nitrogen-containing compounds, principally creatinine, in the blood. The condition is the result of kidney failure, except in cases where there is failure of the circulation from any cause, when the state is described as pre-renal uraemia; such cases may recover when the circulatory collapse is remedied. The uraemic patient suffers from headache, may be anaemic, loses appetite and is dyspeptic; in some cases there may be bleeding from the nose, the stomach or the intestines. There may be drowsiness or fits, and uncontrollable hiccuping; if untreated the patient sinks into a coma. The symptoms may be insidious or acute, according to the cause of renal failure; the treatment is that of the disease responsible for the renal failure, and of the renal failure itself. The normal value for blood urea is 2.5–6.7 mmol/l (15–40 mg/100 ml).

Urates: salts of uric acid, the result of the breakdown of purines, which are compounds which play a very important part in metabolism. Urates are normally present in the blood, but when the blood level is too high crystals may form; in the joints they give rise to gout, and in the kidneys to stones. The normal blood level of uric acid in men is 210–480 μmol/l (3.5–8 mg/100 ml). It is a little lower in women.

Ureter: the muscular tube that connects the kidney to the bladder.

Urethra: the tube that connects the bladder to the exterior through which urine is discharged from the body. It is subject to inflammation in gonorrhoea and non-specific urethritis (q.v.), and may conduct micro-organisms such as *Escherichia coli* from their normal habitat on the perineum into the bladder to set up infection there. This is much more likely to happen in women, for the female urethra is only about 4 cm long while the male urethra is about 20 cm long. The male urethra, however, passes through the prostate gland, and when this is enlarged, as may happen in later life, the urethra may be blocked. The male urethra is also liable to injury, with the possible formation of obstructive strictures, and it is more difficult to pass instruments such as catheters and cystoscopes into the bladder in the male than the female.

Urethritis: inflammation of the urethra.

Uric Acid: *see* Urates.

Urine: the fluid excreted by the kidneys, passed down the ureters into the bladder, where it is stored, and discharged to the exterior through the urethra. In health it is of constant composition within well-defined limits, being about 96% water and containing the waste products of the metabolism of muscles, proteins and nucleic acid and the breakdown products of hormones. The examination and analysis of urine is an invaluable aid to the diagnosis of illness. Specimens can be tested easily for the presence of protein, blood and sugar, of which there should be none, and for the pH, the acid–base reaction: it is normally slightly acid. The appearance is important, for it may be discoloured in frank bleeding from the urinary tract or in the abnormal excretion of bile pigments. In the laboratory the urine can be centrifuged and the sediment examined under the microscope; it can be cultured to detect the presence and identity of infecting organisms, and many chemical analyses can be carried out. The early presence of a pregnancy can be detected. The amount of urine excreted in 24 hours is between one and two litres, but it of course depends on various factors such as the amount of drink taken and the weather. If normal urine is allowed to stand, it may become cloudy with the precipitation of phosphates; this is of no significance, and disappears on boiling.

Urology: the branch of medicine that deals with diseases of the urinary tract in both sexes, and those of the genital organs in the male.

Urticaria (nettle-rash): swelling and redness of the skin, usually with itching; the swellings may disappear, only to reappear in another place. They may affect the face or the whole body. The cause is often an allergic reaction which results in the liberation of histamine in the skin; direct contact with some substances has the same effect, for example the swelling caused by contact with stinging nettles or jelly fish; some insect bites cause urticaria. Reactions to various drugs or foods, for example aspirin, penicillin, strawberries or shellfish can result in widespread urticaria; but in some cases no reason can be found, and while urticaria normally disappears in a short time, such cases can be chronic. The treatment is by antihistamines such as terfenadine or astemizole by mouth, and obviously avoidance of the precipitating factor, if it can be identified.

Application of antihistamine creams to the skin is not useful. Severe cases may call for the injection of adrenaline.

Uterus (the womb): a hollow pear-shaped organ about 7 cm long, 5 cm in breadth and 2–3 cm thick; the muscle of the wall is about 1 cm thick. It is divided into cervix or neck, body, and fundus. The cervix is traversed by a canal which communicates with the vagina at the external os and the body of the uterus at the internal os. The body of the uterus is flattened, so that the cavity is a slit when seen from the side; when seen from in front it is a triangle with the apex at the internal os and the angles at the cornua, where the cavity communicates with the Fallopian tubes at each side. The Fallopian tubes extend out towards the ovaries. The part of the uterus lying above the level of the opening of the tubes is the fundus. The cervix projects into the upper part of the front wall of the vagina, and is flexed slightly forwards. The uterus lies normally almost vertically behind the bladder, being inclined slightly forwards, and the outside is covered by peritoneum. From each side the broad ligament reaches out to the side wall of the pelvis. The uterus may be inclined more forward than usual (anteverted), or be inclined backwards (retroverted), but these positions are not of consequence. For a description of the tissue lining the uterus and its function *see* Menstruation. The uterus is supported in position by the muscles of the pelvic floor. In pregnancy the size of the organ increases enormously, and the muscles become lax, so that in the years following childbirth the uterus may become displaced downwards, undergoing a prolapse, and control of the bladder may be difficult (stress incontinence). These troubles may be greatly helped by operations designed to support the front wall of the vagina and the neck of the bladder, or failing that a pessary may be used. Benign tumours of the muscular wall called fibroids may develop in the uterus, and cause bleeding which necessitates operative removal. Malignant tumours may also develop, some in the cervix; but the practice of periodic cervical smears, in which a specimen of the membrane lining the cervix is taken and examined under the microscope, has enabled cervical cancer to be recognised and treated in its early stages with every hope of success. The examination should be carried out every three or four years on women up to the age of 60 or 65. Cancer of the body of the uterus commonly develops after the menopause and shows itself by bleeding, discharge and sometimes pain; it is treated by surgery and radiotherapy.

Uveitis: inflammation of the uveal tract, the name given to the choroid, ciliary body and iris of the eye (q.v.).

Uvula: the prolongation of the soft palate which hangs down in the middle of the throat over the base of the tongue.

V

Vaccination: vaccinia is a disease of cows – cowpox. In 1774 Benjamin Jesty (1737–1816), a Dorset farmer, having noticed that milkmaids who had been infected with cowpox did not contract smallpox, took the bold step of inoculating his family with matter from a cowpox sore on a cow's udder during a local outbreak of smallpox. The family did not get smallpox. In 1796 Edward Jenner, a physician in Gloucestershire, inoculated one James Phipps with matter from a cowpox vesicle on a milkmaid's hand. He subsequently inoculated him with matter from a smallpox case, and demonstrated that Phipps had acquired a resistance to the infection. He published his observations, and became recognised as the originator of the process of vaccination; the term was later extended to mean the process of active immunisation in general. Immunisation is now carried out against a number of diseases, but is no longer necessary against smallpox, which has been eradicated.

Vaccines are prepared by modifying micro-organisms or their toxins so that when subjects are inoculated with them the disease itself is not produced, but an immunity to the disease or toxin is provoked. When living organisms are used, in general a single dose is sufficient, but in the case of poliomyelitis three doses are required. If the organisms are inactivated, the first dose is followed by a reinforcing dose or doses. In Britain infants are inoculated against diphtheria, tetanus, whooping cough and poliomyelitis at three months, then again six to eight weeks later and again four or six months after that. During their second year they are immunised against measles, mumps and rubella; after three years immunisation against diphtheria, tetanus and poliomyelitis is repeated, and between the 10th and 14th years those who show a negative reaction to tuberculin testing are given the BCG vaccine against tuberculosis, and all girls are offered further immunisation against rubella. On leaving school, immunisation against tetanus and poliomyelitis is repeated. In adult life, immunisation against tetanus can be reinforced every five years, and against poliomyelitis if the subject is travelling to a place where the disease is known to occur. Primary immunisation against tetanus and poliomyelitis can be undertaken in adults who have never been immunised, and women of childbearing age can be tested for immunity against rubella and if negative can be immunised, providing they are not pregnant and do not become pregnant for at least a month after the injection.

Vaccines are prepared every year for use against influenza, following recommendations given by the World Health Organization, but may prove disappointing; they are recommended for the elderly and those with heart, kidney or lung disease, or severe diabetes. Immunisation against anthrax is available for those who may come into contact with infected carcases or hides, or other infected materials. Immunisation against cholera and typhoid is available for travellers, who should have the first injection of two at least a month before they intend to travel. Immunisation against hepatitis B, recommended for those who may come into contact with the disease, takes six months to be fully effective and is given in three doses, the second one month after the first and the third six months later; rabies vaccine is given at similar intervals. Vaccine against meningococcal meningitis is available for travellers to many parts of Africa, to New Delhi and Nepal, and Mecca. Immunisation may be required for those visiting Saudi Arabia before and during the time of the annual pilgrimage to Mecca. Yellow fever vaccine is essential for those travelling to countries where the disease exists; one injection is necessary, and protection lasts for ten years. Those who intend to stay for over a month in Africa, Asia, Central or South America and who have not been vaccinated against tuberculosis should consider immunisation, particularly if they are going to be in close contact with the indigenous population. The skin test and vaccination should be carried out three months before travelling. It is not needed for a short visit.

Vagina: the female genital passage.

Vaginismus: a spasm of the muscles of the vagina on

attempted sexual intercourse. It may be due to pain from a local condition, but may also be due to psychological causes.

Vaginitis: inflammation of the vagina. The commonest causes are infection with *Trichomonas vaginalis* or *Candida albicans* (*see* Candidiasis and Trichomonas). Another common cause is the atrophy that occurs with age as the result of lack of oestrogen; the treatment is with a cream containing the hormone, commonly in the form of dienoestrol, oestriol or conjugated oestrogens.

Vagotomy: the surgical division or partial division of the vagus nerve as it supplies the stomach and duodenum, used in cases of duodenal ulceration. Selective vagotomy diminishes the gastric secretions, but leaves the emptying mechanism of the stomach intact. Complete vagotomy may be accompanied by a pyloroplasty or gastro-enterostomy to ensure emptying of the stomach.

Vagus: the tenth cranial nerve, which forms a very important part of the parasympathetic nervous system (*see* Nervous System). It carries autonomic fibres to the organs of the abdomen and thorax, and also supplies motor fibres to the oesophagus, larynx and pharynx and sensory fibres to the larynx, pharynx, tongue and ear.

Valerian: the root of *Valeriana officinalis*, a plant common in Europe, made into a tincture or extract, was once much used in the treatment of hysteria. There is little evidence that it had any pharmacological effect, but the smell of it is appalling.

Valgus: genu valgus is knock-knee; in talipes valgus, a variety of club-foot, the heel is turned outwards from the midline of the body.

Valvular Heart Disease: the heart has valves to control the flow of blood from the atria into the ventricles, on the right called the tricuspid and on the left the mitral valve, and others to control the flow out of the ventricles, the pulmonary and aortic valves (*see* Heart). Disease of the valves results in incompetence, in which the blood is allowed to regurgitate, or stenosis, where the orifice of the valve is narrowed and impedes the flow of blood. The main causes of valvular disease are rheumatic fever, congenital abnormality and infective endocarditis, and the condition leads to heart failure; but the outlook for patients with valvular heart disease has greatly changed in the last 35 years with the advent of open-heart surgery, for diseased valves can now be reconstructed or replaced.

Varicella: chicken-pox (q.v.).

Varicocele: a varicosity of the pampiniform plexus, a plexus of veins lying round the spermatic cord and draining the testis. The cause is not known, and the condition rarely gives rise to discomfort. It usually occurs on the left side. Varicoceles are found in one-third of cases of infertility, and have been taken as a factor in that condition, but operation to tie off the dilated veins may be disappointing.

Varicose Veins: these occur to some degree in one out of every two women and one out of every four men over the age of 40, but often make their appearance in younger people. They are to a certain degree one of the penalties of standing upright, for then the difficulty of returning blood to the heart from the legs against the pull of gravity becomes greater. Normally this is helped by contraction of the muscles of the legs, which pump the blood upwards through deep veins which have one-way valves so that blood can only flow upwards. The superficial veins drain into the deep veins by communications which also have non-return valves. Varicose veins are superficial veins which have become dilated, and the valves in the communications fail; the blood can no longer flow the right way, and the dilatation becomes worse. It is thought that there is an hereditary tendency towards the development of varicosities, and conditions may not help; pregnancy, obesity and prolonged standing all encourage the veins in the legs to dilate. Varicose veins are unsightly, and may make the ankles swell and the legs ache; in some cases the sluggish venous drainage, allied to the fact that the supply of arterial blood to the skin at the junction of the upper two-thirds of the leg with the lower third is notoriously poor, provokes the formation of varicose ulcers from the slightest injury. The surgical treatment of varicose veins ranges from injections of irritating solution and compression of the veins, so that the walls adhere and the vein is obliterated, to removal of the long saphenous vein; this operation is however unpopular with vascular surgeons, who use the saphenous vein for grafting operations on blocked arteries. Varicose ulcers of any size are best treated by rest in bed, which relieves the engorged and sluggish venous drainage of the legs; but this is often not practical, and compression bandages are used. Most cases of varicose veins are more unsightly than painful, and treatment is not really needed: even if they become uncomfortable, elastic stockings are usually sufficient to give relief. Occasionally varicosities are injured, and bleed profusely. If the patient lies down and the leg is elevated the bleeding stops, and a dressing applied with a pressure bandage controls the haemorrhage.

Variola: smallpox (q.v.).

Varus: genu varus is bow-legs; in talipes varus the club-foot is turned with the heel inwards.

Vas: a hollow tube carrying fluid in the body; when unqualified refers to the vas deferens, the tube that carries spermatozoa from the epididymis into the abdominal cavity and so through the prostate gland at the base of the bladder to the urethra. The vas deferens has thick muscular walls which make it feel like whipcord; it has an outside diameter of 2.5 mm, of which the muscular coat accounts for 2 mm, and is some 45 cm long.

Vascular Surgery: a growing field of surgery in which blocked, injured or diseased arteries and veins are treated. Examples are the repair of aneurysms (q.v.) and the clearance of stroke-producing blockages in the carotid arteries.

Vasectomy: strictly speaking, removal of the vas deferens; the operation carried out for male sterilisation is in fact a partial vasectomy, in which the two vasa are tied off and a portion removed. The operation is a simple one because the vasa run under the skin in the groin. It is however in most cases irreversible.

Vasodilator: a drug which causes the blood vessels to dilate. Vasodilators are commonly used in cases where the vessels have become narrowed through disease, causing a poor circulation in the tissues, in the hope that alternative channels will dilate and add to the blood supply, or in cases where the vessels go into spasm, as for example in Raynaud's disease. Vasodilators used to treat poor circulation include nicotinic acid and its derivatives, cinnarizine, oxpentifylline and thymoxamine, but results are liable to be disappointing. In cases of heart failure, however, a wide range of drugs may be used to dilate the arteries in order to decrease the resistance to the heartbeat, and lower the strain on the heart. These drugs also dilate the veins so that the blood pools in the peripheral veins, the venous return to the heart is diminished, and congestion of the lungs is relieved. The drugs counteract physiological reflexes brought into action by heart failure which increase the tone of the blood vessels.

Vasomotor Rhinitis: a condition causing a clear discharge from the nose, neither allergic nor inflammatory. It resembles hay fever, but is distinguished from it by the fact that it occurs in winter as well as summer. There is persistent congestion of the nasal mucous membrane causing discharge from the nose and in severe cases obstruction of the airways, possibly with sinusitis and the formation of nasal polyps. No one causative agent is found but it may be made worse by central heating, pollution of the air, alcohol, smoking and emotional factors. The condition can be divided into two groups; one shows eosinophil white blood cells in the discharge while the other does not. The first responds to antihistamines such as terfenadine or astemizole, nasal sprays of corticosteroids, or ipratropium bromide; the other group responds to ipratropium bromide. Neither group responds to decongestants or sodium cromoglycate. Sinusitis may be treated with antibiotics and polyps by surgical removal.

Vasovagal Attack: the patient feels hot and cold, yawns and has a 'sinking feeling'. The blood pressure falls and the patient faints, and the pulse is very slow. The symptoms are those of unopposed action of the parasympathetic system; hence the name, for the vagus nerve is the principal nerve in the parasympathetic nervous system. Such a faint can be caused by a number of factors: it may happen in young men on having an injection or having blood taken. Recovery is quick if the patient is laid flat with the legs raised, or sat down with the head lowered between the knees. *See* Fainting.

VDRL: a blood test for syphilis named after the Venereal Disease Research Laboratories.

Vector: an animal carrying infective organisms, for example the mosquito in malaria (q.v.).

Veins: the blood vessels in which the blood drains from the tissues back to the heart. Venous blood has lost the bright red colour of oxyhaemoglobin, for oxygen has been given up to the tissues to be replaced by carbon dioxide, and is much darker than arterial blood. The walls of the veins, like the walls of the arteries, have three coats, but there is much less elastic and muscular tissue and the walls are thin and collapse easily. The pressure in the veins is not sustained by the heartbeat, and is about 5 mm of mercury at the level of the heart. In a subject standing erect and still, the venous pressure in the head is negative, while in the feet the hydrostatic pressure brings the value up to about 100 mm mercury. To enable the veins to return the blood to the heart they have in them one-way valves; when the veins are squeezed by the action of the muscles the blood can only travel towards the heart. The return of blood in the superior vena cava, the great vein in the thorax, is further assisted by inspiration, when the pressure in the chest becomes negative. There are two venous systems in the body, the systemic, where the veins accompany the arteries to the limbs and muscles of the chest, head and abdomen and return the blood directly to the heart, and the portal system in which the veins that drain blood from the gastro-intestinal tract, the pancreas, spleen, and gall-bladder join to form the portal vein which conveys the blood to the liver, where it passes through sinusoids, dilated venous spaces, before being collected in the hepatic veins which join the inferior vena cava. This is the great vein which drains the legs and passes up through the abdomen and diaphragm into the thorax and the heart. The bulk of the blood in the body is in the veins; they fulfil the function of a reservoir for the circulation. Disorders of the veins include varicosities (*see* Varicose Veins) and thrombosis (*see* Thrombophlebitis and Thrombosis). The veins can be outlined for radiography by the injection of a radio-opaque medium, a technique called phlebography.

Vena Cava: the two largest veins in the body are the superior vena cava, into which blood drains from the head, neck, arms, and chest, and the inferior vena cava which receives blood from the legs and abdomen. Both veins empty into the right atrium of the heart.

Venepuncture: the puncture of a vein for the purpose of withdrawing blood or making an intravenous injection.

Venereal Disease: *see* Sexually Transmitted Disease.

Venesection: the cutting of a vein to draw off blood or, more usually, to insert a cannula for intravenous therapy.

Ventilator: artificial breathing machine.

Ventricle: a small cavity, for example the ventricles of the heart or the ventricles in the brain.

Ventricular Fibrillation: a condition in which the muscle of the ventricles of the heart contracts in a continuous uncoordinated way, so that there is no effective heartbeat. The only treatment is defibrillation (q.v.).

Ventricular Septal Defect: normally the ventricles of the heart are separated by a partition or septum (*see* Heart), but a congenital defect can occur in which there is an opening in the septum, a 'hole in the heart'; the treatment is surgical.

Ventriculography: a technique in brain surgery in which air is introduced into the ventricles of the brain through a cannula passed through a burr-hole in the skull in order to make a ventriculogram, an outline of the ventricles on an X-ray plate. It is now rarely used, having been replaced by computerised axial tomography (*see* CAT).

Verruca: a wart (q.v.).

Version: in obstetrics, a manipulation carried out in order to change the position of the foetus in the uterus, converting an abnormal into a normal lie.

Vertebra: one of the bones of the spinal column (q.v.).

Vertigo: giddiness, in which the world seems to be revolving round the patient, who cannot keep a balance and may fall. It is usually caused by disease of the inner ear, for example Ménière's disease (q.v.), or vestibular neuronitis, in which vestibular function (*see* Ear) is disturbed by a virus infection. In severe cases of neuronitis the patient must be put to bed, and told to keep the head still, for the vertigo is set off by head movements. Vomiting, which is caused by vertigo, may be treated with prochlorperazine by intramuscular injection or by mouth, and continuing vertigo is commonly treated with cinnarizine or betahistine hydrochloride; it usually clears up in under a month, but sometimes may persist.

Vesical: to do with the bladder.

Vesicle: a small blister.

Viable: capable of living. The term is applied to a foetus which is capable of living outside the womb; this was taken to be in the 28th week of pregnancy, but recent advances in the care of premature babies have resulted in some surviving at a slightly earlier age.

Vibrio: a Gram-negative genus of bacteria which includes the organism causing cholera, *Vibrio cholerae*. Another less important vibrio causing diarrhoea and abdominal pain is *Vibrio parahaemolyticus*, which lives in the sea in warm climates and infects fish, crabs and prawns; the illness only lasts for a day or two.

Villus: a small protrusion from the surface of a membrane.

Vincent's Angina (trench mouth): a bacterial infection of the mouth and gums, which ulcerate and bleed. The infection is mixed, with *Borrelia vincentii* and *Fusobacterium fusiformis* predominating. It is caused by poor dental hygiene and general ill health, and characterised by a foul breath. The treatment is penicillin or metronidazole, with such dental attention as is necessary. If oral hygiene is allowed to lapse the disease may recur.

Virilism: the appearance of masculine characteristics in the female, which include the overgrowth of hair on the body, acne, baldness of the temples and forehead, deepening of the voice, overgrowth of muscle and loss of the periods. The cause is excess of the androgenic male hormones such as testosterone, which are present normally only in small amounts. They may be produced in excess by abnormalities of the adrenal glands or of the ovaries; the excess may be the result of taking drugs such as anabolic steroids, testosterone or corticosteroids.

Virus: a micro-organism so small that most cannot be seen under the light microscope, consisting only of a nucleic acid, either DNA or RNA, in an envelope of protein. It lives inside the host cell and has to use the host's biochemical resources to multiply. Viruses can be divided into groups according to their hosts, which may be plants, bacteria or animals; they are named after their origins, e.g. rhinovirus from the nose, the way they are transmitted, e.g. arbor virus, which is arthropod-borne, the place where they were first isolated, e.g. Coxsackie virus, or the disease they cause, e.g. poxvirus or herpes virus. Viruses cause many diseases; they are resistant to antibiotics and other similar drugs, but the protein coat bears recognisable antigens, and there are differences between the biochemistry of viruses and their host cells which offer the possibility of disturbing one without the other. Some drugs have been found which

677

exploit these differences, such as acyclovir which is active against herpes virus and zidovudine which inhibits the human immunodeficiency virus. Other drugs will follow. Interferons (q.v.) are being used in cases of hepatitis; but the main defence against viruses is the use of vaccines to produce active immunity, and in this way poliomyelitis and yellow fever have come under control, and smallpox has been eradicated. *See* Vaccination.

Viscera: the large internal organs of the body, for example lungs, liver and intestines.

Visual Purple: rhodopsin (q.v.).

Vitamins: a group of substances which are essential for the normal functioning of the metabolic processes of the body. They were identified by Gowland Hopkins (1861–1947) working in Cambridge in 1912 Deficiencies result in various diseases, but vitamins are present in sufficient quantities in a normal diet. Vitamin A is present in green vegetables and fruit, dairy products and fish liver oil; it is responsible for normal vision, especially in dim light, for the light-sensitive pigment in the eye, rhodopsin or visual purple, contains the vitamin. It is also responsible for the upkeep of the skin and mucous membranes. Vitamin B is a combination of different substances. Vitamin B_1 is thiamine, deficiency of which results in the disease beri-beri (q.v.). Vitamin B_2 is riboflavin, without which the skin of the lips cracks, the mouth becomes sore and the skin of the genitalia is subject to itching dermatitis; various other troubles have been described, but only afflict those whose diet is very poor. Vitamin B_3 is niacin, and the deficiency disease is pellagra (q.v.). Vitamin B_5 is pantothenic acid, and deficiency is very rare; vitamin B_6 is pyridoxine, and again deficiency is rare but causes peripheral neuritis. Vitamin B_{12}, cyanocobalamin, is essential for the formation of red blood cells with folic acid, which is included in the vitamin B complex, and deficiency causes megaloblastic anaemia (*see* Pernicious Anaemia). Vitamin C is ascorbic acid, present in fruit and vegetables, and deficiency leads to scurvy (q.v.). Vitamin D is a number of substances, of which vitamin D_2 is calciferol and vitamin D_3 cholecalciferol; the deficiency disease is rickets (*see* Osteomalacia), and the vitamin is found in fish liver oils, herrings and mackerel and dairy products, and is formed in the skin by the action of sunlight. Vitamin E, tocopherol, is found in vegetable oils, egg yolk, liver and cereals, and deficiency may cause skin changes, anaemia, and oedema, for the vitamin is responsible for the integrity of cell membranes. Vitamin K is found in spinach, cabbage and egg yolk, and is essential for the normal clotting of blood. There are a number of other vitamins which do not seem to be of practical consequence. Because vitamins are contained in adequate quantities in a normal diet, there is no point in taking any vitamin supplements. Indeed, overdoses of vitamin A are harmful during pregnancy, too much pyridoxine is toxic and overdoses of vitamin D can cause nausea and vomiting and other ill effects, as can high doses of vitamin E.

Vitiligo: a skin condition in which there are white patches where the pigment cells have been lost as the result of an auto-immune reaction. The patches are often on the face and neck, and on the genitals; they may be symmetrical, and may affect people with light or dark skin, obviously being more distressing in the latter. The only harm it does is cosmetic. About a third of cases improve; the patches can be disguised by using a covering cream, and the use of psoralens to sensitise the skin followed by exposure to sunlight or UVA radiation has been in some cases effective. Vitiligo may run in families.

Vitreous Humour: a transparent thin jelly that fills the posterior chamber of the eye, between the retina and the lens. *See* Eye.

Vocal Cords: two folds covered with mucous membrane that lie in the larynx. They can be approximated and made tense or relaxed by the muscles of the larynx; by their vibration, when air is forced through, they produce the voice. The muscles are supplied by branches of the vagus nerve, the tenth cranial nerve, which also supplies sensory fibres to the larynx.

Volvulus: condition in which a loop of bowel twists round itself, producing intestinal obstruction and cutting off the blood supply with consequent mortification of the affected bowel.

Vomiting: a reflex protective reaction to the presence in the stomach of irritating matter, controlled by the vomiting centre in the brain. The vomiting centre can be excited by a variety of stimuli, by no means all connected with the stomach; acute fevers, especially in children, are often accompanied by vomiting. It may occur in early pregnancy, and in disorders of the brain such as meningitis, or increased pressure inside the skull caused by tumours or other space-occupying lesions; motion sickness produces vomiting through sensations received by the eyes and the balancing organ of the inner ear, and disturbances of the inner ear inducing vertigo are accompanied by nausea and vomiting. Various drugs can produce vomiting, such as morphia and the cytotoxic drugs used in the treatment of malignant disease, and it occurs in radiation sickness. The treatment of vomiting produced by infective disease of the gastro-intestinal tract, obstruction of the intestines, peritonitis or other abdominal disorders is the treatment of the underlying disease, with attention being paid to the possible excessive loss of fluid and electrolytes in the vomit, particularly if it is accompanied by diarrhoea. Metoclopramidine may be used in vomiting caused by gastro-intestinal disorders. The vomiting of motion sickness and disease of the inner ear is helped by hyoscine or antihistamines such as cinnarizine or prochlorperazine, which can be given by injection or suppositories; there are a number of similar drugs. Vomiting caused by drugs or radiation is counteracted by nabilone, metoclopramide or domperidone. In general, drugs should not be used to control vomiting unless a firm diagnosis has been made of the cause of the vomiting; and drugs should not be used at all in the vomiting of early pregnancy because of the danger to the developing foetus.

Vulva: the external female genitalia, which includes the mons pubis and the labia majora and minora, which enclose the vestibule of the vagina, the external urethral orifice and the clitoris. The mons pubis is formed by a pad of fatty tissue lying over the pubic bone, and is covered by hair. The outer surfaces of the labia majora, two folds of skin and subcutaneous fat, are also covered with hair, but the inner surfaces are smooth. The labia minora are smooth folds of skin, one on each side of the opening of the vagina; in front they unite to form a hood or prepuce over the clitoris, a small and highly sensitive erectile structure which is homologous with the male penis. The hymen at the orifice of the vagina may be in the form of a complete or incomplete membranous ring.

W

Warfarin: named after the Wisconsin Alumni Research Foundation, warfarin is a compound that prevents the clotting of blood by counteracting vitamin K. It is given by mouth and is used in the treatment of deep vein thrombosis, pulmonary embolism, in arterial disease and after vascular surgery including the replacement of heart valves and grafting. It may be used in cases of hip replacement and operations for fractures of the femur to prevent post-operative deep vein thrombosis. In all cases the dose is governed by laboratory blood tests, which must be undertaken at regular intervals. Patients on anticoagulant treatment should carry cards with them and avoid a range of drugs which can cause an increased risk of bleeding, in particular aspirin. Warfarin is also used as a rat poison.

Warts: caused by infection of the skin by the human papilloma virus, warts can affect many parts of the skin. Those on the fingers can be treated with a mixture of salicylic and lactic acids in collodion, or by the use of liquid nitrogen. If left they disappear in time. Small filiform warts can affect the beard area in males, and are treated with liquid nitrogen; if possible the man should stop shaving. Warts on the soles of the feet can be painful, and are very common, the infection being picked up by bare feet in swimming pools, changing rooms and similar places. They are common in schoolchildren; they can be treated by salicylic and lactic acid in collodion, but if left they disappear spontaneously. Warts caused by the human papilloma virus type six can affect the genital organs of both sexes, and are usually sexually transmitted. They can be treated with a paint containing podophyllin resin. This can be toxic if used over large areas of skin, and it should not be used during pregnancy.

Wassermann Reaction: a serological test used in the diagnosis of syphilis, introduced by the Berlin bacteriologist August Paul von Wassermann (1860–1925).

Waterbrash: regurgitation of acid fluid from the stomach into the oesophagus and mouth, associated with heartburn, pain behind the breastbone. It may occur in cases of duodenal ulcer or hiatus hernia (q.v.).

Wax: quite frequently waxy secretions collect in the external auditory meatus, the ear-hole, and deaden the hearing. It is not safe to try to pick the wax out; it must be syringed by a professional. If the wax is hard it can be softened by putting a few drops of olive oil into the ear twice a day for a day or two before the syringing.

Weber's Test: introduced by Freidrich Weber, a German otologist (1832–91), the test is used in cases of deafness. The foot of a vibrating tuning-fork is placed on the forehead or the top of the skull in the midline; if the noise seems to be coming from the middle of the head, the test is normal; but if it seems to be coming from one ear or the other, it is abnormal or positive. In disease of the middle ear the sound is referred to that side because bone conduction is better than conduction of sound in the air. If there is disease of the inner ear the sound is best heard on the normal side. *See* Ear, Rinne's Test.

Weights and Measures: in 1960 units of scientific measurement were agreed as the Système International d'Unités, the International System of Units, abbreviated to SI units. They are now used in medicine. The basic units are: second (s) for time, metre (m) for length, kilogram (kg) for mass, Kelvin (K) for absolute temperature, ampere (A) for electric current, candela (cd) for luminosity, mole (mol) for amount, radian (rad) for plane angles and steradian (st) for solid angles. Defined in terms of these basic units are derived units, of which the most frequently used in medicine are: for force, newton (N), for pressure, pascal (Pa), for energy, joule (J), for power, watt (W), for temperature, Celsius (°C), for radioactivity, becquerel (Bq), for absorbed dose of radioactivity, gray (Gy), for magnetic flux density, tesla (T) and for frequency, hertz (Hz). Some equivalents are: 1 kg force = 10 N, 1 mm mercury = 133 Pa, 1 calorie (energy) = 4.2 J, and

1 kilocalorie (rate of work) = 70 W. In order to avoid a number of figures before or after decimal points, metric prefixes are used, if possible representing 10 raised to a power that is a multiple of three. Examples are: tera (T), 10^{12}, giga (G), 10^9, mega (M), 10^6, kilo (k), 10^3, hecto (h), 10^2, deca (da), 10, centi (c), 10^{-2}, milli (m), 10^{-3}, micro (μ), 10^{-6}, nano (n), 10^{-9}, and pico (p), 10^{-12}. The term mole is applied to ions, molecules and atoms, and is abbreviated mol; the definition of mole is the amount of a substance which has a mass in grams equal to its relative molecular weight. In medicine, the unit of volume is the litre (l); mg per 100 ml is expressed as mg per decilitre (dl). Decimal multiples of the kilogram are written by attaching a prefix to g and not kg. Blood pressures are still given in mm mercury

Weil's Disease: severe form of infection by *Leptospira interrogans*, a spirochaete which infects rats and other animals and is passed on to man mainly by contact with rats, their urine, or water contaminated by their urine. There are a large number of types of the spirochaete, and the type commonly responsible for Weil's disease is *Leptospira icterohaemorrhagica*; it causes damage to the liver and the kidneys. The incubation period is from one to three weeks, and there is headache, fever, shivering and pain in the muscles. The disease progresses to jaundice and kidney failure, sometimes with signs of involvement of the central nervous system such as a change of consciousness. There may be a collapse of the circulation. Treatment is with penicillin or tetracycline; streptomycin or erythromycin may be used, but early treatment is essential. The kidney failure may require renal dialysis. A similar but less severe illness may be produced by *Leptospira canicola*, which may be found in the urine of pigs, dogs and cattle. *See* Leptospira.

Weir–Mitchell Treatment: a regime consisting of absolute rest and a nourishing and easily digested diet, formerly used in the treatment of neuroses; the patients got well out of boredom.

Wen: a sebaceous cyst (q.v.).

Whiplash Injury: in an automobile accident that involves sudden acceleration or deceleration the head may be jerked forwards and backwards, the neck flexing and extending like a whiplash, causing injury to the cervical spine and its muscles. A headrest helps to minimise this type of injury.

Whipworm: *see* Worms.

Whites: a popular name for white vaginal discharge.

Whitlow (felon): a purulent infection of the end of the finger involving the pulp. Cf. Paronychia.

Whooping Cough: pertussis (q.v.).

Windpipe: trachea (q.v.).

Wireworm: *see* Worms.

Wisdom Teeth: the last teeth to erupt, the third molar teeth at the back of the mouth.

Witches' Milk: the milk secreted from the breasts of a newborn baby in response to the hormones of its mother.

Witch-hazel: made up into a lotion or ointment, witch-hazel is mildly astringent. It is sometimes recommended as hamamelis suppositories for use in haemorrhoids.

World Health Organization (WHO): set up by the United Nations in Geneva in 1948 with the aim of helping all countries to improve the health of their people through education and information and practical assistance with mass vaccination programmes, public health schemes and medical facilities. It was largely responsible for the eradication of smallpox from the world.

Womb: the uterus (q.v.).

Worms: these can be divided into three groups: round-worms or nematodes, tapeworms or cestodes and flukes or trematodes. The following list gives the common worms that infest human beings, their length, the type of disease they cause, the method of transmission and the usual treatment.

ROUNDWORMS:

Ascaris lumbricoides	15–25 cm	Inflammation of the intestines and lungs; Eating contaminated food; Levamisole, piperazine.
Enterobius vermicularis (Pinworm, threadworm)	5–15 mm	Itching anus; Contaminated fingers and food; Mebendazole, piperazine, pyrantel.
Trichuris trichiura (Whipworm)	1–2 cm	No symptoms or mild enteritis; Contaminated fingers and food; Mebendazole, pyrantel.
Trichinella spiralis	1.5 mm	Muscular pain and weakness, swelling of face; Undercooked pork; Mebendazole.
Ancylostoma duodenale Necator americanus (Hookworms)	2 cm	(Tropical, subtropical) Anaemia, nutritional disorders; Through skin from infected water or by mouth; Mebendazole, pyrantel, bephenium compounds.
Wuchereria bancrofti Brugia malayi	4–10cm	(Tropical) Elephantiasis, filariasis (q.v.); Mosquitoes; Diethylcarbamazine citrate, ivermectin.

Loa loa	4–7 cm	(Tropical Africa) Filariasis; Mangrove flies (*Chrysops*); Diethylcarbamazine citrate.
Onchocerca volvulus	5–50 cm	(Tropical Africa and America) Filariasis, African river blindness; Blackfly (*Simulium*); Ivermectin.
Strongyloides stercoralis	3 mm	(Tropical) Enteritis and skin eruptions; Contaminated food, larvae can penetrate skin; Thiabendazole.
Dracunculus medinensis (Guinea Worm)	70–120cm	(Tropical) Ulceration and infection of skin; Contaminated water; Removal, thiabendazole, metronidazole.

TAPEWORMS:

Taenia solium	1–2 m	Enteritis, cysticercosis (q.v.); Undercooked pork; Prazantiquel, niclosamide.
Taenia saginata	10 m	Enteritis; Undercooked beef; Praziquantel, niclosamide.
Diphyllobothrium latum	5–25 m	Anaemia, enteritis; Raw fish; Praziquantel, niclosamide.

Echinococcus granulosus	3–9 mm	Hydatid disease (q.v.); Food contaminated by dogs; No specific treatment.

FLUKES:

Schistosoma japonicum *mansoni* *haematobium*	10–15mm	(Tropical and subtropical) Bilharziasis (q.v.); Praziquantel.
Paragonimus *westermani*	8–16 mm	(Far East) Cysts of lung; Undercooked freshwater crabs and crayfish; Praziquantel, bithionol.
Clonorchis sinensis	10–25 mm	(Far East) Liver disease; Raw fish; Praziquantel.
Fasciola hepatica	20–30 mm	Liver disease; Water infected by sheep; Praziquantel, bithionol, chloroquine.

There are a great number of other flukes which can infect man, many of which flourish in the Far East, India and China. Most are acquired from undercooked or raw fish or shellfish, and have various animals as well as man for their definitive hosts.

Wounds: disruption of the tissues by external agents of a mechanical nature which may be classified as incised, punctured, contused, lacerated, perforating and penetrating. Incised wounds are made by cutting, as with a knife; they tend to bleed freely and gape. After such a wound has been cleaned, and the bleeding stopped, the edges can be brought together by stitches or, in the case of minor injuries, by adhesive tapes. Unless they become infected, or a blood clot forms, they will heal quickly. The length of an incised wound is not a factor in healing, for it heals from side to side and not from end to end. Punctured wounds can be dangerous, for it is usually impossible to tell from the appearance how far the puncturing instrument has penetrated. If there is any question of deep penetration, as there must be in wounds of the abdomen or chest, the patient must be observed carefully for any signs of internal damage. The size of the wound in the skin bears no relation to the possible depth of the puncture. In the same way severe contusions or bruises caused, for example, by being run over may indicate serious underlying injury. The extent of the contusion may become apparent relatively slowly; patients with crush injuries can lose a great deal of blood and tissue fluid, and go into shock. Injuries in which the tissues are torn, lacerated injuries, are the most likely to become infected and require thorough surgical cleaning with removal of all dead and damaged tissue; it may be impossible to close such wounds easily, and plastic techniques may have to be used. Through-and-through wounds caused by bullets or fragments of metal are called perforating, and show a small entry wound but a much larger exit wound. The tissues in between are extensively damaged, and arteries go into spasm. Penetrating wounds are caused by foreign bodies that are retained in the tissues; in both cases surgical exploration is carried out to remove damaged and dead tissue and any foreign material in the wound. Complications of wound healing are bleeding, infection and necrosis, the death of tissues; in all cases the possibility of tetanus must be kept in mind and if necessary tetanus vaccine given. In dealing with wounds in the first instance antiseptics should not be used, but the wound covered with a sterile or at least clean dressing, with pressure used to stop the bleeding if it is profuse.

Wrist: the complicated joint between the bones of the forearm, the radius and ulna, and the bones of the hand, the metacarpals. There are eight small bones in the wrist joint, one of which, the scaphoid, may be fractured. The common broken wrist, the Colles' fracture, is a fracture of the radius just above the joint. Sprains of the ligaments of the wrist are not uncommon, nor are inflammations of the tendons passing over the joint, especially in rheumatoid arthritis. *See* Carpal Tunnel Syndrome.

Writer's Cramp: an inability to write, similar to the occupational cramps suffered by pianists, typists and others whose work involves repetitive movements of the hands. It was thought that such cramp had a psychological basis, but treatment founded on this theory has not been successful; it is more likely that the disability is due to a form of dystonia, a neurological disorder of the motor nervous system. Unfortunately this is not well understood, and treatment is disappointing.

Wryneck: *see* Torticollis.

Wuchereria: *see* Filariasis, Worms.

X

Xanthoma: a small deposit or plaque of yellow material sometimes found in the skin and on tendons, particularly the Achilles tendon and the tendons passing over the knuckles, in cases where there is an abnormality of metabolism of fatty substances.

Xenopus Test: a test for pregnancy involving the injection of urine into an African toad, *Xenopus laevis*. Simpler tests have rendered the toads redundant.

Xeroderma: a disorder of the skin in which there is the formation of scales on a dry rough surface. In xeroderma pigmentosum there is an hereditary defect which prevents the repair of DNA after damage by ultraviolet light; skin exposed to sunlight becomes inflamed, and skin cancers are likely to develop.

Xerophthalmia: the result of vitamin A deficiency in which the epithelium of the conjunctiva and the cornea in the eyes breaks down, becomes infected and ulcerates; the eyes become dry because the cells of the conjunctiva cease to secrete mucus, and tears cannot wet the eyes. Blindness follows repeated infection; worst affected are young children. The condition is found in the Far East, where there are few green vegetables in the diet.

Xeroradiography: a method of producing radiographs by a dry process.

X-rays: electromagnetic waves of a very short wavelength, between 5 nanometres and 6 picometres, longer than gamma rays but shorter than ultraviolet light. They can penetrate matter opaque to light. They were discovered by William Röntgen (1845–1923) in 1895. The absorption of X-rays depends on the nature of the atoms they meet, the heavier the atom the greater being the absorption; a thin sheet of lead will absorb much of a beam of X-rays that will penetrate several feet of wood. A beam of X-rays passing through the body is less easily absorbed by flesh than bone, and on a fluorescent screen or a sensitised photographic plate the bones will be revealed by the shadows they cast. Other parts of the body can be made opaque to X-rays by injecting or otherwise introducing appropriate substances, such as barium to outline the gastro-intestinal tract or iodine compounds to outline the gall-bladder or kidneys. X-rays are used in the treatment of many types of cancer and other diseases. *See* Radiation.

Xylocaine: the trade name for lignocaine (q.v.), a widely used local anaesthetic.

Y

Yaws: a chronic disease of the tropics caused by *Treponema pertenue*, a spirochaete almost identical to *Treponema pallidum*, the organism that causes syphilis. Yaws is not a sexually transmitted disease, but is passed on by contact with a papilloma or ulcer on a person suffering from the disease. A pimple develops at the site of inoculation, and enlarges until it looks rather like a raspberry; this gives the disease the alternative name frambesia. The lesion may ulcerate and become infected. About two to six months later a secondary stage follows in which there are multiple excrescences on the skin, particularly in moist places and skin folds and on the palms of the hands and the soles of the feet, which are tender; moreover the bones of the legs may become inflamed and painful, and so walking may be difficult. After about six months the papillomas heal, but may recur. Later in the third stage of the disease granulomas develop, resembling the gummas of the third stage of syphilis; they may affect the face and ulcerate to produce disfiguration. The treatment is penicillin, tetracycline or erythromycin.

Yellow Fever: an acute and severe disease found in Central Africa and Central and South America; it is caused by a virus carried by the mosquito *Aedes aegypti*. The incubation period is less than a week; the patient suddenly develops a fever with a headache and muscular pains. Vomiting follows, with bleeding from the gums and the intestines; the pulse becomes slow and the blood pressure falls. There is albumin in the urine, and progressive kidney failure. In fatal cases death occurs in a week or 10 days. The mortality rate may be as low as 5%, but may be as high as 25%. During convalescence jaundice develops because of damage to the liver. There is no specific treatment for yellow fever, but a vaccine is available which gives protection from the disease for 10 years. Control of the disease depends on control of mosquitoes both on the ground and in aircraft and ships travelling to countries where the fever exists. Travellers to these countries should be protected by the vaccine. There are reservoirs of infection among monkeys in Africa and South America, and infection can spread from monkeys to human beings through mosquitoes.

Z

Zinc: one of the essential trace elements which are needed for enzyme systems in the body. It is normally present in the diet, but deficiency results in stunted growth, skin disease and inadequacy of the immune system. Zinc salts are used externally in medicine for their mildly astringent and antiseptic action; zinc oxide with 0.5% ferric oxide is calamine, used in lotions, and zinc oxide is made up in paste, creams and ointments for use in irritating skin conditions; zinc sulphate lotion, lotio rubra, is used as a dressing for indolent ulcers; zinc undecenoate is used for fungus infections of the skin.

Zoomorphism: a belief that human beings can change into animals, which has been persistent for many centuries. In Greek legend there are instances of men changing into wolves; the wolf in ancient Rome brought up Romulus and Remus, and werewolves appear in Pliny, Herodotus and Virgil. In Ireland, St Patrick is said to have cursed a king, turning him into a wolf. In the fifteenth and sixteenth centuries lycanthropy was a subject of popular belief in Europe; however there were those who recognised that transmogrification was not possible, but that the devil made a man believe he was a wolf. By the seventeenth century the condition had been described as a form of madness. In the Far East different animals, including the tiger, fox, crocodile and hyaena, have been the subject of beliefs similar to lycanthropy.

Zoonosis: any disease of animals which may be transmitted to human beings. Examples are plague and rabies; anthrax, Q fever and salmonella infections; all kinds of worm infestations, and various virus, rickettsial, leptospiral and fungus infections; brucellosis, ornithosis, and glanders. There are many others. Fleas from infested animals will feed on human beings, and infestation may occur with mites of various species, producing symptoms that resemble scabies. Animal lice do not infest humans.

Attention to personal hygiene, for example washing the hands after handling animals, their excreta or bedding, lessens the risk of infection; in particular, pregnant women should be careful how they handle animals (*see* Toxoplasmosis).

Zygomatic Bone: the cheekbone. It forms the prominence of the cheek, and part of the outer wall and floor of the eye-socket, the orbit.

Zygote: the fertilised ovum.